Orthopaedic Trauma Protocols

Orthopaedic Trauma Protocols

EDITORS

Sigvard T. Hansen, Jr., M.D.
Professor
Department of Orthopaedics
University of Washington
Harborview Medical Center
Seattle, Washington

Marc F. Swiontkowski, M.D.
Professor and Vice Chairman
Department of Orthopaedics
University of Washington
Chief of Orthopaedics
Harborview Medical Center
Seattle, Washington

ILLUSTRATOR

Kate Sweeney
Seattle, Washington

Raven Press New York

Raven Press, Ltd., 1185 Avenue of the Americas, New York, NY 10036

Made in the United States of America

Library of Congress Cataloging-in-Publication Data
Orthopaedic Trauma Protocols / edited by Sigvard T. Hansen, Jr., Marc F. Swiontkowski.
p. cm.
Includes bibliographical references and index.
ISBN 0-88167-994-1
1. Orthopaedic emergencies. 2. Musculoskeletal system—Wounds and injuries—Treatment. 3. Fractures—Treatment. 4. Orthopaedic surgery. 5. Medical protocols. I. Hansen, Sigvard T. II. Swiontkowski, Marc F.
[DNLM: 1. Fractures—therapy. 2. Orthopaedics. 3. Wounds and Injuries—therapy. WE 168 07693]
RD750.078 1993
617.4'7044—dc20
DNLM/DLD
for Library of Congress 92-48788

The material contained in this volume was submitted as previously unpublished material, except in the instances in which credit has been given to the source form which some of the illustrative material was derived.

Great care has been taken to maintain the accuracy of the information contained in the volume. However, neither Raven Press nor the editors can be held responsible for errors or for any consequences arising from the use of the information contained herein.

10 9 8 7 6 5 4 3 2 1

To Beverley Esther Means Hansen (1908-1992)
and Sigvard T. Hansen, Sr. (1903-   )
for the "good constitution and good outlook on life" promised
to me as a child and necessary for the work leading to this book
S.T.H.

To Beth, Timothy, Jeffrey, and Ellen Rose,
their support and sacrifice made this work possible
M.F.S.

Contents

Contributing Authors ix
Preface xi
Acknowledgments xii
Introduction xiii
Sigvard T. Hansen, Jr.

Part I: General Considerations

1. The Evolution of Musculoskeletal Traumatology at Harborview Medical Center 3
Sigvard T. Hansen, Jr.
2. The Role of the Trauma Surgeon in the Management of Orthopaedic Trauma 9
Gregory J. Jurkovich
3. Nursing Standards for the Orthopaedic Trauma Patient 17
Jack S. Olsen and Joan S. Rhodes
4. The Psychological and Social Implications of Multiple Trauma 21
Billie Z. Lawson and Lynn Carrigan
5. Anesthetic Considerations in the Traumatized Patient 27
Edward G. Pavlin
6. Protocols for Posttrauma Analgesia 31
F. Peter Buckley
7. Rehabilitation Treatment Strategies 43
Barbara J. de Lateur
8. Rehabilitation: Occupational Therapy 51
Anne Birge James, Carole A. Lossing, Shelly Gruber Sailer, and Robin Irish
9. Acute Physical Therapy 61
Tracey L. Varga
10. Rehabilitation: Nonacute Physical Therapy 65
Kevin Olson

Part II: Regional Fracture Management

11. Shoulder 75
Keith A. Mayo and Marc F. Swiontkowski
12. Humeral Shaft Fractures 91
M. Bradford Henley

13. Elbow 97
M. Bradford Henley

14. Forearm Fractures 115
M. L. Chip Routt, Jr.

15. Wrist 125
Allan W. Bach

16. Hand 153
Thomas E. Trumble and John T. Sack

17. Soft-Tissue Injuries in the Upper Extremity 187
Marc F. Swiontkowski

18. Spine 193
Paul A. Anderson

19. Pelvic Fractures 225
M. L. Chip Routt, Jr.

20. Hip Dislocations and Femoral Head Fractures 237
Marc F. Swiontkowski

21. Hip Joint: Acetabular Fractures 243
Keith A. Mayo

22. Femoral Neck Fractures 255
Marc F. Swiontkowski

23. Intertrochanteric Femoral Fractures 263
Marc F. Swiontkowski

24. Subtrochanteric Femoral Fractures 271
Marc F. Swiontkowski

25. Femoral Shaft Fractures 279
Sigvard T. Hansen, Jr.

26. Knee 291
Stephen K. Benirschke and Marc F. Swiontkowski

27. Tibial Shaft Fractures 331
Marc F. Swiontkowski

28. Foot and Ankle Joint 339
Bruce J. Sangeorzan

29. Associated Fractures 369
Marc F. Swiontkowski

30. Soft-Tissue Injuries in the Lower Extremity 375
Sigvard T. Hansen, Jr.

Subject Index 385

Contributing Authors

Paul A. Anderson, M.D. *Associate Professor, Department of Orthopaedics, Harborview Medical Center, University of Washington, 325 Ninth Avenue, ZA-48, Seattle, Washington 98104*

Allan W. Bach, M.D. *Clinical Professor, Harborview Medical Center University of Washington, 801 Broadway, Suite 701, Seattle, Washington 98104*

Stephen K. Benirschke, M.D. *Associate Professor, Department of Orthopaedics, Harborview Medical Center, University of Washington, 325 Ninth Avenue, ZA-48, Seattle, Washington 98104*

F. Peter Buckley, M.B., F.F.A.R.C.S. *Attending Physician, Pain Relief Service, Harborview Medical Center, Associate Professor of Anesthesiology, University of Washington, Medical Director, Pain and Toxicity Program, Fred Hutchinson Cancer Center, 325 Ninth Avenue, ZA-14, Seattle, Washington 98104*

Lynn Carrigan, A.B.J., M.S.W. *Community Mental Health Center, Harborview Medical Center, University of Washington, 325 Ninth Avenue, ZA-57, Seattle, Washington 98104*

Barbara J. de Lateur, M.D. *Professor, Department of Rehabilitation Medicine, Harborview Medical Center, University of Washington, 325 Ninth Avenue, ZA-57, Seattle, Washington 98104*

Sigvard T. Hansen, Jr., M.D. *Professor and Chief, Department of Orthopaedics, Harborview Medical Center, University of Washington, 325 Ninth Avenue, ZA-48, Seattle, Washington 98104*

M. Bradford Henley, M.D. *Associate Professor, Department of Orthopaedics, Harborview Medical Center, University of Washington, 325 Ninth Avenue, ZA-48, Seattle, Washington 98104*

Robin Irish, M.S., O.T.R. *Division of Occupational Therapy, Harborview Medical Center, University of Washington, 325 Ninth Avenue, ZA-49, Seattle, Washington 98104*

Anne Birge James, M.S., O.T.R. *School of Occupational and Physical Therapy, University of Puget Sound, 1500 North Warner, Tacoma, Washington 98416*

Gregory J. Jurkovich, M.D., F.A.C.S. *Associate Professor, Department of Surgery, Harborview Medical Center, University of Washington, 325 Ninth Avenue, ZA-16, Seattle, Washington 98104*

Billie Z. Lawson, M.A., M.S.W., A.C.S.W. *Department of Social Work, Harborview Medical Center, University of Washington, 325 Ninth Avenue, ZA-70, Seattle, Washington 98104*

Carole A. Lossing, M.S., O.T.R. *Rehabilitation Medicine, Children's Hospital and Medical Center, 9500 Sandpoint Way, Seattle, Washington 98105*

Keith A. Mayo, M.D. *Clinical Associate Professor, Department of Orthopaedics, Harborview Medical Center, University of Washington, 325 Ninth Avenue, ZA-48, Seattle, Washington 98104*

Jack S. Olsen, P.T. *Department of Orthopaedics, Harborview Medical Center, University of Washington, 325 Ninth Avenue, ZA-79, Seattle, Washington 98104*

Kevin Olson, P.T. *Supervisor, Outpatient Clinic, Department of Physical Therapy, Harborview Medical Center, University of Washington, 325 Ninth Avenue, ZA-56, Seattle, Washington 98104*

Edward G. Pavlin, M.B., F.F.A.R.C.S. *Associate Professor, Department of Anesthesiology, Harborview Medical Center, University of Washington, 325 Ninth Avenue, ZA-14, Seattle, Washington 98104*

Joan S. Rhodes, R.N., B.S.N., O.N.C. *Medical Surgical Clinical Instructor, Nursing Education, Harborview Medical Center, University of Washington, 325 Ninth Avenue, ZA-33, Seattle, Washington 98104*

M. L. Chip Routt, Jr., M.D. *Assistant Professor, Department of Orthopaedics, Harborview Medical Center, University of Washington, 325 Ninth Avenue, ZA-48, Seattle, Washington 98104*

John T. Sack, M.D. *Clinical Professor, Department of Orthopaedics, University of Washington, 600 Broadway Medical Center, #440, Seattle, Washington 98122*

Shelly Gruber Sailer, O.T.R. *Division of Occupational Therapy, Harborview Medical Center, University of Washington, 325 Ninth Avenue, ZA-49, Seattle, Washington 98104*

Bruce J. Sangeorzan, M.D. *Associate Professor, Department of Orthopaedics, Harborview Medical Center, University of Washington, 325 Ninth Avenue, ZA-48, Seattle, Washington 98104*

Marc F. Swiontkowski, M.D. *Professor and Vice Chairman, Department of Orthopaedics, University of Washington, Chief of Orthopaedics, Harborview Medical Center, University of Washington, 325 Ninth Avenue, ZA-48, Seattle, Washington 98104*

Thomas E. Trumble, M.D. *Associate Professor, Department of Orthopaedics, Harborview Medical Center, University of Washington, 325 Ninth Avenue, RK10, Seattle, Washington 98104*

Tracey L. Varga, P.T. *Department of Physical Therapy, Harborview Medical Center, University of Washington, 325 Ninth Avenue, ZA-56, Seattle, Washington 98104*

Preface

In the early 1970s, Harborview Medical Center was entering into the era of aggressive stabilization of fractures in multiply injured patients. The clinical faculty and residents in training were in need of a decision-making structure that could be taught in a straightforward manner to aid in decision making, but there was no precedent to build upon. Thus, the operating hypotheses in treatments of the day were coalesced into "protocols." For the next 10 years, these protocols were passed on via conferences and the spoken word. In 1983, Robert Foster, then one of the full-time group at Harborview, began the task of getting these protocols down in writing. He completed the section on the upper extremity, as it stood in those days, but the project fell by the wayside in the disarray of high faculty turnover.

In 1988 rapidly expanding knowledge of the importance of soft-tissue management generated new enthusiasm for the project and it was revitalized. Since that time our protocols have been under continuous assessment, some by prospective randomized trials and others by observation and discussion. They have demonstrated remarkably low infection rates, low morbidity rates in hospital and, considering the severity of the injuries, good return to final function. This book provides the reader with our basic premise for managing the injured appendicular and axial skeleton as we see it in 1993. Protocol assessment is an ongoing process that will be greatly enhanced in the years to come by functional assessments and patient-oriented outcomes.

This book should prove useful to senior house officers assigned to orthopaedic trauma services and all attending orthopaedic surgeons who are either frequently or occasionally called upon to manage severely injured patients.

Acknowledgments

The authors would like to acknowledge the critical role of Kathey Alexander of Raven Press in seeing that this important project be completed. Her dedication to the concept of the book is impressive. Dalia Hansen's excellent editorial work and persistent dogging of the majority of authors lead to the thorough and complete chapters you see before you. Ed Kohnstamm applied his vast photographic talents to producing the radiographs for the book, and Kate Sweeney's talents are apparent in the line drawings.

Our work in the Orthopaedic Department at Harborview Medical Center could not be carried out without the critical role of the Medic One and Airlift Northwest programs, both directed by Michael Copass. His unfaltering dedication to the institution and its mission is an inspiration to us all. The excellent care that is delivered by our ICU and orthopaedic nursing staff and the occupational and physical therapists of our institution is truly remarkable and in a large part is responsible for the renown in which our department shares. Fredrick A. Matsen III, the chairman of our department, went to great effort to recruit and retain the majority of the members of our group. David Jaffe, the CEO of Harborview, continues to be very supportive of our group, a tradition that began under Andrew McCulloch's interim rein. James P. LoGerfo, the medical director, is unfaltering in his clear and consistent leadership of this medical center; the orthopaedic group is one of many beneficiaries.

Karen Morton handled the important aspects of the timetable and budget for which we are thankful. Finally, this project could not have been completed without the essential contributions of Rebecca Lessard who coddled the authors, begged the contributors, sorted each and every illustration, and handled the numerous phone calls regarding details that the authors were not prepared to handle.

This book is a group effort. The thoughtfulness and thoroughness it reflects is represented in the daily patient care delivered by the 12 members of this orthopaedic group, the many Fellows in Orthopaedic Traumatology, and the chief residents from the general residency program. We would be remiss not to specifically acknowledge the efforts of the junior residents for their long hours spent caring for severely injured patients and their dedication to mastering the very difficult skills required in this care.

Editorial assistance for this book was supported by a grant from Veterans Rehabilitation Research and Development contract #V663P-3049-91.

Orthopaedic Trauma Protocols, edited by
Sigvard T. Hansen, Jr., and Marc F. Swiontkowski.
Raven Press, Ltd., New York, ©1993.

Introduction

Sigvard T. Hansen, Jr.

The subject of this book is orthopaedic traumatology, a subspecialty of orthopaedic surgery that is distinctly different from fracture care. Orthopaedic traumatology involves the care of approximately 2% to 5% of all fracture patients who have sustained musculoskeletal injuries from high-energy accidents. The severity of these injuries and their secondary complications can threaten these patients with loss of a limb or even their lives.

The importance of well-organized trauma teams is reflected in the cost of trauma to our society. In 1988, over $150 billion were spent in the United States on caring for victims of accidental injuries—one third of this cost was consumed by hospital care and two thirds for out-of-hospital costs, including lost productivity due to disability and loss of life. Although the number of traumatology patients is small compared with the total number of fracture patients, this population is responsible for a very large percentage of this huge monetary loss. The cost of care and the resultant disability and death can be reduced approximately 50% by efficient trauma teams and hospitals using the type of aggressive treatment proposed in this book.

Unfortunately, the survival rate of most traumatologists and even of trauma hospitals is very short. Whether it is a section of general surgery, orthopaedics, or any other department, traumatology is extremely demanding on the individual surgeon and, in many states and hospitals, has been a financial drain on the institution. The intensely challenging patient care and surgery tend to attract talented and confident individuals who make serious commitments to their profession. Unfortunately, the satisfaction of performing complex trauma surgery often becomes overshadowed by dissatisfaction with the conditions under which it is performed. Trauma surgeons perform the most difficult surgeries with irregular schedules and long hours, factors that place additional stress on their families. They face a much higher personal risk of acquiring hepatitis and HIV than their colleagues, receive lower pay, and usually gain slower academic advancement than their peers. Their colleagues are unsympathetic to these discrepancies because trauma surgeons usurp scarce operating room time without scheduling and frequently perform long operations on patients who are uninsured or inadequately insured, forcing the colleagues' well-prepared, fully-funded elective patients to be rescheduled or cancelled. Arguments for the need for urgent surgery to preserve a young patient's ability to work are rarely persuasive in this situation. Surgical colleagues are angered at having their schedules disrupted, even when a 75-year-old patient who needs a total hip replacement to walk without a cane is displaced for a traumatology patient (average age, 34 years) who is employed, responsible for a young family, and has 30 years of productive life ahead.

Skilled traumatologists require at least 3 years after residency and fellowship to become optimally comfortable and efficient with traumatology, but usually put up with these circumstances for only approximately 5 years. They then switch to private general orthopaedic practice, possibly specializing in posttraumatic reconstruction or another related field, and are exceedingly competent and financially successful because of the high levels of skill they developed in traumatology. However, their departure represents an enormous loss to the community, as all trauma team members are extremely valuable regional resources in the areas where they practice.

Another innate difficulty of trauma surgery is that it requires complete multidepartmental cooperation and the total involvement of major hospital services. This means that hospital administrators, medical school deans, and at least 4 or 5 departmental chairmen must have identical goals and closely coordinated functions with regard to the trauma team. In many schools and teaching hospitals this degree of cooperation would be unprecedented, and in others, it is at best a tenuous and volatile situation that is subject to complete disruption with the change of any key person. Departments can be expected to subjugate other interests to the needs of traumatologists only if everyone concerned real-

Department of Orthopaedics, Harborview Medical Center, University of Washington, Seattle, Washington 98104

izes and appreciates the teaching value for students and residents and the tremendous service and economic benefits a first-rate trauma hospital provides.

The cost–benefit ratio of all medical and surgical treatments is presently under intense study, and I am confident that the conclusion will be reached that greater commitment to traumatology and a decreased emphasis on restorative surgery in the elderly is a much better use of scarce resources. This is not to say that surgery in the elderly should be eliminated or even curtailed, but that its runaway costs must be contained by stabilizing technology, implant design, and surgical fees. The inequities borne by those who choose traumatology as a career must be reduced, which will result in enormous direct benefits to severely injured patients and indirect economic benefits to our communities in general.

The major difference between traumatology care and fracture care is the need for immediate attention. Traumatology care is very time dependent because many of these injuries are open fractures or have a high potential for compartmental syndrome or other severe soft-tissue decompensation. Moreover, they are frequently associated with injuries to the chest, the head, and the abdomen. Proper attention to all these injuries can be provided only by a trauma team working in a hospital with all support facilities operating 24 hours a day.

Many excellent books can be found that concern fracture care, and many of the principles of fracture treatment they espouse are applicable to traumatology. Parts of this book will reflect these common principles, but the emphasis throughout the book is treatment of very severe injuries and the special needs of multiply injured patients. Traumatology protocols are warranted whenever a musculoskeletal injury occurs together with other regional injuries or with head or chest injuries. The fractures most obviously associated with traumatology include displaced pelvic and acetabular fractures, femoral shaft fractures, subtrochanteric and supracondylar femoral fractures, proximal tibia and tibial shaft fractures, and pilon fractures. Open tibial fractures particularly warrant traumatology care because they usually result from high-energy injuries and present difficult challenges in dealing with injured soft tissues. Some of the topics in this book are not obviously relevant to traumatology, particularly postoperative pain, spinal fractures, foot and ankle fractures, and hand injuries. I would like to add some comments to explain their presence in a text on traumatology.

POSTOPERATIVE PAIN

The deleterious effects of postinjury and postoperative pain are often underestimated and, as a result, pain in multiply injured patients is sometimes poorly managed. The relatively recent development of pain management services by anesthesiologists is long overdue and very welcome.

Clinical observations of the "stress response" to injury or multiple organ failure in severely injured patients indicate that patients' perceptions of severe pain significantly increase the debilitating physiologic effects of these reactions. From extensive past experience operating on patients with meningomyelocele, I have observed that major operations carried out in areas of the body devoid of sensation produce minimal, if any, stress response on the part of the patient. More recently, I have observed a similar absence of stress response immediately after surgery in patients who were given long-acting sciatic and femoral local anesthetic blocks for major foot reconstructions. Clearly, the overall effects are far less severe even 14 to 16 hours after surgery, when pain sensation returns and some stress response develops, than when patients awaken from general anesthesia and experience the onset of severe pain. Elderly patients treated with intramuscular opioids for postoperative pain after hip fractures or other injuries demonstrated a very high incidence of complications. These included constipation, atelectasis and pneumonia, urinary obstruction, stasis, infection, and bed sores. We have seen the rate of these complications plummet when opioids were used alternately with nonsteroidal anti-inflammatory drugs (NSAIDs) on a diurnal basis after the first 36 postinjury hours. Opioids are given at night and NSAID medications, occasionally combined with stimulant drugs, are given during the daytime to encourage normal diurnal physiology and activity.

Younger trauma patients experience fewer complications, but diurnal drug variations after the first 36 to 48 postoperative hours decrease habituation and dependency. Patients learn to cope with lower levels of postacute pain through activities and mental distractions. Regional anesthesia with local anesthetics is more appropriate for postacute surgical procedures such as bone grafting, delayed closure, and delayed internal fixation than for acute procedures because compartmental syndromes are less likely to occur at that time and because regional anesthesia is associated with an overall lower incidence of complications.

For musculoskeletal traumatologists, the most effective method for limiting the debilitating effects of the stress response to severe pain is to carry out the earliest possible atraumatic skeletal stabilization. When this is done, significant acute pain usually resolves after 36 to 48 hours. As Dr. Buckley notes in his chapter on *Protocols for Posttrauma Analgesia,* scientifically sound and aggressive pain control by modern techniques is used during this time. Pain control is not just a humanitarian concern; it also shortens the catabolic period, facilitates restoration of normal physiology, and enhances eventual rehabilitation.

SPINAL FRACTURES

The treatment of spine-injured patients at Harborview evolved much more slowly than treatment of other skeletal injuries. In the 1970s, laminectomy was regarded by North American neurologic surgeons as the definitive procedure for decompression of the spinal cord. At Harborview, neurologic surgeons who were called to the emergency department for consultations on patients with spinal cord injuries often insisted on performing this procedure, even though the orthopaedic team at that time believed that reduction and stabilization of the spine was the most effective method of spinal cord decompression and that laminectomy should be reserved for rare occasions when laminar fractures were displaced into the canal.

Over the past 8 years or so, management of patients with spinal injuries has changed dramatically at Harborview. Care of these patients has come under the combined jurisdiction of neurologic surgery and orthopaedic surgery, and early reduction and surgical stabilization has become standard treatment. Two factors brought about this change: neurologic surgeons in North America embraced a new treatment philosophy, and the Neurological Surgery Department at Harborview was reorganized under new leadership. Consequently, our two departments cooperated closely by formulating a philosophy of care, managing virtually all spine-injured patients jointly, and attending combined conferences. The new protocols, calling for the earliest possible reduction and stabilization of skeletal deformities, markedly simplified the general care of patients, the treatment of other injuries, and the management of complications. As a result, patients with spinal injuries now spend far less time in the hospital and are transferred to rehabilitative services much sooner.

Actual salvage of useful neurologic function with early operative stabilization has not been uniformly successful. The functional result is determined for the most part by the primary insult that occurs at the time of the initial injury. In many cases, early reduction of spinal canal deformity has resulted in a dramatic return of function. Although this might be expected in cases of peripheral nerve compression, such as cervical root or cauda equina lesions, it is rare in complete cord compression injuries.

Whether early surgery of the cervical region in patients who can be reduced nonoperatively aggravates swelling and neurologic damage is still unclear. However, this issue should not deter early operative reduction in patients with fractures that cannot be reduced by traction within 6 to 12 hours of injury. Certainly, an unreduced spine presents more risk to the spinal cord and ultimate functional recovery than postoperative swelling, especially when swelling is caused by the primary insult rather than by surgery.

FOOT AND ANKLE FRACTURES

Foot and ankle fractures seldom affect a patient's survival. Only occasionally, when multiple injuries include a severe foot or ankle injury with associated soft-tissue necrosis, does an injury in this area have systemic significance. More often, traumatology philosophy and techniques are required to ensure optimal functional recovery in high-energy foot and ankle injuries. Soft-tissue coverage in the foot is meager and circulation is vulnerable. Foot compartmental syndromes are uncommon, but when they occur, they can be devastating and can lead to significant dysfunction (when they are associated with calcaneal fractures) or amputation of the forefoot (when they are associated with tarsometatarsal fracture–dislocations). Appropriate weight-bearing distribution, overall alignment, and motion in hindfoot and metatarsophalangeal joints are critical to normal foot function and gait.

A chapter on foot and ankle injuries is necessary in a textbook on traumatology. Patients brought to trauma centers for treatment of life-threatening injuries to the head, torso, and proximal extremities may also have high-energy injuries in the ankle and foot. These injuries require early treatment with anatomic skeletal stabilization and the greatest respect for soft tissues and circulation.

I would like to include a comment about postoperative care for foot and ankle fractures. Because the foot is both dependent and peripheral, poor circulation (primarily venous and lymphatic return) is virtually guaranteed. Rehabilitation must include elevation, motion, and weight-bearing to ensure maximal venous return and circulation to prevent articular atrophy, regional swelling leading to chronic edema, and arthrofibrosis. Ideally, rehabilitation combines partial weight-bearing, early motion, and intermittent elevation after stable internal fixation to reduce edema and to maximize nutrition of the articular cartilage. Short-leg casts or removable, short-leg walking boots are generally used and weight-bearing is restricted to "weight-of-leg," or 15 to 20 pounds. Walking boots are used after 10 to 20 postoperative days to allow range-of-motion exercises after the soft tissues have healed.

When treatment requires casting, patients are encouraged to actively move their toes and to do gentle isometric exercises several times a day in lieu of actual weight-bearing or exercises out of cast. Total nonweight-bearing, in which a patient ambulates on crutches with the knee bent and the foot elevated, is contraindicated in virtually all cases. This practice produces significant edema in the foot and is considered dangerous for elderly patients and those with upper body weakness or poor balance.

HAND AND WRIST INJURIES

Injuries to the hand and the wrist frequently require traumatology care, not because they are life-threatening, like major long-bone and axial skeletal injuries, but because they require very specialized and technical care to restore hand function. At other times, hand and wrist injuries occur as components of multiple trauma, and the sum of the injuries' severity demands care by a trauma team. Like the foot, the hand contains a very large number of bones, joints, muscles, tendons, and vessels in a small space. Unlike the foot, however, motion is essential in virtually all the joints in the hand for normal function. Therefore, optimal acute treatment might require multiple technical skills, including precise open reduction and stabilization of intraarticular fractures and microsurgical repair of nerves and vessels. During the postoperative period, specialized warm rooms, monitoring equipment, and occupational and physical therapy modalities are needed for optimal care. All these specialized services should be available in a high-level trauma hospital.

Two lessons can be gleaned from our experiences. First, close cooperation and a common philosophy of care by the core group of services managing multiply injured patients simplify treatment, maximize results, and minimize costs. Second, as with all trauma, early restoration of skeletal integrity facilitates mobilization, promotes soft-tissue healing, and relieves pain, thereby eliminating the need for excessive amounts of medication, particularly sedative and narcotic medications that suppress normal physiologic functions.

General Considerations

Orthopaedic Trauma Protocols, edited by
Sigvard T. Hansen, Jr., and Marc F. Swiontkowski.
Raven Press, Ltd., New York, ©1993.

CHAPTER 1

The Evolution of Musculoskeletal Traumatology at Harborview Medical Center

Sigvard T. Hansen, Jr.

HISTORICAL PERSPECTIVE

Until the 1940s and 1950s, fracture care in the northwest region of the country consisted primarily of nonoperative procedures, often carried out by family practitioners or general surgeons. Fracture care was established as the province of orthopaedic surgery only after World War II, when innovative surgeons including Drs. John LeCocq, Roger Anderson, Harry Emmel, John Stewart, Ernest Burgess, and others were practicing in this area. Roger Anderson, who worked as a clinical faculty member at Harborview (known then as King County Hospital) in addition to running a private practice, introduced his aluminum external fixation devices and a very sophisticated fracture table with built-in mechanisms to reduce and hold fractures while they were stabilized by external or internal fixation. Dr. Anderson also introduced a device called the well-leg splint to treat fractures in one leg with countertraction from the other. In 1958, Dr. Kay Clawson became the first full-time surgical faculty member to assume the position as Chief of the Orthopaedic Division at the University of Washington. One of Dr. Clawson's accomplishments at that time was the development of the sliding hip screw, a device he designed with the Richards Company and which was based on a European design he had seen during his Fellowship with Professor Seddon in London.

King County Hospital, founded in 1877, was originally located in the county poor house. During 1930 a new facility was constructed, the hospital was renamed Harborview Hospital, and its doors opened in 1931 to care for indigent patients. During the 1950s and 1960s, the Orthopaedic Service at Harborview was run by orthopaedic residents from the University of Washington, who were supervised by many of these same clinical and full-time faculty members. At that time, all patients with fractures were admitted directly to the Orthopaedic Service, and appropriate services were consulted if injuries were found in other systems. Many of these orthopaedic patients were elderly and had primary and secondary medical problems in addition to hip fractures. Although hip fractures were commonly managed operatively, operative treatment was uncommon for many other fractures until the early 1960s. Internal fixation devices at that time consisted of Lottes nails, Richards plates, Webb bolts (for tibial plateau fractures), and straight cloverleaf intramedullary nails (for femoral fractures). Before the Richards screw became the standard fixation device for intertrochanteric fractures, this fracture was stabilized with devices such as the Jewett nail, the Pugh nail (also a sliding device), the Smith–Petersen nail, the McLaughlin side plate, and the Massie nail. Fixation with Deyerle pins and Haigie pins was used for intracapsular fractures, and even Richards screws were tried experimentally but were unsuccessful at that time. Many intracapsular fractures were treated by the classic Moore hemiarthroplasty and a variety of long-bone fractures were treated with Rush pins because Harry Emmel was particularly adept in this technique.

Complications were commonplace, including pneumonia in elderly patients with hip fractures, urinary obstructions in patients with prostate problems, and urinary tract infections associated with catheterization. Open bed sores, muscle atrophy, stiffness, chronic edema, and constipation were common with prolonged traction and casting.

The advent of Medicaid and Medicare in 1965, which funded patients rather than hospitals, changed the focus of patient care at Harborview from treatment of routine injuries to treatment of much more severe injuries. Given a choice of hospitals, most patients with fractures preferred to be taken to private hospitals, leaving Harborview to treat the indigent and

Department of Orthopaedics, Harborview Medical Center, University of Washington, Seattle, Washington 98104

those with multiple injuries. In response to losing funded patients, the Orthopaedic Service initiated more personal patient care and introduced unique services to attract new patients. The medical services trained emergency medical technicians through the Fire Department and a paramedic system emerged in 1970. Because the paramedics were able to stabilize severely injured patients at the site of accidents and thus prevent early death, they began bringing patients with very serious injuries to Harborview. In 1968, Dr. Donald Gunn, formerly the Professor of Orthopaedics in Singapore, joined the department as Chief of the Orthopaedic Service at Harborview and proved up to the task of developing more organized and supervised care for our changing patient population. The Orthopaedic Service was redirected in 1970 to treat relatively younger patients with very severe injuries caused by high-energy road traffic and industrial accidents. In addition to fractures, these patients often sustained injuries to multiple systems and required complex care.

Dissimilarities between fracture care and musculoskeletal traumatology were noted early. For example, we knew by the early 1970s, from experience with hip fracture fixation in the elderly and a brief experience with closed intramedullary nailing, that early operative fixation of open fractures and early closed intramedullary nailing of femoral fractures facilitated the overall management of severely injured patients. This assumption was strongly endorsed by others, including Dr. William Horton, an anesthesiologist who ran the surgical Intensive Care Unit at that time. In 1972, I assumed leadership of the Orthopaedic Service and initiated protocols that called for immediate operative stabilization of major long-bone fractures and open fractures in multiply injured patients.

Events that prepared the way for organization of a trauma team were soon to follow. In approximately 1975 a new surgical team with a very strong interest in trauma was assembled at Harborview. They requested to take over the care of all patients with injuries to more than one system and were in agreement with the objectives of the Orthopaedic Service. Orthopaedic guidelines called for operative fixation for all major long-bone fractures and fractures with open wounds immediately after patients were stabilized within general surgical guidelines. The primary care team soon came to include anesthesiologists accustomed to dealing with severely injured patients, and later, neurological surgeons. These four services—General Surgery, Orthopaedic Surgery, Anesthesiology, and Neurological Surgery—became the core of the traumatology team. The hospital's administration supported this endeavor by providing around-the-clock operating rooms, adequate intensive care units, and specialty surgical wards. A designated orthopaedic ward with an efficient and well-trained staff was established to provide optimal care for high-energy fracture patients in postoperative and post-ICU phases.

After patients' survival was guaranteed, problems with postsurgical complications and prolonged rehabilitation were addressed. In contrast to patients with isolated or low-energy fractures, severely injured patients require long hospitalization and extensive rehabilitation. The orthopaedic nursing staff addressed the needs of severely injured fracture patients, mobilizing them early to prevent secondary complications, caring for massive open wounds and injured soft tissues, and monitoring patients for signs of compartmental syndrome and infections. In addition to providing traditional instruction in bed exercises, crutch walking, muscle strengthening, and joint motion, physical therapists assumed responsibility for water-pick cleansing of severe open wounds before skin grafting and, occasionally, for whirlpool management of severe wounds. Occupational therapists managed positioning and self-care training in patients with upper extremity, head, and spinal cord injuries.

Next, attention was turned towards improving the surgical management of traumatized soft tissues. The standard techniques and instrumentation used in fracture care were obviously inadequate for dealing with very contused and stripped soft tissue, and their use resulted in unacceptably high rates of wound complications and infections. We began grading injuries to evaluate soft-tissue damage in open and closed injuries even when no fracture had been sustained. Grading injuries led to the important observation that the size of the open wound and the amount of visible contamination were not nearly as important to the ultimate prognosis as the amount of energy that was absorbed at the time of injury. High-energy injuries are characterized by displacement and comminution of the fracture, stripping and contusion of soft tissues and, occasionally, laceration of major neurovascular structures. A large zone of injury or a multiple-level fracture implied a grave prognosis and the need for early and highly skilled care.

The limitations of salvaging high-energy injuries with large zones of injury, especially those with damage to important vascular structures, became progressively more obvious. The "freeway syndrome" was identified and its ominous portent was recognized. The freeway syndrome occurs in high-energy open fractures, usually in the tibia, when vascular repair is required across a 4 in- to 8 in-long zone of injury. A long vein is grafted or an intact, stripped, and isolated artery traverses the injured area. This vessel (the freeway) might produce a pulse in the foot and elicit a triumphant response from the vascular surgeon, but it has no "off and on ramps" or tributaries within the zone of injury. Consequently, the local region is susceptible to progressive muscle necrosis, infection, and bone nonunion, and late amputation is often inevitable. Sepsis in a peripheral injury can cause secondary organ failure and sometimes leads to death. Once the patterns of deterioration leading to inevitable amputation were recognized, objective criteria were established to accurately direct treatment towards attempted salvage of the limb or to early amputation. Like immediate long-bone stabilization, immediate amputation prevents pulmonary complications, sepsis, and narcotic overload, which facilitates patient care and hastens rehabilitation.

Technological developments further advanced trauma care. Patients with complex fractures in the pelvis, the acetabulum, and the spine experienced the same problems resulting from recumbency and pain that were solved so effectively by early femoral stabilization, but in some cases the risks of very early surgery outweighed the gains. These risks decreased markedly after computerized tomography (CT) scanning became available to define the fracture patterns and allow safe early stabilization. Advanced magnetic resonance imaging (MRI) techniques were used to reveal more information about soft-tissue damage. New fixation devices, such as the locked intramedullary nail, made possible earlier mobilization of patients with comminuted or unstable femoral fractures.

Table 1. *Schematic for grading and triage*

C-O C-I O-I	C-II O-II	C-III O-IIIA O-IIIB O-IIIC
Fracture care	**Gray zone**	**Musculoskeletal traumatology**
Triage to personal physician or to a general hospital	Triage to general orthopaedist with good fracture skills or to a trauma center	Triage to a trauma center offering immediate response and access to traumatology specialists

TRAUMA CARE TODAY

Evaluation

Sophisticated evaluation of an injury is based on grading the magnitude of soft-tissue damage in open or closed injuries, with or without fracture, and relating this information to an accurate prognosis and a guide to treatment. A patient's age and general medical condition, the length of time between injury and treatment, and the presence of other systemic injuries are factors that must be taken into consideration before deciding whether treatment should be directed primarily towards maximizing rehabilitation, saving a limb, or saving a patient's life. Because the severity of a musculoskeletal injury is an important factor in the choice of treatment, a framework is needed to distinguish fracture care from traumatology. Injury severity scores, which have been used predominantly by general surgeons, help to predict mortality and morbidity. Fracture grading is used by musculoskeletal traumatologists to define the severity of the injury, to indicate treatment, and to provide a prognosis for functional outcome. Many evaluation systems are available, some so complex that they are almost unusable and others so simplistic that they are useless.

The system we presently use, which is probably familiar to most orthopaedic surgeons, is functional and practical. It is based on Gustilo's classification of open fractures (1) and Tscherne's classification of closed fractures (2). Both systems have been commonly used for several years in the United States and Europe and their parameters overlap (Table 1). Closed injuries are classified into four grades from 0 to III, and open injuries into five grades from I to IIIC. Fracture grading is based on several factors: the amount of energy absorbed during the injury, the presence of a closed or open injury, the fracture pattern, and the amount of damage to the circulatory system, as well as the subsequent potential for tissue or bone necrosis.

Energy Absorption

The amount of energy absorbed by the fracture is determined by the mechanism of injury. For example, a fall onto an outstretched arm is a relatively low-energy injury, whereas an impact by a fast-moving vehicle is a high-energy injury. In addition, the force must be identified as direct or indirect. For example, a direct force is applied when an automobile bumper strikes a tibia, but indirect force is responsible for a spiral tibia fracture caused by a twisting fall on skis.

Closed and Open Injuries

In closed injuries, factors to be taken into consideration are the amount and rapidity of swelling, the amount of fracture instability, torn ligaments, and obviously contused skin. In open injuries, relevant factors include the size of the open wound, the amount of contusion or necrosis around the wound edges, the amount and type of visible contamination, and the extent of soft-tissue stripping. The size of the zone of injury and the amount of injured soft tissue are the most pertinent factors related to grading.

Fracture Patterns

Fracture patterns are also associated with the amount of energy absorbed during injury. Highly comminuted or segmental fractures usually imply high-energy injuries, higher injury grading, and less favorable prognoses. Displacement of the fracture fragments seen on initial radiographs can help to estimate the energy absorbed during the injury.

Circulatory Damage

Circulatory damage includes not only arterial lacerations, contusion, and stripping but also damage to veins and lymphatics. Repairing lacerated arteries is useless if venous return and lymphatic drainage are inadequate or absent. For example, venous and lymphatic return may be damaged by circumferential degloving. Transection of named vessels, loose particles of bone that are completely denuded of soft tissue, and complete degloving are indicative of severe injuries.

Closed Injuries

According to these parameters, *closed grade 0* (C-0) fractures are relatively mild injuries causing minimal local soft-tissue damage. Representative fractures include greenstick fractures in children and some pathologic fractures in adults, as well as minimally displaced lateral ankle fractures and epiphyseal fractures.

Closed grade I (C-I) fractures cause moderate discomfort and early swelling but are relatively stable fractures that exhibit no skin contusion. These injuries occur from falls and other low-energy mechanisms and include most intracapsular and intertrochanteric fractures in the elderly, as well as many athletic injuries. Epiphyseal injuries in large joints, such as the knee, are also included in this category. Injuries in both these grades can usually be managed without hospitalization.

Closed grade II (C-II) fractures are relatively high-energy injuries and are common in multiply injured patients. They are often caused by direct application of force from contact sports, severe falls, and road traffic accidents. They usually produce displaced or comminuted fracture patterns and significant associated soft-tissue injuries. Fractures of this severity are very unstable and closed reduction cannot be maintained. They require reduction and stabilization by external or internal fixation, followed by a short period of elevation in the hospital.

Closed grade III (C-III) injuries include the most severe closed injuries. Injuries in this classification are almost always caused by significant application of direct force and result in severe soft-tissue injuries, fracture displacement, or joint dislocation. Common complications include degloving, extensive stripping of the skin from underlying fascia, large hematomas or large areas of necrotic tissue, vascular injuries, and other deep injuries requiring surgical repair. The prognosis for C-III injuries is guarded even when hospitalization and good surgical care have been provided. An example of an injury of this severity is a knee dislocation with an associated popliteal arterial injury.

Open Injuries

Gustilo's schema for grading open fractures uses the same parameters that are applied to potentially devitalized tissue and bone in closed fractures, but it includes the amount of contamination and the size of the open wound. The grading system consists of five fracture types; although none is as benign as C-0, they are otherwise numerically comparable up to the most severe open injury grades, which have no counterparts in closed injuries. This schema reflects injury severity scoring and establishes the foundation of triage principles used by paramedics to transport patients to the appropriate hospital.

Open grade I (O-I) fractures are caused by relatively low-energy injuries from indirect forces. Laceration of the skin may be due to a bone spike penetrating the skin from within or from a small-bore, low-energy gunshot wound, usually in the upper extremity. Minimal soft tissue is stripped from bone and crushing is not present. Injuries in this grade correspond to C-I fractures in severity and prognosis.

Open grade II (O-II) injuries are caused by higher-energy, directly applied force, most commonly from road traffic accidents and contact sports. The open wounds are associated with no skin or soft-tissue loss and little contusion or contamination of the wound edges. Fractures of this type may be slightly comminuted but are not significantly displaced. Hospitalization is required for careful debridement and skeletal stabilization to protect the soft tissues from further damage. In general, injuries are graded *after* debridement.

Open grade IIIA (O-IIIA) fractures correspond to C-III fractures and are caused by significant violence. The forces producing this injury are strong enough to cause marked bone displacement and comminution, as well as significant soft-tissue injury. The zone of injury is larger than 4" and some soft tissue and skin are usually lost during debridement. The open wound is usually large and obviously contaminated. Muscle compartments may be open and the muscle may be crushed and separated from bone, but the muscle belly is not completely transected. The incidence of complications, including infection and nonunion, is high, especially when the fracture is not treated by traumatologists. Injuries of this severity are usually caused by road traffic accidents and often occur as components of multiple-injury complexes.

Open grade IIIB (O-IIIB) injuries occur from violent injury, usually from directly applied forces. The skin edges are extremely contused and soft tissue is stripped from bone fragments. A zone of injury over 6" is characterized by significant swelling but no major named vessels are transected. Management of the fracture may be complicated by marked bone displacement, severe comminution, and possibly complete stripping and loss of bone fragments up to 4" long. The size of the open wound and the amount of contamination and crushed tissue often warrant extensive debridement and subsequent skin grafting or free-tissue transfers to cover exposed bone and vital soft tissues. One or more muscle bellies may be completely transected or may have sustained full-thickness contusion.

Open grade IIIC (O-IIIC) injuries are similar to O-IIIB injuries but also involve loss of major vascular, neural, muscle, or bone continuity over a zone of injury that is 6" or larger. These severe injuries require early vascular repair to maintain viability in the distal limb. Partial and complete traumatic amputations are included in this category, as well as severe intercalary injuries requiring amputation for definitive treatment. Although injuries with cavitation from high-energy gunshot wounds or close-range shotgun wounds are included in this category, the most common mechanisms are road traffic accidents and major industrial accidents. A more extensive overview of the pathophysiology of severe trauma can be found in Border et al. (3).

Treatment

Through careful evaluation, the treatment of musculoskeletal injuries can be classified into one of two categories: fracture care or musculoskeletal traumatology. Injuries relegated to fracture care can be adequately managed by any orthopaedist in any general hospital. Musculoskeletal traumatology, on the other hand, is vastly different from fracture care. The care of C-III, O-IIIA, O-IIIB, and O-IIIC injuries is highly demanding, very technical, and team-oriented, and should be done in trauma centers where diverse specialists and facilities are available. When musculoskeletal trauma is not treated in a trauma center, the rate of complications is significantly higher. Injuries falling within the gray zone, C-II and O-II, require care by orthopedists who devote half their practice to trauma and who have ongoing experience with common problems such as hip and ankle fractures.

The Trauma Team

Long experience with trauma has taught us that as the severity of an injury increases, care must become more aggressive in terms of both timing and atraumatic fracture stabilization. The trauma team must be available to carry out complex procedures at all hours, working under the leadership of the trauma team captain. The specialty training of trauma team captains is not as important as their constant presence in the Emergency Department and their total commitment to the role. Specialists from at least four services should be members of the trauma team: an anesthesiologist with skills to induce anesthesia in patients with head injury, flail chest, ruptured viscus, or open fractures immediately after injury; a general surgeon with urgent surgical skills as well as intensive care skills; a neurological surgeon with an interest in trauma and skills in CT and intracranial bolt monitoring; and an orthopaedic surgeon with expertise in managing contused and otherwise severely damaged soft tissues and experience with diverse skeletal stabilization techniques. Severely injured patients often require specialized orthopaedic care for injuries to the spine, the hand, and the foot. The scope of musculoskeletal trauma demands that orthopaedic traumatologists keep abreast of technology and advances within these subspecialties. When sufficient numbers of traumatologists practice in the same facility, these subspecialty skills can be developed as a second interest. Alternatively, individuals with these skills should become affiliated with the trauma center and be available for consultation. Support services, including radiology, angiography, urology, ophthalmology, and otolaryngology should also be available at short notice.

Early Fracture Stabilization

The importance of stabilizing long-bone and axial skeletal fractures early is now well documented, particularly for femoral fractures (4). Early alignment, reduction, and stabilization of open fractures, especially open fractures in joints, decreases the incidence of infection and significantly improves functional outcome. Early stabilization is defined as surgery occurring within 8 to 16 h of injury in closed fractures and within 4 to 6 h of injury in open fractures. Early care performed within these time frames also reduces the cost of care by decreasing morbidity and mortality, ICU time, hospital time, and the amount of disability.

Postoperative Management and Rehabilitation

After early stabilization, patients are managed by surgical intensivists for fluid retention, pulmonary decompensation, and other organ vulnerability for the first few postoperative days and are moved to the orthopaedic ward soon thereafter. Here, the orthopaedic team begins rehabilitation and instigates measures to ward off secondary complications. Complications are treated early and aggressively to avoid unnecessary expense, disability, and frustration (see Chapter 6).

Pain Management

The earliest major postsurgical problem is pain. Stable fixation and careful handling of soft tissues usually resolves intense pain within approximately 2 days postoperatively. Postoperative regional nerve blocks or epidural anesthesia provide pain relief for 4 to 96 h after surgery, but these measures must be avoided if compartmental syndrome is present or suspected. Regularly administered or patient-controlled analgesia (PCA) may be required for 1 or 2 days postoperatively. In early trials, a new injectable nonsteroidal drug, Ketorolac, seems to be very effective in relieving pain and preventing the nausea and physiologic depression that are associated with heavy narcotics. A diurnal medication regimen must be implemented within 24 to 48 h postoperatively. Narcotic analgesia or strong medications are administered only at night and their dosage is decreased considerably during the daytime, when patients are distracted from their pain by activities such as bed exercises, breathing exercises, television viewing, and visitors. By avoiding strong medications during the day, patients return quickly to diurnal sleep patterns, normal elimination, eating, and are able to perform deep breathing exercises.

Support Services

Mobility during the day prevents atelectasis, pneumonia, constipation, urinary stasis, bed sores, depression, and other complications that commonly are caused by a prolonged recumbency. During the first 2 postoperative days, ward nurses supervise mobilization. By the third day, a physical therapist takes over direction of all the activities patients must master before returning home. The services of social workers are essential for many patients. Because trauma often affects people who are having difficulties in their lives, social workers may be needed to find living accommodations, assist interaction with other family members, solve financial problems, and take care of a multitude of other problems. In the immediate postinjury phase, social workers may be needed to advise distressed family members and help them cope with their loss. Many details of a patient's life are often unknown to the surgeon but can affect subsequent rehabilitation. After discharge from the hospital patients are followed in the appropriate outpatient departments. Most ongoing problems affecting multiply injured patients are musculoskeletal, and these are usually followed in the Orthopaedic Department or its divisions.

Documentation

The details of a patient's treatment and progress are entered into a documentation system, in which information on treatment used for particular types of problems is compiled. For a documentation system to function optimally, computer technicians must work closely with nurses in the outpatient department, physical therapists, and physicians, all of whom monitor a patient's progress and watch for complications.

Note: Harborview is now entering its third decade as a trauma center and I am beginning my fourth decade as a physician with a major interest in traumatic musculoskeletal injuries. Through my experiences at Harborview, I have formulated a strong philosophy about evaluation, treatment, and rehabilitation of musculoskeletal injuries and how these factors relate to overall patient care. The treatment of high-energy traumatic injuries is usually, but not always, different from that of low-energy fractures. Sometimes only the timing of the operation differs; at other times, treatment varies within the context of the injury. For example, treatment for a severe local injury might be different from treatment for an injury that threatens the limb or life of a multiply injured patient. The objective in the first case is to maximize rehabilitation of the affected limb; the goal in the second is to save the patient's life. The purpose of this book is twofold: to present our management protocols for treating patients with high-energy injuries and multiple potential complications and to define musculoskeletal traumatology as a distinct subspecialty of Orthopaedic Surgery apart from fracture care.

REFERENCES

1. Gustilo RB, Mendoza RM, Williams DM. Problems in management of type III open fractures. A new classification of type III open fractures. *J Trauma* 1984;24:742–746.
2. Tscherne H, Oestern H-J. Pathophysiology and classification of soft tissue injuries associated with fractures. In: Tscherne H, Gotzen L, eds. *Fractures with soft tissue injuries.* Berlin: Springer-Verlag; 1984: 1–9.
3. Border JR, Allgöwer M, Hansen ST, Rüedi TP, eds. *Blunt multiple trauma. Comprehensive pathophysiology and care.* New York: Marcel Dekker; 1990.
4. Bone LB, Johnson KD, Weigelt J, Scheinberg R. Early versus delayed stabilization of femoral fractures. A prospective randomized study. *J Bone Joint Surg* 1989;71A:336–340.

Orthopaedic Trauma Protocols, edited by Sigvard T. Hansen, Jr., and Marc F. Swiontkowski, Raven Press, Ltd., New York,© 1993.

CHAPTER 2

The Role of the Trauma Surgeon in the Management of Orthopaedic Trauma

Gregory J. Jurkovich

Trauma is the leading cause of death and disability in young Americans and the fourth leading cause of death (after heart disease, cancer, and stroke) in all age groups. The National Safety Council estimates that of the nearly 60 million injuries that occur annually in the United States, 50% require medical care and 10% require hospital admission. An accidental death occurs every 6 min and an injury every 4 s. In 1987, approximately 146,000 deaths in the United States resulted from trauma and for each death there were approximately three permanently disabling injuries. In 1986, deaths and disability cost the nation approximately $118 billion dollars (1).

Motor vehicle accidents are the major cause of death and injury in the general population; falls are the major cause of injury and death in the elderly. As might be expected from these mechanisms of injury, fractures make up a large percentage of these injuries. In 1986, 47% of the 1.8 million work-related injuries that occurred in the United States were disabling injuries to the extremities (1). Approximately 3,000 patients with isolated and multiple traumatic injuries are admitted each year to Harborview Medical Center, a tertiary referral level I trauma center. Of the trauma victims admitted to Harborview in 1989, 36% had sustained orthopaedic injuries: 15% had isolated orthopaedic injuries and 21% had orthopaedic injuries with concurrent head, face, neck, or torso injuries.

Virtually all major trauma centers in the United States have adopted a team approach to care for victims of multiple trauma. The membership of the team is dictated by the availability of personnel and hospital resources but typically includes several physician specialists whose activities are coordinated and directed by a general surgeon specially trained and experienced in trauma care. In contrast, trauma care in Europe is assumed by a traumatologist, who is responsible for the primary management of all the injuries.

The focus of this chapter is on the team approach to trauma care, particularly on the principles of initial triage and the emergency treatment of multiply injured trauma patients. Specific aspects of care will be reviewed and current concepts of regional trauma system development will be outlined.

Department of Surgery. Harborview Medical Center, University of Washington, Seattle, Washington 98104

TRAUMA TEAM ORGANIZATION

The components of a trauma team are dictated in part by the availability of physicians and hospital resources and by the level of trauma care that can realistically be provided by an institution. Recognizing these limitations, the American College of Surgeons (ACS) suggested a three-tiered classification of centers that provide trauma care:

Level I: regional trauma centers providing the most comprehensive trauma care,
Level II: community trauma centers, and
Level III: rural trauma hospitals providing initial treatment and triage (2).

Although the dedication of the participating physicians is essential for providing effective trauma care, the commitment of the hospital and the community are equally important. The trauma team must educate hospital administrators and the community about the importance of having adequate physical space, good nursing care and ancillary personnel, and adequate material resources to provide trauma care to the community. Educating the community and hospital administrators about these important aspects of trauma care is an important aspect of trauma team leadership.

Trauma Team and Team Captain

Trauma care is complex and has many confusing facets. Successful treatment of multiply injured patients requires concise thinking and practiced execution. The management of multiply injured patients is best provided by a trauma team consisting of primary care physicians, consulting physicians, nurses, allied health professionals, and ancillary support staff (Table 1). Although the care of these patients requires the expertise of many individuals, the importance of identifying a single individual as the team leader or captain cannot be overemphasized. Effective leadership is critical to coordinating the activities of individual physicians who might tend to focus on specific problems without paying attention to a patient's overall status. The team captain's responsibilities are to: (i) assess the patient's overall status, (ii) determine the need for specific diagnostic tests and to delegate these activities to team members, (iii) coordinate the activities of ancillary services and specialty consultants, and (iv) make critical treatment and triage decisions. The team captain must be willing to accept the responsibility of leadership, and the other team members must acknowledge and accept that individual as their leader (Fig. 1). Conversely, the team captain must have a clear understanding of how each team member's capabilities contribute to overall patient care.

Ideally, the team captain should be a senior general surgeon on the hospital's trauma service, although an emergency physician may assume this role until the surgeon is available. Overall patient assessment and management decisions are made by the team captain, but technical procedures are delegated to other team members whenever possible. Delegating tasks allows the team captain to continually oversee resuscitation, thus ensuring that the resuscitation is appropriately focused and that no details are neglected or overlooked.

Table 1: *The Trauma Team*[a]

Team Captain
Primary Emergency Care Physicians:
Head
Right side
Left side
Foot
Consulting Physicians:
Anesthesiology or anesthetist
Orthopaedics
Neurosurgery
Otolaryngology/Head and neck
Oral/Maxillofacial surgery
Plastic surgery
Urology
Nurses:
Scribe
Right side
Left side
Transportation monitor
Allied Health Professionals:
Radiology technician
Respiratory therapist
Blood-draw technician
Support staff:
Clerk/secretary
Transportation
Houskeeping

[a]The number of members on a trauma team depends on the size of the institution, the availability of the house staff, and the level of designation of the trauma center. The team members appearing in bold type are considered essential for the initial evaluation of all victims of major trauma. The position designations refer to the location of each team member relative to the patient. Each position has specific, predetermined responsibilities.

Trauma Team Physicians

The members of the physician trauma team must be identified and their duties designated before the arrival of a trauma victim. Although available manpower clearly depends on the resources of the medical institution, sufficient personnel must be preassigned and available for trauma resuscitations. In teaching institutions, general surgery and emergency medicine residents provide adequate manpower while they receive excellent training in initial trauma care. In community hospitals, primary care physicians, on-call surgeons, nurse

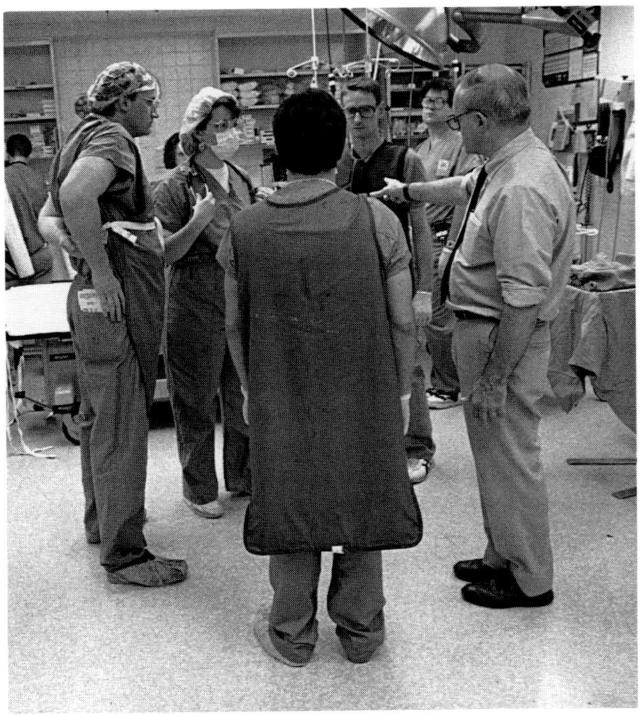

FIG. 1. The team captain is in charge of the evaluation and resuscitation. Delegation of duties prior to patient arrival expedites care. (Photo credit: Rex Ziak. Used with permission.)

anesthetists, or emergency department physicians must assume this role.

Preassignment of team members' duties by their positions around the patient streamlines resuscitation (Fig. 2). For example, the physician assigned to the head of the gurney is responsible for airway control, C-spine stabilization, and nasogastric tube insertion, while the physician assigned to the patient's right side is responsible for intravenous access, Foley catheter insertion, and tube thoracostomy or diagnostic peritoneal lavage. Preassignment of responsibilities has the additional advantage of minimizing noise and confusion during a complex resuscitation, allowing the team captain to focus on directing the resuscitation and planning diagnostic and treatment strategies. Physician team members are expected to provide the team captain with valuable clinical information but they must refrain from making independent clinical decisions. Their primary role is to execute the therapeutic and diagnostic maneuvers ordered by the team captain.

Nurses and Ancillary Personnel

Trauma team nurses provide invaluable assistance during the initial resuscitation. Their primary responsibility is to measure and record vital signs and to report these findings to the team captain. Other responsibilities include administering fluids and drugs, drawing blood or assisting in blood drawing, and assisting with procedures when directed to do so by the team captain. Documenting resuscitation activities may require an individual's full attention, and having a well-organized flow sheet to record data is essential (Fig. 3). A myriad of related activities, such as removing clothing and transporting materials, are dependent on nursing organization and preparation and these functions should be performed without direct orders from the team captain.

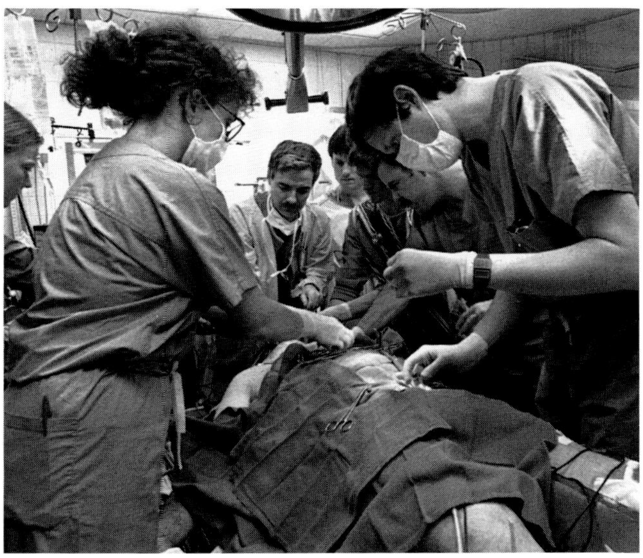

FIG. 2. The duties of each member of the trauma team are designated by position around the patient. (Photo credit: Rex Ziak. Used with permission.)

The organized responses of technicians, assistants, and aides should make resuscitation more efficient, not more noisy, chaotic, or confusing. Radiology technicians must produce good-quality radiographs and should be prepared to obtain a prearranged set of trauma films, including lateral views of the cervical spine, an AP view of the supine chest, and an AP of the pelvis, in the midst of a trauma resuscitation. Respiratory technicians must be ready to administer supplemental oxygen, provide suction, perform mechanical ventilation, and monitor pulse oximetry. The blood bank must be prepared to dispatch necessary blood products. Sufficient aides or clerks must be available to expedite seemingly endless laboratory requests, phone calls, and errands.

The Emergency Department is the portal into the hospital's services, not the site of definitive care. Definitive care of trauma victims often involves a surgical procedure and the team captain must not delay an essential operative procedure by attempting minor therapeutic procedures or performing nonessential diagnostic maneuvers. This type of delay is common when a house officer with inadequate experience acts as the team captain and does not prioritize care appropriately. Coordinating and triaging the treatment plans suggested by the trauma team specialty consultants (e.g., orthopaedists and neurosurgeons) is one of the team captain's critical responsibilities, and the specialty consultants must respect the team captain's directives. The team captain should be able to set limits on operating time and blood loss for a given orthopaedic procedure, e.g., stabilization of a long bone, knowing that the orthopedist is familiar with several techniques that can be applied to a given situation.

Trauma Care Quality Assurance

The team approach to trauma care requires a forum for discussing problems, reviewing adverse outcomes, disseminating information, and implementing new programs or protocols. Regularly scheduled meetings of physician members of the trauma team, including primary physicians, consultants, and team captains, is essential for a harmonious team effort. This type of trauma council also serves as a quality assurance control by which quality of care is documented, outcome is assessed and warranted changes in protocols are implemented. A weekly surgical morbidity and mortality review is also well suited to trauma care assessment. Quantitative factors of quality care, such as emergency department and operating room response times for physicians and ancillary personnel, unplanned repeat operations, and the length of time to perform diagnostic tests, should be reviewed on a regular basis. Internally defined

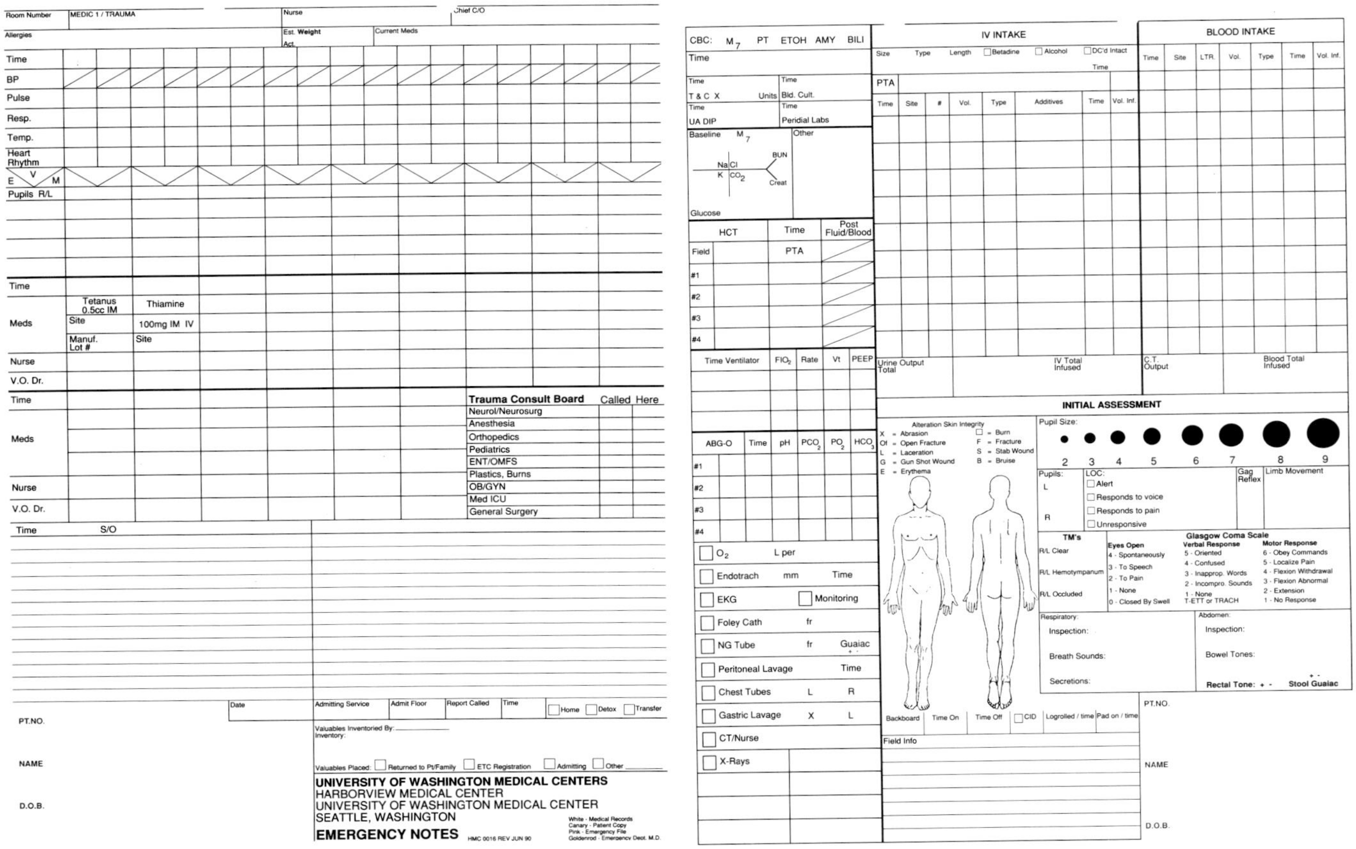

FIG. 3. A,B: A sample flow sheet.

criteria can be used to supplement the standards established by the ACS Committee on Trauma (3). The management of individual patients should be reviewed by the trauma council or by a similar review group.

The trauma registry, which provides a catalogue of patients and procedures pertaining exclusively to trauma, has become an essential component of a trauma center. The registry can be screened to find patients who were treated outside the established guidelines for quality care and to define the trauma population that is served by the hospital. It is also a valuable resource for reviewing trauma outcome retrospectively. Virtually every member of the trauma team must participate in providing information to the trauma registry, although the complexity of the recorded data will vary according to each institution's needs. At present, no single nationally accepted registry exists. Several software packages are commercially available for hospital-based trauma registries and all are designed for personal microcomputers. Some states (Pennsylvania, Virginia, Oregon) and individual institutions (Harborview Medical Center) have designed and developed unique registries.

The Major Trauma Outcome Study (MTOS) group was established in 1982 to collect data on demographics, etiology and severity of injury, as well as outcome from a number of trauma centers, then pool this information to provide national outcome standards for trauma (4). Although more than 100,000 trauma patients are currently entered into this database, information on the patients is incomplete because participation by institutions was voluntary. Nevertheless, this database is a reliable starting point for institutional self-evaluation and comparison to national norms. Recognizing the limitations of the MTOS and the need for data that can be interpreted on a national level, the ACS Committee on Trauma is presently developing a national trauma registry and software package with well-defined minimal and optimal data-entry criteria. Central storage and data processing will be located at the ACS office in Chicago, but participating institutions will have access to the information and data-analysis capabilities.

PRINCIPLES OF INITIAL MANAGEMENT OF THE MULTIPLY INJURED PATIENT

Triage Priorities

Successful resuscitation of a trauma victim is predicated on treating injuries in the order of their importance. For this approach to succeed, two assumptions must be accepted as true: (i) the patient might have more than one injury, and (ii) the obvious injury might not be the most serious one. Four categories of injury are identified:

1. *Exigent:* the most life-threatening conditions requiring instantaneous intervention (e.g., airway obstruction, tension pneumothorax)
2. *Emergent:* conditions requiring intervention within the first hour after injury (e.g., subdural/epidural hematoma, ongoing intraabdominal hemorrhage, suspected torn aorta)
3. *Urgent:* conditions requiring early intervention within the first few hours of injury (e.g., open fracture, femoral fracture in a multiple-trauma patient, hip dislocation)
4. *Deferrable:* conditions that are neither life threatening nor immediately apparent but which will require treatment or further evaluation (e.g., contusions/abrasions, facial fractures, distal extremity fractures)

Thus, resuscitation requires a deliberate and regimented approach yet one with enough flexibility to change priorities if they are warranted by diagnostic disclosures that are discovered during resuscitation. Maintaining a balance between a structured resuscitation protocol and a possible sudden change in priorities is the responsibility of one person, the team captain.

Initial Resuscitation

The principles of initial assessment and management described in the ACS Advanced Trauma Life Support (ATLS) course have been widely accepted as guidelines for early trauma care (5). The key to initial care is treatment of injuries in the order of their life-threatening potential. The priorities of initial trauma care are often called the ABCs of trauma resuscitation.

Airway

Brain function is permanently impaired after 3 min of anoxia. Therefore, the first priority in trauma care is to ensure an adequate airway, followed by adequate ventilation and oxygenation. Mechanical removal of oral debris and chin-lift or jaw-thrust maneuvers can be attempted first in less severely injured patients. However, if adequacy of the airway is in question because of shock or severe head, facial, or thoracic trauma, more definitive airway control is indicated. In most cases this involves endotracheal intubation.

No trauma patient should expire from lack of an airway because of concern over a possible cervical spinal injury. Endotracheal intubation in an unconscious or intoxicated patient with a possible cervical spinal injury warrants gentle maneuvers to restore the airway and injudicious movements of the neck should be avoided. Nasotracheal intubation can be performed in a patient who has not sustained a midfacial injury and who is breathing spontaneously. Rarely, surgical establishment of an airway (tracheostomy) may be required.

Breathing

The three most common reasons for ineffective ventilation after successful placement of an airway are malposition of the endotracheal tube, pneumothorax, and hemothorax. Although chest radiographs usually cannot be obtained before invasive therapeutic procedures in patients with profound hemodynamic instability or suspected tension pneumothorax, needle-catheter decompression can be used both to make a diagnosis and to initiate therapy. Under these circumstances, rapid decompression of the chest with tube thoracostomy or a flutter valve is appropriate before a radiograph is obtained. Assisted ventilation may also be necessary in the presence of decreased respiratory drive (e.g., in a head injury) or an unstable chest wall.

Circulation

Control of obvious hemorrhage, placement of intravenous lines, and fluid replacement are the next priorities. When possible, control of hemorrhage should precede the placement of intravenous lines. Applying direct external compression to sites of obvious hemorrhage is preferable to blind clamping or placing tourniquets. Traction and splinting of extremity fractures should be maintained during resuscitation. Military antishock trousers (MAST) are often used as a temporary splint for pelvic fractures, although their efficacy in this role is not documented.

At least two large-bore (16-gauge) intravenous cannulas are usually placed percutaneously in the arm or the groin but should not be placed through an injured extremity unless absolutely necessary. Alternative access sites include the saphenous vein via a cutdown in adults and intraosseus infusion in children under the age of 6 years. With the exception of large (8 French) introduction catheters, subclavian venipuncture does not permit rapid fluid administration and is best reserved for monitoring responses to fluid therapy. An initial bolus of 1000 ml of lactated Ringer's solution is administered in adults and 20 ml/kg is administered in children. The response to therapy is monitored by skin perfusion, urinary output, and central venous pressure readings after the line has been placed. Hemodynamic stability is defined as the presence of normal vital signs requiring only maintenance levels of fluid replacement. The need for continuous fluid boluses to maintain normal blood pressure is indicative of ongoing blood loss.

Disability/Neurologic Assessment

A critical component of the initial resuscitation is a brief examination conducted to determine the severity of neurologic injury. This examination includes assessment of the patient's level of consciousness, pupillary response, sensation, and motor activity in all the extremities. The level of consciousness can be assessed and documented by the AVPU system: (A alert; V, responds to verbal stimuli; P, responds to painful stimuli; U, unresponsive.) A more precise measurement of neurologic disability and predicted recovery is provided by the Glasgow Coma Scale, developed by Teasdale and Jennett (Table 2) (6). When we document responses according to the Glasgow Coma Scale, we add the modifiers "T" (intubated) and "P" (paralyzed) to indicate that the score may be inaccurate. Pupillary response can be assessed in a paralyzed patient.

Table 2. *Glasgow coma scale*

Eye Opening	
Spontaneous	E4
To speech	3
To pain	2
Nil	1
Best Motor Response	
Obeys	M6
Localizes	5
Withdraws	4
Abnormal flexion	3
Extensor response	2
Nil	1
Verbal Response	
Oriented	V5
Confused conversation	4
Inappropriate words	3
Incomprehensible sounds	2
Nil	1
Coma Score (E + M + V) = 3 to 15	

Exposure for Complete Examination

By this point, most life-threatening injuries have been identified and treated. The next step is to completely undress (E, exposure) the patient and to perform a thorough but expeditious physical examination. A complete physical examination (F, "ph"ysical) is done typically from head to toe and includes data analyses from appropriate laboratory and radiographic tests. The results of the accumulated data sometimes warrant reevaluation and establishment of new treatment priorities. Additional lines, catheters (nasogastric, Foley), and monitoring devices can be placed during the examination.

After adequate oxygenation, ventilation, and perfusion have been established, subsequent treatment can be planned. If a patient is not adequately resuscitated by this time, the ABCs are reviewed to ensure that no significant injury has been overlooked (G, go back to the beginning). Initial lack of response to resuscitation is usually due to unrecognized cardiac tamponade, delayed development of tension pneumothorax, or unrecognized retroperitoneal bleeding. Continued patient instability in the absence of these conditions requires additional assistance (H, help).

Problem Areas

These well-established priorities of trauma care and resuscitation apply to most trauma victims. The ABCs of resuscitation are simple, straightforward, dogmatic, and effective. They help the emergency physician, the primary care doctor, or the responding surgeon to sort through the complexity of early care and to treat early life-threatening complications in the order of their urgency. As the complexity of the injury increases, the options for treatment also increase, and triage and emergency care may include diagnostic maneuvers and definitive procedures in addition to resuscitation. The trauma team captain retains the authority to establish the priority of diagnostic studies and definitive care after consultations with specialists. At our institution, one general surgery trauma specialist objectively oversees all phases of trauma care. Diagnostic and treatment modalities are prescribed in the sequence of the patient's overall needs, avoiding a narrow focus on specialty problems or considerations of physicians' convenience.

Some problems regarding the care of multiply injured patients arise frequently, and trauma centers respond to these problems by developing their own consistent protocols to minimize confusion, debate, and delay. Examples of potential patient-management problems include uncertainty about the presence of cervical spinal fractures, airway problems, pelvic fractures with intraabdominal bleeding, torso trauma with potential spinal injuries, and combined head-and-torso trauma requiring laparotomy or thoracotomy. Another common problem is lack of clearly defined indications for torso or extremity angiography. Topics for discussion that arise frequently at this institution include: (i) how to determine when a patient needs rapid long-bone fixation rather than optimal fixation aimed at a good long-term functional result; or (ii) when an elaborate work-up is indicated; and (iii) when factors such as increased intracerebral pressure, hypothermia, or coagulopathy might warrant a delay in internal fixation. Making these decisions requires an excellent understanding both of the positive effects of early long-bone stabilization on decreasing systemic problems, including ARDS, and of the modifying factors (operating time, expected blood loss, patient positioning) associated with the various methods of bone stabilization. The postoperative management of multiply injured patients is also a frequent topic of discussion. In most cases the general trauma surgeon remains the patient's primary physician during the postoperative period, particularly when treatment in the Intensive Care Unit is required. The patient is transferred to a specialty service or to another physician's care when the major remaining management problem is a single organ system. As a result, the general surgeon is responsible for much of a multiply injured patient's early postoperative care even when no general surgical procedures were performed.

These discussions are most productive when the relative risks and benefits to the patient are discussed in a calm and reasoned manner by the specialty consultants, the anesthesiologist, and the senior trauma surgeon, who serves as the mediator and the final arbitrator. Clearly, the benefits of the discussion are related to the experience of the participants, and a patient's best interests are served when survival with the least possible morbidity is the common goal.

PREVENTABLE DEATH

Despite the recognition that trauma is the leading cause of death in children and young adults, injury continues to be the most neglected disease of modern society. Development of regional trauma care systems is limited by concerns about need, efficacy, cost, and economic impact on hospitals and physicians. In 1988, West et al. (7) surveyed the state chairmen of the ACS Committee on Trauma and found that 29 states totally lacked a trauma care system, 19 were deficient in one or more components, and only two states satisfied all the requirements of a statewide trauma care system. Nevertheless, it is becoming increasingly obvious that trauma centers and trauma systems save lives. The most striking example of the impact of trauma care systems on our society is expressed by the concept of preventable death. Initially based on subjective impressions and implicit criteria, this concept has evolved over the past three decades into well-defined objective findings based on explicit criteria.

In 1955, Zollinger (8) examined the quality of trauma care that was provided for victims of motor vehicle accidents. Over the next two decades, quality of care became closely associated with outcome as others reviewed fatalities and identified subpopulations of patients who might have survived with optimal care. In 1974, Trunkey and Lim (9) analyzed 425 fatalities in San Francisco. They found that 155 of these patients were alive at the time the ambulance arrived and concluded that 19 of the deaths were preventable. Most notably, they found that the incidence of preventable deaths at the trauma center was disproportionately lower than the incidence of preventable death at other hospitals. Six deaths among 142 patients treated at the designated trauma center were deemed preventable, compared with 13 deaths in 13 patients treated elsewhere.

In 1979, West et al. (10) compared trauma care in two California counties. They found that 39 of 90 deaths should have been prevented in Orange County, whereas only one of 92 was found to be preventable in San Francisco County. They attributed this difference to lack of a trauma system. Orange County trauma victims were brought to the nearest hospital but patients in San Francisco County were brought to San Francisco General, the trauma center for that county.

In 1985, Cales and Trunkey (11) reviewed 22 reports from nontrauma systems and found their average preventable death rate to be 27%. More recently, Dade County, Florida reported a preventable death rate of 21% in trauma patients without central nervous system damage (12). The causes of death were attributed primarily to delayed surgery or to the lack of an appropriate surgical procedure. The rate of preventable death in Dade County's level I trauma center was 12% compared with 26% at the other 22 hospitals in the county. Implementation of a regional trauma system in Orange County reduced preventable mortality by more than 50%. In San Diego County, the implementation of a regional trauma system is credited with reducing preventable mortality from 13.5% to 2.7% (13).

Evidence is mounting from preventable death studies that trauma care systems make a difference. The fact that trauma is the leading cause of lost productive life should serve as a stimulus and a challenge to trauma system development and should help to overcome the legion of obstacles preventing establishment of regional trauma care systems. The key components of a regional or state trauma system have been identified and several working trauma system models currently exist (Pennsylvania, Oregon, San Diego). The implementation and management of such systems has been outlined step by step (7).

REGIONAL TRAUMA SYSTEM ORGANIZATION

Designation of a hospital as a trauma care facility implies a coordinated three-phase response to trauma. Each phase (prehospital, hospital, and rehabilitation) is an important step in providing optimal care (14). The importance of prehospital care is well documented. Ornato et al. (15) noted that the number of deaths due to trauma in Nebraska declined by 24% from 1972 to 1982 after improved prehospital emergency medical services were established. The components of prehospital care include a committed medical director, established lines of communication, tested triage criteria, effective transportation, and a cadre of prehospital care providers who are trained in specific field interventions.

Hospital care comprises care provided in the emergency department, the operating room, and the acute wards, and involves a tremendous dedication and coordination of hospital resources. Although the impact of improved rehabilitative services within a trauma system has not been adequately examined, the National Research Council's white paper, *Injury in America,* highlights rehabilitation as an integral factor in returning an injured patient to a productive life (16). Coordination of these three phases of trauma care is essential because deficiencies in one component can negate the benefits in care derived from the others. Local, regional, and state councils have been established in some states to oversee trauma system development. These councils are usually under the direction of the State Department of Health or its equivalent or of an independent trauma foundation, such as the one that exists in Pennsylvania.

The concept of regional medical care is neither new nor unique to trauma care. Luft and colleagues (17) argued for concentration of resources and presented data on 12 complex general surgical procedures, demonstrating a decreased mortality rate with larger numbers of patients. As noted earlier in the discussion about preventable death, several other studies have also demonstrated the value of regional civilian trauma care. Studies from diverse geographic and demographic areas report similar incidences of preventable deaths (24–35%) in areas without regional trauma systems and less than half those rates after system deployment (11).

The goals of regional trauma care systems are to decrease mortality and to minimize disability and morbidity resulting from injury. Trunkey (18) and others have suggested that trauma deaths follow a trimodal distribution: immediate, early, and late. Most immediate deaths (from severe head injuries or transected aortas) can be prevented only by public education and new insights into preventing injuries. Patients who die early often have sustained a severe but correctable injury, such as an epidural or subdural hematoma, hemopneumothorax, spleen or liver fractures, or blood loss from fractures and multiple injuries. Trauma center hospitals and coordinated prehospital care benefit these patients the most dramatically. Trauma victims who die later usually succumb to infection, sepsis, or multiple organ failure, often as a consequence of complications from their initial management. These patients also benefit from regional trauma centers because patients with the most difficult problems are concentrated in specially equipped and staffed centers that are prepared to deal with them.

The lack of care for disabled patients represents perhaps the most significant single deficiency in trauma care in the United States today. With the exception of a few excellent spinal cord rehabilitation centers, inadequate effort has been expended on incorporating rehabilitation into regional trauma care systems. The efficacy of rehabilitation, especially for spinal cord injuries, is well documented. Approximately 85% of patients who are rehabilitated after spinal cord injuries are able to live independently, with fewer complications and subsequent hospitalizations. Moreover, the cost of rehabilitation is less than one tenth the cost of custodial care and repeated hospitalizations (16).

Establishment of regional trauma care throughout the United States requires excellent cooperation among governments, insurance agencies, hospitals, physicians, and other health-care providers. Proof that such a drastic alteration in the current care of trauma is truly beneficial must be provided before resources are committed. Data are needed from regional trauma care systems that clearly show a decrease in mortality and morbidity rates at a reasonable cost. It is the responsibility of physicians currently practicing in regional trauma centers to demonstrate the advantages of such systems and to educate the public, political leaders, and health-care administrators about the advantages of modern trauma care.

REFERENCES

1. National Safety Council, ed. *Accident facts.* Chicago: 1990.
2. Committee on Trauma, American College of Surgeons, eds. *Resources for optimal care of the injured patient.* Chicago: 1990.
3. In: *Resources for optimal care of the injured patient.* Committee on Trauma, American College of Surgeons, eds. Quality assurance in trauma care. Chicago: 1990.
4. Champion H, Copes W, Sacco W, Flanagan M. Injury severity scoring. In: Moore EE, ed. *Early care of the injured patient.* Toronto: B C Decker; 1990.
5. Committee on Trauma, American College of Surgeons, eds. *Advanced trauma life support manual.* Chicago: American College of Surgeons; 1989.
6. Teasdale G, Jennett B. Assessment of coma and impaired consciousness: a practical scale. *Lancet* 1974;81–4.
7. West J, Williams M, Trunkey D, Wolferth C. Trauma systems. Current status—future challenges. *JAMA* 1988;259:3597–3600.
8. Zollinger R. Traffic injuries: a surgical problem. *Arch Surg* 1955;70:694–700.
9. Trunkey D, Lim R. Analyasis of 425 consecutive trauma fatalities: an autopsy study. *J Am Coll Emerg Phys* 1974;3:1364–69.
10. West J, Trunkey D, Lim R. Systems of trauma care: a strudy of two counties. *Arch Surg* 1979;114:455–60.
11. Cales R, Trunkey D. Preventable trauma deaths: a review of trauma care systems development. *JAMA* 1985;254:1059.
12. Kreis D, Plasencia G, Augenstein D, et al. Preventable trauma deaths: Dade County, Florida. *J Trauma* 1986;26:649–54,
13. Shackford S, Hollingsworth-Friedlund P, Cooper G, Eastman A. The effect of regionalization upon the quality of trauma care as assessed by concurrent audit before and after institution of a trauma system. *J Trauma* 1986;26:812–18.
14. Eastman A, Lewis F Jr, Champion H, Mattox K. Regional trauma system design: critical concepts. *Am J Surg* 1987;154:79.
15. Ornato J, Craren E, Nelsonk N, Kimball K. Impact of improved emergency medical services and emergency trauma care on the reduction in mortality from trauma. *J Trauma* 1985;25:575–79.
16. Committee on Trauma Research, ed. *Injury in America. A continuing public health problem.* Washington, DC: National Academy Press; 1985.
17. Luft H, Bunker J, Enthoven A. Should operations be regionalized? The empirical relation between surgical volume and mortality. *N Engl J Med* 1979;301:1364.
18. Trunkey D. Trauma. *Sci Am* 1983;249:28–35.

Orthopaedic Trauma Protocols, edited by
Sigvard T. Hansen, Jr., and Marc F. Swiontkowski,
Raven Press, Ltd., New York, ©1993.

CHAPTER 3

Nursing Standards for the Orthopaedic Trauma Patient

Jack S. Olsen and *Joan S. Rhodes

INTRODUCTION

Patients with high-energy orthopaedic trauma have complex, diverse injuries and unplanned hospitalizations. These circumstances present unique challenges to orthopaedic nurses. Nurses usually encounter their patients after discharge from the recovery room and must focus on their postoperative and rehabilitative care. Because of the traumatic nature of these patients' problems, the nursing staff must provide physical and emotional support in addition to assessing their needs, planning their care, evaluating their progress, and acting as patient advocates. Expertise is acquired through preceptorial orientations, routine nursing rounds, and nursing education leading to certification by the National Association of Orthopedic Nurses. Attendance at daily rounds, during which representatives of all the disciplines take part in each patient's care, greatly helps to coordinate care. Multidisciplinary rounds foster collegiality among nurses, physicians, physical therapists, occupational therapists, social workers, and dieticians, and are vital for achieving optimal functional patient outcomes.

The nursing standards of care for specific diagnosed problems that are commonly encountered during the care of traumatic orthopaedic injuries are discussed below. These standards ensure optimal care and prevention of potential complications for all orthopaedic patients and are particularly relevant to orthopaedic trauma patients(1).

PAIN

Nursing Diagnosis: Pain

Pain may be the greatest single problem for orthopaedic trauma patients and, consequently, for the nursing staff. Pain management requires a collaborative effort by the entire health-care team and the cooperation of the patient(2). The nurse must be the patient's advocate, believe the patient's reports about pain, and strive to explore techniques that work to relieve pain for individual patients. With assistance from a pain relief service and the introduction of new techniques and strategies to relieve pain, nurses are becoming more proficient at assessing and managing postoperative and traumatic pain (see Chapter 6).

All patients are assessed continuously for the presence of pain, factors that precipitate and alleviate pain, and the manner in which they express pain. Orthopaedic nurses must be skilled at comparing normal responses to trauma and surgery with signs of impending complications, such as compartment syndrome, progressive neurological deficit, hematoma, or dislocation of an injured joint or a prosthesis. Pain assessment is documented in the medical record at least every 4 h. A pain assessment tool is used to help the patient describe and measure the level of pain that is experienced. All affected extremities must be elevated and positioned for comfort and function. Patients are instructed about the expected duration and the type of pain to be expected from their injuries.

Pain medications are administered before the pain level peaks and approximately 30 min before physical therapy or mobilization. During the interim, nonpharmacological pain-relieving measures such as icing, rest, distraction, cutaneous stimulation, relaxation, discussion, and teaching are employed. Patients with active substance-abuse problems are treated non-judgmentally, with the goal of achieving pain relief without attempting withdrawal. An individual's care may include receiving regularly scheduled large doses of analgesics and subsequent referral for rehabilitation after hospitalization.

At discharge, all patients receive instructions on pain management, comfortable positions, and stimuli that are likely to increase or decrease pain. Patients who do not experience satisfactory relief from pain are referred to the pain relief service.

Departments of Inpatient Orthopaedics and *Nursing Education, Harborview Medical Center, University of Washington, Seattle, Washington 98104

NEUROVASCULAR COMPLICATIONS

The postoperative assessment of each patient includes a complete examination of incisions, skin, drains, and appliances, as well as an assessment of the musculoskeletal and neurovascular systems, respiratory function, and mental status. Patients arriving on the ward are also examined for blood loss or previously undiagnosed injuries. Suspected fractures are splinted or immobilized. Neurovascular evaluations are done immediately postoperatively, followed by examinations every hour for 4 h, every 2 h times 2, every 4 h times 4, then every 8 h. Patients immobilized in a cast or a splint are assessed for potential neurovascular complications or bleeding at least every 4 h.

An injured extremity is assessed by comparing it to the opposite side. Circulation, sensation, and motion are assessed by the following parameters:

Circulation: color (pink, pale, or cyanotic)
Temperature: warm, cool, cold
Pulse: strong, weak, not palpable; or by Doppler
Capillary refill: normal (1–3 sec), rapid, sluggish, or absent
Edema: absent, mild, moderate; degree of pitting
Sensation: light touch (normal, numb, tingling, absent)
Motion: movement distal to the fracture (normal range of motion, painful, minimal)

Injured extremities are elevated to the level of the heart with the distal joint positioned higher than the more proximal joint. All patients are assessed for compartment syndrome at least every 4 h. Assessment parameters include pain out of proportion to the severity of the injury, localized pain, pain on passive stretch, localized edema, muscle weakness, and numbness or tingling in the area of the compartment.

IMPAIRED MOBILITY

The mobility of patients who experience traumatic orthopaedic injuries may be impaired by activity restrictions, pain, or anxiety. The goal is to mobilize each patient as early as possible to maintain or improve function and to avoid complications. In general, patients are mobilized for maximal activity at least twice a day. Pain is managed to allow for maximal activity. A physical therapist coordinates activities, which are individualized according to the severity of each patient's injuries, flexion restrictions, weight-bearing status, and general condition. Noncompliant patients are instructed in activities, encouraged to be active, and provided with care and equipment to minimize harm associated with the type of noncompliance they manifest (e.g., a mattress overlay is provided for a patient who refuses to be mobilized). Patients restricted to bed are turned at least every 2 h. A respiratory assessment is documented every 8 h; respiratory exercises are used for patients who are at risk for respiratory complications.

MOBILITY AND SELF-CARE

Many patients are unfamiliar with the process of healing and may need instruction in learning the new skills that are essential for therapy. They must be made to understand that effort, stamina, and temporary discomfort are necessary to achieve optimal functional outcomes. The rationale behind encouraging mobilization, gaining strength, maintaining function, and preventing side effects must be clearly explained. Patients should be made aware of plans for their care and mobility. Such instructions are repeated and reinforced as needed.

Self-care (e.g., toileting, grooming) may be compromised secondary to neurologic status, pain, anxiety, or loss of function. Patients are encouraged to care for themselves within their physical limitations. Occupational therapists are consulted to assist with techniques and devices to support self-care. Each patient's requirements for assistance after discharge from the hospital are assessed at the time of admission and appropriate support is arranged. Families or significant others are instructed how to assist the patient with the activities of daily living and with specific treatments. Patients who require intensive rehabilitation are referred to Rehabilitation Medicine.

SKIN BREAKDOWN

Skin integrity may be compromised by immobility, casts, orthotics, edema, dressings, previous time on a backboard, poor nutritional status, severe injuries, or loss of sensation. Elements to consider in the assessment of skin breakdown include the general appearance, insensitivity, color, vascularity, lesions, edema, moisture, temperature, texture, thickness, and turgor of the skin. Each patient's skin is assessed at least every 8 h for signs of impending decubitus ulceration, such as redness that does not fade in 15 min, warmth, skin depression, or the presence of a hard or spongy lump. Daily assessments, interventions, evaluations of the effectiveness of interventions, and revised treatment plans are documented for all patients suffering skin breakdown.

Spinal injuries with subsequent neurologic deficit place patients at high risk for skin breakdown. These patients are supplied with appropriate protective devices (mattress overlays, special beds, padding, dressings) and assessed every 4 h. Patients who are immobile are turned at least every 2 h. Patients who had been immobilized on a backboard after their initial trauma are considered to be at high risk for skin breakdown. Their skin and scalp are assessed every 4 h for 1 week. The length of time spent on a backboard must be kept to a minimum.

All patients with new casts are assessed for skin breakdown every hour for 4 h, every 2 h times 2, every 4 h times 4, then every 8 h. Patients in a thoracolumbar sacral orthotic (TLSO) device are examined for redness, especially at the iliac crests, the lateral chest wall, the axilla, and the back. The jacket is removed and assessment is performed 2 h after the TLSO is applied. After the initial examination, the time between each examination is increased by 30 min until the device remains in place for 24 h, except for bathing. After tolerance is attained, the skin of insensate patients is inspected every 8 h and the skin of sensate patients is inspected every 12 h. After the device has been worn for 1 to 3 weeks, the skin can be inspected once daily. Patients with halo-vest devices must have their skin cleansed and inspected daily and pressure-sensitive areas must be inspected as often as necessary.

The condition of all patients with skin breakdown is documented daily with respect to assessment, interventions, evaluation of the effectiveness of the interventions, and revised plans. Supine patients are transferred by lifting or with the aid of a slider board to prevent shearing and friction. Patients with casts or orthotics are instructed how to inspect their own skin and to be responsible for their own hygiene, and are advised to avoid lotions, ointments, or powders other than cornstarch.

RESPIRATORY COMPLICATIONS

Prevention of posttraumatic and postoperative respiratory complications [ARDS] fat emboli, pulmonary emboli, pneumonia) is an important aspect of nursing care. Patients are assessed continuously for respiratory, cardiac, neurologic, and integumentary changes and complications during their postoperative course. Mobilization is begun as soon as possible to avoid atelectasis and pneumonia. All postoperative patients and those at risk of impaired gas exchange are instructed and encouraged to breathe deeply and to cough, with the assistance of an incentive spirometer, every hour or two. Prophylactic devices, including antiembolic stockings, an inspirometer, and venous pumps, are used for patients at risk for impaired gas exchange. Those at risk of emboli are assessed for signs and symptoms of impending complications at least every 8 h. Assessment of respiratory function is documented every 8 h.

INFECTION

Factors that increase the risk of infection include open fractures, crush injuries, extended surgery time, nutritional compromise, vascular compromise, poor dressing technique, and indwelling devices or lines. Prevention of the devastating effects of long-term osteomyelitis is the goal of good nursing care.

Body fluid and secretion precautions are practiced to minimize cross-contamination and to protect the caregiver. Sterile technique is used whenever contact is made with nonintact skin or indwelling lines. Sites of line insertion, incisions, and other nonintact skin are assessed and documented at least every 8 h for signs and symptoms of infection. Each patient's temperature is taken and recorded at least every 8 h when the temperature is normal and every 4 h when it is elevated. The pin tracts of external fixator, halo, and traction pins are cleansed with half-strength hydrogen peroxide at least every 12 h or more frequently in the presence of infection or exposed tissue. Patients are encouraged and instructed to begin self-care of pin sites as early as possible.

Patients who will be responsible for changing their own dressings after discharge are instructed in the appropriate techniques. All patients are taught to recognize the signs and symptoms of infection and when to report suspicious findings to a physician.

INEFFECTIVE COPING

Trauma victims may have concerns or experience life disruptions related to changes in their body image or function, loss of independence, domestic disruption, lack of financial resources, employment, or legal matters. Many trauma patients have histories of substance abuse, poor impulse control or personality disorders.

On admission, patients are assessed for a history of substance abuse or psychiatric illness. All patients are assessed for signs of posttraumatic response on an ongoing basis. Nurses support their patients' emotional needs by listening to them nonjudgmentally. A psychiatric clinical nurse specialist or a social worker is consulted to assist patients who require additional emotional support and to provide additional input into the nursing care plan. Referrals for long-term emotional support are appropriate concerns in the discharge plan.

Victims of high-energy trauma face increased life stresses, serious injury, and unplanned hospitalization, and present great challenges to their care providers. Frequent personal contact with patients puts nurses in a unique position to provide a great deal of emotional support, counseling, assessment, and teaching, in addition to providing the technical aspects of care.

REFERENCES

1. Pellino TA, ed: *N.A.O.N. core curriculum for orthopaedic nursing.* NJ Anthony J. Jannetti; 1986.
2. McCaffery M, Beebe A: *Pain clinical manual for nursing practice.* St. Louis: CV Mosby; 1989.

Orthopaedic Trauma Protocols, edited by
Sigvard T. Hansen, Jr., and Marc F. Swiontkowski,
Raven Press, Ltd., New York, ©1993.

CHAPTER 4

The Psychological and Social Implications of Multiple Trauma

Billie Z. Lawson and *Lynn Carrigan

INTRODUCTION

Trauma victims experience fear, discomfort, anxiety, and depression, the same reactions typical for people undergoing planned surgical procedures. In addition, the emotional distress they suffer as a result of the accident intensifies their responses to their injuries and to the people around them. Characteristic stresses have been identified at each stage of hospitalization that can compromise a trauma victim's recovery. Correlation exists between a patient's negative psychological reactions after surgery and the incidence of postoperative medical complications. Knowing these psychological transitions, the physician and hospital staff can anticipate them, intervene, and lessen the intensity of their ramifications.

This chapter discusses the emotional, psychological, and social factors that affect patients undergoing surgery. These factors are important to consider in trauma patients undergoing delayed reconstruction procedures. We will also examine the unique psychological repercussions experienced by victims of trauma.

FACTORS THAT INFLUENCE EMOTIONAL RESPONSES TO SURGERY

Personality Traits and Coping Styles

Personality traits are patterns of thought, feeling, and behavior that enable an individual to adapt to changing physical and social environments and to the internal tensions they produce (1). These traits are predictable even when an individual must cope with a new situation. For example, the coping mechanisms employed by children during hospitalization are typical of their personalities before hospitalization (2). Similarly, persons who become newly dependent on others can be expected to exhibit behaviors typical of their interaction with authority figures in the past. An individual who copes with stress by abandoning responsibility or by abusing drugs is likely to be difficult to manage when these coping patterns are restricted by hospital regulations.

Lazarus and Launier (3) identified four major modes of coping: direct action, information seeking, fantasy or denial, and inhibition. By determining a patient's coping strategies, the health-care team can assist recovery more effectively. Questioning patients about previous stressful experiences will often identify their predominant coping strategies.

Previous Experiences with Injury and Hospitalization

People who demonstrate undue anxiety over a situation are often responding to fears based on previous experiences. Every reaction to each situation is understandable if the factors that account for it can be discovered (4). These dynamics often become evident during good family medical and psychiatric histories. Sometimes, the patient knows someone who suffered a similar injury or illness that had an unfavorable outcome. Some patients identify with media reports of similar situations. For example, geriatric patients are often susceptible to postoperative depression because they fear continued institutionalization after surgery.

Predilections to death must be uncovered. Postoperative mortality rates are exceptionally high for patients who are convinced that they will die as a result of surgery (5) and for those who have negative outlooks or who lack an orientation towards the future (6). Patients might relate to the outcomes of other situations that have no realistic bearing to their individual situations. Once such identifications are discussed,

Department of Social Work and *Community Mental Health Center. Harborview Medical Center, University of Washington, Seattle, Washington 98104 patients are usually more able to understand the details of their specific conditions (7).

Significance of Affected Body Parts

Cultural and social values influence individuals' perceptions of particularly important body parts and functions. Certain kinds of injuries elicit major emotional reactions, although the responses differ according to cultural expectations (8). In the United States, for example, cultural importance is placed on performance and achievement. Impairment of the ability to work in one's chosen career often requires significant psychological adjustment. Injury to the sexual organs, to the face, or the potential loss of sexual function is also extremely threatening (9).

Human beings ascribe symbolic meanings to various parts of their bodies in highly idiosyncratic ways; the emotional perception of an injured body part can drastically affect an individual's self-image. A particular part of the body might be associated with family identity and therefore will be symbolically important. Surgical alteration of such an area results not only in grief for the loss of that attribute but also in a need for major readjustment of the self-image. Impairment of any visible body area may potentially limit an individual's ability to communicate. A person's occupation, hobbies, recreational interest, family, culture, social roles, and responsibilities can identify which physical features and functions are central to self-image. Determining the significance of a body part can be helpful in understanding what at first might appear to be a paradoxical reaction or an overreaction to a surgical procedure.

Cultural Considerations

Ethnic and cultural beliefs and practices influence how patients and their families will cope with an illness or injury, make medical decisions, and comply with medical treatment. Cultural beliefs can determine pain behavior, concern over appearance, functional priorities (work, food, sleep), faith in the capacity for rejuvenation, and illness behavior (cooperation, resistance, pessimism, despair, optimism) (10). For example, if an illness or injury is regarded as a punishment for a sin, patients and their families will react differently than if the injury is thought to have happened to an innocent victim.

Religion, language, dietary habits, and family living patterns may also influence patients' relationships with their health care providers (11). Communication in hospital settings is often hurried and intrusive, and traditions of modesty, manners, spatial distance, touch, respect for elders, or even the correct pronunciation of names are often overlooked or disregarded (12). Failure to understand and respect cultural distinctions frequently results in avoidance and frustration, which can cause abrasive relationships between patients and staff.

Social Support Systems

An individual's family and community provide three basic kinds of support: emotional (intimacy, reassurance, encouragement); tangible (direct aid, services, loans, gifts); and informational (advice with problems, feedback concerning behavior). These support systems can influence a patient's progress substantially by influencing how the event is initially appraised, by moderating anxiety with calmness and reassurance, by encouraging the patient to increase efforts to get well, and by encouraging health-promoting behavior (13). A high level of social support has been correlated with increased longevity, physical mobility, productivity, and compliance with medical orders. Conversely, negative events such as separation, divorce, or the illness of another family member can have deleterious effects on a person's sense of well-being (14).

Some individuals can utilize their support systems effectively in times of crisis, whereas others may turn to them prematurely before attempting to solve their own problems. There are patients who fail to turn to others when it would be beneficial for them to do so and those who alienate their support system by seeking attention in ways that are destructive (15). The amount of help a patient can expect to receive and whether it will be utilized must be determined. Patients with few established social supports will require more staff planning and community involvement after discharge from the hospital.

Preparatory Instruction

In his psychoanalytic and behavioral studies of surgical patients, Janis (16) showed that patients who are instructed about their operations remember both the surgery and its sequelae more favorably than patients who are not well informed. He designed a study to investigate the effects of preoperative instruction on patients scheduled to undergo elective intraabdominal surgery. The experimental group of patients was visited by an anesthesiologist and given information about the recovery room, the amount of pain to be expected postoperatively, and medication options which would be available to them. This group required less than half the usual postoperative narcotic medication and was discharged from the hospital an average of 2.7 days sooner than patients in the study who did not receive preoperative information.

Preoperative instruction has beneficial effects on patient compliance, satisfaction, and postoperative management when the decision to perform surgery is made by negotiation between the patient and the physician rather than as an authoritarian decision (17–20).

THE ACCIDENT PROCESS

Accident-Prone Individuals

In 1919, Greenwood and Woods (21) reported that a small number of individuals appeared to sustain the majority of industrial accidents. Since then, many studies have proposed the existence of "accident-prone" personalities—people with traits that make them vulnerable to accidents (22). Common characteristics among accident victims include aggressiveness, paranoid ideation, unmet dependency needs, risk-taking behavior, and a tendency towards depression (23–25).

Hirschfeld and Behan (26) reviewed 300 industrial accidents and defined the accident process as "events captured by the personality for the purpose of solving an individual's life problem." The accident process therefore begins when anxiety or conflict builds up before the accident. If the accident or resulting injury resolves the conflict, the patient will very likely become dependent on the ongoing disability and will not respond to rehabilitation or pain management. However, being prone to accidents might not be a lifelong or chronic condition but a transient syndrome that involves a variety of personality traits and recent life stresses. This concept of the accident process seems consistent with observations made from discussions with trauma victims about stressful events that were present before the injury. Several studies acknowledge that professional and personal stresses, recent emotional upsets, and a number of recent life changes can contribute to traffic or industrial accidents (27).

The Role of Alcohol

The relationship between alcohol and vehicular accidents is well known, but a strong link also appears to exist between alcohol and all forms of trauma. Lowenfels and Miller's (28) collective review of alcohol and trauma cites evidence that alcohol is a significant factor in pedestrian injuries, burns, hypothermia and frostbite, aquatic injuries, aviation accidents involving private pilots, homicides, and suicides. The use of alcohol has important management implications and should be recognized at the time of admission. Alcohol abuse may have significant bearing on a patient's support system. Friends and family may be dysfunctional themselves or alienated from the patient, who may have been disrupting their lives. Individuals skilled in the management of alcoholism and who are familiar with alcohol and drug treatment resources in the community are essential for effective management of these patients.

PSYCHOLOGICAL REPERCUSSIONS EXPERIENCED BY TRAUMA VICTIMS

Reactions to Victimization

Disaster studies and studies of rape victims indicate that the occurrence of an external life-threatening event is of such psychological magnitude that most people who experience these events will respond in predictable ways, regardless of personality or situational variables (29).

Bard and Sangrey (30) have labeled the initial responses experienced by victims the "impact-disorganization" phase. This stage is characterized by disorientation, denial, feelings of loneliness, depression, and vulnerability. The initial trauma is followed by sleep disturbances accompanied by episodes of fear, anxiety, and panic (31). Individuals experiencing this phase of victimization are emotionally numb and disoriented and may seek a great deal of reassurance and direction from health-care providers. Hospital staff may view these behaviors as excessively dependent and may resist responding to patients' requests for assistance, assuming that doing so will reinforce regressive and unhealthy behavior. Another common reaction at this time is to attempt to reestablish control over all aspects of one's life. Hospital personnel must provide ample opportunity for trauma victims to be actively involved in as many aspects of their care as possible. However, dependence in trauma victims is usually temporary, and once the need for direction and reassurance is satisfied patients can move successfully through this phase.

The "recoil" phase appears later for many victims and frequently involves mood swings in which emotions shift from fear to anger. The most common reactions expressed by people who have experienced injury are fear of the event being repeated, feelings of being responsible for it, and rage at the source of the trauma (32). Expressions of guilt, anger, apathy, and sadness, which frequently appear during the recoil phase, can be emotionally wearing on family and health-care providers. During this time, victims need to relive and retell the trauma incident in detail. By apportioning the storytelling between shifts and among caregivers, victims can tell their stories over and over without having important support people withdraw because of boredom or discomfort with the repetitions.

Family Management

Trauma victims are often unconscious on arrival at the hospital and the legal next of kin become the main source of medical consent and information about prior medical history. Thus, families often are the initial "patients" who must receive psychological support from trauma personnel. Initially family members experience shock and denial while they struggle to understand the effects of the trauma on the patient and themselves. They face the possible loss of someone who plays important roles and has serious responsibilities, perhaps a devastating change in financial status, a disruption in routine, and a potential loss of morale or even family unity if the injury is conflict-related, as might occur in a suicide attempt or a crime (33).

The goals of crisis intervention are to help the patient and the family adapt to the changes inflicted on their lives and to return them to the maximal level of functioning by educating them about realistic expectations, exchanging information on a regular basis, and countering the negative impacts of the event with appropriate resources (34). Families may exhibit cognitive confusion, disorganized behavior, increased tension, and inability to retain information or make decisions (35). Initial family management should include an introduction to the critical care unit and its staff, an explanation of the physical status of the patient, and a description of the visible equipment and supplies being used. They should be oriented to the rules and floor plan of the hospital as well as to resource personnel available to them (e.g., chaplain, social workers, psychologists). Identifying the circumstances of the injury is particularly critical information, since the circumstances of accident, assault, or self-harm are pivotal in the reactions of patient, family, and staff. The family should also receive information about any other individuals involved in the trauma, their conditions, and their locations.

The family should be prepared for the initial visit to the patient's bedside with a description of the patient's physical appearance and how it may change over time. Their emotional state may interfere with their comprehension of the actual situation, and critical information should be repeated frequently. Brief visits with the patient must be allowed to confirm that the patient is alive, and the family must be assured that they will be notified should the patient's condition change.

Fear of Death

Fear of death or disfigurement is uppermost in the minds of both patients and families, and trauma staff may be forced to discuss these extremely sensitive issues before having established any relationship with the persons involved. The most frequently unasked question in patients' minds is whether they will live, yet expressing this thought may be impossible. Families may be quicker to ask for this dreaded piece of information but may fear and reject any negative answers.

When facing death, patients employ the same coping strategies they have used throughout life. One patient may be terrified, whereas another will be resigned, struggle, or exhibit remarkable calm. Each individual will have unique concerns to address, and both patient and family must receive truthful information about the patient's medical condition.

Near-Death Experiences

The experience of having survived what one had expected to be certain death can be a dramatic psychic event, but people are often reluctant to disclose any unusual experiences to treatment personnel for fear they might be diagnosed as psychotic. Anecdotes of near-death experiences and altered states of consciousness in trauma victims should alert health-care professionals to the possibility that a patient may have experienced a phenomenon during trauma that could have important psychological repercussions. Insomnia, anxiety, restlessness, and irritability may follow such an experience. A friend or family member may comment that the patient seems transformed or more peaceful. The best way to elicit information about such an experience is to ask the patient directly.

Reevaluation of Care

Although transfer of patients from an intensive care unit to an acute ward is a milestone for both patients and families, it often leaves patients psychologically vulnerable. They must begin accepting the changes in appearance, physical abilities, and self-concept. A high level of expectation is placed on the patient for increased independence while prolonged pain, fatigue, and exhaustion may precipitate emotional and behavioral problems such as withdrawal, outbursts of anger, noncompliance with hospital regulations, uncontrollable crying, or violent resistance (36).

Normal and temporary reactions must be distinguished from chronic symptoms and patterns that may negatively affect recovery. Expressing grief over the loss of a meaningful body part or function or the loss of one's occupation is considered normal and diminishes in time. Many patients become distressed in a trauma setting, experiencing loss of control or feelings of rejection by changes in staff, unavailability of doctors, failure to obtain immediate pain relief, or inconsistent schedules. In attempting to regain autonomy and control over their situations, they often express anxiety, pain, or anger. Most patients respond well to time, information, and negotiation, but others may require specific and well-coordinated management of their behavior.

Behavior Management

Positive reinforcement is usually more effective than criticism or threats for influencing behavior changes. Special requests such as for cigarettes, passes, or time off from treatment can be negotiated as rewards for complying with medical orders. Families are crucial in influencing patients to adhere to health-care regimens through their approval of compliance with hospital rules and disapproval of inappropriate or destructive behavior. It is therefore important to acquaint them with any behavior modification attempts the staff has implemented.

Patients must be encouraged to keep their hospitalization in perspective and to maintain their orientation and sense of identity. Making graphs or progress charts, furnishing the hospital room with familiar objects, and scheduling activities all can help.

Pain Control

Pain is a multidimensional phenomenon that incorporates cognitive, affective, behavioral, and sensory intensity components (37). Pain assessment attempts to determine the amount of pain experienced, factors that influence its quality and duration, and recommendations for treatment. In pain assessment, allowances should be made for the patients' perceptions of pain and the adaptive and maladaptive coping mechanisms they employ (38).

The primary psychological and social interventions in the comprehensive treatment of pain are to provide information about the procedures being performed and to erase unrealistic myths and fears (39). By participating in decisions about their pain medications, choosing their rest periods, and taking part in wound care, patients avoid learned helplessness (40). Pain management techniques involve deep breathing, muscle relaxation or meditation, positive suggestion, and distracting activities such as music, reading, or anticipation of pleasant activities in the future. Guided imagery and hypnosis are also useful in pain management (see Chapter 6).

Rehabilitation

The transition from an inpatient to a home setting transfers the responsibility for ongoing care from the hospital to the community. Financial concerns are very important at this stage, and information about disability payments, medical assistance, food stamps, home services, social security, and vocational rehabilitation should be made available to patients before they leave the hospital. Support groups, home visits, clinic follow-up appointments, and communication with local caregivers can assist patients and their families through this transition (41). Arrangements must also be made for the treatment of premorbid conditions, such as alcohol or drug addiction, psychiatric disorders, and family dysfunction, which might have contributed to the hospitalization. It should be noted that physicians are viewed by patients and families as the final authority on treatment decisions. Without physician support for a comprehensive discharge plan, patients and families often hold fast to the sick role and cannot begin to move towards recovery.

In summary, an individual's response to injury and surgery and the ability to recover are determined by personality and cultural values. Victims of trauma are subject not only to these variables but also to specific reactions to victimization, unexpected disability, long and difficult rehabilitation, and possibly drastic changes in social roles. Trauma patients and their families require intervention and assistance by trained professionals to regain their emotional and social stability and to be able to function independently once again. A multidisciplinary approach that includes social workers, psychologists, chaplains, vocational rehabilitation counselors, and other health-care providers ensures comprehensive treatment and discharge planning.

REFERENCES

1. Titchner JL, Levine M. *Surgery as a human experience: the psychodynamics of surgical practice*. New York: Oxford University Press; 1960.
2. Prugh D, Staub S, et al. A study of the emotional reactions of children and families to hospitalization and illness. *Am J Orthopsychiatr* 1953;23:70–106.
3. Lazarus RS, Launier R. Stress-related transactions between person and environment. In: Arnold WJ, ed. *Perspectives in interactional psychology*. New York: Plenum Press; 1978:287–327.
4. Hackett TP, Weisman A. Psychiatric management of operative syndromes II: Psychodynamic factors in formulations and management. *Psychosom Med* 1960;22:356–72.
5. Weisman AD, Hackett TP. Predilection to death and dying as a psychiatric problem. *Psychosom Med* 1961;23:232–56.
6. Kimball CP. A predictive study of adjustment to cardiac surgery. *J Thoracic Cardiovasc Surg* 1969;58:891–96.
7. Abram HS, Benjamin G. Predictions of postoperative psychiatric complications. *N Engl J Med* 1961;265:1123–8.
8. Adamson JD, Hershberg D, et al. The psychic significance of parts of the body in surgery. In: Howells JC, ed. *Modern perspectives in the psychiatric aspects of surgery*: Brunner/Mazel; 1976:20–47.
9. Renneker R, Cutter M. Psychological problems of adjustment to cancer of the breast. *JAMA* 1952;148:833–8.
10. Strelzer J, Wade TC. The influence of the cultural group on the undertreatment of postoperative pain. *Psychosom Med* 1981;43:397–403.
11. Meleis A, Jonsen A. Ethical crises and cultural differences. *Western J Med* 1983;138:893.
12. Graison B, O'Leary L, Wagner J. Cultural assessment: how well do we know our patients? *J Nephrol Nursing* 1984;Nov/Dec: 132–4.
13. Wortman CB. Social support and the cancer patient: conceptual and methodologic issues. *Cancer* 1984;53(suppl):2339–60.
14. Cobb S. Social support as a moderator of life stress. *Psychosom Med* 1976;38:300–14.
15. Dean A, Lin N. The stress-buffering role of social support: problems and prospects for systematic investigation. *J Nerv Ment Dis* 1977;165:403–417.
16. Janis IL. *Psychological stress: psychoanalytic and behavioral studies of surgical patients*. New York: Wiley; 1958.
17. Lazare A, Eisenthal S, Wasserman L. The customer approach to patienthood. *Arch Gen Psychiatr* 1975;32:553–8.
18. Lazare A, Eisenthal S, Frank A, et al. Studies on a negotiated approach to patienthood. In: Gallagher EB, ed. *The doctor-patient relationship in the changing health scene*. DHEW Publication No (NIH) 78–183. Washington, DC: Dept. of Health, Education and Welfare; 1978:119–39.
19. Stimson G. Obeying doctors' orders. *Soc Sci Med* 1974;18:97–104.
20. Davis M. Variations in patients' compliance with doctors' advice. *Am J Pub Health* 1968;58:274–88.
21. Greenwood M, Woods IM. A report on the incidence of industrial accidents upon individuals with special reference to multiple accidents. *Rep Indust Fat Res Bd (London)* 4:1919.
22. Schmidt CW. The accident-prone syndrome. In: Howells JG, ed. *Modern perspectives in the psychiatric aspects of surgery*. New York: Brunner/Mazel; 1976:61–76.
23. Rosenbaum JE. The accident victim. In: Hacket TP, Cassem N, eds. *Massachusetts General Hospital handbook of general hospital psychiatry*. St. Louis: CV Mosby; 1978:380–91.

24. Tillman WA, Hobbs GE. The accident-prone automobile driver: a study of psychiatric and social background. *Am J Psychiatr* 1949;106:321–31.
25. Conger JJ, Gaskill HS, et al. Personal and interpersonal factors in motor vehicle accidents. *Am J Psychiatr* 1957;113:1069–74.
26. Hirschfeld A, Behan R. The accident process I. Etiological considerations of industrial injuries. *JAMA* 1963;186:193–9.
27. Selzer ML, Vinokur A. Life events, subjective stress, and traffic accidents. *Am J Psychiatr* 1974;131:903–6.
28. Lowenfels AB, Miller TT. Alcohol and trauma. *Ann Emerg Med* 1984;13:1056–60.
29. Newman GG. Children of disaster: clinical observations at Buffalo Creek. *Am J Psychiatr* 1976;133:306–12.
30. Bard M, Sangrey D. *The crime victim's book.* New York: Basic Books; 1979.
31. Frederick C. Effects of natural vs. human-induced violence. In: Kivens L, ed. *Evaluation and change: services for survivors.* Minneapolis: Minneapolis Medical Research Foundation; 1980:71–75.
32. Kilpatrick DG, Resnick PA, Veronen LJ. Assessment of the aftermath of rape: changing patterns of fear. *J Behav Assess* 1979;133–148.
33. Moonilal JM. Trauma centers: a new dimension for hospital social work. *Social Work Health Care* 1982;7:15–25.
34. Golan N. Social work intervention in medical crises. *Hosp Community Psychiatr* 1972;Feb: 25–29.
35. Epperson MM. Families in sudden crisis: process and intervention in a critical care center. *Social Work Health Care* 1977; 2(No.3):265–73.
36. McCartney JR. Management of refusal of medical treatment. *Int J Psychiatr Med* 1985–86;15:31–6.
37. Wolfer JA, Davis CE. Assessment of surgical patients' preoperative emotional condition and postoperative welfare. *Nursing Res* 1970; 19:402– 14.
38. Turk DC, Kerns RD. Conceptual issues in the assessment of clinical pain. *Int J Psychiatr Med* 1983–84;31.
39. Shipley RH. Behavioral management of acute anxiety and pain of stressful medical procedures. In: Boudewyns PA, Keefe FJ, eds. *Behavioral medicine in general medical practice.* Menlo Park, CA: Addison Wesley; 1982.
40. Kelley ML, et al. Decreasing burned children's pain behavior impacting the trauma of hydrotherapy. *J Appl Behav Anal* 1984;17:147–58.
41. Scanlon-Schilpp A, Levesque J. Helping the patient cope with the sequelae of trauma through the self-help group approach. *J Trauma* 1982;21:135–9.

Orthopaedic Trauma Protocols, edited by Sigvard T. Hansen, Jr., and Marc F. Swiontkowski, Raven Press, Ltd., New York, © 1993.

CHAPTER 5

Anesthetic Considerations in the Traumatized Patient

Edward G. Pavlin

Before administering anesthesia to an acutely injured patient, the anesthesiologist must know the physiological consequences of the injuries, establish priorities, and rapidly effect appropriate treatment and medical support. Like the surgeon, the anesthesiologist may have little initial knowledge of a patient's previous medical history or use of medication or drugs. Indeed, when little is known about the patient beyond the mode of injury, ongoing physiological assessment and rapid response to critical organ dysfunction become imperative. As a member of a trauma team comprising many surgical and nonsurgical specialties, the anesthesiologist must respect the surgeon's judgment and treatment plan for the various injuries sustained by the patient. Optimal care by many diverse specialists requires good communication among those administering treatment. This chapter outlines the priorities and interventions used by anesthesiologists to manage life-threatening problems.

AIRWAY

An adequate airway is always the first and most important priority in patient management. The decision to place an endotracheal tube can be made at the site of injury, in the emergency department, or in the operating room immediately before surgery. The indications for emergency endotracheal tube placement include:

1. real or incipient airway obstruction due to loss of consciousness, mechanical injury to the oral cavity, or upper airway or oropharyngeal swelling;
2. inadequate ventilation secondary to head injury or drugs, mechanical problems with the airway or the thorax, or muscle weakness;
3. pulmonary aspiration of gastric contents or blood;
4. inadequately resolved hypoxemia from oxygen applied by a face mask; and
5. hypotension and shock.

Several important differences exist between victims of trauma and patients presenting for elective surgery: the presence of extremely severe injuries that make airway access difficult; hypovolemia or shock that makes the administration of anesthetic and opioid drugs dangerous; the need for rapid intervention; and the presumption of significant gastric filling that places the patient in danger of pulmonary aspiration of regurgitated material during the establishment of an airway.

In general, our approach to establishing an airway includes:

1. having the patient breathe a high concentration of oxygen for 5 min before induction of anesthesia (this pulmonary reservoir prolongs the time an apneic patient will remain oxygenated);
2. administering an anesthetic agent such as thiopental (the correct dosage of this type of drug is determined by the patient's cardiovascular status, but its administration may be contraindicated by shock);
3. applying cricothyroid pressure (this method effectively prevents regurgitation of gastric contents into the oral cavity);
4. administering a muscle relaxant, usually succinylcholine, to effect paralysis; and
5. placing an endotracheal tube through the vocal cords under direct vision (proper placement is confirmed by clinical observation and, most important, by the amount of carbon dioxide measured in the expired breath).

Most patients involved in decelerating injuries are presumed to have sustained cervical spinal trauma. Because

Department of Anesthesiology, Harborview Medical Center, University of Washington, Seattle, Washington 98104 manipulating the head may injure the cervical spinal cord, some modifications to the above approach are required. In-line traction is applied to the head by someone familiar with this technique (viewing the larynx is more difficult with the head in this position). Provisions for extralaryngeal access to the airway are made if establishment of an oral airway proves difficult. This technique includes high-pressure ventilation through a large-bore needle inserted in the cricothyroid membrane after equipment and personnel are assembled for a rapid cricothyrotomy (1).

VENTILATION

Acute trauma can have both immediate and delayed effects on the ability to ventilate a patient's lungs. Once an airway has been established, ventilation and oxygenation are defined by the arterial blood gas values of PaO_2 and $PaCO_2$. Inadequate oxygenation may be due to either extraalveolar or intraalveolar causes. Extrapulmonary problems include pneumothorax, hemothorax, abdominal distention, or diaphragmatic rupture. Difficulty in maintaining ventilation in the presence of hypoxemia also suggests an extraalveolar problem. Complications associated with intraalveolar problems include immediate alveolar collapse secondary to airway damage and aspiration of gastric contents or blood. Diagnosis is made and treatment is directed by the results of a clinical examination and a chest radiograph.

Adult respiratory distress syndrome (ARDS) is a frequent complication of traumatic injuries. In a study conducted at this institution, the following risk factors for ARDS were identified: massive blood loss (>12 units in 24 h), fracture of the pelvis or the long bones, and sepsis (2). The incidence of ARDS was 18% when one risk factor was present, 43% for two risk factors, and 78% when all three risk factors were present. Moreover, 75% of ARDS was diagnosed within 24 h of injury, indicating that noncardiac pulmonary edema with hypoxemia evolves early enough with acute injuries to be a factor in the anesthetic management. Treatment with positive end-expiratory pressure (PEEP) may have to be considered.

Breathing is monitored noninvasively by pulse oximeter (for oxygen saturation), end-tidal CO_2 values, tidal volumes, minute-ventilation, and arterial blood gas measurements obtained from indwelling arterial lines, and pulmonary inflation pressures in mechanically ventilated patients.

CIRCULATION

Hemorrhage and the potential for hypovolemic shock are serious complications of both penetrating and blunt trauma. Fluid resuscitation is usually carried out in the form of component therapy. The individual components include *volume* (crystalloid or colloid solutions), *red blood cells* (exogenous or salvaged), and *coagulation factors* (including platelet suspensions).

Volume

The end-points of volume resuscitation are determined by monitoring arterial pressure with an arterial cannula, central venous pressure (CVP), and urinary output (a minimum output of 50 ml/h is indicative of adequate volume resuscitation). Although there is a discrepancy between left and right atrial pressures in some patients, the use of pulmonary arterial catheters is often impractical in acutely traumatized patients. Central venous pressure monitoring can be useful if 500-ml boluses of crystalloid solution are used and the effects on CVP and mean arterial pressure are noted. If hypotension and elevated CVP persist, other causes, such as pericardial tamponade, hemothorax, tension pneumothorax, or acute cardiac failure must be considered.

Three to four liters of crystalloid solution, in the form of a balanced salt solution, are used in the initial resuscitation of shock. Continued volume replacement can be carried out with either crystalloid or colloid solutions. Most studies comparing the efficacy of both solutions on lung function or the formation of pulmonary edema have shown no advantage of colloid over crystalloid for either lung function or renal function. In view of this, the advisability of increasing the cost and risk to a patient by adding colloid, which contains, e.g., albumin, plasma, or hetastarch, must be questioned. Crystalloid is used for volume replacement at this institution. When a crystalloid solution is used, the amount of replacement fluid must equal at least three times the amount of blood loss and usually will result in significant peripheral edema.

Red Blood Cells

Two problems are associated with red blood cell replacement: determining the amount to give and deciding on the source. With supplies decreasing and demands increasing, less blood is available in many centers. Increased concern about blood-transmitted diseases has led to caution in administering blood products. A National Institutes of Health (NIH) Consensus Conference (3) has proposed the following recommendations regarding red blood cell transfusions for perioperative bleeding:

1. transfusing to a hematocrit over 30% offers few advantages for the patient;
2. allowing the hematocrits of otherwise healthy patients with acute hemorrhage to drop below 20% is associated with increased rates of morbidity and mortality; and
3. determining where to maintain hematocrits between 20–30% depends on whether a patient is able to increase oxygen delivery with increased cardiac output, whether oxygen utilization will be increased postoperatively, and whether a patient's bone marrow is capable of increasing the production of red blood cells in the event of anemia.

Scavenged shed blood is being used more frequently to minimize transfusion-borne diseases. The Haemonetic Cell

Saver (Haemonetics, Braintree, MA) effectively collects and washes red blood cells in operatively shed blood and allows autotransfusion in the operating room (4). In orthopaedic cases, this device has been particularly useful in surgery involving the spine or the pelvis.

Coagulation Factors

Studies at this institution and others have established that dilution of platelets is the initial coagulation defect in hemorrhage. The circulating platelet count in the average adult decreases significantly after a loss of 10 units of blood. Therefore, platelets can be administered after 10 units of volume have been lost. Further bleeding or the presence of disseminated intravascular coagulation may require the administration of fresh frozen plasma or cryoprecipitate. Indications for infusion of coagulation factors include prothrombin times greater than 17 s and clinical nonsurgical bleeding.

HEAD INJURY

Closed head injuries are often seen after blunt or decelerating trauma. The diagnosis and treatment of intracranial injuries are the next priority after establishment of an airway, adequate ventilation, and control of hypotension and shock. The Glasgow Coma Scale (see Chapter 2) assesses a trauma victim's eye-opening, verbal, and motor responses to verbal and painful stimuli. Signs of deterioration can be quantified against the initial score. In seriously injured patients, pharmacological paralysis and endotracheal intubation in the field or in the emergency department may preclude adequate assessment. The need for operative intervention is determined in large part by CT scans of the head and by measurement of intracranial pressure (ICP). Emergency intracranial and intraabdominal surgical procedures can be performed simultaneously.

Anesthetic management in the presence of real or suspected head injury can be modified in several ways:

1. Because laryngeotracheal reflexes can raise ICP, 100 mg of lidocaine or 250 mg of fentanyl are administered 2 to 3 min before laryngoscopy and intubation to attenuate the increase in ICP.
2. Devices to monitor ICP are placed in unconscious patients to detect accumulation of intracranial blood (subdural or epidural) or brain edema and to guide therapy for lowering the ICP.
3. Anesthesia is guided by maneuvers that minimize ICP:
   a. using a low concentration of inhaled agents because they are, to a variable degree, cerebrovasodilators;
   b. using narcotics as anesthetic supplements because they decrease cerebral metabolism, lower cerebral blood flow (CBF), and minimize cardiovascular response to noxious stimuli such as laryngoscopy, movement of the endotracheal tube, and the skin incision;
   c. using thiopental with induction or during maintenance of anesthesia to acutely lower ICP;
   d. lowering $PaCO_2$, CBF, and ICP (normal range is 25–30 mm Hg) with alveolar hyperventilation;
   e. decreasing brain edema with mannitol; and
   f. controlling blood pressure.

One difficult aspect of intraoperative care is establishing treatment priority between a head injury and injuries that produce shock. Many maneuvers required to sustain adequate cardiac output and circulate blood volume, such as infusing large volumes of crystalloid solution or using little or no anesthetic agents, are necessary for circulation but are not optimal for brain protection. In such cases, the head injury assumes priority in management only after volume resuscitation and cardiovascular stability are achieved.

HYPOTHERMIA

Hypothermia is associated with trauma. In a study conducted at this institution (5), 25% of trauma victims arrived at the emergency department with core body temperatures of 33.9°C or lower. Many continued to cool during their treatment in the emergency department, the operating room, and the intensive care unit. The degree of hypothermia did not correlate with the patient's age or blood alcohol level, the time of year, or weather conditions. Hypothermia was associated with severe injury in spite of rapid transportation time to the hospital. Positive correlation of trauma with core hypothermia was established by the volume of crystalloid solution and red blood cells that were infused, the injury Severity Score, and the mortality rate. By all indications, severely injured patients lost more blood, got colder, and were more likely to have a fatal outcome.

How much hypothermia contributes to mortality and morbidity is unknown, but certain physiological effects are known to be detrimental to victims of polytrauma. Atrial arrhythmias can occur spontaneously at temperatures below 34°C and ventricular arrhythmias can occur below 31°C in otherwise healthy patients. Furthermore, once ventricular arrhythmias or asystole are established, they are extremely difficult to treat in a cold heart, either pharmacologically or electrically (6). Blood clotting dysfunctions are attributed to cold. Platelet count is decreased due to platelet sequestration in the liver and the spleen (7). Intrinsic clotting activity (measured by prothrombin time, partial thromboplastin time, and thrombin time) is significantly slowed at temperatures below 34°C. Increased blood viscosity accompanies increased peripheral vascular resistance. Fluid shifts from intravascular to intercellular spaces cause a relative polycythemia and low circulating blood volume. Shivering increases oxygen requirements up to 600% and may be accompanied by metabolic acidosis. In the presence of lung injury, hypoxia may occur secondary to venous desaturation.

Prevention and treatment of hypothermia are considered very important in the overall care of acutely injured victims of polytrauma. Techniques to prevent heat loss include:

1. heating inspired gases to 42°C and humidifying them to almost 100% water saturation;
2. heating all infused fluids (crystalloid and blood products) (efficient blood warmers using countercurrent heaters are preferred to contact-type heaters);
3. placing warming blankets on top of the patient (placing warming blankets under a patient offers little advantage over using a foam mattress; the new warm air generator, the Bair Hugger [Allied Medical, Cincinnati, Ohio], is particularly useful);
4. performing active warming maneuvers when hypothermia is severe or unresponsive to conventional treatment (peritoneal lavage with warm saline solution may be helpful; direct blood rewarming without the use of cardiopulmonary bypass has been described and used clinically); and
5. aggressively stopping shivering (administration of small doses [25 mg/70 kg/patient] of intravenous Demerol is very effective, whereas morphine and fentanyl are ineffective) (8).

ALCOHOL AND OTHER DRUGS

The association between trauma and alcohol or drug intake is well established. A study from this institution has shown that 60% of traumatized patients had positive blood alcohol levels over 100 mg at the time of admission (9). Over 50% of all victims of homicide and traumatic injuries have positive blood alcohol levels. Alcohol and cocaine are the drugs most frequently associated with injury. The logical conclusion from these statistics is that the cerebral effects caused by these drugs are at least in part responsible for the traumatic event.

The presence of these drugs in the circulation presents potential anesthetic problems in a high percentage of patients undergoing emergent or urgent surgery. Patients under the influence of these substances may not cooperate during their examinations or radiographic assessments and such noncompliance may precipitate the need for early intubation and pharmacological restraint. For the same reasons, regional anesthesia may also be precluded. Alcohol decreases the amount of anesthetic required, produces vasodilation and hypotension, and acts as a cardiac depressant. In addition, alcohol exacerbates the morbidity and mortality associated with cardiac tamponade. Acute cocaine toxicity in young people is associated with coronary vasospasm, cardiac ischemia, and ventricular arrhythmias, and may result in cardiac arrest. Thus, acute drug intoxication in polytraumatized patients interferes with making an accurate diagnosis and assessment of their injuries and increases the pharmacologic complexity of administering anesthesia.

POSITION OF PATIENT

Patients with multiple or complex fractures require prolonged surgery that often lasts 8 h or longer. The anesthetized patient is susceptible to injury from malpositioning or from having assumed one position for a long time. Decubitus ulceration is common, particularly in patients who have periods of hypotension and decreased skin blood flow. Frequently, trauma victims are stabilized on a backboard in the case of spinal injury and at times this splinting is maintained during surgery. Every effort should be made to rule out spinal injuries and to remove this potential source of ulceration over bony prominences. Brachial plexus injuries due to arm extension may occur from lying in the prone position for a prolonged time. When the patient is prone, the arm should be abducted no more than 90° from the side with the head turned to the abducted arm. If one arm cannot be tucked alongside the body, the head should be positioned to look forward to minimize tension on the brachial plexus. Appropriate padding and support for the upper extremities (particularly the elbows) helps to lower the incidence of compressive neural injuries.

Traumatized patients are both interesting and complicated subjects for anesthetic management. Many problems that occur in the operating room require knowledge of the pathophysiology of injury and the ability to quickly diagnose and assess changes in organ functions. This knowledge is gained by communication and cooperation among the physicians and surgeons involved in the patient's care as well as both clinical and academic interest in the care of multiply injured patients.

REFERENCES

1. Weymuller EJ, Pavlin EG. Management of difficult airway problems with percutaneous transtracheal ventilation. *Ann Otol Rhinol Laryngol* 1984;93:34–7.
2. Pepe P, Holtman-Reus DH, Pilcher SL, et al. Clinical predictors of ARDS. *Am J Surg* 1982;144:124.
3. NIH Consensus Conference. Perioperative red cell transfusion. *Transfusion Med Rev* 1989;3:63–8.
4. Huth JF, Maier RV, Pavlin EG, Carrico CJ. Utilization of blood recycling in nonelective surgery. *Arch Surg* 1983;118:626–30.
5. Luna G, Maier RV, Pavlin EG, et al. Incidence and effects of hypothermia in seriously injured patients. *J Trauma* 1987;27:1014–18.
6. Pickering BG, Bristow GK, Craig DB. Core rewarming by peritoneal irrigation in accidental hypothermia with cardiac arrest. *Anesth Analg* 1977;56:574–77.
7. Hessel EA, Schmer G, Dillard DH. Platelet kinetics during deep hypothermia. *J Surg Res* 1980;28:23–9.
8. Macintyre PE, Pavlin EG, Dwerstag JF. The effect of meperidine on the oxygen consumption, carbon dioxide production and respiratory gas exchange in postanesthesia shivering. *Anesth Analg* 1987;66:751–5.
9. Huth JF, Maier RV, Simonowitz DA, Herman CM. Effect of acute ethanolism on the hospital course and outcome of injured automobile drivers. *J Trauma* 1983;23:494–6.

Orthopaedic Trauma Protocols, edited by
Sigard T. Hansen, Jr., and Marc F. Swiontkowski,
Raven Press, Ltd., New York, © 1993.

CHAPTER 6

Protocols for Posttrauma Analgesia

F. Peter Buckley

INTRODUCTION

The International Association for the Study of Pain (IASP) defines pain as "the sensory and emotional experience associated with actual or potential tissue damage, or described in terms of such damage." This reflects current thinking that a variety of factors, in addition to tissue damage, contribute to the genesis of pain complaints, and encompasses the view that the experience of pain is a multidimensional experience. The model developed by Loeser (Fig. 1) is useful in considering current thinking on pain. Central to the model is nociception (neurophysiological signals from peripheral receptors indicating tissue damage), which one assumes occurs, for it is unmeasurable in clinical circumstances. At the next level is the processing of this information by the central nervous system (CNS), which results in the human experience, comprising both sensory and emotional components—that forms "pain." This "pain" then leads to the distress that the patient suffers and which is probably influenced by cognitive—environmental, societal, emotional, and other factors. Finally, this compendium of pain and distress, which are subjective and therefore unmeasurable, emerges to be expressed as pain behaviors (complaints, actions, requests for pain relief) which constitute the only piece of the system that can be directly observed by the clinician.

That much of the system is subjective, and not directly observable, means that the clinician cannot exactly know what is going on inside the system. However, it is possible to observe and quantify the system's output—the patient's complaint of pain—and to use that as an approximation of what is going on inside the system. Thus, in the clinical setting we take pain as being "what the patient says hurts," to the degree the patient says it hurts.

Department of Anesthesiology, Harborview Medical Center, University of Washington, Seattle, Washington 98104

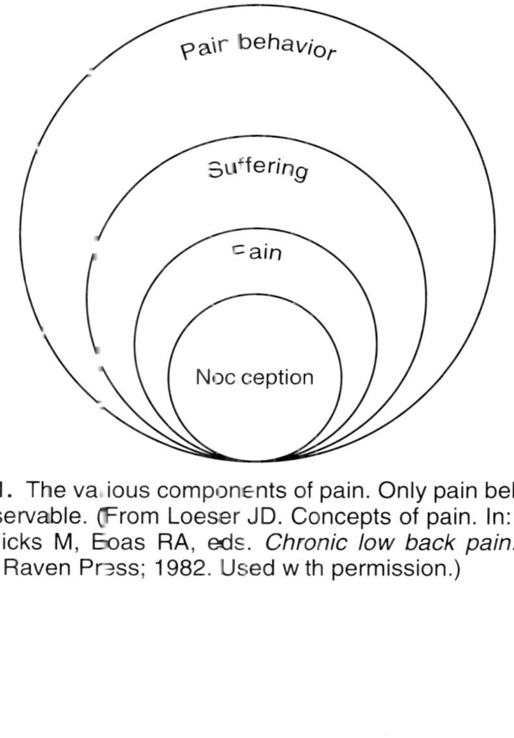

FIG. 1. The various components of pain. Only pain behavior is observable. (From Loeser JD. Concepts of pain. In: Stanton Hicks M, Boas RA, eds. *Chronic low back pain.* New York: Raven Press; 1982. Used with permission.)

MEASURING PAIN

In the clinical setting it is useful to have a method that quantifies pain complaints, so that therapies can be selected and their efficacy evaluated. The system in use at Harborview is a 10-point scale, 0 = no pain to 10 = excruciating pain. Inevitably there are patients who score their pain as being greater than 10. This does not indicate that the patient is "faking" the severity of the pain but rather that the patient is distressed and needs a way to express that distress. As an aid to evaluating pain and effectiveness of treatment, we have developed a Nursing Pain Management Flowsheet (Fig. 2).

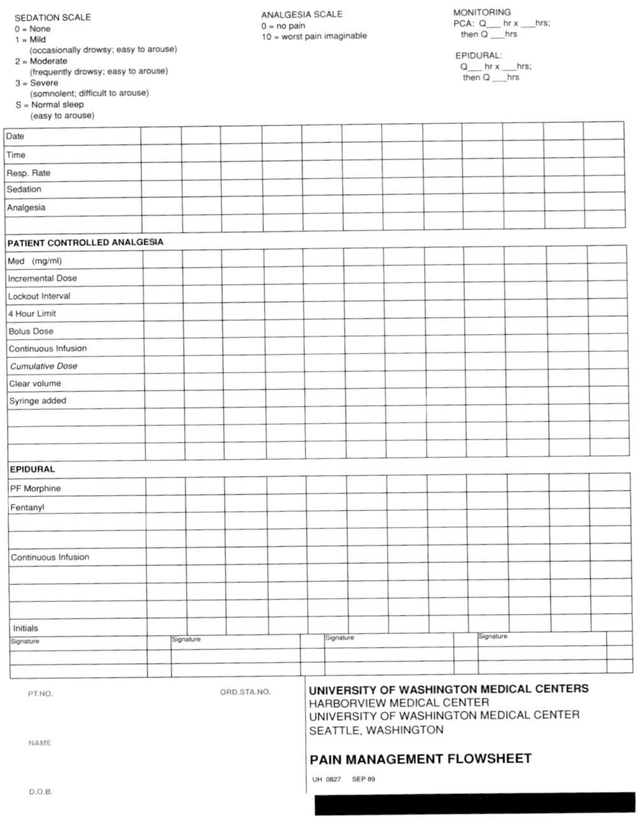

FIG. 2. Pain management flowsheet from Harborview Medical Center.

How Much Pain Do Victims of Extremity Trauma Suffer?

In the acute situation, victims of extremity trauma obviously suffer tissue damage and, presumably, activation of nociceptive pathways. In the acute circumstance the average amount of pain they complain of correlates with the degree of injury. However, both clinical observation and studies tell us that some recently badly injured patients will complain of little pain, whereas others with modest injuries will complain of severe pain. This implies that in even the recently injured the amount of pain complained of is influenced by factors other than nociception alone. In the healing phase, when nociception is decreasing, persisting pain complaints are increasingly more likely to be due to factors other than nociception.

There are clear ranking hierarchies of the amount of pain postsurgical patients suffer (thoracotomy > upper abdominal > lower abdominal > body surface), but no similar data exist for the extremity trauma victim. Extremity trauma patients may complain of more pain than elective surgery patients. Certain characteristics of extremity trauma patients may account for this difference:

1. they have tissue damage to more than one body area;
2. they have experienced an unexpected, very stressful event and find themselves in a stressful, threatening environment;
3. they have a high incidence of substance use, both licit and illicit; and
4. they tend to be young and either have more active nociceptor systems or do not cope with pain as well as the old.

Table 1. *Incidence of therapeutic failures for conventional intramuscular injections of opiates*

Reference	Number of patients	"Insufficient analgesia"; "Moderate or severe pain" (%)
Papper et al. (1952)	286	33
Lasagna and Beecher (1954)	122	33
Keeri-Szanto and Heaman (1972)	106	20
Cronin et al. (1973)	100	42
Banister (1974)	437	12–26
Tammisto (1978)	100	24
Cohen (1980)	109	75
Tamsen et al. (1983)	56	38
Donovan (1983)	200	31
Sriwatanakul et al. (1983)	82	41
Donovan et al. (1987)	350	58

How Well Do We Treat Trauma Patients' Pain?

No exact data on this topic exist. Data on the efficacy of the usual p.r.n. i.m. opioid regimen in postoperative patients do exist and paint a dismal picture (Table 1), with 30% to 40% of patients suffering moderate to severe pain, an incidence that has changed little in 30 years. It is likely that p.r.n. i.m. opioid regimens are similarly lacking in extremity trauma patients. There are many obstacles to providing effective analgesia—educational, systematic, and cultural—some of which are detailed in Table 2.

Why Worry About Treating Pain?

Why worry about providing analgesia? After all, before the introduction of analgesic regimes in the 19th century human beings had, for millennia, survived traumatic insults. Even with the less than perfect p.r.n. i.m. analgesic regimens patients seem to survive well.

The first reason for treating pain, an overwhelmingly obvious one, is for humanitarian reasons. However, there are other less obvious reasons. The experience of postoperative pain and therefore, in all likelihood, extremity trauma pain, is associated with a number of deleterious effects that contribute to morbidity. Some of these may be mitigated by analgesia:

1. Metabolic: reduction in the "stress response" with less catabolism;

2. Cardiovascular: reduction in the amount of cardiac work secondary to catecholamine and other stimuli;
3. Respiratory: improvement in pulmonary function;
4. Rheologic: reduction in thromboembolic phenomena;
5. Overall morbidity and mortality: reduced, particularly in extensive surgical procedures in the elderly and unfit;
6. Rehabilitation: early return to normal function militates against the patient "learning to hurt" and learning a disabled role; and
7. Reduction in duration of hospital stay: aggressive pain management in association with early mobilization.

Whether extremity trauma patients accrue similar benefits from analgesia is not clear; studies are lacking. However, as there are many shared traits between the postoperative patient and the extremity trauma patient, similar benefits seem likely.

Recent Changes in the Analgesic Armamentarium

In recent years there have been many developments which are likely to improve analgesia delivery:

1. awareness of the inadequacies of current regimens and of the factors which contribute to those inadequacies (see Table 2);
2. availability of new techniques that permit the delivery of systemic analgesics in a pharmacokinetically and pharmacodynamically rational fashion, (e.g., patient-controlled analgesia [PCA]);
3. the direct application of potent analgesics onto specific targets within CNS (e.g., epidural and subarachnoid opioid analgesia, continuous nerve plexus blocks); and
4. the emergence of postoperative pain relief services, staffed by those with an interest and expertise in the area, which has stimulated the development of analgesia protocols that allow the safe and routine use of potent new techniques.

Table 2. *Potential barriers to effective pain control*

Lack of knowledge of:
Pathophysiology of posttraumatic pain
Pharmacology of opioid and nonopioid analgesics
New analgesic techniques—pharmacologic and others
Differences between tolerance/habituation/addiction
Effects of fear and anxiety on pain
Benefits of psychological strategies for analgesia
Regional anesthetic/analgesic techniques
Low incidence of risks of opioids
Attitudes:
Beliefs that:
Some pain is a good thing
Complete analgesia is not a goal
Patients cannot safely self-administer opioids
Analgesia may mask underlying process
Patients are not in pain, just seeking opioids
Analgesia is not a priority
Overconcerns about:
Risks of addiction
Incidence of respiratory depression
Inaccuracy of patient's pain scores
Contacting MDs if analgesia is inadequate
System Factors:
Analgesia assigned a low priority
Analgesia the responsibility of junior personnel
All analgesic techniques need MD approval
No audit of analgesia delivery or efficacy
Inadequate education in analgesic techniques
Lack of pain management resource

ANALGESIC TECHNIQUES AND PROTOCOLS IN USE AT HARBORVIEW

Nonpharmacologic Techniques

A wide variety of such techniques (e.g., relaxation, guided imagery, self-hypnosis) are of benefit in the elective surgery population, for whom preoperative instruction, training, and coaching are possible. Extremity trauma patients do not have the luxury of such circumstances. One technique, self-hypnosis, taught and coached by a clinical psychologist, has been used with some success at Harborview for the management of incident-related pain, such as dressing changes.

Nonopioid Analgesics

When studied in double blind clinical trials, many of these agents produce analgesia as effectively as some opioids. However, both patients and physicians view their usefulness with skepticism. Nonopioids are OK for "nonhospital" and "minor" pain but "hospital," "trauma," and "operation" pains are believed to require the use of stronger analgesics. Nonopioids may not be capable of providing satisfactory analgesia on their own but, when combined with opioids, they can provide analgesia superior to that of opioids alone and can reduce the need for opioids.

To provide analgesia with nonopioids, adequate and stable therapeutic blood levels of these drugs must be achieved and maintained. After an initial loading dose, subsequent doses are given on a time-contingent (i.e., q 4, 6, 8 h) basis consistent with the drug's pharmacokinetics, rather than on a symptom-contingent (p.r.n.) basis.

This class of drugs has certain liabilities which limit their use in the trauma patient. First, they are primarily oral preparations. Extremity trauma victims may be unable to take them by mouth or may have slowed gastric emptying. Second, all of these agents affect platelet function and can potentially cause hemostatic abnormalities.

A wide variety of nonopioid analgesics is available. The oral drugs most commonly used at Harborview, as well as

Table 3. *Nonopioid drugs for adults at Harborview Medical Center*

Drug	Loading dose (mg)	Dose (mg)	Dose interval (h)
Aspirin	975	325–650	4
Aceta-minophen	975	325–650	4
Ibuprofen	800	400–600	6–8
Naproxen	500	250	6–8
Piroxicam	20	10–20	16–24

their doses and dosage intervals, are listed in Table 3. These drugs are commonly given in combination with oral opioids for reasons previously described. The recently introduced injectable drug Ketorolac, with 30–90 mg i.m. as a loading dose followed by 15–30 mg i.m. at 6-h intervals for maintenance, appears to have promise.

Systemic Opioids

These drugs modulate nociceptive information within the CNS. They can be given by any route (oral, rectal, intravenous, subcutaneous, or intramuscular). To be effective, the blood level of the drug must be within the effective range for an individual patient and yet not in the toxic range (Fig. 3). The blood level of drug at which the patient finds analgesia to be inadequate, therefore requiring another dosage of the drug, can be defined experimentally and is termed the minimum effective analgesic concentration (MEAC) (Fig. 4) of that drug. Within any one patient the MEAC is remarkably constant, but between patients individual MEACs vary widely. In the study shown in Fig. 4, the range of individual MEACs of methadone in 16 patients ranged from 34 to 80 ng/ml with a mean of 58 ng/ml, and a mean variance of 20%.

It follows that for any one patient, doses of drug, by whatever route, must be individualized, the aim being to achieve and maintain blood levels above MEAC that are within the effective range and yet do not stray into the toxic range. This can be achieved with some difficulty with i.v., i.m., and p.o. routes but more easily with PCA machines (see Fig. 3).

Opioid analgesics can be divided into those that exert opioid agonist effects (primarily the more classic opioids morphine, meperidine, methadone, hydromorphone, codeine, oxycodone) and those that possess both opioid agonist and antagonist effects and are termed mixed agonists/antagonists. The latter group is exemplified by nalorphine, which,

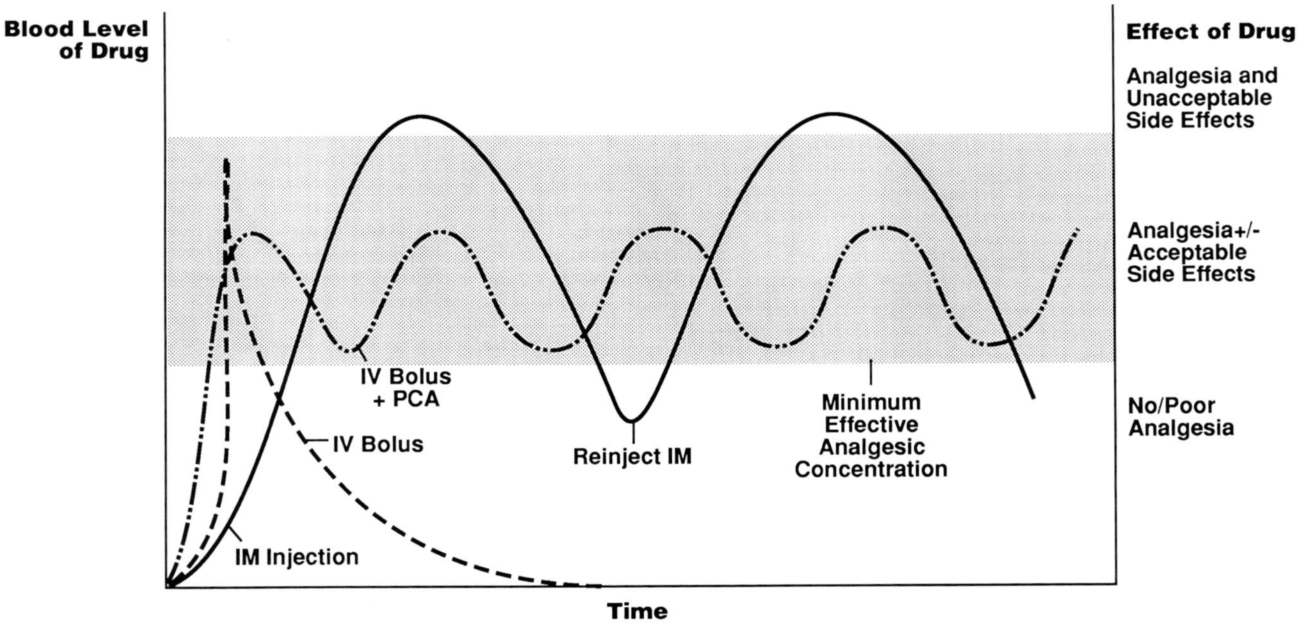

FIG. 3. Blood levels of drug that result from i.v. bolus (dashed line) i.m. (solid line) injections of opioid, and from PCA (dotted line). Opioids have a narrow window of effectiveness. Blood levels of drug below the MEAC result in inadequate analgesia. As blood levels of drug rise above MEAC there is a range that provides effective analgesia and an acceptable incidence of side effects. At blood levels of drug above this range; analgesia occurs but is associated with unacceptable or dangerous side effects. After i.v. boluses of drug, blood levels of drug rise quickly, may enter the toxic range then fall quickly, passing out of the effective range, and thus providing analgesia of only short duration. After i.m., injection blood levels of drug take time to reach the effective range, then rise into the toxic range, and then fall relatively slowly until the next i.m. injection, when the sequence is repeated. Using the patient as the sensor of need for more analgesia or drug, PCA has the ability to deliver small amounts of drug at a high frequency, thus maintaining blood levels of drug within the effective range, without blood levels of drug rising into the toxic range.

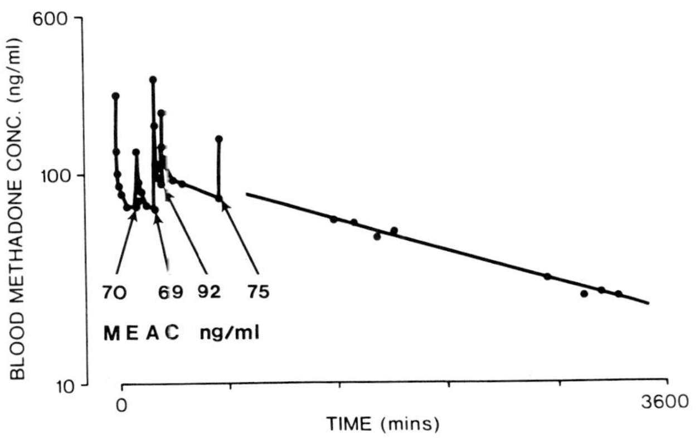

FIG. 4. After cholecystectomy an initial i.v. bolus of 20 mg methadone is administered. Each time the patient requests further pain relief a blood sample is drawn for methadone levels and further i.v. boluses of methadone 5 mg are administered. The patient's blood levels of methadone at the time of request for further pain relief are indicated by arrows. The blood level of drug when the patient requests further analgesic is termed the Minimum Effective Analgesic Concentration (MEAC). Note that within this individual patient the scatter of MEACs is very narrow. (From Gourlay G, Willis RW, Wilson P. Postoperative pain control with methadone. *Anesthesiology* 1984;61:18–25. Used with permission.)

when given alone, has agonist analgesic effects, but when given in the presence of another agonist reverses, to some extent, the other agonist's effects. The efforts of the pharmaceutic community to develop new opioid analgesics usually result in mixed agonist/antagonists (butorphanol, nalbuphine, buprenorphine) which behave similarly to nalorphine. Two drugs, naloxone and naltrexone, are pure antagonists with virtually no activity in the absence of an agonist drug, yet both will reverse an agonist.

All opioid analgesics show a similar profile of side effects (e.g., respiratory depression, sedation, nausea and vomiting, pruritus) and it is often the side effects that limit how much drug the patient will tolerate (see below). The practice at Harborview is to use agonist analgesics almost exclusively, as it seems to make little sense to use drugs with intrinsic competing effects. Of all the new drugs available, almost none show truly significant advantages over the older and cheaper drugs.

Opioids possess certain properties that are of concern to physicians and that make physicians cautious or unwilling to use them. These properties are:

1. Tolerance: with persistent use the patient becomes tolerant, needing progressively larger doses to achieve a given effect. Tolerance is a purely drug-related phenomenon and can occur in any individual exposed to an opioid. Tolerance may be a problem in providing analgesia, as doses may need to be escalated to provide a satisfactory effect, but tolerance carries no other sinister connotations.
2. Habituation: also termed dependence. With repeated exposure patients come to rely, unwillingly and unconsciously, on the drug to feel well both physically and psychologically. Abruptly ceasing the opioid may precipitate an abstinence, or withdrawal, syndrome. Like tolerance, habituation is a drug-related phenomenon and similarly does not carry sinister connotations.
3. Addiction: a state in which the individual's existence revolves around the seeking, acquisition, and consumption of the drug of choice. Addiction is an individual's problem rather than a drug problem and has complex physical, psychological, social, and environmental correlates.

Whereas addicts are certainly tolerant and habituated to opioids, the reverse is not true, i.e., those who are opioid-tolerant and habituated are not necessarily addicts. An absolutely normal non-addict may become both tolerant and habituated to opioids with repeated exposure but, after being weaned from the drug, will return to the previous drug-free status and will not become an addict. There are pervasive fears among the community at large, and specifically amongst the medical community, of patients becoming iatrogenically addicted through the therapeutic use of opioids. Studies of medical and surgical populations with no previous substance abuse history, who are therapeutically exposed to opioids cite subsequent addiction rates of 1:3,000–1:5,000, a very low incidence.

It is possible that the incidence of iatrogenic addiction among that segment of the trauma population without a substance-abuse history may be higher than the figures cited above, given that the trauma population may have a longer exposure to opioids. However, no such data on the trauma population exist. As a group, trauma patients have a high incidence of previous substance abuse. Those with such a history constitute a different category from those without such a history. The previous users may be tolerant to opioids, possibly habituated, and will have higher than usual opioid requirements to provide satisfactory analgesia.

The essential message is that although iatrogenic habituation and addiction can occur, the incidence of addiction is so low that opioids should not be withheld from the traumatized patient for fear of producing such a state.

Oral Opioids

Oral opioids can provide satisfactory analgesia provided the dose regimes ensure that the MEAC is achieved and maintained. Adequate doses must be given at appropriate intervals, taking into consideration the oral/systemic bioavailability ratios (Table 4).

The use of oral opioids at Harborview is closely tied to the needs of the patients, bearing in mind the potencies, speeds of onset, and duration of action of the various drugs. In changing a patient from a systemic to an oral opioid the information given in Table 4 is used. For maintenance analgesia with relatively minor degrees of injury, codeine and

Table 4. *Approximate analgesic equivalents to 10 mg morphine (MS) intramuscularly (IM) and oral/parenteral bioavailability*

Drug	Onset of action (min)	Peak action (min)	Duration (h)	Oral/parenteral bioavailability	Equivalent to 10 mg MS IM	
					p.o.	i.m.
Morphine	60	60–90	4–5	0.17–0.33	60	10
Slow-release morphine	60	180	8	0–18	45	—
Hydromorphone	15–30	30	3–4	0.2	7.5	1.5
Meperidine	40–60	60–120	2–4	0.25	300	100
Methadone	60	120	6–8	0.5	15	10
Codeine	45	60	3–4	0.6	200	130
Oxycodone	45	60	3–4	0.5	30	15

oxycodone are used. For maintenance analgesia in more severe injuries, one of the longer-acting agents such as methadone, morphine, or slow-release morphine is used. For rapid-onset analgesia of short duration (e.g., dressing changes), hydromorphone is used. Oral Demerol is infrequently used.

Oral opioids have a special role in humanely and safely tapering the doses of analgesics. After patients have been taking opioids they may become tolerant and perhaps habituated and, if the drug is abruptly reduced or stopped, they may manifest withdrawal syndrome. The frequency with which withdrawal occurs can be greatly reduced by gradually tapering the dose of oral opioid over 5 to 7 days. This can be achieved by evaluating the patient's total opioid intake, by whatever route, over a 24-h period and converting that dose into an equivalent amount of oral opioid (see Table 4). That dose is administered in divided doses at specific time intervals over a 24-h period. This can be achieved with pills, gradually reducing the number of pills given each day, but this technique may lead to anticipatory anxiety on the part of the patients, who fear that with fewer pills they may feel more pain. To circumvent this anticipatory anxiety, the "pain cocktail" strategy is often adopted. For this the 24-h opioid dose is put into 40 ml of a liquid vehicle, 10 ml of which are administered every 6 h. The next day the 24-h opioid dose is reduced 15% to 20% but given in the same 40-ml volume of vehicle, 10 ml being administered every 6 h. This strategy is repeated until the patient is no longer taking any opioid. Classically, methadone is the drug used in the "pain cocktail" but, just as alcoholic cocktails can contain a variety of ingredients, so may the "pain cocktail" (e.g. codeine, oxycodone). A specimen prescription sheet for the "pain cocktail" is shown in Fig. 5.

Conventional Intramuscular Opioids

Although intramuscular opioids have been the mainstay of analgesic regimens for many years, they have distinct liabilities. The blood levels of drug that result from a given injection vary with the site of injection and the perfusion of that site (i.m. injections may be dangerous in the hypoperfused patient because an injection may not be absorbed from a hypoperfused area, giving poor analgesia at that time, only to be absorbed, unpredictably, when perfusion is reestablished). The blood levels that are produced by i.m. injections are cyclic and may rise above the toxic threshold or all below the MEAC (see Fig. 3). There are inevitable delays associated with the i.m. technique. The patient detects the need for further analgesia and calls the nurse, the nurse evaluates the patient's request, gets the drug, checks it with a colleague and administers the drug, which takes about 20 min. The drug takes 30 to 40 min to be absorbed into the systemic circulation in sufficient amounts to become effective, leaving

GENERAL DIRECTIONS: 1. PLEASE SPECIFY HOW MANY DOSES ARE NEEDED UNDER "DOSES ORDERED". IF NO NUMBER IS SPECIFIED, THE PHARMACY WILL SEND ONLY A 48-HOUR SUPPLY.
2. MEDICATIONS, SHOULD BE TAPERED ACCORDING TO PROTOCOL.
3. NORMAL PAIN COCKTAIL COMPOUNDING TIMES ARE BETWEEN 0900 AND 1900 HOURS.
4. ALL REFILLS MUST BE REWRITTEN AND SIGNED.
5. SEE PAIN COCKTAIL PROTOCOL ON BACK.

INGREDIENTS	DOSE FOR THIS PATIENT	STANDARD DOSE RANGE
*METHADONE	mg/10ml	0-10 mg/DOSE
HYDROXYZINE	mg/10ml	25-50 mg/DOSE
PHENOBARBITAL	mg/10ml	0-30 mg/DOSE
ACETAMINOPHEN	mg/10ml	650 mg/DOSE
PLEBEX® (OPTIONAL MASKING AGENT)	ml/10ml	0.1 or 0.2 cc/DOSE
OTHER**		

*METHADONE IS A C II NARCOTIC AND ALL NARCOTIC REGULATIONS MUST BE FOLLOWED.
**THE FOLLOWING DRUGS ARE UNSTABLE IN AQUEOUS SOLUTION: ASPIRIN, VALIUM®, DALMANE®, LIBRIUM®.

ADD ABOVE TO THE FOLLOWING VEHICLE: (CHECK APPROPRIATE BOX).

☐ CHERRY SYRUP
☐ MAALOX®
☐ MYLANTA®
☐ SORBITOL 10% (LOW CALORIE)
☐ OTHER ______

DOSING SCHEDULE
GIVE 10 ml EVERY ______ HOURS

DOSES ORDERED (MAXIMUM 25 DOSES/250 ml)

SPECIAL INSTRUCTIONS

PHYSICIAN'S SIGNATURE	DEA NO.	DATE	TIME

PHARMACY USE ONLY

PAIN COCKTAIL NUMBER	AMOUNT DISPENSED	PHARMACIST'S INITIALS	DATE

UNIVERSITY OF WASHINGTON HOSPITALS
HARBORVIEW MEDICAL CENTER
UNIVERSITY HOSPITAL
SEATTLE, WASHINGTON

PAIN COCKTAIL ORDERS

WHITE—Medical Chart
CANARY—Pharmacy
PINK—Nursing Unit

UH 0686 REV JUN 82

FIG. 5. Example of a pain cocktail order form.

the patient in pain for an hour or so. Because of these inadequacies, the use of i.m. injections as an analgesic regimen is waning at Harborview, giving way to the more sophisticated PCA systems which address many of the deficiencies of i.m. regimens.

Intravenous Opioids

Single boluses of opioids produce blood level profiles as shown in Fig 3. By virtue of the rapid fall in blood levels they have a very limited duration of analgesic effect. Intravenous doses are a good means for rapidly bringing blood levels of drug to therapeutic levels, where they can be maintained by an infusion of drug or by conversion to a PCA regimen. If an individual patient's MEAC and the pharmacokinetic parameters of the drug within the patient could be defined, i.v. opioid infusions would be a logical way to maintain therapeutic blood levels of drug. Attempts have been made to achieve this, but at present these are experimental.

At Harborview, i.v. opioids are used in the acute circumstance to rapidly achieve therapeutic blood levels of drug, titrating small increments to the desired end-point and against side effects, before going on to the use of other modes of drug delivery. They are also used to provide brief but intense analgesia for incident-related pain, such as dressing changes. Intravenous infusions of opioids are used in intubated, ventilated patients in the ICUs, the necessary dose being titrated against the desired analgesic effect. For i.v. use morphine is the drug of choice, with fentanyl being increasingly used for incident-related pain.

Patient-Controlled Analgesia

This particular technique of analgesia rests on several premises (see Fig. 3). First, opioids have a therapeutic window, i.e., they will produce acceptable analgesia at blood levels above MEAC. Second, blood levels of drug must rise substantially beyond the MEAC before undesirable effects become troublesome. Finally, when patients are permitted to self-administer small doses of opioids they will titrate the amount of drug they consume to maintain blood levels above MEAC but below the toxic threshold, as in PCA.

What began as a theory has been translated into practice with the availability of PCA machines. These machines are power-driven syringes with control systems that permit the patient to self-administer a physician-determined dose of drug, at a physician-determined minimum interval. The usual setting for the device is to deliver 1.0 mg of morphine at a minimum interval of once every 10 min, although the doses and the intervals vary widely from individual to individual. Such devices enable each patient to determine his or her individual needs. For individual patients the rate of opioid use is very stable over time. Concerns that patients would use the drug intemperately have not been realized. The technique has an excellent safety record and a high level of patient acceptance.

Despite its many virtues, PCA also has some vices. If a patient falls asleep for several hours while using PCA, the blood levels may fall below MEAC and the small incremental doses available from PCA machines may not allow the patient to "catch up." Attempts have been made to remedy such deficiencies by developing devices that provide a baseline infusion of drug, even when the patient is asleep, in addition to manual PCA. Studies of such a technique have shown that the analgesic outcome is similar to that of regular PCA. Although PCA meets with a high degree of patient acceptance patients rarely titrate themselves to a perfect level of analgesia (with pain levels of 0–2/10): more often, they titrate to pain levels of 2–4/10. It appears that patients titrate their dosage to produce acceptable analgesia, balancing that against the side effects of the drug.

Harborview widely uses the Abbott PCA machines. Patients receive a loading dose of drug in the ward or in the recovery room, and the PCA device is set up. Patients are instructed to push the PCA button whenever they feel that they need further analgesia. The most commonly used drug is morphine, with Demerol following a distant second. However, it is possible to use any injectable opioid. A formalized order sheet is used, categorizing the device parameters that must be initially set (Fig. 6). For dressing changes or other

1. PCA PRESCRIPTION:

MODE:	☐ PCA Only	☐ PCA + Continuous Infusion		☐ Continuous Infusion only
DRUG:	☐ Morphine 1 mg / ml	☐ Meperidine 10 mg / ml	☐ Hydromorphone 0.2 mg / ml	☐ Other: ____ ____ mg - mcg / ml
PCA MODE: Incremental Dose	____ mg	____ mg	____ mg	____ mg - mcg
Lockout	____ minutes	____ minutes	____ minutes	____ minutes
4 Hour Limit	30 mg (Adult) or ____ mg (Pediatric)	300 mg (Adult) or ____ mg (Pediatric)	6mg (Adult) or ____ mg (Pediatric)	____ mg
OPTIONAL INFUSION MODE: (Recommended starting rate)	____ mg/hr Adult (0.5 mg/hr) Pediatric (0.007 mg/kg/hr)	____ mg/hr Adult (5 mg/hr) Pediatric (0.1 mg/kg/hr)	____ mg/hr Adult (0.1 mg/hr) Pediatric (1.5 mcg/kg/hr)	____ mg - mcg/hr (Consult PRS)
Instructions for infusion:	☐ Continuous ☐ Infuse from 2200 to 0600 nightly	☐ Continuous ☐ Infuse from 2200 to 0600 nightly	☐ Continuous ☐ Infuse from 2200 to 0600 nightly	☐ Continuous ☐ Infuse from 2200 to 0600 nightly
LOADING DOSES: (via PCA pump when block recedes or for breakthrough pain)	____ mg q 5 min to a maximum of ____ mg	____ mg q 5 min to a maximum of ____ mg	____ mg q 5 min to a maximum of ____ mg	____ mg - mcg q 5 min to a maximum of ____ mg - mcg
FOR INADEQUATE RELIEF: after 1 hr with initial pump settings:	Increase Incremental Dose to ____ mg	Increase Incremental Dose to ____ mg	Increase Incremental Dose to ____ mg	Increase Incremental Dose to ____ mg - mcg
FOR INADEQUATE RELIEF: after 1 additional hr:	Decrease lockout to ____ min	Decrease lockout to ____ min	Decrease lockout to ____ min	Decrease lockout to ____ min

2. No systemic narcotics or other CNS depressants to be given except on direct one-time order from HO/PRS.

3. MONITORING: Respiratory rate, Pain Level (0-10), Sedation Scale (0-3) - q2 hr for 8 hrs; then q 4 hr while patient is on PCA. Document on "Pain Management Flowsheet".

4. TREATMENT OF SIDE EFFECTS:

A. Call HO/PRS for Sedation Scale = 3, RR < 8 per min or < 50% of normal RR.

B. For Sedation Scale = 3 and RR < 8 per min or < 50% of normal RR, give Naloxone ____ mg IV stat. May repeat x ____ q 5 min. Call HO/PRS.

C. METOCLOPRAMIDE ____ mg IV q 4 hr prn for nausea / vomiting. In addition, TRANSDERMAL SCOPOLAMINE PATCH to either mastoid area (1/2 patch for 12 > age > 60 yrs). Change q 72 hr prn. Not recommended for children < age 6 yrs.

D. DIPHENHYDRAMINE ____ mg, IV or PO q 6 hr for severe itching.

E. For urinary retention, "in and out" catheter prn

5. For sleep ____

6. For inadequate analgesia or other problems related to PCA, call HO/PRS.

DATE	TIME	PHYSICIAN
		M. D.

PT.NO.

NAME

D.O.B.

UNIVERSITY OF WASHINGTON MEDICAL CENTERS
HARBORVIEW MEDICAL CENTER
UNIVERSITY OF WASHINGTON MEDICAL CENTER
SEATTLE, WASHINGTON

INTRAVENOUS PATIENT CONTROLLED ANALGESIA (PCA)
PHYSICIANS ORDERS

WHITE - MEDICAL RECORDS
CANARY - PHARMACY
PINK - NURSE'S COPY

HMC 0564 REV MAR 92

FIG. 6. Prescription form for patient-controlled i.v. analgesia.

painful maneuvers, PCA devices can also be used to deliver boluses of drug greater in size than the usual incremental doses.

SPECIALIZED TECHNIQUES

Pain Relief Service

The techniques described thus far are used by surgeons and have improved analgesia delivery. However, for certain groups of patients, or for patients with certain injuries, these techniques may not provide effective analgesia. To achieve analgesia in these patients and injuries, more potent analgesic techniques are available (e.g., neuraxial opioids, continuous local anesthetic [LA] blocks). However, as in other circumstances, potency is accompanied by an array of side effects and potential complications. Therefore, the use of these specialized techniques mandates expert delivery and monitoring. At Harborview, this has been achieved by the formation of a Pain Relief Service, staffed by the Department of Anesthesiology. This service, in concert with surgeons and nursing staff, has been responsible for developing the protocols for specialized analgesic techniques and bringing those techniques into routine clinical use.

Neuraxial Opioid Analgesia (Epidural Opioid Analgesia: EOA)

In the early 1970s, specific opioid receptors were found in the dorsal horn of the spinal cord. These were shown to be capable of modulating the afferent nociceptive traffic while exerting few other effects. Clinically, relevance was established when it was shown that the introduction of very small amounts of opioid into human CSF produced profound and long-lasting analgesia. For example, injection of 0.2 mg of morphine into the subarachnoid space (CSF) produced analgesia that lasted 10 to 15 h. Furthermore, the quality of analgesia was more profound and long-lasting than that obtained by systemic administration of opioids.

To gain access to the dorsal horn, opioids must reach the CSF, either by direct subarachnoid injection or by injection into the epidural space, where the drug diffuses across the dura/arachnoid into the CSF. In clinical practice the subarachnoid route is rarely used except for single–shot dosage, epidurals via indwelling catheters forming the vast majority of practice. For epidurals, a catheter is placed in the epidural space close to the center of the segments through which the nociceptive traffic enters the spinal cord. Correct catheter placement is confirmed by producing a discernible epidural block with a small dose of LA or by performing a metrizamide epidurogram. The catheter is taped in place or, if it will be needed for a prolonged period of time or the skin of the back is potentially contaminated, the catheter is tunneled subcutaneously from the site of insertion, exiting the skin some distance away.

There is considerable dispute about how opioids behave in the epidural space and the CSF. The prevailing theories are illustrated in Fig. 7. Injected epidurally, the drug crosses the dura/arachnoid layer by diffusion, enters the CSF, and binds to the opioid receptors in the dorsal horn. The speed and the mass of drug that crosses the dura/arachnoid is probably a function of the fat solubility of the drug. Fat-soluble drugs such as fentanyl cross quickly in large amounts, whereas water-soluble drugs such as morphine cross slowly in small amounts. However, fat-soluble drugs are removed quickly by the spinal cord vasculature, resulting in a short duration of action, whereas the water-soluble drugs are removed slowly, resulting in a long duration of action. The long duration of action of a drug such as morphine is clinically desirable, but this long duration results from persistent drug in the CSF. In so doing, the drug may diffuse throughout the CSF as far as the medulla, where it can produce the medullary effects of sedation and respiratory depression. In practice, the doses used and the frequency at which they are administered must strike a balance between providing enough drug at the spinal level to produce satisfactory analgesia and yet not so much that spread to the medulla, with resulting sedation and respiratory depression, is likely to occur.

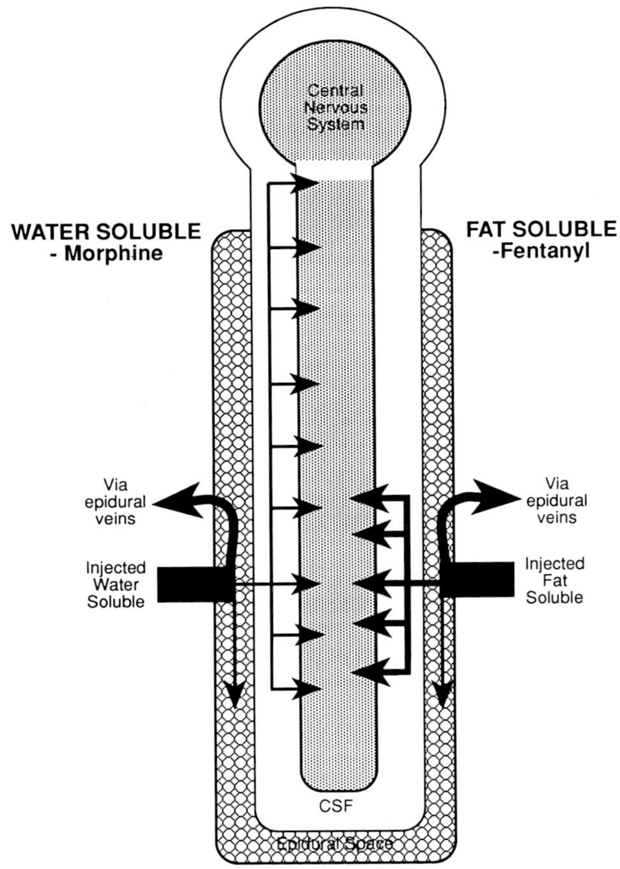

FIG. 7. The migration of fat-soluble and water-soluble opioids into the CSF after epidural injection. See text for details.

In practice, respiratory depression after EOA does occur, with a cited incidence of 0.1% to 0.5% of patients. The patients in whom it does occur are usually the elderly and those who have received substantial amounts of parenteral opioids. It is unclear whether the incidence of clinical respiratory depression is greater or less than that which occurs when analgesia is provided by systemic opioids. The worrying aspect of respiratory depression after EOA is that it may occur some hours after drug administration, presumably reflecting the time required for the drug to ascend through the CSF to the medulla. The respiratory depression resulting from EOA can be reversed, without unduly affecting analgesia, by naloxone. Epidural opioids have other troublesome but less serious side effects. Pan-body itch, nausea, and urinary retention each occur in about 30% of patients, and can be so severe that the technique must be abandoned in 5% to 10% of patients.

Epidural opioids provide very effective relief of the constant background pain in the trauma patient. However, they are not as effective in relieving the sharp pain associated with movement, either patient-initiated or produced by constant passive motion (CPM) machines. If it is anticipated that a large part of the pain will be related to movement, an alternative choice of technique may be appropriate (e.g., LA with or without opioid, or a continuous LA block).

Because of safety concerns, the EOA protocol in use at Harborview initially called for all patients to be cared for and monitored in an ICU. Subsequently, the further development of the protocol by the Pain Relief Service and in-service teaching of the nursing staff about the technique have permitted the expansion of the technique into the wards. Patients who are old, ill, unstable, or complex are still cared for in the ICU. The current protocol at Harborview mandates a number of safeguards, which are reflected in the physicians' order sheet (Fig. 8). Morphine is the standard drug used: the guidelines for dosage used at 6-h intervals are given in Table 5. Provision exists for the use of small doses of a short-acting opioid, fentanyl, for the relief of breakthrough pain. No other opioids or sedatives are permitted except after consultation with the pain relief service, because such drugs may interact synergistically with the EOA and produce a confusing picture with regard to sedation or respiratory depression. Constant i.v. access and availability of naloxone are mandated to treat any excessive sedation and respiratory depression, and orders are given for immediate administration of naloxone by a nurse if the need should arise. Continuous oxygen administration is required. Monitoring of respiratory rate, sedation, pain levels, and side effects is done hourly and recorded on the Pain Assessment Flowsheet (see Fig. 1). Standing orders for routine treatment of side effects such as nausea, itching, and urinary retention are included.

Although morphine and fentanyl, given by bolus injection, are the standard drugs used for EOA at Harborview, a provision exists within the protocol and order sheet for the use of continuous infusion of fentanyl, but this technique is rarely used.

A huge variety of other opioids have been administered epidurally and have produced satisfactory analgesia, though none have been shown to possess significant advantages over the current drugs. Mixtures of low concentrations of bupivacaine (0.1–0.2%) and fentanyl (2–4 µg/ml) given by epidural infusion at rates of 8 to 12 ml/h, produce excellent analgesia and have been occasionally used on patients in the ICU at HMC. However, their routine use requires a specific protocol for administration and monitoring, as a consequence of the neuraxial effects of LAs (see below). Such a protocol has yet to be developed at Harborview.

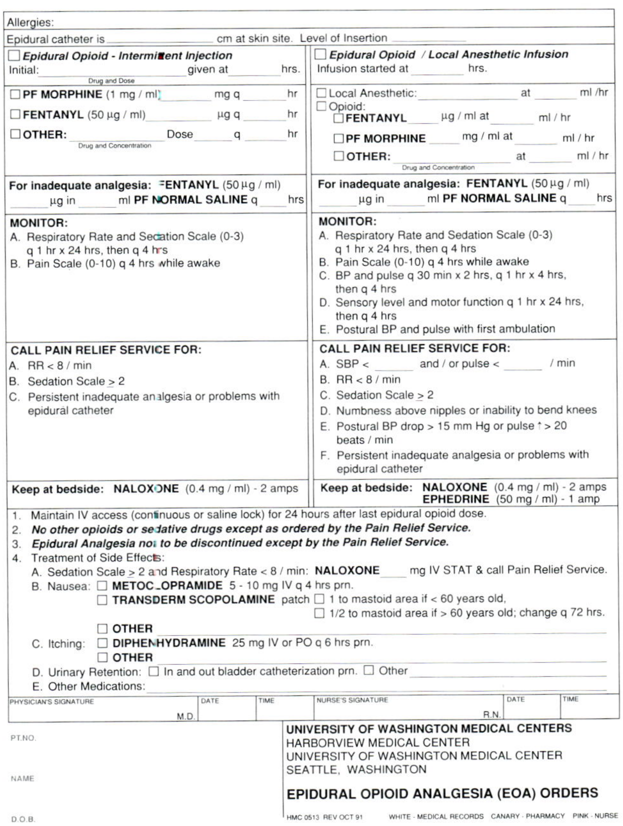
Allergies:
Epidural catheter is ______ cm at skin site. Level of Insertion ______

☐ *Epidural Opioid - Intermittent Injection*
Initial: ______ given at ______ hrs.
Drug and Dose
☐ **PF MORPHINE** (1 mg / ml) ______ mg q ______ hr
☐ **FENTANYL** (50 µg / ml) ______ µg q ______ hr
☐ **OTHER:** ______ Dose ______ q ______ hr
Drug and Concentration

For inadequate analgesia: **FENTANYL** (50 µg / ml) ______ µg in ______ ml **PF NORMAL SALINE** q ______ hrs

MONITOR:
A. Respiratory Rate and Sedation Scale (0-3) q 1 hr x 24 hrs, then q 4 hrs
B. Pain Scale (0-10) q 4 hrs while awake

CALL PAIN RELIEF SERVICE FOR:
A. RR < 8 / min
B. Sedation Scale ≥ 2
C. Persistent inadequate analgesia or problems with epidural catheter

Keep at bedside: **NALOXONE** (0.4 mg / ml) - 2 amps

☐ *Epidural Opioid / Local Anesthetic Infusion*
Infusion started at ______ hrs.
☐ Local Anesthetic: ______ at ______ ml /hr
☐ Opioid:
☐ **FENTANYL** ______ µg / ml at ______ ml / hr
☐ **PF MORPHINE** ______ mg / ml at ______ ml / hr
☐ **OTHER:** ______ at ______ ml / hr
Drug and Concentration

For inadequate analgesia: **FENTANYL** (50 µg / ml) ______ µg in ______ ml **PF NORMAL SALINE** q ______ hrs

MONITOR:
A. Respiratory Rate and Sedation Scale (0-3) q 1 hr x 24 hrs, then q 4 hrs
B. Pain Scale (0-10) q 4 hrs while awake
C. BP and pulse q 30 min x 2 hrs, q 1 hr x 4 hrs, then q 4 hrs
D. Sensory level and motor function q 1 hr x 24 hrs, then q 4 hrs
E. Postural BP and pulse with first ambulation

CALL PAIN RELIEF SERVICE FOR:
A. SBP < ______ and / or pulse < ______ / min
B. RR < 8 / min
C. Sedation Scale ≥ 2
D. Numbness above nipples or inability to bend knees
E. Postural BP drop > 15 mm Hg or pulse ↑ > 20 beats / min
F. Persistent inadequate analgesia or problems with epidural catheter

Keep at bedside: **NALOXONE** (0.4 mg / ml) - 2 amps
EPHEDRINE (50 mg / ml) - 1 amp

1. Maintain IV access (continuous or saline lock) for 24 hours after last epidural opioid dose.
2. ***No other opioids or sedative drugs except as ordered by the Pain Relief Service.***
3. ***Epidural Analgesia not to be discontinued except by the Pain Relief Service.***
4. Treatment of Side Effects:
   A. Sedation Scale ≥ 2 and Respiratory Rate < 8 / min: **NALOXONE** ______ mg IV STAT & call Pain Relief Service.
   B. Nausea: ☐ **METOCLOPRAMIDE** 5 - 10 mg IV q 4 hrs prn.
   ☐ **TRANSDERM SCOPOLAMINE** patch ☐ 1 to mastoid area if < 60 years old, ☐ 1/2 to mastoid area if > 60 years old; change q 72 hrs.
   ☐ **OTHER** ______
   C. Itching: ☐ **DIPHENHYDRAMINE** 25 mg IV or PO q 6 hrs prn.
   ☐ **OTHER** ______
   D. Urinary Retention: ☐ In and out bladder catheterization prn. ☐ Other ______
   E. Other Medications: ______

PHYSICIAN'S SIGNATURE ______ M.D. DATE ______ TIME ______ NURSE'S SIGNATURE ______ R.N. DATE ______ TIME ______

PT.NO.
NAME
D.O.B.

UNIVERSITY OF WASHINGTON MEDICAL CENTERS
HARBORVIEW MEDICAL CENTER
UNIVERSITY OF WASHINGTON MEDICAL CENTER
SEATTLE, WASHINGTON

EPIDURAL OPIOID ANALGESIA (EOA) ORDERS

HMC 0513 REV OCT 91 WHITE - MEDICAL RECORDS CANARY - PHARMACY PINK - NURSE

FIG. 8. An order form for epidural opioid analgesia.

Table 5. *Guidelines for selecting epidural opioid dose* [a]

Age (yr)	Nonthoracic Surgery	Thoracic surgery	
	Lumbar cath[b]	Thoracic cath[b]	Lumbar cath[b]
15–44	4	4	5
45–65	3	3	4
66–75	2	2	3
76+	1	1	2

[a] Initial dose (mg) of 0.1% preservative-free morphine.
[b] cath, catheter.

Epidural Local Anesthetics

Local anesthetics administered into the epidural space diffuse across the dura arachnoid layer and produce a nonselective conduction block of the spinal nerves at the nerve root level. Although such a technique produces superb deafferentation, it can also produce a sympathetic and parasympathetic block and a variable degree of motor block. Therefore, when this technique is used the patient may experience some degree of lower extremity paresis and may be at risk for hypotension because of the sympathetic blockade. The extent of motor block and the risk of hypotension can be minimized by a judicious choice of catheter placement and drug concentration. However, to be used safely the technique requires a specific management and monitoring protocol and should probably only be used in the setting of the ICU. At Harborview a specific protocol for this technique has not yet been developed, although the technique is occasionally used on a one-off basis.

Peripheral Nerve Blocks

When applied to a nerve, LAs produce a nonselective block of neural traffic that continues until the concentration of LA falls below a critical level, at which time neural function returns. Therefore, LA blocks can produce deafferentation, which can contribute to posttraumatic analgesia.

Single-Shot Nerve Blocks

Single-shot nerve blocks with long acting LAs such as bupivacaine, either by wound infiltration or by a peripheral nerve block, provide analgesia of the blocked area for the duration of the drug's action. The duration of analgesia after infiltration with bupivacaine is 4 to 6 h and after peripheral nerve block is 8 to 20 h. Evidence is emerging that single-shot nerve blocks at the time of surgery not only provide analgesia for the duration of action of the drug but may also lead to less pain and less analgesic need when the block has worn off. The precise mechanism of such an effect is unclear.

While the peripheral block works, the blocked area is both insensate and paretic. It is imperative to manage the patient so that the insensate and paretic limb will not be inadvertently damaged and will not damage other parts of the body. When the clinical circumstances are such that pain might be a warning of ongoing pathology, (e.g., a compartment syndrome), peripheral nerve blocks should be used with caution and the affected limb properly monitored. Although nerve blocks provide good analgesia in the blocked area, patients should have access to other sources of analgesia (PCA) to deal with discomfort outside the blocked area (i.v. sites, NG tubes) and to provide a smooth transition to alternative sources of analgesia when the block wears off.

At Harborview, about 20% to 30% of patients receive regional anesthesia for operative procedures. The usual maximal doses of bupivacaine plus epinephrine 1:200,000 are on the order of 3.0 mg/kg.

Continuous Peripheral Nerve Blocks

When applied to a nerve, LAs unselectively block neural traffic and, provided that a blocking concentration of LA is maintained around the nerve, both afferent and efferent traffic can be blocked on a long-term basis. With very judicious choice of administered mass of drug, it is sometimes possible to produce differential block (i.e., a primarily afferent block of the nerve), yet still retain some motor function. However, this differential block cannot predictably be achieved, and any patient with a continuous local anesthetic block is highly likely to have a paretic, as well as an analgesic, limb. Therefore, any patient with a functioning continuous block must be managed, with regard to protection of the blocked area and a potential compartment syndrome, as a patient with a single-shot nerve block.

In practice, continuous blocks are achieved by placing a catheter close to the appropriate nerve and either infusing sufficient LA to maintain local blocking levels or repeatedly injecting LA at intervals appropriate to the kinetics of the drug used. The common anatomic sites at which this can be accomplished are the brachial plexus (interscalene, supraclavicular, and axillary routes), the femoral nerve at the groin, and the sciatic nerve, either at the buttock or in the popliteal fossa. Such catheter placement is done under sterile conditions in the OR.

A major concern with continuous LA blocks is to keep the blood levels of the drug within safe, nontoxic limits. When LAs are injected they are absorbed from the injection site, producing a peak blood level of drug about 20 to 40 min after the injection. The LA is then cleared systemically with progressive falls in blood levels of drug. In maintaining a continuous nerve block, three circumstances give cause for concern. First, when the block is maintained by continuous infusion and the rate of drug administration exceeds the rate at which the drug is cleared systemically, the blood levels of drug will slowly rise, perhaps reaching toxic levels and resulting in convulsions. Data concerning the rate at which LAs used for continuous blocks are cleared systemically are sparse. Those data available show the clearance values to be highly variable, and safe dosage schedules for LAs used in continuous nerve blocks do not exist. Second, when a block is maintained by periodic bolus injection and the overall rate of administration exceeds the clearance rate, similar effects of LA on blood levels and potential side effects, as for continuous infusions of LA, can occur. However, the time at which such a situation is most likely to occur is 30 to 40 min after an injection, as the drug is absorbed from the site of injection and reaches the peak blood levels of drug attributable to the injection. Finally, when a block is being maintained by either of the above methods there is the risk that the catheter may erode into a blood vessel. If this event is not recognized, any drug given via the catheter will be directed into the systemic circulation, with potential side effects.

The speed and the quantity of LAs absorbed from any site, and therefore the resulting blood levels of drug, can be reduced by the addition of epinephrine to the injectate. It is not clear whether the long-term use of epinephrine results in greater neural morbidity. There are concerns that the use of epinephrine in and around large arteries might cause arterial constriction and accentuate peripheral ischemia. However, causing a large artery to constrict is unlikely, and the systemic effects of the amount of epinephrine used are a rise in cardiac output and a fall in peripheral resistance, both of which would be likely to improve peripheral perfusion.

The protocol in use for continuous local anesthetic blocks at Harborview has been designed to accommodate all these uncertainties. The initial block is performed with a maximum dose of bupivacaine 3 mg/kg plus epinephrine 1:200,000. Repeated injections are given by the Pain Relief Service, or by other anesthesiologists, at 8-h intervals, using a bupivacaine dose of 1.5 mg/kg. Usually, between six and eight reinjections are done. The reinjections are given in the Post-Anesthesia Recovery Unit (PARU) with all appropriate equipment available to deal with local anesthetic toxicity. The patients are observed for 30 to 40 min, i.e., beyond the time when peak blood levels of local anesthetic are likely to occur, and then returned to the floor. Patients are kept NPO for the 4 h before the catheter reinjection. All patients receiving a continuous nerve block also have access to other modes of analgesia because, even though the traumatized area is anesthetized, the patient may have other sources of discomfort, (e.g., sore i.v. site, sore buttocks and heels). An order sheet has been developed to assist in the protocol (Fig. 9).

☐ 1. STANDARD DURATION OF TREATMENT SHALL BE 48 HOURS; 6 REINJECTIONS AT 8 HOUR INTERVALS

DAY / DATE:	TIME: ☐ PTS' ROOM ☐ PACU	TIME: ☐ PTS' ROOM ☐ PACU	TIME: ☐ PTS' ROOM ☐ PACU
DAY / DATE:	TIME: ☐ PTS' ROOM ☐ PACU	TIME: ☐ PTS' ROOM ☐ PACU	TIME: ☐ PTS' ROOM ☐ PACU
DAY / DATE:	TIME: ☐ PTS' ROOM ☐ PACU	TIME: ☐ PTS' ROOM ☐ PACU	TIME: ☐ PTS' ROOM ☐ PACU

☐ 2. OTHER

DAY / DATE:	TIME: ☐ PTS' ROOM ☐ PACU	TIME: ☐ PTS' ROOM ☐ PACU	TIME: ☐ PTS' ROOM ☐ PACU
DAY / DATE:	TIME: ☐ PTS' ROOM ☐ PACU	TIME: ☐ PTS' ROOM ☐ PACU	TIME: ☐ PTS' ROOM ☐ PACU
DAY / DATE:	TIME: ☐ PTS' ROOM ☐ PACU	TIME: ☐ PTS' ROOM ☐ PACU	TIME: ☐ PTS' ROOM ☐ PACU

☐ 3. THE PATIENT SHALL BE NPO FOR 4 HOURS PRIOR TO EACH REINJECTION

DAY / DATE: ______ TIME: ______, ______, ______
DAY / DATE: ______ TIME: ______, ______, ______
DAY / DATE: ______ TIME: ______, ______, ______

☐ 4. PATIENT TO RECEIVE SUPPLEMENTAL PAIN MEDICATION PER SURGEON'S ORDERS

PHYSICIAN'S SIGNATURE | DATE | TIME

PT.NO.
NAME
D.O.B.

UNIVERSITY OF WASHINGTON MEDICAL CENTERS
HARBORVIEW MEDICAL CENTER
UNIVERSITY OF WASHINGTON MEDICAL CENTER
SEATTLE, WASHINGTON

CONTINUOUS BRACHIAL PLEXUS / FEMEROL SCIATIC NERVE BLOCK STANDING ORDERS

HMC N 0594 AUG 91

FIG. 9. Standing orders for patient receiving continuous brachial plexus/femoral sciatic nerve block.

Continuous Perineural Infusion of Local Anesthetic

Evidence is emerging that a period of differentiation around the time of an elective amputation results in a decreased incidence of stump and phantom limb pain. At Harborview, this is being achieved by placing a 20-gauge catheter close to the major nerves supplying the amputated area at operation and then infusing bupivacaine postoperatively for 3 to 4 days. Because of accurate placement of the LA, the dose required is less than with a conventional percutaneous catheter block, but the same caveats apply.

SPECIAL CIRCUMSTANCES

The Opioid Addict

Addicts use opioids for reasons other than their analgesic effects, both to get high and to enable them to cope with the world around them. Their life revolves around their addiction and they are both tolerant and habituated to their drug of choice. Addicts suffer nociceptive input after trauma and are deserving of physicians' efforts to modulate that nociceptive input. When opioids are prescribed for the addict, physicians should not feel that they are producing the addicted state (which already exists), nor that they are sanctioning the use of such medications. Physicians should use the tools at their disposal to provide patient comfort, although this is frequently a thankless and frustrating task.

What Analgesic Options Are Available for the Addict? Systemic Opioids (i.v., i.m., PCA)

Addicts are tolerant and habituated and therefore require greater than normal doses of opioid to provide effect. Perhaps the best way to manage this is with PCA. For some patients this provides satisfactory analgesia, whereas others, while appearing objectively to achieve satisfactory analgesia (e.g., slow heart rate, low blood pressure) will relentlessly complain of pain. This may be an example of a patient communicating distress using the language of pain.

Table 6. *Specimen analgesic systems and durations of use following trauma*

Upper extremity	Simple	Single-shot axillary block 8–12 h → PCA 2–4 days → oral opioids 5–7 days → oral nonopioids
	Complex	PCA 4–6 days → oral opioids 5–7 days → oral nonopioids or Continuous axillary block + PCA 2 days → PCA 2–4 days → oral opioids 5–7 days → nonopioids
	Reimplants	Continuous axillary block + PCA 2 days → PCA 2–4 days → oral opioids 5–7 days → oral nonopioids
	Amputations	Perineural LA infusion + PCA 3–4 days → PCA 2–4 days → oral opioids 5–7 days → oral nonopioids
Spinal		PCA 5 days → oral opioids 5–7 days → oral nonopioids
Pelvic		Initially PCA until ORIF After ORIF: epidural opioids + LA 3–4 days → PCA or oral → oral nonopioids
Lower extremity	Proximal femur	PCA 3–4 days → oral opioids 5–7 days → oral nonopioids
	Distal femur, knee, proximal tibia	PCA ± continuous femoral block 2 days → PCA 2 days→ oral opioids 3–5 days → PCA 2 days → oral opioids 3–5 days → oral nonopioids
	Tibia	PCA 3–5 days → oral opioids 3–5 days → oral nonopioids
	Foot	Single-shot sciatic block + PCA 1 day → PCA 2–4 days → oral opioids 4–6 days → oral nonopioids

Epidural Opioid Analgesia

When EOA is used the addict's tolerance must be taken into account. The technique may fail to provide satisfaction, for similar reasons to PCA. It may be helpful to use EOA for its antinociceptive effects and to use other techniques to provide sedation, in a closely monitored environment.

Deafferentation with LA Blocks

The doses of LA needed in the addict are similar to those for normal patients. Even providing perfect deafferentation may not change the addict's complaints. PCA should also be used.

The Recovering Opioid Addict

The opioid addicts' self-help program, Narcotics Anonymous, has the policy of encouraging complete avoidance of opioids, even in therapeutic circumstances. This policy is based on the belief that the addict so desires the psychic state produced by opioids that even a single exposure will set the recovering addict back into addiction. If the physician encounters members of NA he should honor their wishes to avoid opioids and, if the NA policy is correct, should consider avoiding opioids in all previous addicts, members of NA or not.

SUMMARY

The provision of adequate analgesia after extremity trauma is not unimportant. There are a variety of ways in which such analgesia may be provided, either by the orthopaedic team caring for the patient or by others.

Specific schemata for the provision of analgesia at Harborview in a variety of situations are given in Table 6.

SELECTED READINGS

American Pain Society. *Principles of analgesic use in the treatment of acute pain and chronic cancer pain: a concise guide to medical practice.* 2nd ed. Skokie, IL: 1989.

Melzak R, Wall PD. *The challenge of pain.* New York: Penguin USA; 1991.

Oden RV, ed. Management of postoperative pain. *Anesthesiol Clin North Am* 1989;7.

Stevens DS, Edwards WT. Management of pain in the critically ill. *J Intensive Care Med* 1990;5:258.

US Department of Health and Human Services, Public Health Service, Agency for Health Care Policy and Research. *Clinical practice guideline: acute pain management: operative and medical procedures and trauma 1992.* Center for Research Dissemination and Liason, AHCPR Clearinghouse, PO Box 8547, Silver Spring, MD 20907.

Orthopaedic Trauma Protocols, edited by
Sigvard T. Hansen, Jr., and Marc F. Swiontkowski,
Raven Press, Ltd., New York, ©1993.

CHAPTER 7

Rehabilitation Treatment Strategies

Barbara J. de Lateur

INTRODUCTION

Rehabilitation of patients with high-energy injuries begins soon after definitive treatment and lasts until patients can function as independently as possible. The rehabilitation medicine service includes specially trained physicians and nurses as well as physical and occupational therapists who work with patients in the hospital and with those who have been discharged. The general goals of therapy are to prevent secondary disability, to enhance the functions of both affected and unaffected systems, and to help patients adapt to their physical and social environments by means of physical restoration and adaptive devices. The strategies used to accomplish these goals are explained and specific protocols are described for both physical and occupational therapies.

PREVENTING SECONDARY DISABILITY

Prevention of secondary disability and complications is extremely important in the management of acute trauma. Treatment of one injury must not compromise other systems or parts of the same system. For example, the uninjured hand of a patient whose shoulder is immobilized can develop edema and residual stiffness when it is left in a dependent position. Knowing that "edema is glue," a therapist applies hand mobilization techniques within a patient's physical limitations to prevent stiffness. When a patient is capable of full, active range of motion, edema can be prevented by performing hand exercises hourly during waking hours. When a patient is supine with the shoulder immobilized, active exercise with the hand elevated above the level of the heart is still possible to prevent edema. Conversely, if the hand is immobilized in a cast, active shoulder range-of-motion exercises are necessary to prevent stiffness in the shoulder.

Department of Rehabilitation Medicine, Harborview Medical Center, University of Washington, Seattle, Washington 98104

The Bed-Bound Patient

Patients restricted to bed are susceptible to contractures and to vascular, integumentary, and neural compromise. For example, patients with weak internal rotators of the hips tend to position the hips in external rotation and slight flexion, a position that subsequently causes flexion and external rotation contractures of the hip. Moreover, prolonged positioning in external rotation can lead to compression neuropathy of the peroneal nerve at the neck of the fibula. These complications can be prevented by applying a derotational splint, which prevents external rotation of the hip, protects the peroneal nerve, and prevents plantarflexion contractures of the ankle and foot.

Vascular System

Deep-vein thrombosis can occur when the lower extremity is immobilized. Thrombosis can be prevented mechanically, physiologically, or pharmacologically. Rhythmic isometric exercises can be performed in cast to promote circulation and to prevent pooling of blood in the veins. Sequential compression devices are useful for patients without casts or external skeletal fixators who are confined to bed for prolonged periods of time. Although administration of preventative doses of heparin (5,000 units subcutaneously twice daily) is left to the judgment of the clinician, this treatment should be considered for patients who are confined to bed for a prolonged time, particularly for those with neurologic impairment in the lower limbs.

Contractures

Contractures are caused primarily by positioning (1). A joint or a muscle that is immobilized in a shortened position for 23 h a day will develop contractures even when range-of-motion exercises are performed for half an hour twice daily.

Proper positioning is relatively simple. For example, the muscles and ligaments in the lower extremity always follow the path of least resistance when a patient is supine. The iliofemoral ligament becomes taut in internal rotation and extension but lax in flexion, external rotation, and abduction. Therefore, supine patients rarely develop internal rotation or extension contractures of the hip and derotational splints can be used to properly position the foot, ankle, and hip (Fig. 1).

Pressure Sores

Patients who lie in one position for a prolonged time are susceptible to pressure sores, particularly in the area of the sacrum. Susceptibility to pressure sores increases in a semiconscious patient or one with sensory impairment (e.g., from a spinal injury). Pressure is relieved by changing the patient's position at least every 2 h. Patients with good sensation and strength usually manage to relieve the pressure themselves.

Some hospital beds and certain positions predispose patients to pressure sores of the sacrum. A bed in which the patient can be raised to a seated position applies shear forces to the sacrum during elevation of the backrest and concentrates pressure on the sacrum once the patient is sitting up. Similarly, patients with cervical traction in rotating beds are subjected to constantly repeated shear forces even though the direction and magnitude of the forces change. A gel cushion can be placed under the sacrum to ease shear.

Dependence on Pain Medications

Administration of powerful, short-acting, narcotic analgesics (such as oxycodone) as needed for longer than 72 h can result in substance dependence, especially in individuals who misuse alcohol or other drugs. Ironically, dependence can be produced when a patient does not receive enough medication to alleviate pain. In an often-used but ill-advised strategy to reduce the intake of narcotic analgesics, patients are asked to go without medication as long as possible. Medication is requested only after pain is well established and patients are very uncomfortable. Sometimes the medication is not delivered for another 15–30 min and the patient becomes distraught. When it is finally administered, a short-acting medication not only relieves pain but also provides a certain amount of euphoria, reinforcing the link between experiencing discomfort and asking for a narcotic each time this cycle is repeated.

A better plan for the administration of narcotic medications that will be required for longer than 72 h is to add a long-acting medication, such as methadone, as an ingredient in a taste-masking liquid called a "pain cocktail." A pain cocktail is given on a time-contingent rather than symptom-contingent (p.r.n.) basis, and the dosage of methadone can be increased or decreased without creating drug dependence. This strategy weakens the link between experiencing pain and taking medication because pain is not allowed to become established and the patient does not have to ask for medication or wait for relief. Pain cocktails are described in detail in Chapter 6.

ENHANCING FUNCTION OF THE AFFECTED SYSTEMS

Traditional medicine and surgery are directed towards reducing pathology and enhancing the functions of the affected systems. Contractures and weakness caused by

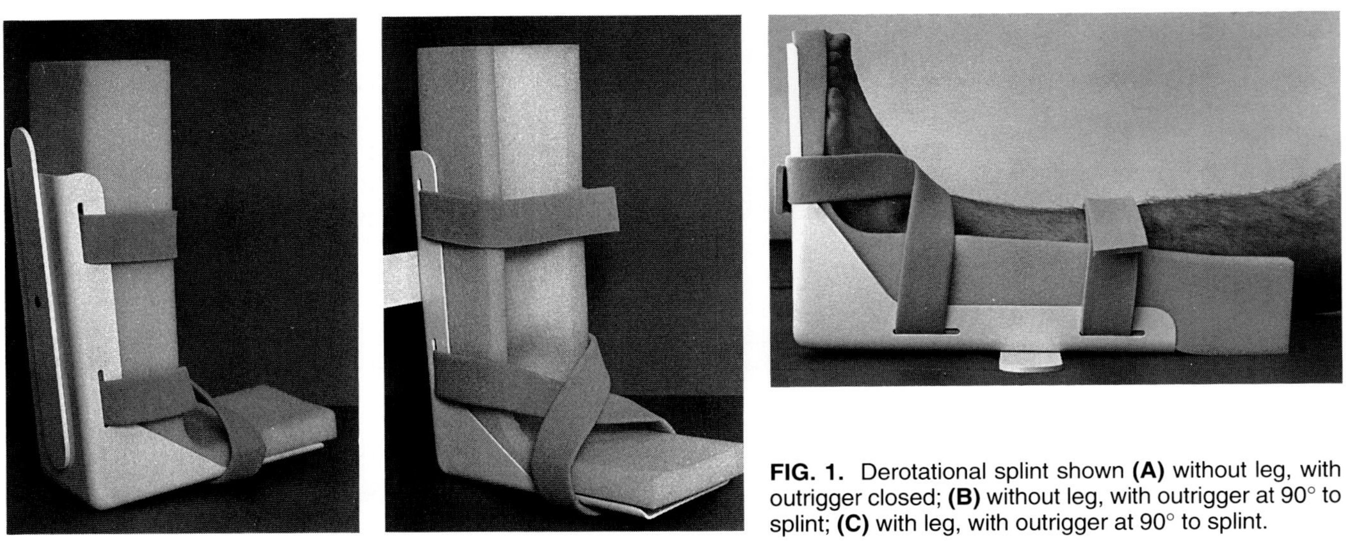

A,B C

FIG. 1. Derotational splint shown **(A)** without leg, with outrigger closed; **(B)** without leg, with outrigger at 90° to splint; **(C)** with leg, with outrigger at 90° to splint.

disuse, pain inhibition, or neural injury are treated by physical therapy protocols.

In managment of contractures, the soft-tissue structures that limit range of motion must be identified so that stretching exercises can be combined with heat or cold. For example, when a joint capsule is the structure preventing full range of motion, stretching should be combined with heat. A capsule located deep in the shoulder or the hip joint must be heated by ultrasound, the only form of heat that can reach the appropriate level. Ultrasound is applied for at least 5 min but can be continued for as long as 20 min. The temperature required to temporarily increase the elasticity of collagen and produce greater residual length is at the upper limits of the therapeutic temperature range. (Therapeutic temperature range is between 40°C and 45°C; the upper limits are between 43°C and 45°C.) The timing and the type of stretch are also important because collagen is elastic for the first 2 min at subtherapeutic temperatures, such as normal body temperatures. Stretching must be performed concurrently with heating or, if this is impossible, immediately after heating, to take advantage of this short-lived benefit. Ideally, stretches are done with weights and pulleys because a therapist cannot apply a steady pull with one hand for 20 min while applying ultrasound to the joint with the other (Figs. 2 and 3).

For stretching the hip flexors or the anterior aspect of the hip joint capsule and the reinforcing ligaments, the patient should be placed in the Thomas-test position, i.e., with the knee opposite the hip being treated raised to the chest (see Fig. 3). For stretching the rectus femoris, the hip is extended and the knee is flexed; for stretching the tensor fascia lata and the iliotibial band, the patient is placed in the Ober-test position, i.e., lying on the normal side with the involved hip extended as far as possible, the knee flexed, and allowing gravity to pull the thigh towards adduction. After the patient is positioned appropriately, ultrasound is applied for as long as 20 min for a single field of application. The joint is allowed to cool down in the stretched position. If muscle is the structure limiting range of motion, the stretch is prolonged as long as possible. With this technique, a shortened muscle can be stretched with serial casting or a resting orthosis. Whether true neurologically determined spasticity exists in a muscle must be ascertained. In the presence of true neurologic spasticity, the muscle must be cooled for 20 to 30 min before stretching. When spasticity is absent the muscle should be warmed up by active rhythmic and relatively prolonged exercise to promote circulation. Thus, muscles with normal innervation (upper motor neuron and lower motor neuron) should not be stretched while cold, whereas muscles with true spasticity should be cooled before stretching (2–4).

Range of motion is usually limited by two-joint muscles, rarely by one-joint muscles. Muscles that are typically tight after immobilization include the gastrocnemius, the rectus femoris, the medial and lateral hamstrings (long head of the biceps femoris), and the pectoralis major. Although the pectoralis major is sometimes considered a one-joint muscle, it crosses the glenohumeral joint (which in turn is connected to

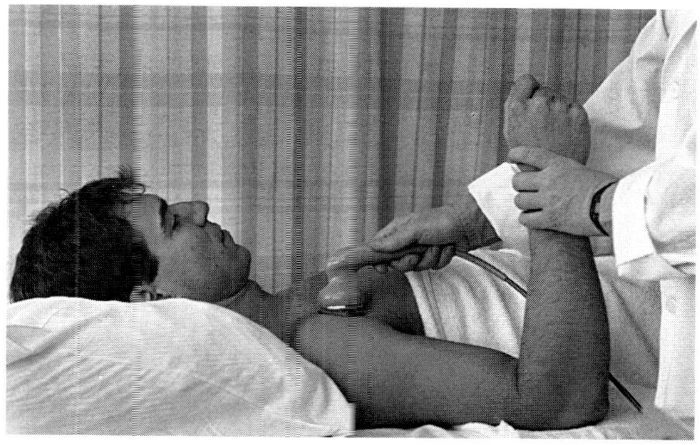

FIG. 2. Ultrasound applied to shoulder joint.

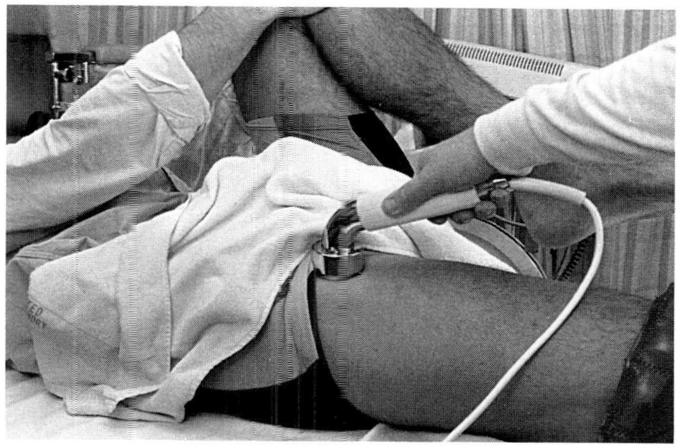

FIG. 3. Ultrasound applied to hip joint with patient in Thomas-test position.

the thorax by the scapulothoracic "joint") and functions essentially as a two-joint muscle. The muscle that limits range of motion can be identified by measuring joint range of motion with the muscle stretched or lax. For example, if the rectus femoris is suspected of being short, the patient is placed first in the supine position, allowing the knee and hip to flex at the same time Full range of knee flexion can be achieved in this position. Next, the patient is turned prone, a position in which hip flexion is prevented (Fig. 4). If the rectus femoris is contracted, i.e., has relatively fixed muscle shortening, flexion will be markedly limited in this position (Fig. 5) (5,6).

The chart in Figure 5 represents progressive knee flexion that was attained in a patient after heating and stretching. The patient complained of chronic benign back pain and allegedly convinced his pharmacist that he had terminal carcinoma. The pharmacist reportedly allowed the patient unlimited access to pentazocine, which the patient and his wife injected repeatedly into all accessible two-joint muscles, particularly the rectus femoris. He experienced severe contractures of virtually every two-joint muscle in his body. On admission he had 16° of knee flexion when lying prone but 135° of knee flexion when lying supine with the

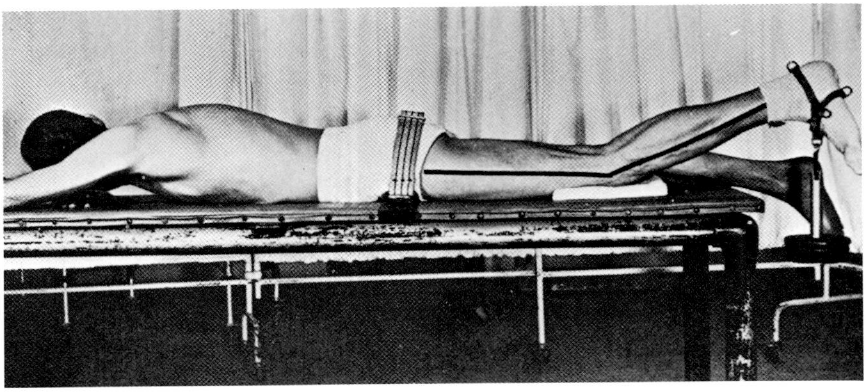

FIG. 4. The individual depicted here is receiving stretching towards knee extension, but the same position would be used for assessing tightness of the rectus femoris. The only difference is that the force would be applied towards flexion of the knee. (From Kottke FJ. Therapeutic exercise to maintain mobility. In: Kottke FJ, Lehmann JF, eds. *Krusen's handbook of physical medicine and rehabilitation.* Philadelphia: WB Saunders; 1990:436–51. Used with permission.)

hip flexed. After several weeks of vigorous stretching without deep heating, knee flexion in the prone position increased to 45° at the beginning of unilateral heat and stretch. Range of motion in the treated rectus femoris improved markedly over the untreated side. After 25 sessions heat was added to the stretching regimen of the untreated leg, and range of motion rapidly caught up with that of the treated leg, which had reached a plateau.

In the shoulder, the structure that limits full range of motion can be determined by observing the glenohumeral joint. Normally, the range of external rotation in this joint is greater when the humerus is abducted to 90° than when it is adducted to the side. When greater external rotation is possible in the adducted position, the limiting structure is the pectoralis major. When a contracted structure is stretched, it should be placed in the same position that was used for testing for contracture.

Choice of Heating Modality

Choice of heating modality is determined by the desirability or nondesirability of producing a vigorous effect and by the location of the site to be heated (superficial or deep). If a muscle is splinting a painful structure and does not actually have a contracture, heating the skin will be sufficient to produce a reflex relaxation of the underlying muscle, and any convenient form of superficial heat may be selected. Hot paraffin wax (125–130°F) is preferable on a well-healed burn scar because it both softens and heats the area. A whirlpool bath can be used for heating as well as buoyancy and cleansing of a limb that has just been removed from a cast. Hydrocollator packs are useful to heat the large surface of the lower back. Short-wave diathermy or microwave diathermy can be used for heating muscles unless these forms of diathermy are *contraindicated* by the presence of metal implants, fluid-filled blebs, or cardiac pacemakers.

Only ultrasound can raise the temperature of a contracture in a deep joint or joint capsule, such as the shoulder or the hip, into the therapeutic temperature range. However, ultrasound does not penetrate bone or reach the other side of the capsule, and the anterior, lateral, and posterior sides must be treated separately. A prescription for a tight shoulder capsule might read: "Ultrasound to the left shoulder; three fields, anterior, lateral, and posterior; 6 min each field, intensity 1.5 to 2 W/cm^2, stroking technique. While applying ultrasound to the anterior field, stretch toward external rotation and abduction. While sounding the posterior field, stretch toward internal rotation and horizontal adduction."

Heat Versus Cold

Cold therapy should be used very early (minutes to days, depending upon the indication) after traumatic injuries occur. In acute trauma, heat should be avoided or used in mild forms at a distance from the actual pathology. For example, superficial heat can be applied to the skin of the upper trapezius and the posterior neck musculature in a flexion–extension (whiplash) injury.

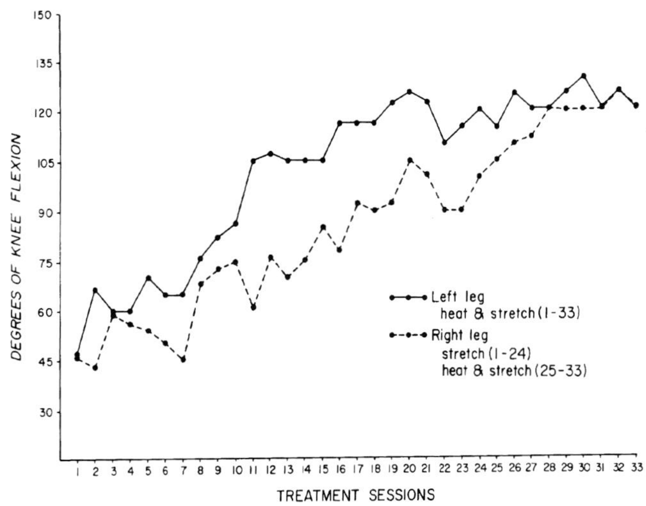

FIG. 5. The degrees of knee flexion due to residual elongation of the right and left rectus femoris muscles before each treatment session. (From de Lateur BJ, Stonebridge JB, Lehmann JF. Fibrous muscular contractures: treatment with a new direct contract microwave applicator operating at 915 MHz. *Arch Phys Med Rehabil* 1978;59:488–90. Used with permission.)

Although application of superficial cold can cool deeply (owing to vasoconstriction), application of superficial heat cannot heat deeply because vasodilatation and increased circulation carry away heated blood and keep the surrounding tissue relatively cool. As mentioned earlier, superficial heat can be used to relax neurologically normal muscle. However, in the presence of true spasticity, cold must be applied long enough to cool the muscle spindles. This modality decreases the sensitivity of the muscle spindles to stretch. For collagenous contractures, the shortened structures should be treated with combined heat and stretch.

Contraindications to Heat and Cold

General contraindications to heat include mentally obtunded patients as well as those with sensory impairment, vascular insufficiency, or cancer in the area to be treated. Specific contraindications to short-wave and microwave diathermy include cardiac pacemakers, metal implants, fluid-filled blebs, and treatment near the eye, the male genitalia, or a pregnant uterus. Ultrasound can be used in the vicinity of metal implants but not near methylmethacrylate. Vigorous heating, in which the site of pathology is rapidly heated close to tolerance levels, should be reserved for chronic disease processes. Contraindications to cold include cold hypersensitivity, cryoglobulinemia, and an exaggerated cold–pressor response. Raynaud's disease is a relative contraindication to cold unless cooling is used as part of a carefully monitored desensitization program.

Disuse Weakness

Strengthening of weakened muscles that cross a painful joint is begun with a relatively mild form of exercise such as "setting" exercises (a subclass of isometric exercises). As the muscle becomes stronger and the painful joint becomes quiescent, motion can be added. The muscle must be strengthened throughout its range of motion without injuring the joint. Special positions, techniques, or devices are sometimes useful to prevent placing undue stress on a joint within its range of motion and thus to avoid producing further injury. For example, quadriceps exercises can be modified to avoid placing unnecessary stress on the patellofemoral joint (Figs. 6–8) (7,8). Deep knee bends provide strengthening stress to the quadriceps muscles but may injure the patellofemoral joint. Placing weight on the limb, particularly at right angles

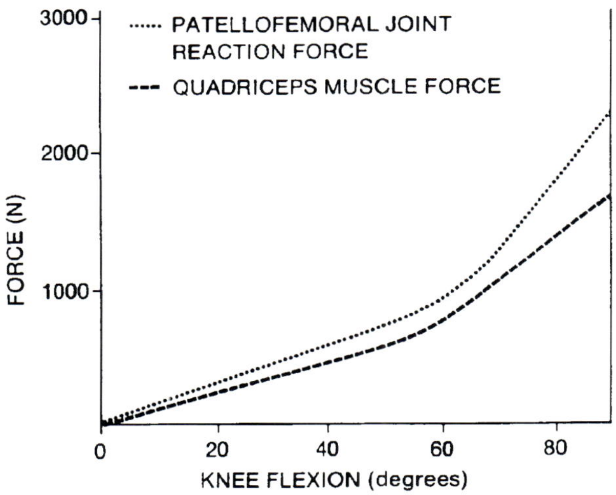

FIG. 6. Patellofemoral joint reaction force and quadriceps muscle force during knee bend to 90° (three subjects). This exercise should be avoided in patients with patellofemoral impairment. (Adapted from Reilly DT, Martens M. Experimental analysis of the quadriceps muscle force and patellofemoral joint reaction force for various activities. *Acta Orthop Scand* 1972;43:126–37, by Nordin M, Frankel VH. *Basic biomechanics of the skeletal system, 2nd ed.* Philadelphia: Lea & Febiger; 1989. Used with permission.)

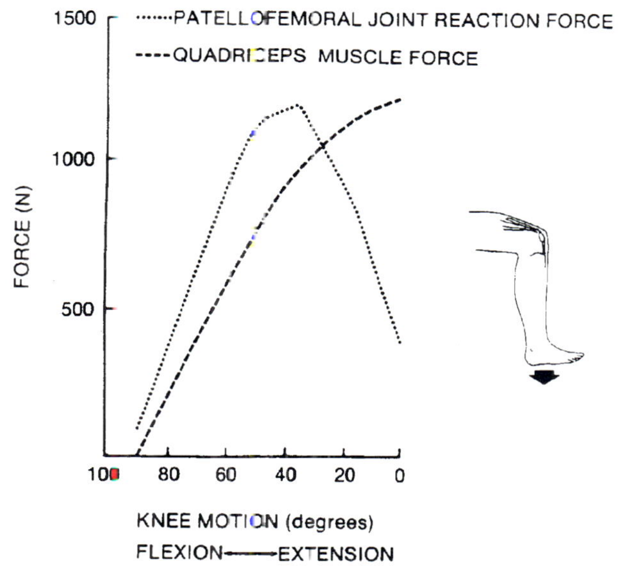

FIG. 7. Patellofemoral joint reaction force and quadriceps muscle force during knee extension against resistance provided by a 9-kg-weight boot with the subject sitting and the lower leg free-hanging (three subjects). (Adapted from Reilly DT, Martens M. Experimental analysis of the quadriceps muscle force and patellofemoral joint reaction force for various activities. *Acta Orthop Scand* 1972;43:126–137, by Frankel VH, Nordin M. *Basic biomechanics of the skeletal system.* Philadelphia: Lea & Febiger; 1980. Used with permission.)

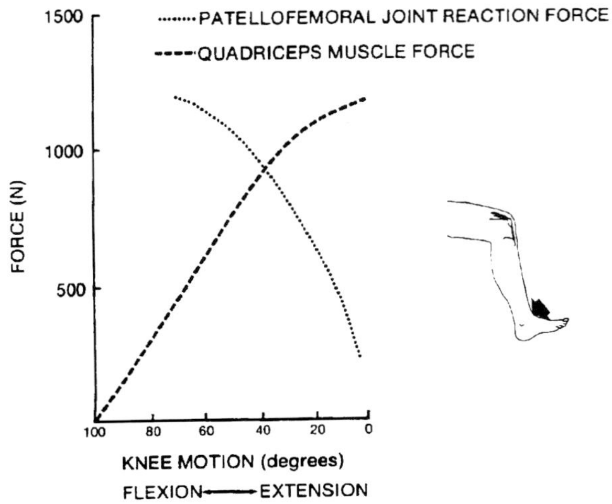

FIG. 8. Patellofemoral joint reaction force during extension with resistance provided at a right angle to the long axis of the lower limb throughout knee extension. This is a preferred way of performing weighted quadriceps training, especially if the exercise is confined to the last 40° of extension. (From Frankel VH, Nordin M. *Basic biomechanics of the skeletal system.* Philadelphia: Lea & Febiger; 1980. Used with permission.)

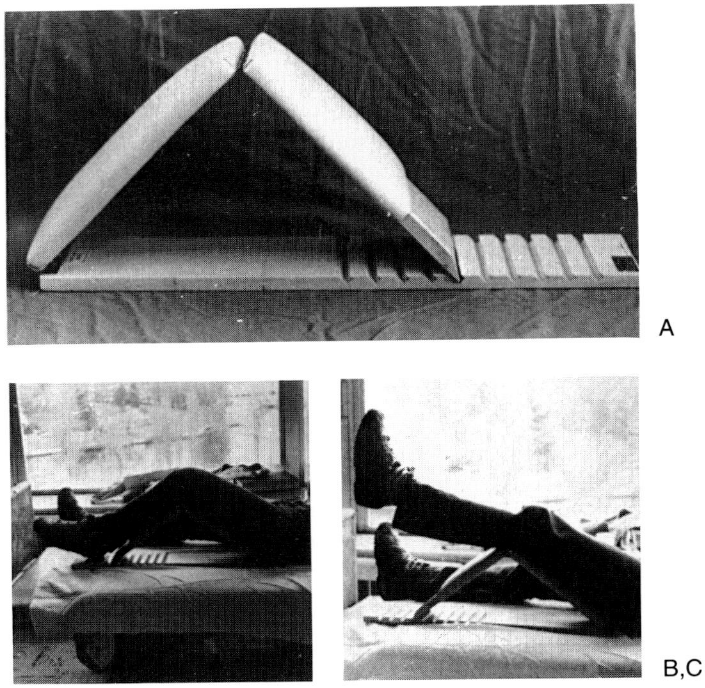

FIG. 9. The quadriceps board or fracture board. **A:** The angle of the knee is determined by the slot in which the distal portion of the board is placed. **B:** Subject using fracture board, knee flexed. **C:** Subject using fracture board, knee extended. (From de Lateur BJ, Lehmann JF. Strengthening exercise. In: Leek JC, Gershwin MA, Fowler WM Jr, eds. *Principles of physical medicine and rehabilitation in musculoskeletal diseases.* Orlando, FL: Grune & Stratton; 1986:26–60. Used with permission.)

to the tibial and straight knee, reduces the patellofemoral reactive force while it allows excellent stressing of the quadriceps. Depending on how load is applied, the knee can be safely extended from the last 10° to 40° of extension. Extension devices range from simple terminal knee-extension boards (fracture boards or quadriceps boards) to expensive computerized equipment (Fig. 9) (9).

ENHANCING THE FUNCTION OF UNAFFECTED SYSTEMS

Sometimes strategies must be devised to compensate for lost function in injured limbs. For example, muscle strength in the upper limbs must be increased in patients with long-lasting impairment in the lower limbs. The upper extremity muscles of paraplegics can be strengthened to support the weight of the entire body with one arm.

A less obvious but equally important strategy is to improve the function of the unimpaired lower limb in an amputee. Unless prosthetic fitting is optimal (and sometimes even when fitting is optimal) a great deal of stress is placed on an amputee's sound limb. A piston-like effect occurring on the residual limb in the prosthesis makes the side with the prosthesis functionally or even anatomically too long during swing phase. To clear the prosthetic side during swing phase, the patient may resort to vaulting on the sound limb. The calf musculature on the sound side may not be equal to the task, especially in the presence of vascular insufficiency. Although it is often neglected, a thorough evaluation of strength, motor control, and vascularity in the sound limb is indicated before fitting of a patient with a prosthesis.

A similar problem arises when a patient with skeletal, ligamentous, or neuromuscular insufficiency is fitted with a knee–ankle–foot orthosis (KAFO) or any type of brace that restricts free knee flexion. The presence of the brace makes that side functionally too long and various adaptive maneuvers are required to clear the braced leg during swing phase. The problem can be solved by adding a lift to the shoe on the sound side. Similarly, rising from a chair in an orthosis that locks the knee in extension may stress the musculature of the unaffected side, particularly if the chair has no arms and the patient is using only one crutch or a cane. In such cases, the quadriceps and hip extensors of the unaffected side should be strengthened.

USING ADAPTIVE DEVICES

Adaptive devices should be chosen to promote maximal immediate and long-term function. If a patient is expected to recover full function, devices can be selected to promote short-term comfort and improve immediate function without consideration for permanent use. For example, a trapeze (monkey bar) and an overhead frame can be installed for a fracture patient with heavy external immobilizing devices that make bed mobility difficult. This type of bar greatly improves immediate function without compromising long-range function. However, such a device would not be used by a paraplegic, who must learn permanent techniques that can be used for all types of beds, both with and without a trapeze. Developing a reliance on a trapeze would limit the activities of a paraplegic, who could never travel or stay in hotels in which such devices are unavailable. The same considerations apply to wall rails, which are appropriate on an orthopaedic ward but, in the opinion of the author, would be inappropriate on a rehabilitation ward.

The activities of daily living can be made easier by prescribing a variety of orthoses for the upper and lower limbs and the trunk, within certain guidelines. When prescribing devices for the lower limb, the physician or surgeon should specify whether the purpose of the device is simply to maintain skeletal alignment or also to restrict weight bearing. To maintain alignment, the three-point principle or the hydraulic principle can be used. The three-point principle applies pressure on three locations in the limb, e.g., the posterior thigh, the kneecap, and the posterior distal leg. A hydraulic device works like a sausage casing that is flaccid when not filled but resists the forces of gravity when filled. Some devices combine these two principles. Many spinal orthoses and some lower limb orthoses use the hydraulic principle. For example, the chair-back brace and many other spinal orthoses are fitted with abdominal pads that support the spine by compressing the abdominal contents.

To relieve weight bearing, a device that transfers weight from the skeleton and places it more proximally must be built into the orthosis, e.g., a patellar tendon-bearing brace or an ischial weight-bearing brace. For these devices to be effective, the length of the weight-bearing upright supports of the brace must clear the sole of the foot and the inner side of the shoe. They are most effective when they are used with rocker-bottomed soles and a lift on the opposite shoe. Considerable coordination and balance are required to walk safely in such a device (10–12).

Physical therapy management of fractures immediately after fracture stabilization through fracture consolidation and occupational therapy considerations are discussed in Chapters 8, 9, and 10.

REFERENCES

1. Stolov WC. The concept of normal muscle tone, hypotonia and hypertonia. *Arch Phys Med Rehabil*, 1966;47:156–168.
2. Lehmann JF de Lateur BJ. Application of heat and cold in the clinical setting. In: Lehmann JF, ed. *Therapeutic heat and cold*. 4th ed. Baltimore: Williams & Wilkins; 1990:633–44.
3. Lehmann JF de Lateur BJ Cryotherapy. In: Lehmann JF, ed. *Therapeutic heat and cold*. 4th ed. Baltimore: Williams & Wilkins; 1990:590–632.
4. Lehmann JF de Lateur BJ: Therapeutic heat. In: Lehman JF, ed. *Therapeutic heat and cold*, 4th ed. Baltimore: Williams & Wilkins; 1990:633–44.
5. de Lateur BJ, Halliday WR. Pentazocine fibrous myopathy: report of two cases and literature review. *Arch Phys Med Rehabil* 1978;59:394–7.
6. de Lateur BJ, Stonebridge JB, Lehmann JF. Fibrous muscular contractures: treatment with a new direct contact microwave applicator operating at 915 MHz. *Arch Phys Med Rehabil* 1978;59:488–90.
7. Frankel VH Nordin M. Basic biomechanics of the skeletal system. Philadelphia Lea & Febiger; 1980.
8. Reilly DT, Martens M. Experimental analysis of the quadriceps muscle force and patellofemoral joint reaction force for various activities. *Acta Orthop Scand* 1972;43:126–37.
9. de Lateur BJ, Lehmann JF. Strengthening exercise. In: Leek JC, Gershwin ME, Fowler WM Jr, eds. *Principles of physical medicine and rehabilitation in musculoskeletal diseases*. New York: Grune & Stratton, 1986;25–60.
10. Lehmann JF, de Lateur BJ. Lower extremity orthotics. In: Kottke FJ, Lehmann JF, eds. *Krusen's handbook of physical medicine and rehabilitation*. 4th ed. Philadelphia: WB Saunders; 1990;602–46.
11. Bartelink DL. The role of abdominal pressure in relieving the pressure on the lumbar intervertebral disk. *J Bone Joint Surg* 1957;39B:718–25.
12. Lucas DB, Jacobs RR, Trautman P. Spinal orthotics for pain and instability. In Redford JB, ed. *Orthotics etcetera*. 3rd ed. Baltimore: Williams & Wilkins; 1986;122–52.

Orthopaedic Trauma Protocols, edited by
Sigvard T. Hansen, Jr., and Marc F. Swiontkowski.
Raven Press, Ltd., New York, ©1993.

CHAPTER 8

Rehabilitation: Occupational Therapy

Anne Birge James, *Carole A. Lossing, †Shelly Gruber Sailer, and Robin Irish

INTRODUCTION

The goal of occupational therapy is to protect the patient's physical integrity by promoting early functional activity. Independent activity contributes positively to hastening patients' transition from the intensive care unit (ICU) to an acute care unit, their progression through rehabilitation and discharge from the hospital, and subsequently their return to work and normal activities.

Communication between therapists and physicians is facilitated by using clearly defined protocols for assessment and intervention strategies, which include precautions related to specific diagnoses or medical treatments. Because precautions, which are based on diagnosis and physician preference, can vary significantly, therapists must be aware of factors that preclude the use of specific evaluation or treatment techniques. The justifications for all precautions must be clearly understood so that they can be safely generalized to a variety of situations. Assessing problems, establishing appropriate goals with the patient and the interdisciplinary team, implementing treatment, and evaluating progress is a dynamic process. Changes in a patient's existing condition, such as medical or surgical intervention, can significantly alter treatment precautions and necessitate corresponding changes in occupational therapy goals and treatment.

Occupational therapy protocols commonly related to orthopaedic trauma are discussed in this chapter. These protocols are to be used as general considerations for determining appropriate precautions, assessment, and management of a patient's injuries from the time of admission to the ICU until discharge from the hospital.

School of Occupational and Physical Therapy. University of Puget Sound, Tacoma, Washington 98416; *Rehabilitation Medicine. Children's Hospital and Medical Center, Seattle, Washington 98105; †Department of Occupational Therapy. Harborview Medical Center, University of Washington, Seattle, Washington 98104

OCCUPATIONAL THERAPY IN THE ICU

Patients who require occupational therapy services frequently have sustained multiple-system injuries that might include brain injury, multiple fractures, abdominal or thoracic injuries, spinal cord injuries, traumatic amputation, acute respiratory distress syndrome (ARDs), acute renal failure, or sepsis. The length of a patient's stay in the surgical ICU can range from a few days to a month or longer. In addition to problems related to their injuries, these patients are often at risk for complications stemming from poor nutritional status, a history of substance abuse, or poor overall health before admission.

Precautions

Before planning or initiating treatment for a patient in the ICU, an occupational therapist must understand the patient's current overall medical condition and stay abreast of any changes that may occur. The therapist must be familiar with the critical-care environment and with the monitoring and life-support systems that are used.

Assessment and Management

Assessment of a multiply injured orthopaedic patient usually begins with a referral from the attending physician, often within 24 h of the patient's admission to the ICU. This initial referral may request a comprehensive assessment of the patient's total needs and occupational therapy goals, or it may focus on a specific problem for immediate resolution. Formal assessment methods, such as manual muscle testing, are often impossible to carry out on traumatized patients because their mental function may be impaired secondary to sedation or a brain injury.

The primary objectives of early occupational therapy intervention in the ICU are to maintain range of motion, to protect the skin against breakdown, and to preserve existing function in spite of serious and possibly unstable medical conditions. These goals are fulfilled by maintaining skin integrity, decreasing edema, and enhancing the patient's mobility, self-care, and communication (1).

Skin

Skin protection is essential during immobility to facilitate overall care and to hasten rehabilitation. Wounds are inspected in conjunction with the nursing assessment. Problem areas such as the occiput, the chin (during cervical stabilization with an orthosis), the elbows, the sacrum, and the heels are protected by cut-out cushions, sheepskin padding, commercially manufactured padding, or gel pads. If access is required for wound care, application of removable splints may be preferable to casting for some extremity injuries. Splints can be easily modified and adjusted to accommodate changes in the size of the extremity due to muscle flaps or edema and to adjust the position of the joints (Fig. 1). Custom-fabricated or commercially made rigid foot splints can be altered to accommodate dressings, edema, or external fixators. They are lined with sheepskin and may have gel pads placed proximal to the Achilles tendon to elevate the heel and prevent the development of pressure sores (see Fig. 1). Patients with fragile skin, ecchymosis, or wounds around the ankle or foot may require positioning devices made of foam to elevate the foot and to eliminate pressure on the heel and the malleoli. All protected areas must be closely monitored by the medical, nursing, and therapy staff to ensure that positioning devices are applied correctly and that any problems are addressed immediately.

Edema

Secondary joint stiffness in the hand can result from the deforming position imposed by swelling. Edema is evaluated by circumferential measurements. Treatment modalities consist of pressure (applied by gloves or pressure wrapping), elevation, and active range-of-motion (ROM) exercises (2).

Mobility

Patients with injured extremities must be properly positioned to protect the injured limbs and prevent contractures. Goniometric measurements are taken to measure joint ROM and mobilization is begun with passive or active ROM exercises (1). Static or dynamic splints and other positioning devices can be used to maintain an optimal position for func-

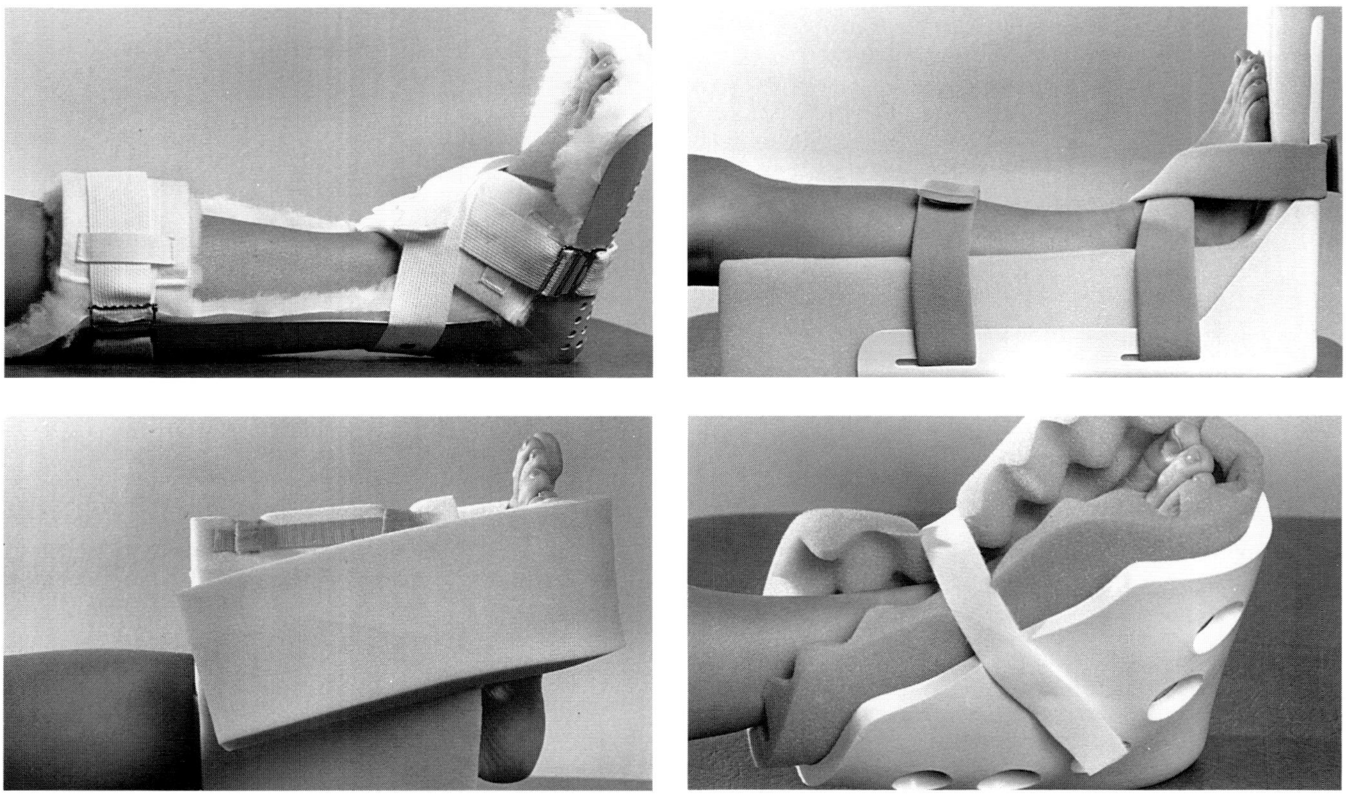

A B C D

FIG. 1. Foot splints. **A:** Posterior foot splint. **B:** Derotational foot splint. **C:** Span-aid. **D:** Spenco boot.

tion between exercise sessions. A variety of upper extremity splints can be fabricated by the occupational therapist to fit a patient's unique needs. A resting hand splint can be used to keep the hand and wrist in a safe position, to prevent joint contractures in the upper extremity (Fig. 2) (2,3). In the lower extremity, dynamic foot splints are used to begin early ankle ROM and posterior foot splints are used for more rigid immobilization (Fig. 3). A posterior foot splint is also useful for maintaining ankle dorsiflexion in a limb with flaccid muscle tone, a condition that without intervention can lead to shortening of the Achilles tendon (see Fig. 1). When the extensor muscles of the lower extremity are hypertonic, a posterior splint or a well-padded cast can be applied to prevent prolonged plantar flexion and subsequent contractures.

Self-Care

A basic self-care assessment is completed to establish a patient's functional status, to determine individual requirements for more independent function in the ICU, and to identify the need for more intensive rehabilitation at a later time. Adaptive equipment (e.g., built-up handles on utensils for self-feeding and devices to extend reach) are provided and special skills are taught to enhance function within medical or physical limitations (1). Patients are encouraged to participate in their own self-care as early as possible to regain a sense of autonomy, to anticipate further rehabilitation, and to increase overall strength and endurance before a more active treatment program is begun.

Communication

An important need of patients in the ICU is to be able to communicate with staff and family members during recovery (4). Assessment of a patient's communication difficulties and implementation of intervention strategies are usually carried out by an occupational therapist together with a speech pathologist and the nursing staff. In the initial examination, the team evaluates the patient's vision and any existing physical, cognitive, or communication deficits. An easily accessible system for the patient to call a nurse for assistance must be devised. Basic communication techniques, such as writing, controlling a communication system with the tongue, lips, or teeth, controlling a switch to activate a call light, or blinking the eyes to indicate yes or no, are evaluated. Intervention systems are then designed to enhance the patient's ability to communicate within the physical limitations of the complex ICU environment. Proper positioning in bed or in a chair is required to promote even limited communication, especially when alternative communication systems are controlled by delicate physical movements (5). Communication can be improved by providing the patient an optional method, e.g., an electrolarynx in addition to paper and pencil.

Communication needs and skills may change rapidly during an ICU stay, and frequent contacts with the patient and staff are necessary to ensure that communication systems remain appropriate. As patients gain greater physical stamina, the number and length of daily therapy sessions are extended to increase their endurance for communication.

SPINAL INJURIES AND LOWER EXTREMITY INJURIES AND AMPUTATIONS

Precautions

An interdisciplinary plan of care greatly facilitates early mobilization and functional retraining. In addition to knowing a patient's overall medical condition, the occupational therapist must be aware of precautions related to specific

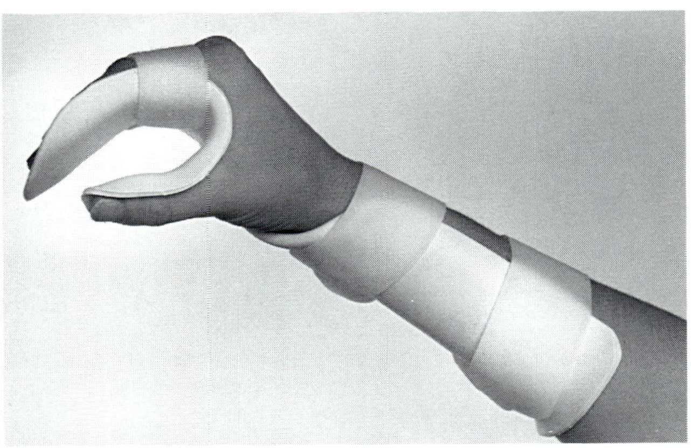

FIG. 2. Resting splints can be used to maintain the hand and wrist in a functional position during immobilization or periods of disuse.

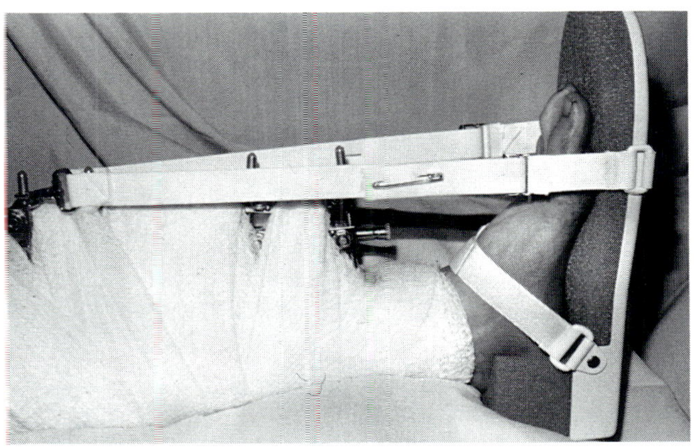

FIG. 3. Dynamic foot splints attach to external fixators and hold the ankle in a neutral position. The dynamic elastic straps allow early active exercise.

injuries of the spine, the pelvis, and the lower extremities. Restrictions in these areas usually consist of mobility and weight-bearing precautions and of limitations imposed by orthotics and prosthetics.

Mobility restrictions are imposed when movement extending into specific ranges or planes of motion would further damage or prevent injured structures from healing. For example, patients with hip fractures may have to limit hip flexion, preventing them from reaching their feet for dressing.

Weight-bearing precautions may be prescribed for specific lower extremity injuries or amputations. Patients must adhere to these restrictions throughout all the activities of daily living.

Orthotics prescribed to stabilize the spine are usually worn at all times. The therapist must be familiar with their application, the prescribed wearing schedule, and their effect on the activities of daily life. The occupational therapist must inform the patient and the family of the wearing schedule of the orthosis and instruct them in self-care tasks that can be done within the limitations of the orthosis.

Prosthetics may include a wearing schedule when they are newly prescribed for patients with lower extremity amputations. A wearing schedule allows the residual limb to build up a tolerance to the prosthesis, but it may impose restrictions on a patient's daily living activities if the prosthesis must be used for ambulation.

Assessment and Management

Before an occupational therapist assesses a patient with a spinal or lower extremity injury, a physician prescribes the appropriate splinting or positioning. These recommendations may be discussed or modified after an assessment of the patient's skin integrity, compliance (cognitive function, neurological status), and the appropriateness of the splint (e.g., the advantages of a dynamic foot splint versus a static foot splint). Alternatives to casting can be explored with the physician if a cast limits a patient's functional potential. At this stage of assessment, the therapist's role is to determine which splint or positioning device supports both the surgical intervention and the patient's acute and long-term needs. Functional mobility must be preserved as much as possible.

The assessment and management of self-care includes an evaluation of a patient's functional capacity. Specific concerns to be addressed include limitations in toileting, bathing, lower extremity dressing, and functional mobility (1). Adaptive equipment and specific training may be required for a patient to perform these activities independently before discharge or on follow-up (Fig. 4). For example, a stationary bath bench may be recommended for safety and a long-handled sponge might be needed to extend reach, within precautions, while bathing. For toileting, a raised toilet seat or wall-mounted grab bars ensure safe transfers, and a toilet aid can be used to extend reach. Patients with limited mobility or range of reach might require a reacher, a sock aid, a dressing stick, and techniques designed by the occupational therapist to assist them with independent dressing. Mobility limitations may interfere with many self-care and homemaking tasks, such as retrieving clothes from a closet or carrying food from the refrigerator. Adaptive equipment (e.g., a walker basket) or alternative techniques can be introduced to increase independence.

Discharge from the hospital is planned early to allow adequate time for training, completing home adaptations, and making referrals. Patients and their families must be informed of the magnitude of the patient's injuries and the precautions associated with them. Training must be provided in the care, donning, and removal of orthoses and prostheses. Competent patients can often appropriately direct their own care for tasks they cannot perform independently. These techniques are demonstrated in the hospital and the patient practices them until all aspects of care can be performed proficiently. Verbal instructions and written materials are reviewed with patients and care providers before discharge. Special services, such as home health aides or home-delivered meals, are arranged as needed. To accurately determine any difficulties a patient might encounter after returning home, a home visit may be required. This can be done by the occupational therapist before discharge or by a home-care agency therapist after the patient returns home. Problems are solved most efficiently in the environment where the patient is experiencing difficulties. Restrictions are removed as healing progresses and function returns.

An occupational therapist also acts as an intermediary with a patient's employer, preparing the transition back to work by making recommendations regarding the patient's capacity for work or necessary changes in the work environment. In some cases a patient may need a referral to a formal return-to-work program or vocational counseling for consideration of alternative employment.

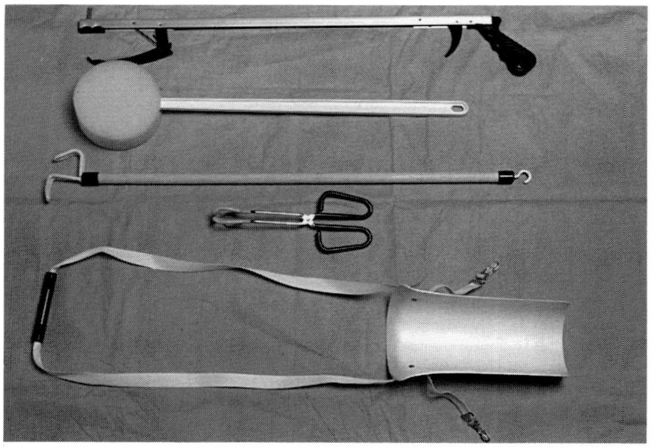

FIG. 4. Adaptive equipment can compensate for limited reach, e.g., after a total hip replacement or for patients wearing a body jacket. From top to bottom: reacher, long-handled sponge, dressing stick, toilet aid, sock aid.

UPPER EXTREMITY INJURIES AND AMPUTATIONS

Upper extremity trauma encompasses a wide range of injuries with diverse precautions and treatment requirements. When a patient sustains a combination of upper extremity injuries and other trauma, such as a head injury or a lower extremity fracture, the complexity of medical and therapeutic management is significantly increased. Because delayed rehabilitation results in decreased mobility and compromised function, evaluation and treatment are initiated early, usually between 1 and 3 days after injury or surgery. To ensure compliance, patients are completely informed about the purpose of any splints or assistive devices that are used and the restrictions that apply to their injuries.

Precautions

Patients with upper extremity injuries or amputations may be subject to precautions regarding mobility, resistance, pressure, and weight-bearing on the upper extremity.

Mobility Restrictions

Passive mobility restrictions are imposed when external forces acting on a joint could further damage or prevent healing of the injured structure. However, movement restrictions are applied only to specific joints and are removed as soon as the extremity has healed and motion can be safely reinstated to avoid compromised joint mobility and function owing to prolonged immobilization.

Active motion restrictions are required when unresisted active motion could further damage or prevent healing of an injured structure. Active unresisted motion does not load the joints and can be initiated early in stable fractures with solid fixation. Depending on the injury, mobility restrictions may include passive motion, active motion, or a combination of both. Creative combinations of restrictions can be devised by the occupational therapist to allow good mobility while protecting injured structures. For example, exercises prescribed for flexor tendon repairs must prevent formation of adhesions without injuring the newly repaired tendon. Both requirements are met by a combination of passive flexion and active extension exercises. Whereas active finger flexion would stress the repair during muscle contracture, passive flexion can be done safely by the patient or therapist. Conversely, passive extension can stress the repair because external forces acting on the tendon are inconsistent. Active extension, which exerts minimal forces on the newly repaired tendon, can be done safely (2).

The following considerations may help guide the physician and the therapist in selecting appropriate mobility restrictions:

1. Which joints or muscles should be restricted? What kind of motion is contraindicated—passive, active, or both?
2. Is all mobility contraindicated or can limited mobility be prescribed? If limited mobility is allowed, what range of motion is safe?
3. Is a positioning device (a splint or cast) needed? What is the wearing schedule?

Resistance Restrictions

Resisted motion, which loads the joints, may be partially or entirely contraindicated. Questions that must be considered before beginning therapy include:

1. Which joints can tolerate manual resistance during activities and exercise? How much resistance?
2. Does the resistive exercise allow good range of motion so that strengthening occurs throughout the range? For example, squeezing rubber balls is usually contraindicated because this activity limits digital flexion.
3. Which functional activities providing safe levels of resistance can be included in a patient's daily routine? Which tasks or task components are too resistive and must be altered or eliminated?
4. Are lifting restrictions necessary?

Resistive activities and exercises are usually initiated in the later stages of rehabilitation. Instructions given to patients must be specific and practical to ensure patient compliance.

Pressure Restrictions

Compressive pressure wraps or garments may be applied to control edema. Splints and adaptive equipment may be required to position or to augment function in an injured limb. However, these devices may be contraindicated in patients with vascular compromise (e.g., recent vascular repairs and muscle or soft-tissue flaps), and therapists must plan assistance within specific guidelines.

Weight-Bearing Restrictions on the Upper Extremity

Upper extremity weight-bearing restrictions may limit the mobility of patients who rely on their arms for activities such as changing position from sitting to standing or ambulating with crutches. Alternative techniques or adaptive equipment may be needed to compensate for functional deficits resulting from this precaution.

Assessment and Management

Like initial occupational therapy management for other injuries, assessment and management of upper extremity injuries and amputations includes protection of the skin, resolution of edema, and enhancement of mobility. In addition, attention must be directed to sensation, strength, and functional use in the hand. Skin, wounds, and scars are examined. The therapist must note trophic changes such as altered skin color, temperature, hydration, hair growth, and fingernail texture. Trophic changes that may be indicative of reflex sympathetic dystrophy must be reported immediately to the treating physician to prevent permanent disability. Photographs are useful for documentation. Wounds are monitored for signs of infection. Hypertrophic scars are managed by pressure garments or wraps, stretching, and massage (2).

Edema is evaluated by means of volumetric and circumferential measurements. Management of edema must be carried out around the clock with elevation, compression (wraps, garments, or intermittent pumps), and active motion to facilitate return flow in the venous and lymphatic systems (2). Excessive compression may produce a rebound effect and must be avoided. Patient compliance and nursing assistance are essential for effective management.

Motion restrictions are determined by the physician, who prescribes casts or splints to ensure appropriate positioning (Fig. 5). Removable splints can be fabricated by an occupational therapist when access is needed for wound care or a supervised exercise program. For example, posterior elbow splints are used for patients with proximal radial or olecranon fractures. A custom-fitted Sarmiento humeral splint can be adjusted to accommodate fluctuating edema and provides better stability than a cast (6). When hand motion is restricted, the hand should be maintained in a safe position unless precautions contraindicate this position in part or entirely. The recommended safe position of the hand is 70° of metacarpophalangeal flexion to prevent shortening of the collateral ligaments, full extension (0°) of the proximal interphalangeal and distal interphalangeal joints to prevent shortening of the volar plate, thumb abduction to maintain mobility of the first web space, and 30° of wrist extension to preserve function and to facilitate finger positioning (7).

Range of motion is evaluated by goniometric measurements (1). Mobility of the uninvolved joints must not be restricted when the hand is immobilized in a cast. For example, wrist casts that limit MCP flexion as well as thumb flexion and opposition can result in joint contractures. Joints are mobilized with passive or active ROM exercises, joint mobilization techniques, or CPM (Figs. 5 and 6). Optimal positioning between treatments can be maintained with static splints or positioning devices. Pronation and supination are often neglected in distal upper extremity injuries, but these motions must be maintained to avoid significant functional deficits. Uninjured joints may also become impaired from abnormal posturing and disuse. For example, the unimpaired shoulder of a patient with tendinous injuries in the hand may become stiff after weeks of disuse. The entire upper extrem ity must be reassessed often to ensure that intervention is initiated in a timely manner.

Primary sensation is determined by assessing a patient's perception of pain, temperature, vibration, and cutaneous pressure (8). Cutaneous pressure is most accurately measured by Semmes–Weinstein monofilaments (2). Areas of hypersensitivity must be noted as well as areas of hyposensitivity. Discriminatory sensation is assessed by measuring two-point discrimination and sterognosis and by functional evaluations such as the Moberg pick-up test. Phantom limb sensation and pain must be noted in patients with amputations. Sensory evaluations must be done periodically in patients with peripheral nerve damage to document returning neural function. Patients with decreased sensation must be made aware of their deficits to prevent injury and may receive sensory retraining to help them utilize remaining sensory functions. Hypersensitivity can be treated by desensitization programs. Pain can be reduced or alleviated by relaxation techniques; however, chronic pain may require the systemic treatment approach of a comprehensive pain management program.

Strength is evaluated by manual muscle testing of isolated muscles or muscle groups and by measuring grip strength and pinch strength (1,2). In addition to general strengthening and endurance programs, graded activity programs can be designed to strengthen targeted muscles through functional activities. When goals are set, the patient's age, occupation, and expected disposition are taken into consideration to ensure the patient's needs are met.

Functional use of the upper extremity must be addressed specifically. Whereas evaluation of sensation, ROM, and strength provides insight into the causes of functional limitations, these parameters do not gauge the impact of impaired upper extremity function on a patient's ability to perform the activities of daily living independently. Factors that influence functional outcome include a patient's personal reactions to the injury, adaptation to the disability, extent of daily needs, and the socioeconomic environment.

Assessment begins in the acute stage of injury and continues until the patient is able to return to work. Hand function is evaluated by noting the patient's prehensile patterns and administering standardized coordination tests. Specific upper extremity functional deficits are treated by individualized activities and exercise programs (Fig. 7). Splinting can compensate for some impaired motor functions; for example, a lumbrical block splint can be used for ulnar nerve palsy or a dynamic MCP extension splint can be used for radial nerve palsy (Fig. 8) (3). A patient's overall function is determined by a self-care assessment, a pre-vocational assessment, a physical capacities evaluation, and a work assessment. When adaptations to a patient's physical environment are anticipated, the patient's home, community, and work place are assessed. Many functional deficits can be remedied by teaching patients alternative methods, providing adaptive equipment, or altering the environment (Fig. 9). Immediately after injury, patients may rely on adaptive equipment or special services to compensate for temporary loss of upper extremity function. However, they must be weaned from equipment as soon as possible to encourage use of the injured extremity as

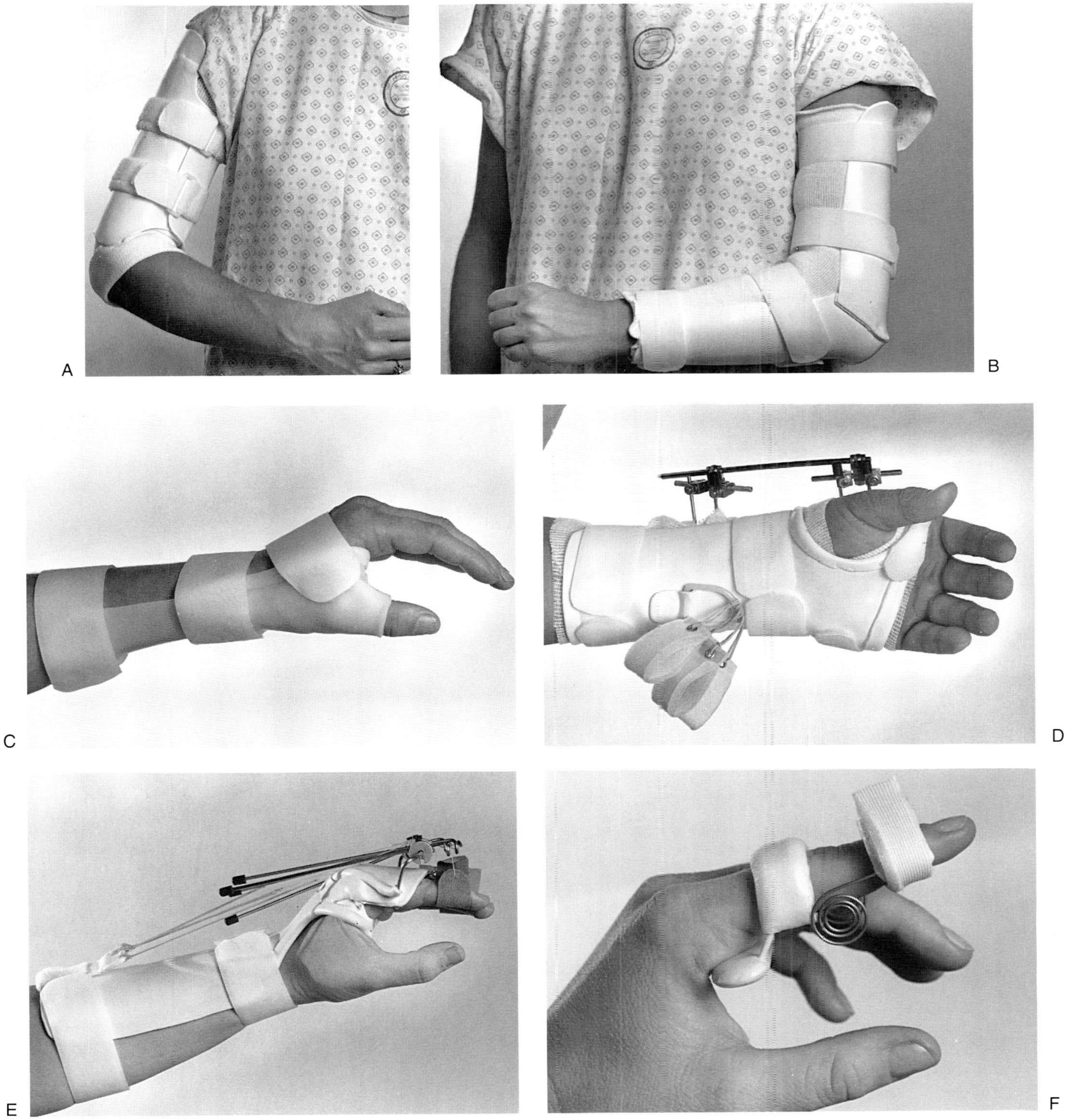

FIG. 5. Upper extremity splints. **A:** Sarmiento humeral splint. **B:** Posterior elbow splint. **C:** Long opponens splint. **D:** Wrist cock-up with dynamic MCP flexion loops. **E:** Dynamic finger extension splint. **F:** LMB spring finger extension splint.

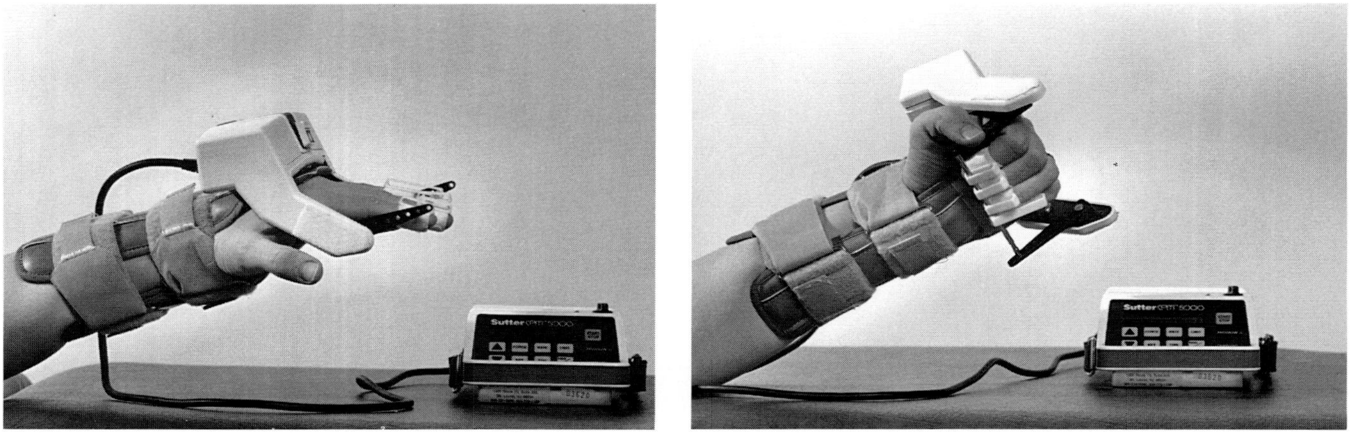

A B

FIG. 6. A continuous passive motion machine passively moves the finger joints through full or partial ranges of motion. **A:** Extension. **B:** Flexion.

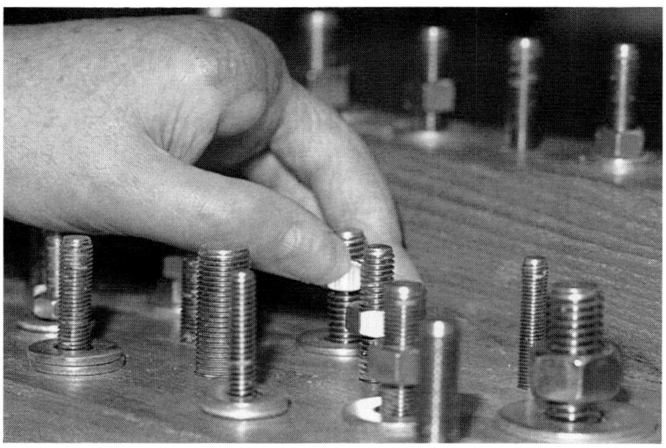

FIG. 7. Functional retraining activities should be initiated early to ensure that gains made in range of motion, strength, and sensation are carried over into functional tasks.

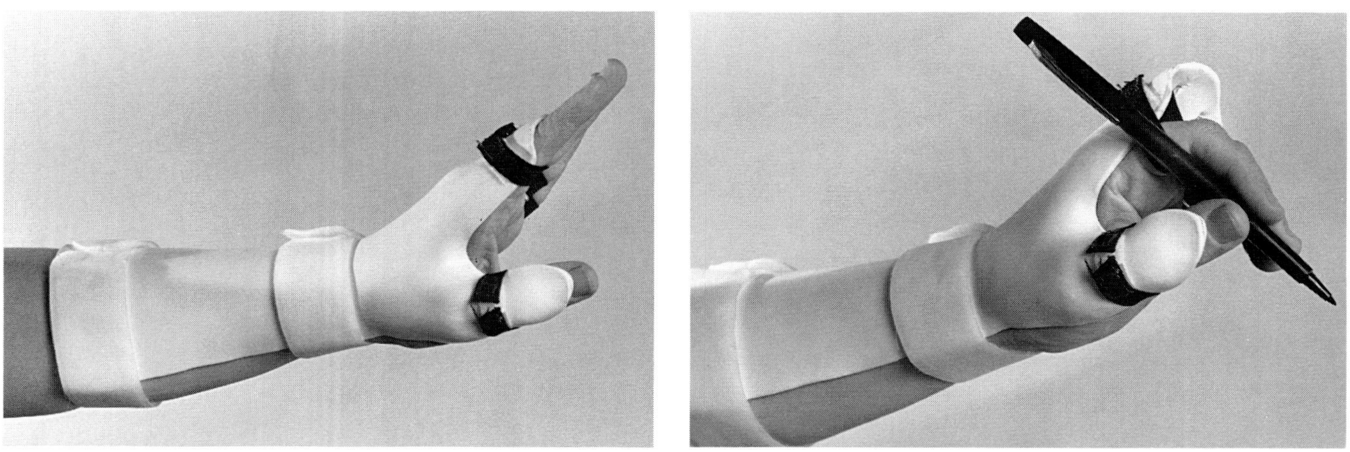

A B

FIG. 8. A,B: Low-profile radial nerve splints support the wrist in a functional position and provide dynamic extension of the MCP joints via elastic straps while allowing the patient to use remaining muscles for functional tasks.

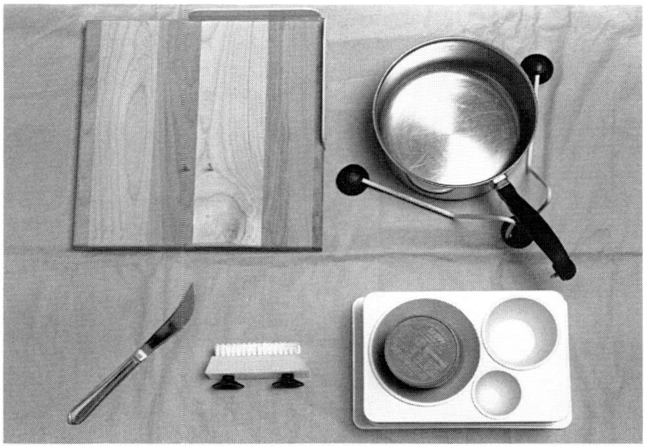

FIG. 9. Adaptive equipment can be used by patients who have lost the use of one upper extremity. From top left, clockwise: one-handed cutting board, pan holder, jar opener, suction brush, rocker knife.

function returns. When activities are no longer restricted by a patient's medical condition, a work-hardening program can be started to redevelop the skills and endurance necessary to return safely and successfully to work.

The physician must decide whether a patient with an amputation at the level of the wrist or higher is a candidate for immediate fitting of a postoperative cast with a terminal device (9). In this case, a cast is applied in the operating room and a terminal device is later fitted by a prosthetist. An occupational therapist assesses the fit of the prosthesis and the patient's ability to operate the specific features of the limb. Function is assessed and treatment is implemented the same as for other upper extremity injuries. Patients with unilateral amputations require few adaptive devices. Those with bilateral amputations require extensive equipment and environmental adaptations for functional independence.

REFERENCES

1. Trombly CA, ed. *Occupational therapy for physical dysfunction.* 3rd ed. Baltimore: Williams and Wilkins; 1989.
2. Hunter JM, Schneider LH, Macklin EJ, Callahan AD, eds. *Rehabilitation of the hand.* 3rd ed. St. Louis: CV Mosby; 1990.
3. Tenney CG, Lisak JM. *Atlas of hand splinting.* Boston: Little, Brown; 1986.
4. Dowden P, Beukelman DR, Lossing CA. Serving nonspeaking patients in acute care settings: intervention outcomes. *Augment Altern Commun* 1986;2:38–44.
5. Halpern AS. Functional communication assessment of adults with neurogenic disorders. In: *Functional assessment in rehabilitation.* Baltimore: Paul H Brookes; 1984.
6. Rockwood CA, Green DP, eds. *Fractures in adults.* 2nd ed. Philadelphia: JB Lippincott; 1984.
7. Fess E, Phillips CA. *Hand splinting: principles and methods.* 2nd ed. St. Louis: CV Mosby; 1987.
8. Dellon AL. *Evaluation of sensibility and re-education of sensation in the hand.* Baltimore: Williams & Wilkins; 1981.
9. Banerjee SN, ed. *Rehabilitation management of amputees.* Baltimore: Williams & Wilkins; 1982.

Orthopaedic Trauma Protocols, edited by
Sigvard T. Hansen, Jr., and Marc F. Swiontkowski,
Raven Press, Ltd., New York, ©1993.

CHAPTER 9

Acute Physical Therapy

Tracey L. Varga

INTRODUCTION

Physical therapy is initiated very soon after definitive treatment of a fracture has been carried out. The goals of physical therapy before fracture consolidation are to increase mobility, maximize function, and prevent secondary complications. When assessing and treating patients with acute orthopaedic injuries, physical therapists take into consideration many physiologic and anatomic factors, such as the extent of soft-tissue injury, the rate of fracture healing, the stability of the fixation, and the deleterious effects of prolonged immobility. Multiple-trauma patients, as well as those with isolated orthopaedic injuries, are educated and trained in rehabilitation techniques to ensure optimal functional outcomes.

The goals of physical therapy intervention for orthopaedic injuries will be outlined in general terms, followed by a discussion of specific acute-care rehabilitation techniques and modalities for intraarticular fractures, joint dislocations, and neurologically intact spinal injuries.

GENERAL CONSIDERATIONS

Overriding all other considerations is to do no harm to the patient. Each therapy regimen is individualized according to the needs and abilities of the patient, the severity of the fracture, the type of fixation, and associated skeletal, soft-tissue, and neurovascular involvement. The plan is approved by the attending surgeon and carried out as a team effort. The physical therapist is an integral member of the health-care team and takes part in daily multidisciplinary rounds, contributing input towards establishing a treatment plan, precautions, and goals.

Many secondary complications can be prevented by physical therapy intervention. Fracture disease and the pain–spasm cycle can be prevented by means of specific modalities such as superficial heat and cold, motion, transcutaneous electrical nerve stimulation (TENS), facilitation–inhibition techniques, and soft-tissue mobilization. Joint stiffness and contractures can be prevented by proper positioning, early range-of-motion (ROM) exercises, superficial heat and cold modalities, joint mobilization techniques, and soft-tissue mobilization. Similarly, edema is prevented by motion, compressive dressings, electrical stimulation, soft-tissue mobilization, and proper positioning (elevating the extremity while at rest and avoiding prolonged dependency of the involved extremity before and after surgery).

Muscle atrophy is prevented by early isometric exercises, electrical stimulation, facilitation techniques, and isotonic, isokinetic, and eccentric training. Disuse osteoporosis is avoided by active range-of-motion (AROM), strengthening, isometric exercises, and weight-bearing as allowed (Figs. 1–4). However, precautions related to specific injuries may contraindicate some of these exercises.

Physical therapists also assist in preventing complications caused by prolonged bed rest by initiating isometric exercises, early AROM strengthening of the uninvolved extremities and joints, continuous passive motion (CPM) of the involved joints and extremities, and by teaching early bed mobility, transfer, and gait techniques. Patients and their families are actively involved early in a patient's care, and self-reliance is stressed. The protocols regarding the use of orthotics, strengthening and endurance training, and isotonic and isokinetic exercises are modified for each patient, as are the precautions related to individual skeletal, neurovascular, and soft-tissue injuries. The exercise and mobility regimens can also be varied to accommodate physician preference and the skeletal stabilization.

Department of Rehabilitation Medicine, Harborview Medical Center, University of Washington, Seattle, Washington 98104

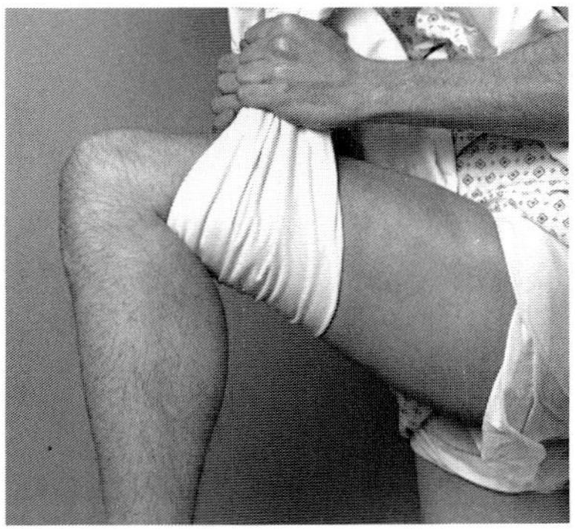

FIG. 1. Hip and knee PROM and AAROM, included in the rehabilitation of the pelvis and the femur.

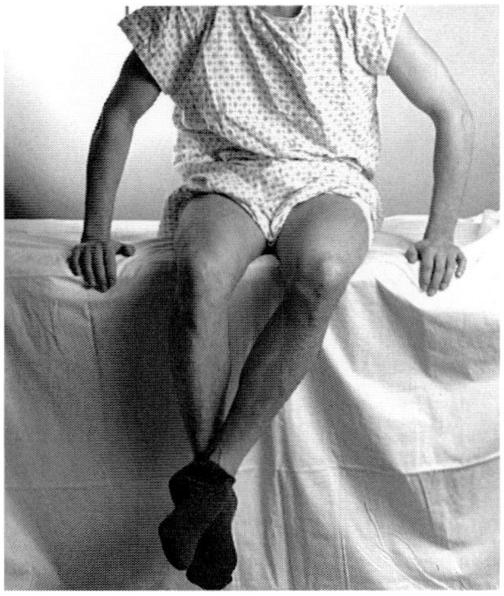

FIG. 2. Knee PROM and prolonged stretch, included in the rehabilitation of the femur and the proximal tibia to regain knee motion. The patient is providing a flexion moment on the right leg with the uninjured left leg.

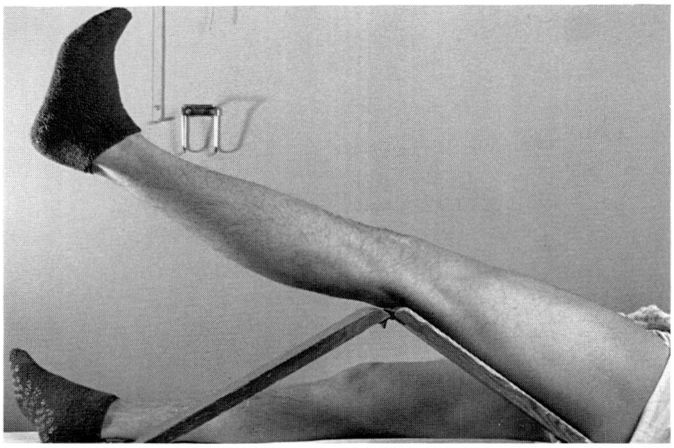

FIG. 3. Terminal knee extension, included in the rehabilitation of the pelvis, the tibia, and the femur after IM nailing to strengthen the quadriceps muscles.

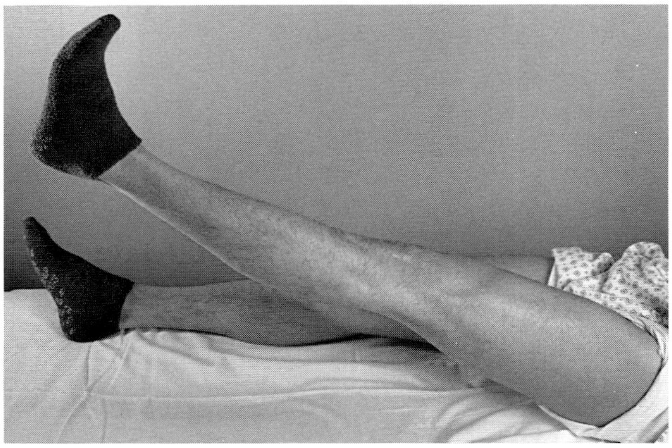

FIG. 4. Straight leg raise (SLR), included in the rehabilitation of the pelvis, the femur, and the tibia to strengthen the hip flexors and the quadriceps muscles.

SPECIFIC ACUTE CARE REHABILITATION

Intraarticular Fractures

The acute management of intraarticular fractures is aimed at preventing the deleterious effects of immobilization and avoiding excessive stress on healing synovial joints. Complications associated with joint immobilization include articular cartilage degeneration, joint adhesions, joint stiffness, pain, muscle atrophy, and disuse osteoporosis (1–3). Early motion is the primary strategy used to decrease the incidence and severity of these complications which, cumulatively, can lead to posttraumatic degenerative changes.

Continuous passive motion is begun on the first postoperative day and the patient's tolerance is increased until the machine can be used for 10 to 12 h per day during the hospital stay. Gentle active-assisted range-of-motion (AAROM), AROM, and isometric strengthening exercises of the involved joint are encouraged. In addition to mobilizing the injured joint, patients perform AROM and strengthening exercises with the uninvolved extremities and joints. Transfer skills and gait training with protected weight-bearing are taught early within the limitations of the fracture fixation. Heat and cold modalities are applied to control pain, relax the muscles, and minimize muscle guarding.

Hip Dislocations

Physical therapy management of hip dislocations is begun within one to three days after injury and consists of a gradual progression of quadriceps sets, ankle AROM, terminal knee extension, knee AROM, gentle hip AAROM, and isometric exercises with range-of-motion limitations. Patients are instructed in bed mobility, transfer, and gait training with the use of assistive devices. In posterior dislocations, hip flexion greater than 60°, hip adduction, and internal rotation past neutral are avoided for the first 4 to 6 weeks. The weight-bearing status of a patient with a posterior dislocation depends on the severity of the dislocation and the stability of the reduction.

Precautions for anterior dislocations always include extremes of motion, external rotation, and abduction. Flexion or extension is limited, depending on the mechanism of injury.

Glenohumeral Dislocations

Anterior dislocations of the glenohumeral joint are the most common. After the shoulder is reduced and stabilized, it is immobilized in adduction and internal rotation in a sling. By the second or third postinjury day, gentle shoulder pendulum exercises, AROM exercises of the elbow, wrist, and hand, and grip strengthening are begun. Isometric exercises aimed at strengthening the shoulder girdle musculature and the deltoid muscle are performed within the limits of pain tolerance and fixation stability. Gentle passive range of motion (PROM) of the shoulder is begun by the second or third postoperative week. By the fourth to sixth week, patients are allowed to progress to AROM and strengthening exercises of the shoulder. External rotation and abduction are to be avoided until 6 weeks after injury. The injured upper extremity is generally not used for weight-bearing activities for 3 to 6 weeks.

Neurologically Intact Spinal Injuries

Physical therapy evaluation and treatment of patients with bone injuries of the spine or ligamentous instability without neurologic involvement are begun before the injury is stabilized. Prestabilization management of cervical, thoracic, or lumbosacral injuries can include AROM and isometric exercises unless they are contraindicated by the location of the injury. The goals of prestabilization management are to prevent excessive stress or injury to the spine, to avoid complications resulting from immobilization and bed rest, and to educate the patient and the family early about precautions, mobility, and recommendations. Poststabilization management includes instructing patients in spinal precautions and training them to use protective body mechanics. Patients are taught to maintain optimal spinal curvature while recumbent, sitting, and standing. Early mobilization includes bed mobility, transfers, and ambulation with assistive devices. Active range-of-motion and strengthening exercises are encouraged within the precautions of the specific injury. Paraspinal, trunk, and abdominal isometric exercises are performed within an orthosis.

General precautions related to spinal injuries include avoidance of twisting, rotation, lifting, and forward flexion of the neck and trunk. An overhead trapeze above the bed is not used during hospitalization. Lifting or pulling with the upper extremities and asymmetrical overhead shoulder motion should be avoided after cervical and upper thoracic spinal injuries; hip flexion greater than 90° and trunk torque are contraindicated after injury to the lower thoracic and lumbosacral spine. Patients who have sustained spinal injuries with partial or complete neurologic involvement receive early physical therapy for range-of-motion and positioning within the limitations of their injuries. The goals of early therapy are to prevent contractures and skin breakdown and to promote early mobility.

REHABILITATION MODALITIES

Traction

In the rare instance when a patient is immobilized in traction, physical therapy is begun to help avoid complications related to bed rest and immobility and to encourage motion within the precautions dictated by the injury. Early instruction in AROM and strengthening of the uninjured extremities, ankle AROM, and isometric exercises of the joints distal to the affected limb are started on the first day after injury.

Continuous Passive Motion

Continuous passive motion is used as an adjunct to trauma rehabilitation. Patients with intraarticular lower extremity fractures and those who have undergone knee reconstructions are the primary postoperative candidates for this device (Figs. 5–8). The general benefits of CPM include restoration and maintenance of normal joint mobility, prevention of contractures, and decreased pain and edema. Specific benefits to the synovial joints include increased synovial fluid circulation, enhanced articular cartilage regeneration, accelerated intraarticular tissue healing, better connective tissue orientation, and a lower incidence of intraarticular adhesions (4).

The protocols for CPM include initiation of the device as early as possible, usually on the first postoperative day. Continuous passive motion can be used on the hip, knee, ankle, shoulder, elbow, wrist, or hand. The degree of joint motion is modified by the type of fracture, the amount of soft-tissue involvement, and the comfort of the patient. Motion is increased by 10° to 20° each day and the time spent on the machine is gradually increased until the patient can tolerate 10 to 12 hours per day on the machine. A CPM machine is normally used for 2 to 3 weeks after injury, depending on patient compliance and ROM limitations.

In summary, physical therapy rehabilitation makes use of diverse procedures and treatment modalities to reach desired mobility goals. Many exercise techniques, modalities, and types of equipment are used to reinforce safety precautions and enhance optimal mobility and function. Early individualized physical therapy intervention conforming to patients' reliability and the availability of outside support are extremely important to achieve optimal functional results. At the time of discharge from the hospital, patients are referred to appropriate advanced rehabilitation services to continue their progress.

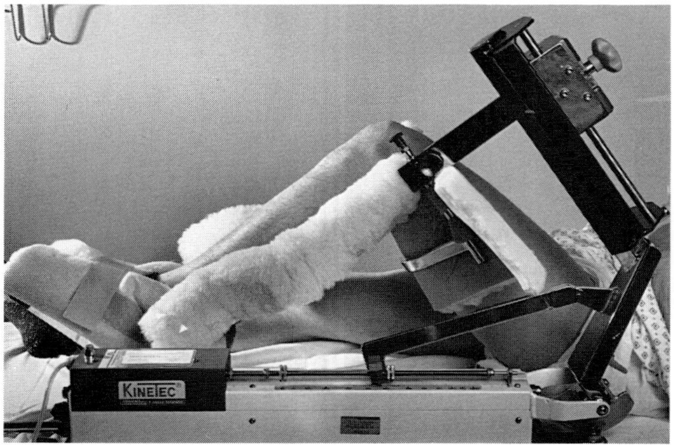

FIG. 5. CPM: isolated hip flexion.

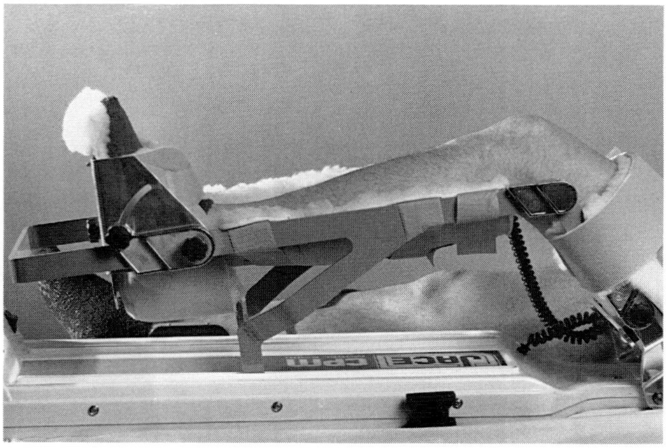

FIG. 6. CPM: knee flexion and extension.

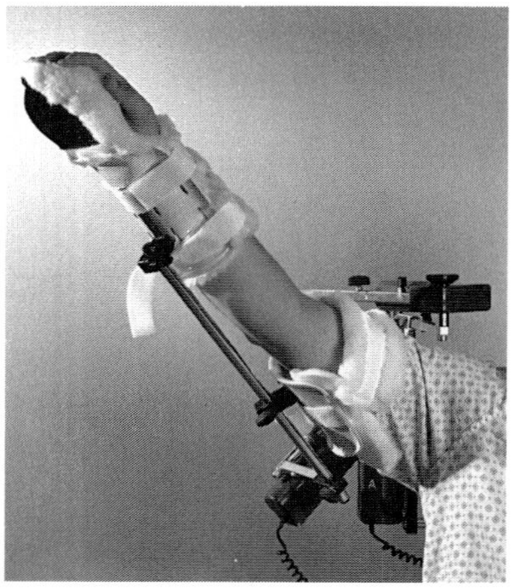

FIG. 7. CPM: shoulder forward flexion.

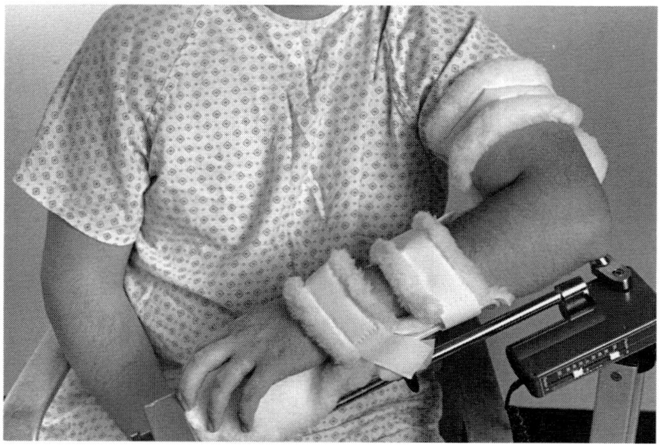

FIG. 8. CPM: elbow flexion and extension with forearm pronation and supination.

REFERENCES

1. Akeson WH, Amiel D, Garfin SR, Woosly. Effects of immobilization on joints. *Clin Orthop,* 1987;219:28–37.
2. Akeson WH, Amiel D, Woosley. Immobility effects on synovial joints: the pathomechanics of joint contractures. *Biorheology,* 1980;17:95.
3. Enneking WF, Horovitz M. The intra-articular effect of immoblized human knees. *J Bone Joint Surg,* 1972;54A:973.
4. Salter RB. The biologic concept of continuous passive motion of synovial joints: the first 18 years of basic research and its clinical application. *Clin Orthop,* 1989;242:12–25.

SELECTED READINGS

Cooksun J, Kent B. Orthopaedic manual therapy, an overview: the extremities. *J Am Phys Ther Assoc,* 1979;59:136.

Cronan T. Effects of immobilization and mobilization on cartilaginous, bony and soft tissue structure: a review of the literature. *J Burn Care Rehab,* 1986;7:54–7.

Frank C, Akeson WH, Woosly. Physiology and therapeutic value of passive joint motion. *Clin Orthop,* 1984;185:113–24.

Gould JA. *Orthopaedic and Sports Physical Therapy,* St. Louis: CV Mosby Co.; 1990.

Shimizu T, Videman T, Shimazak K, Mooney V. Experimental study on the repair of full thickness articular cartilage defects: effects of varying periods of continuous passive motion, cage activity and immobilization. *J Orthop Research,* 1987;5:187–98.

Williams PE. Effect of intermittent stretch on immobilized muscle. *Annals Rheum Disorders,* 1988;1014–16.

Williams PE, Cataneset, Lucey EG, Goldspink G. The importance of stretch and contractile activity in prevention of connective tissue accumulation in muscle. *J Anatomy,* 1988;158:109–14.

Orthopaedic Trauma Protocols, edited by
Sigvard T. Hansen, Jr., and Marc F. Swiontkowski,
Raven Press, Ltd., New York, ©1993.

CHAPTER 10

Rehabilitation: Nonacute Physical Therapy

Kevin Olson

Patients referred to the Outpatient Physical Therapy Clinic are assessed and treated for disabilities related to loss of joint range-of-motion (ROM), soft-tissue mobility, strength, endurance, and ambulation. They also receive functional training and are instructed in home treatment programs. To ensure that appropriate care will be provided, the physical therapist and the surgeon discuss precautions regarding the fracture, the patient's weight-bearing status, associated injuries or soft-tissue involvement, and the amount of healing that has occurred at the time of the referral. This information is used to assist the therapist in setting up a treatment program and outlining safe and realistic goals. Treatment plans consisting of appropriate exercises, modalities, and facilitation techniques are individualized for each patient and are reassessed on a regular basis. The ultimate goal of rehabilitation is to restore maximal function as quickly as possible. Tables 1 through 3 outline the recommended physical therapy protocols for upper and lower fractures.

GENERAL CONSIDERATIONS

Physical therapy management of patients after fracture consolidation covers a wide range of disabilities, and programs are individualized for each patient. As fractures show radiographic evidence of healing, weight-bearing is increased, more aggressive ROM exercises are added, and strengthening as well as functional training are begun. All patients are instructed in home exercise programs through illustrations and written instructions. They are encouraged to participate actively in their own care and to be responsible for their own progress.

Pain and swelling continue to be a problem for many orthopaedic patients after discharge from the hospital. The modalities and treatment techniques that can be applied to these problems are incorporated into individual treatment programs as needed. The primary modalities for treating pain consist of applications of heat or cold, and electrical stimulation. In most fractures, pain can be alleviated by active range-of-motion exercises (AROM) and joint mobilization. Swelling is managed by elevating the extremity and performing AROM within the limitations of the fracture. For example, a patient with a distal radial fracture is instructed to keep the injured arm elevated above the level of the heart as much as possible and to perform finger AROM exercises every hour. Contrast baths are useful for treating subacute or chronic swelling in the ankle, foot, wrist, and hand.

Depending on the stage of fracture healing, active, active-assisted, or passive ROM exercises can be prescribed to increase joint range of motion. Early AROM is especially important for intraarticular fractures. Passive ROM and stretching exercises are prescribed to alleviate joint or capsular tightness. Patients with severe soft-tissue injuries progress slowly, performing ROM exercises in the joints proximal and distal to the fracture but deferring mobilization techniques to increase ROM in the injured joint until the fracture has healed sufficiently to tolerate these techniques. Ultrasound and fluidotherapy are used to warm tissues in preparation for ROM and mobilization exercises. Soft-tissue techniques such as cross-friction or scar massage, myofascial release, and stretching are used to enhance mobility if it is restricted by muscle or fascial tightness or by surgical adhesions. For best results, active and passive ROM exercises must be performed immediately after these soft-tissue techniques.

Strength is often lost in a limb after injury but can be regained through effective exercise and a functional retraining program. Isometric and active exercises are used initially. Functional electrical stimulation (FES) can be used as an adjunct to a strengthening program, especially to a quadriceps strengthening program. Isokinetic strengthening is incorporated into all lower extremity fracture management programs. Isokinetic assessment should be done whenever

Department of Rehabilitation Medicine, Harborview Medical Center, Seattle, Washington 98104

Table 1. *Upper Extremity*

Fracture	Fixation	Mobility Precautions
Scapula scapular body acromion process coracoid process glenoid neck glenoid fossa	screws reconstruction plates tubular plates mini T-plates	**Stable:** WBAT **Unstable:** protected weight-bearing 2–3 months no deltoid isometrics until 6 weeks post-stabilization sling immobilization as needed
Clavicle displaced nondisplaced	reconstruction plates dynamic compression plate (DCP)	**Stable:** WBAT **Unstable:** PWB-NWB 6–8 weeks postinjury sling, figure 8 immobilization as fracture/patient status dictates
Humerus 1. Proximal fractures greater tuberosity lesser tuberosity surgical neck anatomic neck	plate wires (tension-band, K-wire) 2.5-mm Schanz pins screws external fixation hemiarthroplasty (elderly patient)	NWB 8–12 weeks immobilization with sling, abduction pillow, and splint 8–12 weeks
2. Humeral shaft	DCP locked IM nail	NWB 6–8 weeks Sling, splint, plaster immobilization NWB-WBAT as fracture pattern dictates
3. Distal humerus	reconstruction plates tubular plates screws tension-band wire for olecranon osteotomy	NWB 8–12 weeks plaster, splint immobilization
Radius & Ulna 1. Olecranon	tension-band wiring screw, wire fixation	protective plaster splinting 6 weeks NWB
2. Radial head	closed reduction mini-fragment screws mini T-plates	cast, splint, sling immobilization NWB
3. Forearm isolated radius, ulna—both bones Monteggia Galeazzi	closed reduction plates screws (rare) IM nail (rare)	immobilization 8–12 weeks (cast splint) NWB 8–12 weeks
4. Distal radius	closed reduction external fixation ORIF	immobilization 8–12 weeks (cast, removable splint) NWB 8–12 weeks
Wrist & Hand carpal MC phalanx	closed reduction wires mini-plates	cast, splint immobilization NWB-PWB 8–12 weeks

Terminology:

1. (NWB) Nonweight-bearing—patient may *not* use extremity for any weight-bearing activity
2. (TDWB) Touch-down weight-bearing—extremity may touch the ground just during rest, not during ambulation
3. (TTWB) Toe-touch weight-bearing—toe may touch ground just for balance
4. (WOLWB) Weight-of-leg weight-bearing—approximately 20–30 lbs.
5. (PWB) Partial weight-bearing—weight limit specified by M.D.

Table 1. *Upper Extremity (Continued)*

Initial Physical Therapy Program*	Advanced Physical Therapy **
Days 1–5: shoulder pendulum exercises elbow, forearm; wrist, hand AROM; grip strengthening **Weeks 2–3:** gentle PROM-AAROM shoulder; deltoid, rotator cuff isometrics **Weeks 6–8:** AROM shoulder joint **If stable fracture pattern**—shoulder PROM-AAROM initiated 1 week postinjury, ROM, strengthening progressed to tolerance	**Stable:** PROM/strengthening as tolerated **Unstable:** strengthening at 3 months; progress to isometrics, surgical tubing, and free weights
Stable **Day 1 post-stabilization:** early shoulder AROM-AAROM to tolerance; shoulder isometrics; elbow, forearm, wrist, hand AROM; grip strengthening **Unstable:** limit ROM as fracture pattern dictates	**Stable:** PROM/strengthening as tolerated **Unstable:** strengthening at 6–8 weeks; return to activity in 10–12 weeks
Day 1 post-stabilization: elbow, forearm, wrist, hand AROM; grip strengthening **Days 2–5:** pendulum shoulder exercises **Weeks 1–3:** early gentle AAROM shoulder joint within mobility limitations; deltoid, biceps, triceps, isometrics **Weeks 3–6:** AROM, gentle PROM shoulder	**Week 12:** begin strengthening; progress to isometrics, surgical tubing, free weights, isokinetics; scapular stabilization exercises are important
Day 1 post-stabilization: elbow, forearm, wrist, hand AROM grip strengthening **Days 2–5:** Pendulum shoulder exercises **Weeks 1–3:** Early gentle AAROM shoulder joint within mobility limitations: deltoid, biceps, triceps, isometrics **Weeks 3–6:** AROM, gentle PROM shoulder	**Weeks 10–12:** strengthening **Week 12:** progression the same as for the proximal humerus
Day 1 post-stabilization: shoulder AAROM-AROM; wrist, hand active range of motion-CPM (elbow) as M.D. indicates **Days 2–5:** gentle elbow, forearm AROM; deltoid isometrics; grip strengthening **Weeks 8–10:** gentle PROM-AAROM elbow, forearm	**Weeks 10–12:** strengthening **Week 12:** isokinetics
Days 1–7 post-stabilization: early gentle AAROM-AROM forearm, elbow (initiated after 2–3 days); shoulder, wrist, hand AROM; grip strengthening	**Weeks 10–12:** PROM; strengthening
Days 1–7 post-stabilization: early elbow AROM shoulder, wrist, hand AROM; grip strengthening	**Weeks 10–12:** PROM; strengthening
Days 1–5 post-stabilization: immediate shoulder, hand AROM; early, gentle AAROM forearm, elbow, wrist as fracture stability allows; grip strengthening	**Weeks 10–12:** PROM **Week 12:** strengthening
Days 1–5 post-stabilization: immediate AROM shoulder, elbow, fingers; initiation of gentle wrist AROM as immobilization allows (after cast removal then splint); grip strengthening	**Weeks 8–10:** PROM; light activity **Weeks 10–12:** strengthening
Days 1-5 post-stabilization: early AROM-AAROM fingers, wrist, forearm as fracture and stabilization allow; elbow, shoulder AROM; fine motor control, desensitization; techniques as indicated	**Weeks 8–10:** PROM; light activity **Weeks 10–12:** strengthening

6. (WBAT) Weight–bearing as tolerated—patient may bear weight through extremity as tolerated
7. (TKE) Terminal knee extension—short-arc quadriceps strengthening exercises
8. (SLR) Straight leg raises—isometric strengthening exercises with hip flexion

* Post-stabilization to healing
** After fracture healing
Table prepared by Kevin Olson and Tracey Varga

Table 2. *Lower Extremity: Acetabulum to Femur*

Fracture	Fixation	Mobility Precautions
Acetabulum posterior wall; posterior columns; anterior wall; anterior column; transverse; T-shaped; posterior column/posterior wall; transverse/ posterior wall; both column; anterior column with posterior hemitransverse (Letournel classification)	lag screws reconstruction plates	**Kocher-Langenbeck approach:** (posterior), avoid active hip extension, rotation **Ilionguinal approach:** (anterior), avoid active hip flexion, vigorous trunk and abdominal flexion **Extended iliofemoral approach:** (posterolateral), no active hip abduction 6–8 weeks; weight-bearing; TDWB-WOL 8–12 weeks; positioning ROM; posterior wall involvement–no hip flexion greater than 60° for 6 weeks.
Pelvis 1. Anterior ring pubic symphysis rami	plating external fixation lag screws	TDWB-WBAT 10–12 weeks postinjury (depends on associated, posterior ring involvement)
2. Posterior Ring sacrum SI fracture/dislocation iliac wing	screws plating	TDWB-WOLWB 10–12 weeks
Femur 1. Femoral head	screw fixation; hemiarthroplasty THA (in elderly patient as fracture dictates)	Toe-touch weight-bearing 8–12 weeks No straight leg raises (SLR) TTWB, WBAT dependent on prosthesis/ fixation (see femoral neck fracture)
2. Femoral neck	screws dynamic hip screw endoprosthesis (elderly)	TTWB involved side 8–12 weeks TTWB/WBAT as directed by M.D. **ROM precautions:** anterior surgical approach: avoid extreme hip extension; external rotation past neutral; no SLR 6–8 weeks **Posterior surgical approach:** no hip flexion greater than 60°; avoid hip adduction, internal rotation past neutral; no SLR 6–8 weeks
3. Subtrochanteric femur	DHS blade plate IM nail	TTWB; no SLR; no active hip abduction with blade-plate fixation
Intertrochanteric femur	DHS IM nail	
4. Femoral shaft	IM nail dynamic vs. static interlocked nail nonlocked nail DCP, LC, DCP	Interlocked nail/plate TTWB 6–8 weeks nonlocked nail-WBAT avoid hip; inversion and eversion during mobilization **Note:** Knee immobilizer, external support may be needed to allow early crutch training if quad control slowly achieved; DCP fixation same as IM nail protocol
5. Supracondylar, intracondylar femur	condylar blade plate; condylar buttress plate; screws	TDWB 10–12 weeks

Terminology:
1. (NWB) Nonweight-bearing—patient may *not* use extremity for any weight-bearing activity
2. (TDWB) Touch-down weight-bearing—extremity may touch the ground just during rest, not during ambulation
3. (TTWB) Toe-touch weight-bearing—toe may touch ground just for balance
4. (WOLWB) Weight-of-leg weight-bearing—approximately 20–30 lbs.
5. (PWB) Partial weight-bearing—weight limit specified by M.D.

Table 2. *Lower Extremity: Acetabulum to Femur (Continued)*

Initial Physical Therapy Program*	Advanced Physical Therapy**
Day 1 post-operative: immediate CPM (hip flexion, abduction) **Days 2–5:** bilateral UE strengthening; AROM knee, ankle; quad, hamstring isometrics, TKE; early mobilization initiated (exercise instruction, bed mobility, transfer, ambulation training); hip PROM within ROM limitations; lying prone is encouraged in patients with hip flexion precaution to avoid contracture (2–3x/day, 20 min intervals); **Weeks 6–8:** AROM-AAROM hip; hip abductor isometrics	**Weeks 12–14:** WBAT, waen from crutches, gait retraining; strengthen quads, hamstrings, abductors, flexors, extensors, and lower trunk muscles; initiate balance/proprioceptive awareness training; aerobic/fitness training; rehabilitation is tailored to the surgical approach (i.e., extended iliofemoral approach requires more extensive hip abductor strengthening)
Days 1–7 post-stabilization: bilateral UE strengthening; PROM hip joint as fracture stability/pattern allows; quad/hamstring sets, terminal knee extension; AROM knee, ankle	**Weeks 12–14:** WBAT, wean from crutches, gait retraining; strengthen quads, hamstrings, hip adductors, flexors, extensors, and lower trunk muscles; balance/proprioceptive training; aerobic/fitness training
Days 1–7 post-stabilization: bilateral UE strengthening; PROM hip joint as fracture stability/pattern allows; quad/hamstring sets, terminal knee extension; AROM knee, ankle	**Weeks 12–14:** WBAT, wean from crutches, gait retraining; strengthen quads, hamstrings, hip adductors, abductors, flexors, extensors, and lower trunk muscles; initiate balance/proprioceptive awareness training; aerobic/fitness training
Days 1–7 post-stabilization: bilateral UE strengthening; quad/hamstring isometrics, TKE; gentle AAROM hip; involved extremity knee, ankle AAROM; early mobilization/transfer and ambulation training	**Week 8-12:** WBAT, wean from crutches, gait retraining **Week 12:** strengthen quads, hamstrings, and hip abductors; balance/proprioceptive training; closed kinetic chain activities
Days 1–7 post-stabilization: bilateral UE strengthening; knee, ankle AROM; quad/hamstring isometrics, TKE; gentle hip AAROM within precaution limitations; bed mobility, transfers, gait, body mechanics instructions **Weeks 6–8:** hip PROM; hip abductor isometrics	**Week 8-12:** WBAT, wean from crutches, gait retraining **Week 12:** strengthen quads, hamstrings and hip abductors; balance/proprioceptive training: closed kinetic chain activities
Immediate post-stabilization: knee CPM **Days 1–7:** bilateral UE strengthening; hip and knee AAROM—all motions except no abduction with blade plate; quad/hamstring isometrics, TKE; ankle AROM; bed mobility, transfers, gait, body mechanics instructions **Weeks 6–8:** hip ROM; hip abductor isometrics	**Weeks 8–12:** WBAT, wean from crutches, gait retraining **Week 12:** strengthen quads, hamstrings, and hip abductors; balance/proprioceptive training: closed kinetic chain activities
Preoperative: bilateral UE strenthening; unaffected leg LE strengthening; co-contraction quad/hamstring sets on affected leg as fracture pattern/soft-tissue involvement allows; ankle AROM/pumps bilaterally (especially affected leg) **Day 1 postoperative:** CPM (knee); quad sets, ankle pumps; IM nail exercise protocol **Day 2 to discharge:** increase CPM daily (10–20°/day); goal: 90° ROM before discharge; quad/hamstring sets; TKEs, SLR (progress to independent, encourage full knee extension); AAROM-AROM hip flexion, hip abductors, adductors (gravity eliminated); AAROM, PROM stretch to regain knee motion. Use of modalities (heat, ice)	**Weeks 8–12:** WBAT, wean from crutches, gait retraining **Week 12:** strengthen quads, hamstrings, and hip abductors; balance/proprioceptive training: closed kinetic chain activities
Day 1 post-stabilization: bilateral UE strengthening; knee CPM; quad sets, hamstring sets, ankle AROM	**Weeks 8–12:** WBAT, wean from crutches, gait retraining **Week 12:** strengthen quads, hamstrings, and hip abductors; balance/proprioceptive training: closed kinetic chain activities

6. (WBAT) Weight-bearing as tolerated—patient may bear weight through extremity as tolerated
7. (TKE) Terminal knee extension—short-arc quadriceps-strengthening exercises
8. (SLR) Straight leg raises—isometric strengthening exercises with hip flexion
9. (UE) Upper extremity
10. (LE) Lower extremity

* Post-stabilization to healing
** After fracture healing
Table prepared by Kevin Olsen and Tracey Varga

Table 3. *Lower Extremity: Patella to Foot*

Fracture	Fixation	Mobility Precautions
Patella Nondisplaced; displaced	immobilization: cylinder cast, knee immobilizer lag screw (s) tension-band wiring	**Stable:** WBAT **Unstable:** TTWB 4–8 weeks
Tibia 1. Tibial plateau	buttress T-plate DCP screws	TDWB 8–12 weeks NO TKE exercise (avoid excessive end-range anterior tibial glide)
2. Tibial shaft	IM nail reamed and unreamed; plates and screws; external fixator	IM nail-TTWB 6–8 weeks; plates and screws; TDWB 8–12 weeks; external fixator-NWB 8–12 weeks
Ankle 1. Pilon	screws and plates	NWB 12 weeks
2. Medial malleolus, posterior malleolus, lateral malleolus (Weber A, B, C)	screws, plates, and tension-band wiring	TDWB/NWB 8–12 weeks
Foot 1. Calcaneus extraarticular intraarticular	reconstruction plate H-plate; lag screw K-wires	NWB 12 weeks
2. Talus	lag screws K-wires (rare)	NWB 12 weeks
3. Metatarsals and phalanx	screws, wires, and pins	closed reduction immobilization

Terminology:
1. (NWB) Nonweight-bearing—patient may *not* use extremity for any weight-bearing activity
2. (TDWB) Touch-down weight-bearing—extremity may touch the ground just during rest, not during ambulation
3. (TTWB) Toe-touch weight-bearing—toe may touch ground just for balance
4. (WOLWB) Weight-of-leg weight-bearing—approximately 20-30 lbs.
5. (PWB) Partial weight-bearing—weight limit specified by M.D.
6. (WBAT) Weight-bearing as tolerated—patient may bear weight through extremity as tolerated
7. (TKE) Terminal knee extension—short-arc quadriceps-strengthening exercises

possible to objectively determine the extent of compromised function in the injured muscles. The results are compared with an assessment of the unaffected extremity. In bilateral injuries the test can be measured against normative data. Two-speed or three-speed bilateral tests are usually performed. Although many parameters are possible, the primary considerations are peak torque, power, endurance ratios or fatigue index, and agonist/antagonist ratios.

Once a patient is allowed to bear weight as tolerated, assistive devices are used as long as pain or antalgic gait persist. Gait retraining is necessary for patients who have used crutches for at least 3 or 4 months. Endurance or aerobic fitness programs are equally important for patients who have used crutches or other assistive devices for a long time. Balance and coordination training is initiated in patients with proprioceptive deficits secondary to intraarticular fractures or

Table 3. *Lower Extremity: Patella to Foot (Continued)*

Initial Physical Therapy Program*	Advanced Physical Therapy**
Day 1: bilateral UE strengthening; ankle AROM; knee CPM post-op if indicated **Day 2 to discharge:** quad hamstring isometrics†; knee/AROM as fracture pattern allows† ;SLR†	**Weeks 4–8:** strengthening; progress knee A/AAROM; begin quad isometrics and SLR if there was quad mechanism involvement **Week 8:** WBAT, wean from crutches; concentrate on short arc/end range; quadriceps strengthening; closed kinetic chain activities (i.e., cycling, partial squats, leg press); balance proprioceptive training
Immediate: bilateral UE strengthening; knee CPM post-op; ankle AROM **Day 2 to discharge:** quad, hamstring isometrics; SLR; hip, knee/AAROM **Weeks 6–8:** TKE initiated	**Week 12**: WBAT, gait progression; strengthening
Immediate: bilateral UE strengthening; ankle AROM; quad, hamstring isometrics **Day 2 to discharge:** hip, knee AROM; SLR, TKE	**Weeks 6–8:** IM nail fixation; strengthening initiated **Weeks 10–12**: plate, screws, external fixation; strengthening initiated
Immediate post-stabilization: bilateral UE strengthening; gluteal, quad, hamstring isometrics **Day 2 to discharge:** hip, knee, toe AROM; SLR, TKE **Week 2:** ankle subtalar AROM; progressive hip and knee strengthening	**Week 12**: PROM initiated; strengthening; balance/proprioceptive awareness training; WBAT, wean from crutches; closed kinetc chain progam
Same as pilon fracture	**Weeks 8–10:** gait progression after fracture healing; AROM/PROM ankle and subtalar joints; balance/proprioceptive awareness training
Preoperative: UE strengthening; uninvolved extremity strengthening involved extremity hip, knee isometrics; crutch training for short distance (primary elevation of extremity) **Day 1:** UE strengthening; uninvolved extremity AROM/strengthening involved extremity hip-knee isometric, AROM, toe AROM to tolerance **Days 2–3:** crutch training, NWB involved extremity (limited time in dependent position) **Days 4–7:** early ankle, subtalar AROM when surgical incision is sealed **Week 1 to month 3:** continue early AROM ankle, subtalar, toes; gentle PROM toe dorsiflexion and plantarflexion; progress involved extremity; hip-knee conditioning	**Month 3:** gradually increase weight-bearing starting at 20 lbs. to FWB over 1 mo; gradually wean from assistive device as patient tolerates; pool therapy if available; gait training, re-education; desensitization techniques as needed; ankle subtalar AAROM. isometrics; low-impact endurance training **Months 4–6:** gait progression advanced balance and proprioceptive activities; ankle, subtalar scmetric, isotonic strengthening with tubing/theraband; no free weights; soft-tissue immobilization **Month 6:** ankle, subtalar PROM; joint mobilization; isokinetic assessment, strength-endurance training; advanced balance, gait training as indicated
Same as calcaneus	Same as calcaneus
Day 1 post-stabilization: bilateral UE strengthening; hip, knee AROM isometrics; ankle, subtalar, toe AROM as fracture pattern allows	**Weeks 8–12:** WBAT; wean from crutches; proprioceptive/balance training; closed kinetic chain activities

8. (SLR) Straight leg raises—isometric strengthening exercises with hip flexion
9. (UE) Upper extremity
10. (LE) Lower extremity

* Post-stabilization to healing
** After fracture healing
†Note: No active quads if quadriceps mechanisms involved or disrupted
Table prepared by Kevin Olson and Tracey Varga

prolonged immobilization. Because weight-bearing is the primary function of the lower extremities, a closed kinetic chain strengthening program is instituted for all lower extremity fractures. This type of exercise program incorporates functional weight-bearing activities into strengthening exercises. Examples of closed kinetic chain activities are climbing stairs, walking on a treadmill, bicycling, and performing squats, step-ups, and leg presses. These exercises are designed to adapt patients to the demands that will be made on them during daily work or recreational activities.

Specific protocols for rehabilitation of orthopedic trauma injuries are difficult to establish because every fracture and patient is unique. These protocols are to be used as guidelines, keeping in mind that each patient's injury and stage of recovery will determine the appropriate rehabilitation treatment plan.

SPINAL FRACTURES

Thoracic and Lumbar Spine Injuries

After discharge from the hospital, patients with thoracic and lumbar spinal fractures are supervised by the Outpatient physical therapy clinic. During the first 3 to 4 months patients perform all activities within a brace. A physical therapist supervises the patient's progress in isometric trunk exercises and ambulation as tolerated until the patient is able to ambulate independently without assistive devices. To prevent back problems in the future, patients are required to attend a 2-h back school presentation, which focuses on body mechanics, posture and lifting, and flexion limitations. Lifting is limited to 20 pounds for the first 3 months after injury. To maintain cardiovascular fitness while in a brace, patients are instructed in low-impact, low-load fitness exercises. Recommended activities include walking, stationary bicycling, and upper body ergometry (UBE), a bicycling device for the upper extremities. Rowing machines can be used if patients are skilled in good body mechanics. To be effective, the fitness program must be performed four or five times per week for at least 30 min at a target heart rate of 60% to 75% of the patient's maximal heart rate.

Patients are weaned from the brace after the fracture heals, usually in approximately 3 to 4 months. At that time, trunk ROM and trunk-strengthening exercises are added to the fitness program. Strengthening of the thoracic and lumbar spinal extensor and abdominal muscles is emphasized to help prevent reinjury. An endurance program, including swimming, bicycling, jogging, and low-impact aerobics, is started to improve overall fitness. Balance training is added to restore proprioception and coordination, followed by work hardening or conditioning to allow patients to return to work as soon as possible.

Cervical and Upper Thoracic Fractures

Physical therapy for patients with cervical or upper thoracic spinal fractures is initially performed within the brace. Treatment begins with neck isometric exercises performed in front of a mirror for good visual feedback. Symmetrical upper extremity strengthening exercises using low resistance are added, followed by a fitness program consisting of walking, stationary bicycling, and UBE. In upper thoracic fractures, in which increased thoracic kyphosis is of concern, extension exercises are begun to strengthen the thoracic spinal extensors. Like patients with lumbar fractures, patients with cervical and upper thoracic fractures are required to attend a 2-h Back School presentation, which focuses on proper body mechanics and posture.

After the fracture has healed, patients are weaned from the brace over a period of 2 to 4 weeks. At that time the physical therapy regimen is expanded to include neck ROM exercises, a progressive strengthening exercise program for the upper trunk and neck, and an advanced endurance program emphasizing upper trunk fitness (swimming, UBE, a rowing machine, or a cross-country skiing machine). A work conditioning or work hardening program is incorporated to adapt patients to preinjury levels of activity.

SELECTED READINGS

1. Bigos SJ, Battie MC. Acute care to prevent back disability. Ten years of progress. *Clin Orthop* 1987; 221:121–130.
2. Ivers LD, Clawson DK. *Manual of acute orthopaedic therapeutics,* 3rd ed. Boston: Little, Brown; 1987.
3. Robinson, Marx. A nail safe method. *Am J Nursing* 1985;158–161.
4. Evan P. The healing process at cellular level: a review. *Physiotherapy* 1980;66:256–259.
5. Lehmann JF. *Therapeutic heat and cold,* 4th ed. Baltimore: Williams & Wilkins; 1990.
6. Muller EA. Influence of training and of inactivity on muscle strength. *Arch Phys Med Rehabil* 1970;51:449.

Regional Fracture Management

Orthopaedic Trauma Protocols, edited by
Sigvard T. Hansen, Jr., and Marc F. Swiontkowski,
Raven Press, Ltd., New York, © 1993.

CHAPTER 11

Shoulder

Keith A. Mayo and Marc F. Swiontkowski

Sternoclavicular Dislocations

MECHANISMS OF INJURY

Sternoclavicular dislocations result from direct blows to the anterior chest wall or from lateral blows to the shoulder girdle. Anterior impacts usually produce posterior dislocations and are usually caused by high-energy trauma, most commonly by direct impact with the steering wheel during a motor vehicle accident. Lateral injuries may occur from low-energy falls and most commonly result in anterior dislocations. Complete disruption and distraction of the joint may be seen with scapulothoracic dissociations from high-energy trauma to the anterior aspect of the forequarter. This injury complex frequently involves axillary arterial and brachial plexus trauma as well. Anterior sternoclavicular joint disruptions are rarely associated with serious visceral or vascular injuries, whereas posterior sternoclavicular dislocations may be associated with occlusion of the superior vena cava and the esophagus.

ANATOMIC CONSIDERATIONS

The sternoclavicular joint is invested by a strong capsule and ligaments (Fig. 1). The anterior aspect of the joint is covered only by subcutaneous fat and skin; the critical associated anatomy lies posterior to the joint. The major veins in the head and the upper limbs merge to form the superior vena cava, which lies just posterior to the sternoclavicular joint. The esophagus is also in close proximity to this joint.

CLASSIFICATION

Sternoclavicular dislocations are classified by the direction of the dislocation in the coronal plane. According to these criteria, the clavicle lies anterior to the sternum in an anterior dislocation and posterior to the sternum in a posterior dislocation.

Department of Orthopaedics, Harborview Medical Center, University of Washington, Seattle, Washington 98104

ASSESSMENT

Physical Examination

The history of the trauma provides the key to making an accurate diagnosis. Blows to the posterior and lateral aspects of the shoulder are usually associated with anterior dislocations and those to the anterior aspect of the chest are associated with posterior injuries. Typical symptoms of both dislocations include swelling, pain, and tenderness on the medial aspect of the clavicle. In addition, posterior dislocations frequently demonstrate a palpable sulcus on the lateral edge of the involved side of the manubrium. Symptoms produced by visceral or vascular impingement with posterior dislocations include dysphagia, stridor, and upper-extremity venous distension secondary to central venous obstruction syndrome.

Radiographic Evaluation

Sternoclavicular dislocations are difficult to assess from plain radiographs. Anteroposterior radiographic views of the chest and the clavicle rarely reveal a definitive diagnosis. Comparison radiographs of the normal side may be useful for evaluating the relative articular position. Specialized 40° to 45° caudal cranial projections and Hobb's view may provide more detail.

Special Studies

The diagnosis is confirmed by CT scans taken in 1.5-mm

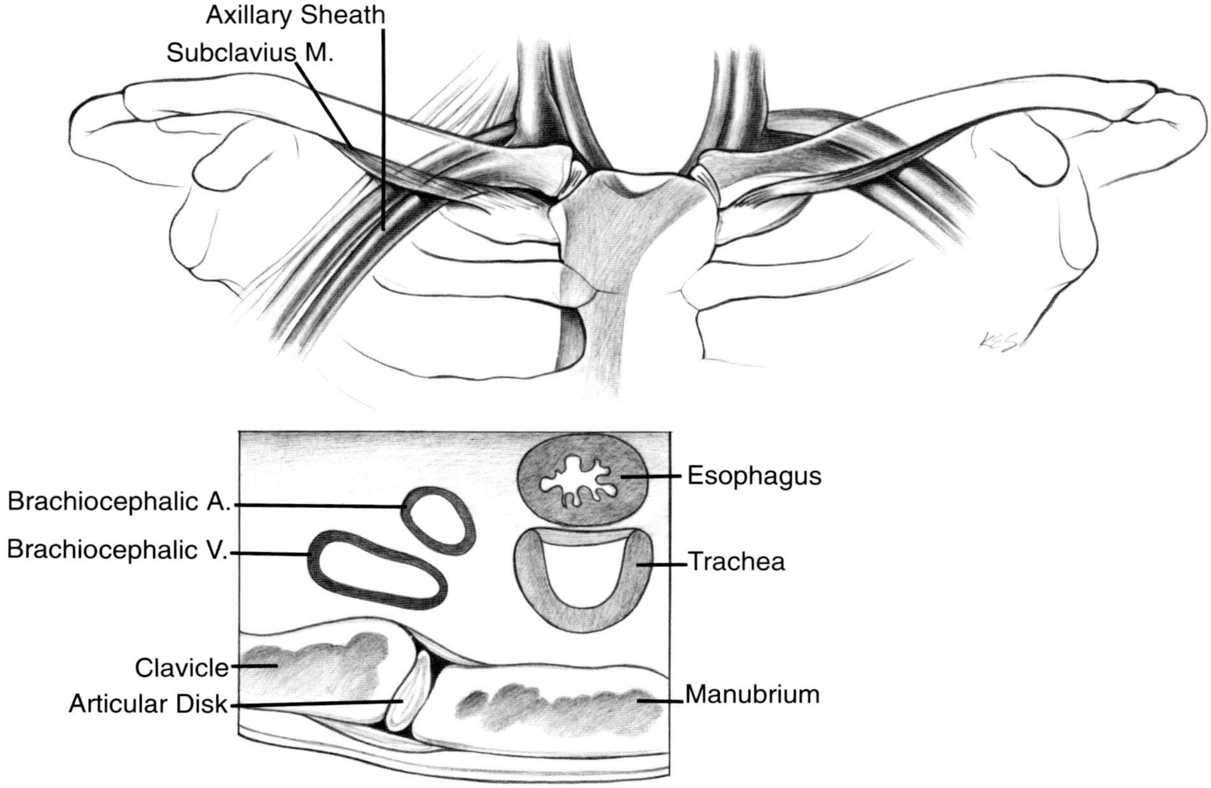

FIG. 1. Anatomy of the sternoclavicular joint. The close proximity to the esophagus and great vessels results in frequent compromise of these structures with posterior dislocations.

intervals through the sternoclavicular joint. The normal side is used for reference.

EMERGENT MANAGEMENT

Posterior dislocations rarely produce a superior vena caval syndrome that requires urgent reduction. Reduction is often achieved by placing a large roll between the scapulae and exerting posterior force simultaneously to the anterior aspects of both shoulders. Failing reduction with this maneuver, direct manipulation of the medial end of the clavicle with a towel clip may be required to extract it from the anterior mediastinum. This maneuver should not be performed without previous consultation with a thoracic surgeon.

DEFINITIVE MANAGEMENT

Most anterior dislocations do not require active treatment. Symptomatic posterior dislocations should be reduced in the operating room under general anesthesia, using the reduction maneuver described earlier. Failure of reduction by manipulation with pointed reduction forceps warrants open reduction, ideally with the assistance of a thoracic surgeon. Pins or screws are not ordinarily used for fixation because they tend to migrate. Instead, the clavicle is stabilized with synthetic suture passed through drill holes. The patient must wear a sling for 3 to 4 weeks. Rehabilitation begins with pendulum exercises and progresses to assisted forward flexion and external rotation. Strengthening exercises can be started at 6 postoperative weeks.

COMPLICATIONS

Posterior dislocations of the sternoclavicular joint may be associated with esophageal, laryngeal, or vena caval obstructions. Inappropriately treated, these conditions can produce serious or even fatal consequences. Stabilization with pins or screws may result in both visceral and vascular penetration from secondary migration.

SKELETALLY IMMATURE PATIENTS

Sternoclavicular injuries are rare in children. It should be remembered that injuries that appear to be sternoclavicular dislocations may, in fact, be medial physeal fractures. They are treated in the same manner as injuries in adults.

Clavicular Fractures

MECHANISMS OF INJURY

Clavicular fractures can result from direct blows or axial load applied to the upper limb. Commonly associated injuries include scapular fractures (articular and nonarticular), rib fractures, long-bone fractures of the ipsilateral upper limb, and scapulothoracic dissociations.

ANATOMIC CONSIDERATIONS

The anterosuperior surface of the clavicle is almost entirely subcutaneous. Therefore, clavicular fractures caused by high-energy mechanisms often result in open injuries. The subclavian vessels and the brachial plexus are located immediately adjacent to the clavicle (Fig. 2).

CLASSIFICATION

No widely accepted classification exists for clavicular fractures. Fractures are described by location and fracture pattern, the same terminology that is used for other long-bone fractures. However, there is some benefit in defining a subclassification for distal-third fractures. In general, these are separated into three categories:

1. Fractures that are located between the intact coracoclavicular and coracoacromial ligaments. These fractures are unlikely to undergo much displacement.
2. Fractures occurring just medial to the coracoclavicu-lar ligament attachments. These fracture maintain position of the distal end of the clavicle in continity with the acromioclavicular joint capsule, as well as the ligamentous attachments to the coracoid. In this situation, the pull of the sternocleidomastoid frequently elevates the medial portion of the clavicle significantly. In a variant of this pattern, the conoid ligament is attached to the medial fragment and is ruptured, and the trapezoid ligament remains intact to the distal segment. Displacement patterns are similar for these two injuries.
3. Fractures involving only the articular surface of the acromioclavicular joint without major ligamentous disruption. These injuries, frequently misdiagnosed as type I acromioclavicular joint injuries, often produce late degenerative changes.

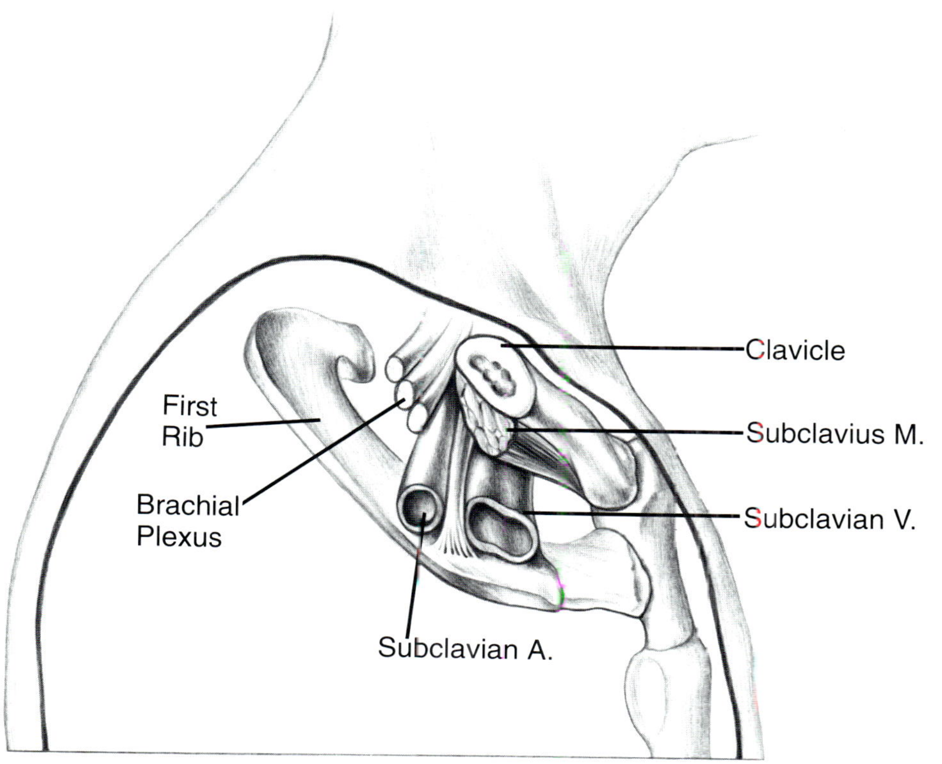

FIG. 2. Clavicular anatomic relationships. The subclavian vessels and brachial plexus are at risk with widely displaced and/or open clavicular fractures as well as with scapulothoracic dissociation.

ASSESSMENT

Physical Examination

Typical symptoms of a clavicular fracture include swelling, crepitus, and tenderness in the clavicular region. The patient is examined for associated vascular injuries and for a brachial plexus injury. The circulatory status is assessed by palpation of pulses, comparison arm blood pressures, ultrasound Doppler, and a careful sensory and motor evaluation. Fracture displacement or associated rib fractures may produce an ipsilateral pneumothorax. The lungs are examined by auscultation, and tenderness in the chest wall must be noted.

Radiographic Evaluation

Clavicular fractures are readily seen on most admitting chest radiographs. If these routine radiographs do not reveal sufficient information about the fracture to complete preoperative planning, a 20° caudal–cranial AP radiograph centered over both clavicles is indicated.

Special Studies

No special studies are required.

EMERGENT MANAGEMENT

Closed injuries require rapid evaluation of sensory, motor, and circulatory status and of pulmonary function. In open injuries, the wound should be evaluated noninvasively and covered with a sterile dressing.

DEFINITIVE MANAGEMENT

Most clavicular fractures are closed injuries and are adequately managed by closed techniques. After closed reduction, the ipsilateral arm is immobilized in a sling or a figure-8 bandage to provide comfort. Shoulder rehabilitation is begun with pendulum exercises 7 to 10 days after injury. This regimen may progress to assisted forward flexion and external rotation exercises as tolerated.

Indications for operative stabilization of midclavicular fractures include open fractures, vascular or neural injuries requiring repair, bilateral fractures, ipsilateral scapular or glenoid neck fractures, scapulothoracic dissociations (Fig. 3), flail chest, and nonunion. Significantly displaced closed fractures that show no evidence of union after 4 to 6 postop-

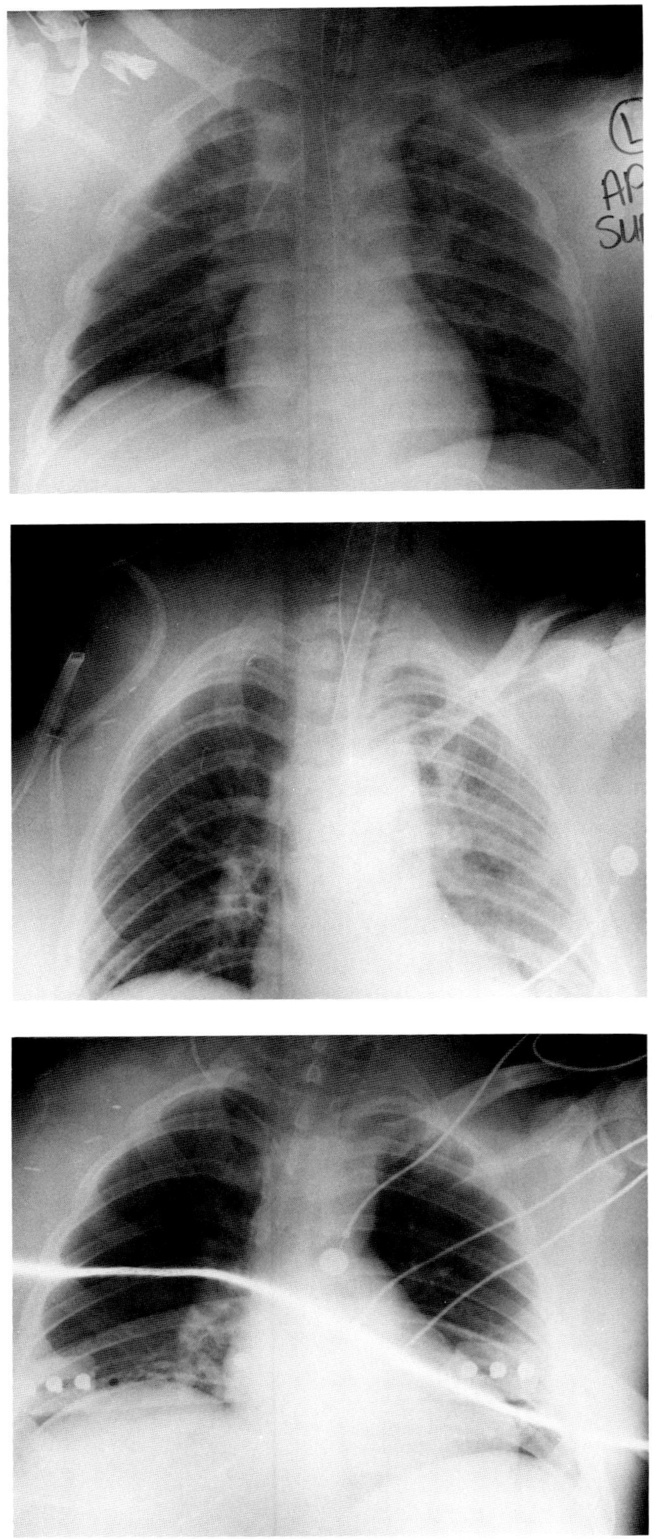

A

B

C

FIG. 3. Severe scapulothoracic dissociation in a 20-year-old motorcyclist. **A:** There is complete disruption of the axillary artery and vein, a brachial plexus avulsion, and disruption of the AC joint (type IV) and the sternoclavicular joint. Note wide displacement of the scapula. **B:** An open forequarter amputation is performed because of severe neurovascular injury. **C:** Following flap closure.

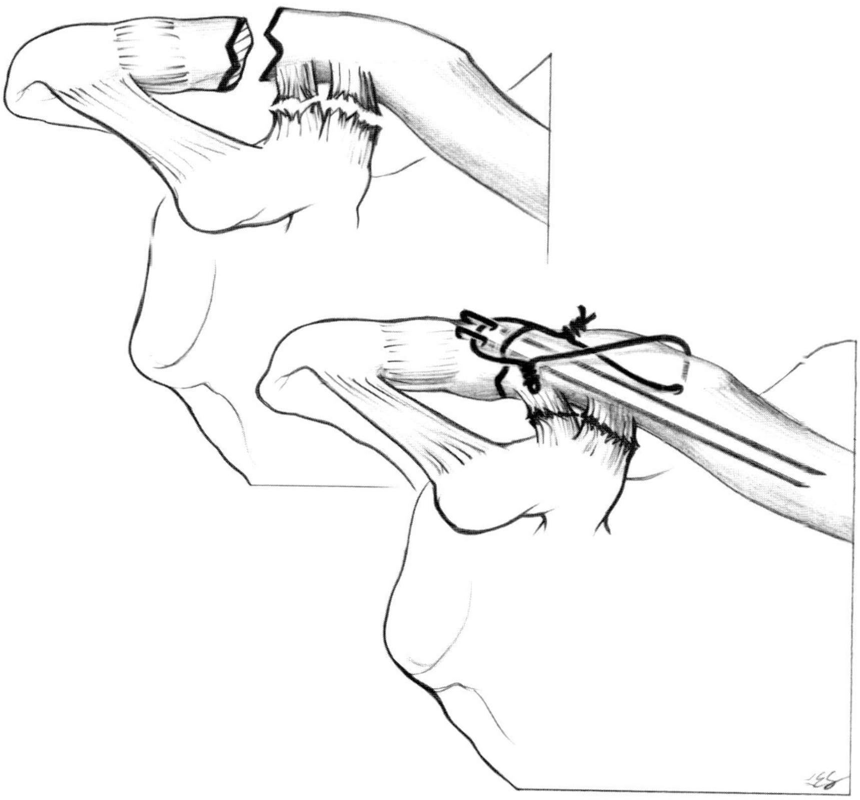

FIG. 4. Fixation of a distal third clavicle fracture. Fractures with marked displacement due to rupture of the coracoclavicular ligament complex are best repaired with a tension band wire. The Kirschner wires should be bent over to prevent migration.

erative months are stabilized surgically. Displaced fractures of the distal third of the clavicle with associated coracoclavicular ligament rupture are best managed with tension band wiring techniques (Fig. 4).

Radiographs are examined to determine the type of implant that is needed. An oblique incision is made over the fracture site and the fracture is stabilized with a 3.5-mm reconstruction plate and screws. Fractures that require a long time to heal (i.e., comminuted, open, or widely displaced fractures) require autogenous bone grafting to supplement the fixation. Alternatively, a Knowles pin can be passed from the lateral into the medial segment visualized from the fracture site, after predrilling from within the fracture laterally in the latent fragment. This technique works well in patients with prominent clavicles and in relatively simple fracture patterns. It also requires minimal soft-tissue stripping at the fracture site.

After stabilization, a shoulder immobilizer is used with concurrent deltoid isometric exercises for 2 to 3 weeks. Pendulum exercises and assisted ROM exercises are started between 3 and 6 postoperative weeks and active exercises are begun between 6 and 12 weeks. A strengthening program is initiated after 12 postoperative weeks.

COMPLICATIONS

Complications, including vascular injuries, nerve injuries, and pneumothorax, may be caused by the initial injury or by surgical intervention. They are managed by vascular or plexus repair, cable grafting, or tube thoracostomy. Clavicular nonunion is managed by the plate stabilization and bone grafting methods described earlier. The incidence of infection after a clavicular fracture is extremely low, but when it occurs the fixation device must be left in place (if it remains well fixed) until fracture union is secure. The fixation device is removed at that time and the local area is debrided.

SKELETALLY IMMATURE PATIENTS

Most clavicular fractures in children, including open fractures, are managed nonoperatively. Open reduction and fixation are warranted only in widely displaced, comminuted open fractures with bone loss. Immature periosteum promotes very rapid healing, and even low-grade open fractures can be managed by wound care and a shoulder immobilizer.

Acromioclavicular Injuries

MECHANISM OF INJURY

Acromioclavicular (AC) injuries are usually caused by application of axial loads to the superior aspect of the adducted shoulder. They commonly result from falls during athletic activities such as rugby, football, and skiing. The same mechanism combined with higher-energy trauma, such as falls from bicycles or motorcycles, produces more extensive injuries.

ANATOMIC CONSIDERATIONS

The AC joint is invested by a joint capsule that is thickened circumferentially. The conoid and trapezoid segments of the coracoclavicular ligaments stabilize the clavicle in relation to the scapula (Fig. 5).

CLASSIFICATION

Acromioclavicular injuries are graded by the severity of the associated soft-tissue injuries (Fig. 6). A grade I injury is a stable capsular injury. In a grade II injury the capsule is totally disrupted but the coracoclavicular ligaments remain partially intact; the coracoclavicular ligaments provide limited stability and the clavicle and the acromion maintain contact. Therefore, grade II injuries may be associated with severe degenerative arthritis of the AC joint. In grade III injuries, both the capsule and the coracoclavicular ligaments are completely disrupted and the clavicle is displaced superiorly. Grade III injuries are sometimes further subdivided into grade IV, in which the distal clavicle is displaced posteriorly and buttonholes through the trapezius muscle, and grade V, in which the clavicle is displaced superiorly by the pull of the sternocleidomastoid. Greater displacement occurs in grade V injuries because the deltoid and trapezius attachments to the distal clavicle are disrupted. Grade VI injuries are rare and are caused by an inferiorly directed force that produces a subcoracoid dislocation in which the distal end of the clavicle becomes entrapped posterior to the conjoined tendon of the biceps and coracobrachialis.

ASSESSMENT

Physical Examination

Swelling, ecchymosis, and tenderness are noted in the region of the AC joint; deformity is seen in severe injuries.

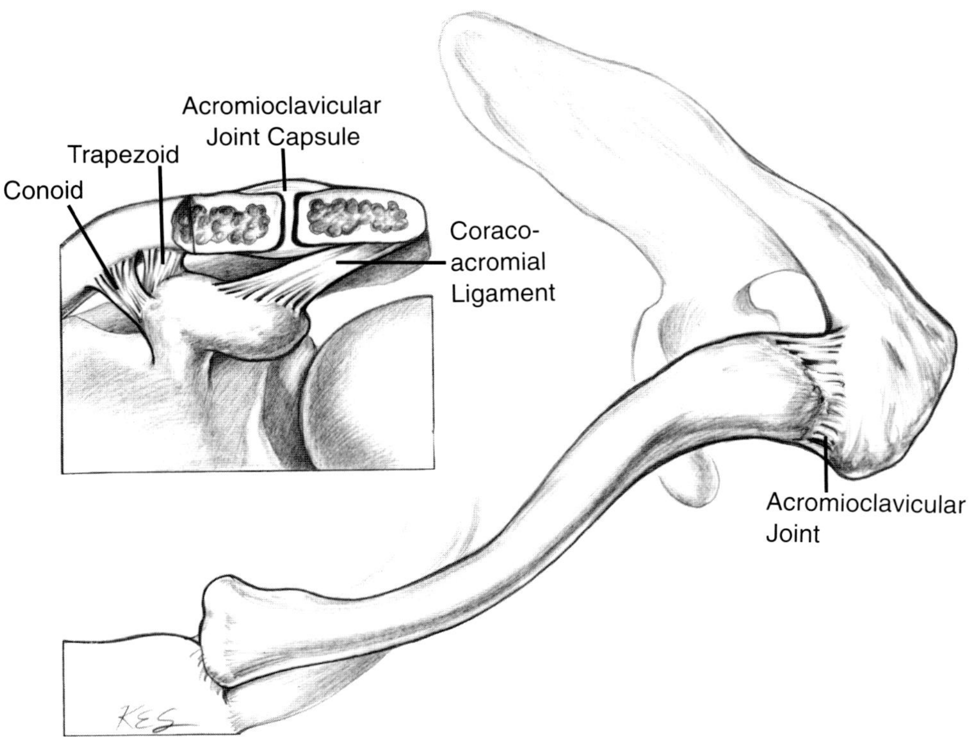

FIG. 5. Acromioclavicular joint anatomy. The relatively thick joint capsule and conoid and trapezoid portions of the coracoclavicular ligament stabilize this articulation.

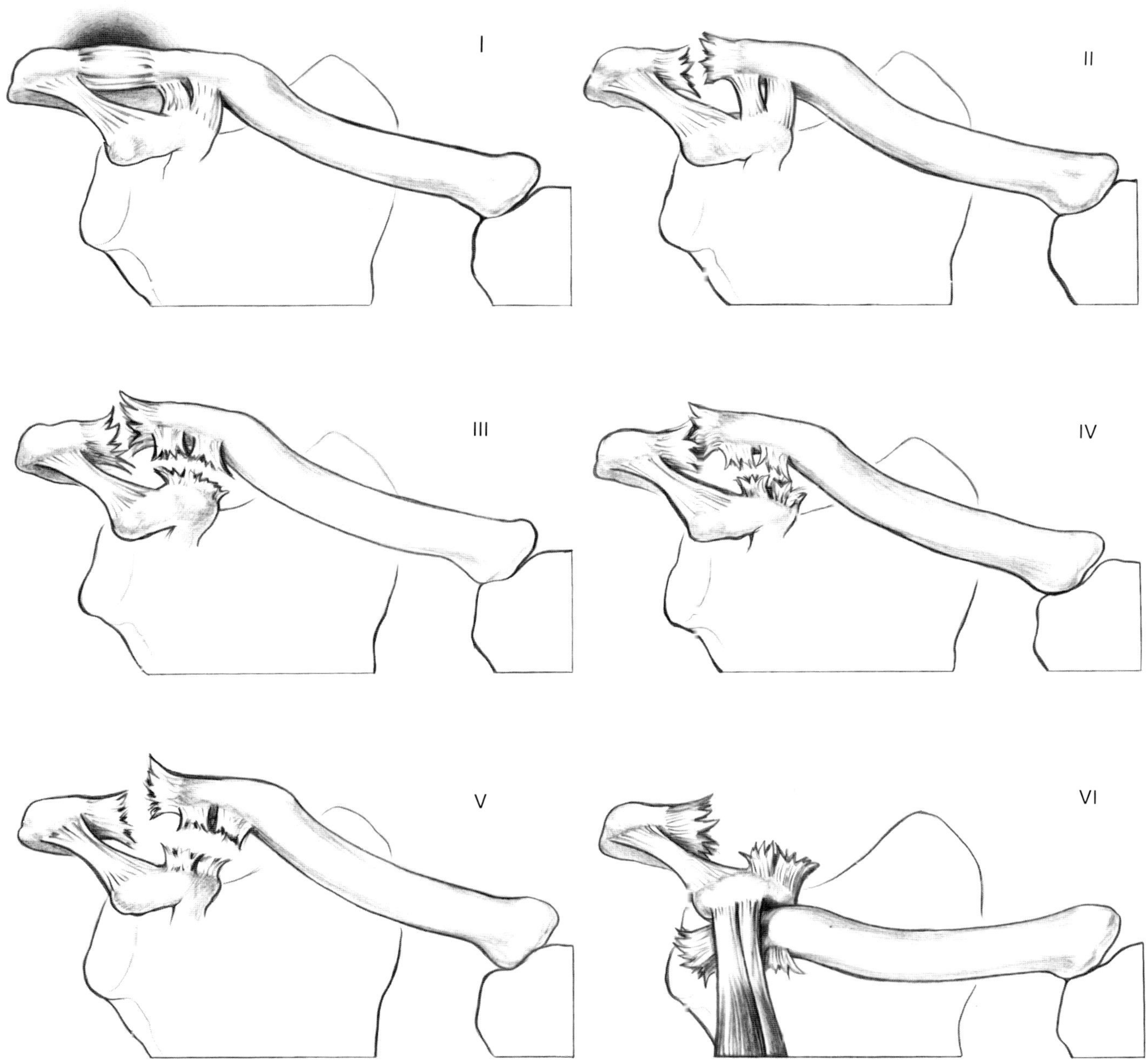

FIG. 6. Classification of acromioclavicular joint injuries (see text). Types IV, V, and VI all represent variants of type III, where both joint capsule and coracoclavicular ligament complex are completely disrupted.

Because the joint is subcutaneous, these findings are readily apparent even in obese patients. The focus of the physical examination is to document the sensory and motor status of the arm and to evaluate the arterial pulses by palpation or a Doppler examination. Injuries to the adjacent chest wall, the scapula, and the proximal extremity are noted.

Radiographic Evaluation

The admitting chest radiograph usually reveals the pertinent pathology. Complete assessment of the AC joint may require a comparison caudal–cranial projection of both clavicles on a single cassette. The distance between the superior

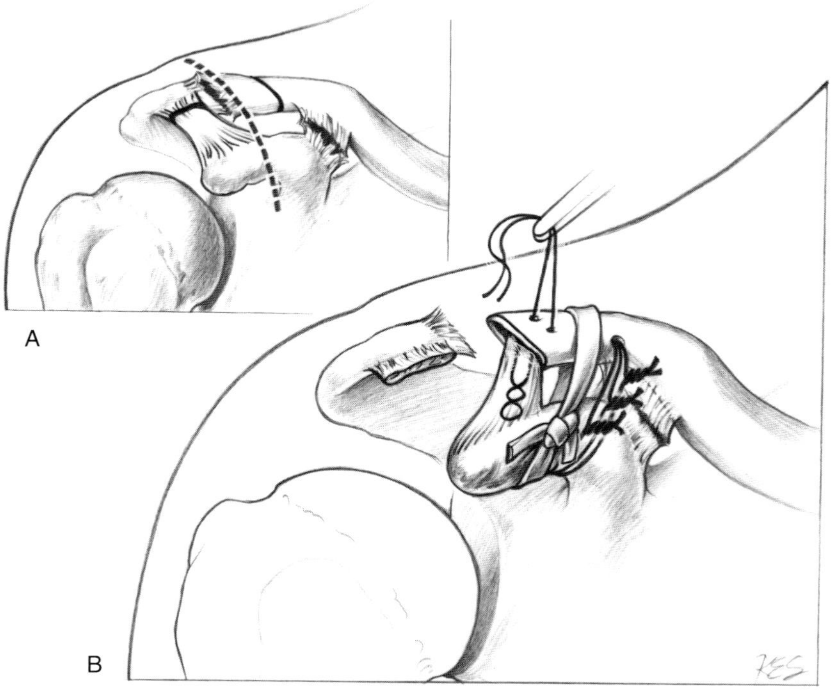

FIG. 7. The Weaver-Dunn reconstruction. **A:** Skin incision. **B:** A Mersilene tape is passed under the coracoid and around the clavicle. After resecting the distal 1.5 cm of clavicle, the coracoacromial ligament is sutured into the clavicle.

aspect of the coracoid process and the inferior aspect (cortical margin) of the clavicle is measured. This radiographic view is repeated as a stress radiograph with 10-lb weights held in each hand. Greater coracoclavicular distances correspond to progressive injury in the capsular and ligamentous structures.

Special Studies

No special studies are routinely indicated for evaluation of the AC joint.

EMERGENT MANAGEMENT

No emergent treatment is required. Associated axillary arterial injuries and severe chest trauma must be carefully ruled out because they require immediate exploration and repair.

DEFINITIVE MANAGEMENT

Most AC joint injuries are treated nonoperatively. However, the issues of cosmetic appearance and function should be discussed with the patient. A patient with a grade II injury must be informed that degenerative arthritis and subsequent pain may require a reconstructive procedure, such as a distal clavicular resection. For a grade III lesion, reconstruction might consist of distal clavicular resection with concurrent clavicular stabilization using the coracoacromial ligament (the Weaver–Dunn procedure) augmented by suture loops around the base of the coracoid (Fig. 7). Screws should not be inserted through the clavicle into the coracoid base.

Ipsilateral chest or periscapular injuries are indications for operative stabilization of grade III acromioclavicular disruptions. Isolated injuries can also be stabilized operatively for better cosmetic results. The operative approach for a grade III injury is determined by the degree of soft-tissue injury. A patient with a scapulothoracic dissociation is placed in the lateral decubitus position on a beanbag with the injured forequarter draped free. For all other injuries, the patient is positioned supine in the beach-chair position.

The subcoracoid-loop technique is preferred for isolated injuries. An oblique incision is made over the AC joint, running along Langer's lines. Three strands of #5 Tevdek suture are passed under the coracoid with curved or right-angled clamps. A hole is drilled through the middle of the clavicle in the dorsal–ventral plane and the three strands of suture are tied separately. This technique is preferred to passing the suture around the clavicle, which causes anterior translation of the clavicle and the AC joint when the sutures are tied. For delayed reconstruction of grade III AC joint separations, this procedure is combined with resection of the distal clavicle and transfer of the coracoacromial ligament (see Fig. 7).

Soft-tissue injuries, as well as associated scapular neck and multiple rib fractures, warrant AC joint reconstruction with a tension-band wiring technique. The reduction is held through the drill holes with two small-pointed reduction forceps, one on the acromial side of the joint and the other on the clavicular side. Two parallel 0.062-inch Kirschner wires are passed across the cephalad portion of the joint from the acromial tip. A loop of 18-gauge wire is then placed superior to the parallel wires in a figure-8 configuration through a sagittal drill hole in the distal clavicle. The wire loop is secured under the Kirschner wires, the tips of which have been bent 180°, cut short, and driven into the acromial tip. Bending the pins prevents complications with pin migration. Associated scapulothoracic dissociations that produce severe soft-tissue injuries may warrant more substantial fixation. In this case, a five- or six-hole 3.5-mm reconstruction plate is applied on the superior aspect of the acromion, the AC joint, and the clavicle with 3.5-mm cortical screws.

The postoperative care of AC joint injuries depends on the severity of injury sustained by the surrounding structures. In moderately severe injuries, a shoulder immobilizer is used for 3 or 4 weeks in conjunction with deltoid isometric exercises. Pendulum and assisted exercises can be started near the end of that time. Active ROM exercises are begun after 6 to 8 postoperative weeks. For severe soft-tissue or skeletal injuries, a shoulder immobilizer is used for 4 to 6 weeks, and the later stages of rehabilitation are delayed accordingly.

COMPLICATIONS

Symptomatic degenerative arthritis of the AC joint after a grade II injury is managed by resection of the distal clavicle. Symptomatic chronic instability of grade III injuries is managed by resection of the distal clavicle and reconstruction of the coracoclavicular ligament.

SKELETALLY IMMATURE PATIENTS

Acromioclavicular injuries in children are rare and usually do not require operative management. When soft-tissue injuries are severe, the figure-8 tension-band wiring technique is used, with appropriate Kirschner wires.

Scapular Fractures

MECHANISMS OF INJURY

Intraarticular and body fractures of the scapula usually result from high-energy trauma during vehicular, athletic, or industrial accidents. The mechanism may be a direct blow or an indirect impact transmitted through the humeral shaft. The only exception to these mechanisms is an anterior fracture of the glenoid lip, which may occur in association with a Bankart's lesion and which is produced by an anterior glenohumeral dislocation.

ANATOMIC CONSIDERATIONS

The scapula is a geometrically complex structure. The scapular body is almost completely encased in muscle. This soft-tissue envelope tends to dissipate energy during the injury, limiting fracture displacement and enhancing healing. The scapular spine and the acromion are contiguous structures. The glenoid surface is relatively flat, and the stability of the glenohumeral joint is dependent on the capsule and muscles. Three critical articulations are found in the scapula: the chest wall, the humeral head, and the clavicle. Because these articulations are important for normal function, operative management is considered when they are involved in the injury.

CLASSIFICATION

Scapular fractures are described anatomically to indicate involvement of the body, the neck, the glenoid, the coracoid, or the acromion. The fracture pattern may include several components. The magnitude and direction of displacement are carefully assessed and are included in the description of the injury.

ASSESSMENT

Physical Examination

Patients are carefully evaluated for head, chest, and abdominal injuries as well as for spinal and pelvic fractures. Contusion, swelling, and tenderness are noted in the area of the shoulder girdle. Associated AC injury and clavicular fracture are noted. Injury to the axillary artery is ruled out by palpation or ultrasound Doppler examination of the distal pulses and verification of symmetric arm blood pressures. In cooperative patients, the sensory distribution of the axillary and musculocutaneous nerves is evaluated by pinprick and light touch. The muscles of the shoulder girdle, particularly the deltoid, the supraspinous, the infraspinous, and the rhomboid muscles, are evaluated. A weak contraction can usually be palpated even with pain inhibition. Associated injury to the brachial plexus must be suspected and ruled out by distal muscle and sensory examinations.

Radiographic Evaluation

The radiographic series for shoulder trauma consists of AP, lateral, and axillary views of the scapula. These radiographs are used to direct operative treatment and to indicate any additional diagnostic studies for complex injury patterns, particularly those involving the glenoid.

Special Studies

Arteriography is required when an axillary arterial injury is suspected. Computerized tomography scans are necessary for adequate evaluation of most scapular fractures; a three-dimensional CT reconstruction is particularly useful. Neural injuries, most commonly neuropraxia, are monitored by electromyography.

EMERGENT MANAGEMENT

Scapular fractures typically occur as closed injuries and require no emergent management except in the presence of an associated vascular injury.

DEFINITIVE MANAGEMENT

Indications for operative management include displaced acromial fractures, which present a risk of nonunion with deltoid activity, displaced (>2–3 mm) glenoid fractures, severely displaced (>2 cm) body fractures, and glenoid neck fractures with ipsilateral clavicular fractures that result in significant medial displacement of the glenoid.

Acromial Fractures

Patients are positioned supine in the beach-chair position with a roll under the scapular body to elevate the injured shoulder from the operating table. The fracture is approached through a superior incision made in line with the acromion. Standard fixation consists of long 2.7-mm or 3.5-mm lag screws neutralized by a superior 2.7-mm or 3.5-mm reconstruction plate acting as a tension band.

Glenoid Fractures

The surgical approach is planned from the CT scan. (Fig. 8) Fractures in the anterior or coronal planes can be approached through a deltopectoral incision; fractures in the horizontal plane or those associated with scapular body or acromial fractures are best approached from a posterior (Judet) exposure (1). For this approach, patients are positioned laterally with the injured shoulder and the arm hanging free. A beanbag is placed under the chest to stabilize the thorax. Articular reduction is done through the muscle interval between the infraspinous and supraspinous muscles or between the infraspinous and the teres major muscles. In severely comminuted cases the infraspinous muscle, and sometimes the supraspinous muscle, can be detached medially and reflected on the suprascapular nerve to allow access to the joint. The joint surface is fixed internally with 3.5-mm or 2.7-mm lag screws. When fracture fragments include a portion of the lateral border of the scapula or when the glenoid neck is fractured, one-third tubular or 3.5-mm or 2.7-mm reconstruction plates are used. Fractures located along the spine are also fixed with these implants.

Fractures of the ipsilateral scapular neck and the clavicular shaft mandate stabilization of the clavicle to indirectly reduce the neck. Early motion is enhanced, and a separate posterior approach is not required because healing is rapid in this area.

Scapular Body Fractures

Surgery is rarely indicated for fractures in the scapular body. An exception is made for grossly displaced fractures of the lateral or medial borders (seen on the transscapular lateral radiograph) which hinder scapulothoracic gliding. The positioning of the patient, the implants, and the approach are the same as those for glenoid fractures. Because areas of the scapula are paper-thin, adequate fixation can be obtained only on the medial and lateral borders and along the scapular spine.

Deltoid isometric exercises are started immediately after surgery. A shoulder immobilizer is used until the wound is healed, and pendulum exercises and assisted ROM exercises are initiated at that time. Active ROM is begun between 4 and 6 postoperative weeks, and strengthening exercises are begun between 6 and 8 weeks.

COMPLICATIONS

The major complication, loss of motion in the scapulothoracic or glenohumeral joints, can be avoided by intense therapy and patient education. Because the scapula is surrounded by muscle, infection and nonunion are rare. Injury to the suprascapular and axillary nerves is avoided by visualization of the nerves during the surgical approach.

SKELETALLY IMMATURE PATIENTS

Scapular injuries are rare in children. An os acromiale should not be mistaken for an acromial fracture. Glenoid fractures in adolescents are managed in the same manner as fractures in adults. Acromial fractures are stabilized by small-fragment implants or by a tension-band wiring technique with supplemental Kirschner wires. The ends of the Kirschner wires are bent at the tips to prevent migration. Shoulder spica casting is appropriate for very young children and does not lead to shoulder stiffness.

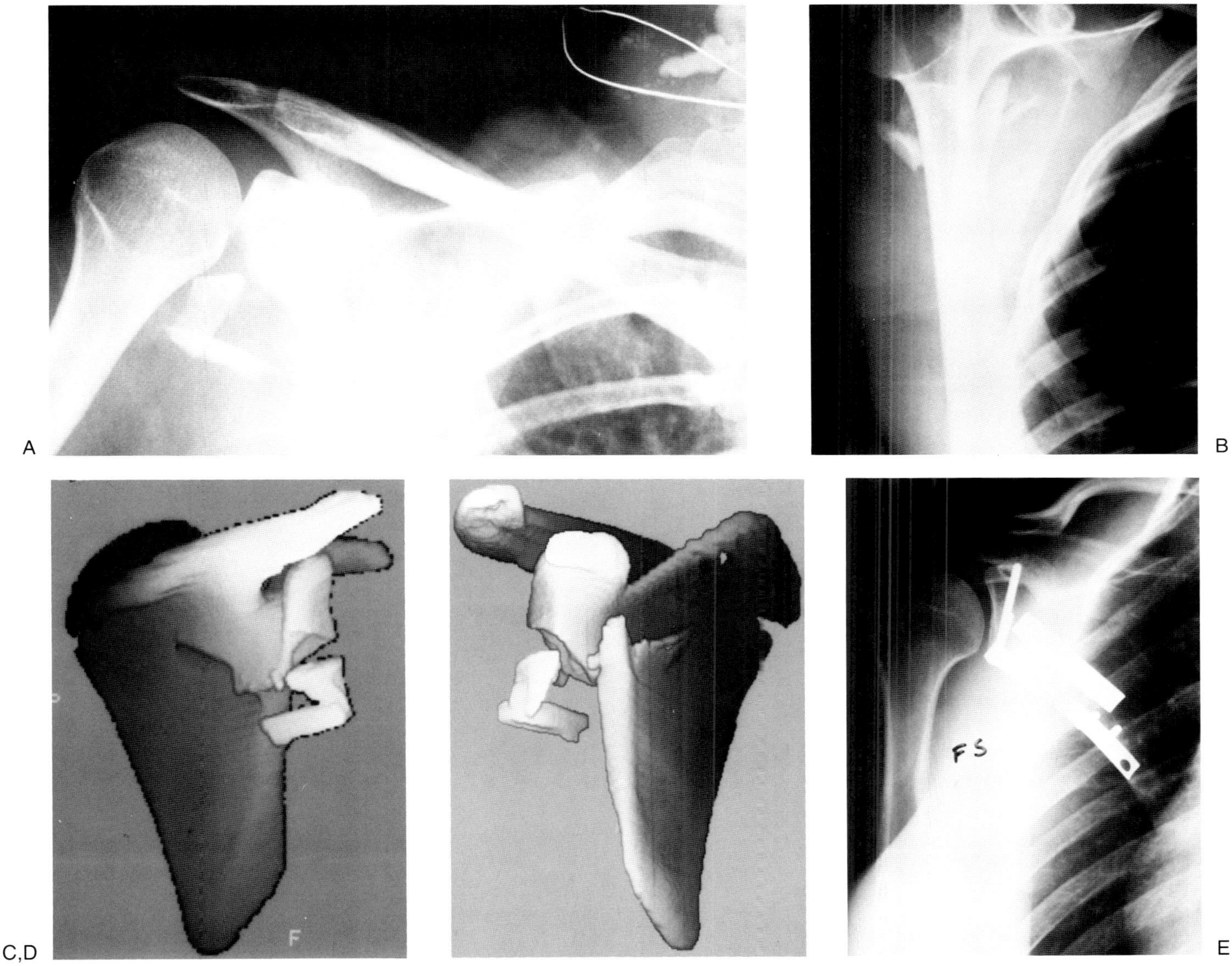

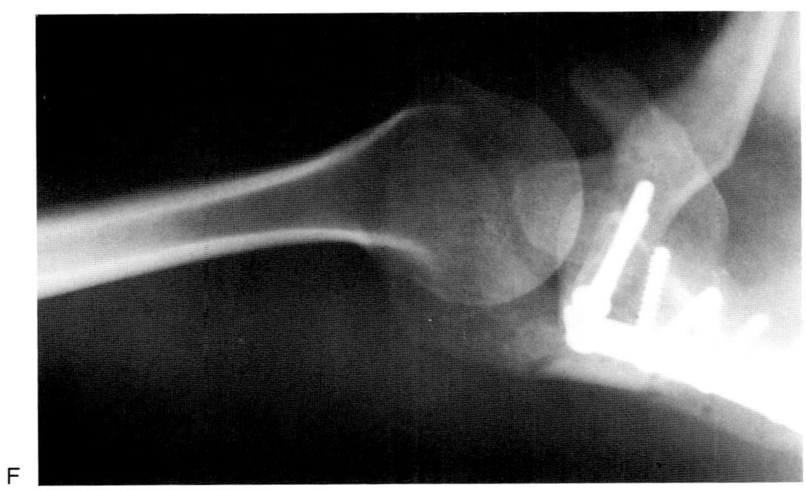

FIG. 8. A–D: Management of a displaced glenoid fracture. Plain radiographs and 3-D CT reconstruction of glenoid fracture also show typical scapular body involvement. **E,F:** Postoperative views show anatomic restoration via posterior (Judet) approach.

Glenohumeral Dislocations

MECHANISMS OF INJURY

Anterior glenohumeral dislocations are usually caused by excessive abduction and external rotation, a common position in sports. Elderly patients may sustain associated axillary arterial injuries and brachial plexus palsy. Common associated injuries in young patients include neuropraxic injuries to the axillary, radial, or musculocutaneous nerves. Posterior glenohumeral dislocations may result from marked internal rotation due to seizure, electrocution or, rarely, from a direct blow. Fractures of the tuberosities can occur with either mechanism.

ANATOMIC CONSIDERATIONS

The glenoid surface is flat and slightly concave. The glenoid labrum, the joint capsule, and the surrounding muscles provide joint stability.

CLASSIFICATION

These dislocations are most accurately described as anterior or posterior, according to the direction of the humeral head displacement. Inferior dislocations may occur but are uncommon.

ASSESSMENT

Physical Examination

A patient with an anterior glenohumeral dislocation complains of significant discomfort and usually holds the injured arm adducted against the side. A palpable or visible deformity may be present. Both active and passive ROM are limited. The circulatory status is evaluated by palpation of the distal pulses and by ultrasound Doppler. Next, a complete sensory examination is conducted, with particular attention paid to the status of the axillary, musculocutaneous, and radial nerves and the muscles they innervate. Although the motor examination may be limited by pain, muscle contractions can usually be palpated. This examination is repeated after reduction.

Radiographic Evaluation

The shoulder trauma series, consisting of AP, lateral, and axillary radiographs of the scapula, is obtained. Assistance is required to hold the arm in position for the axillary view, but this view does not require wide abduction to be useful. Careful evaluation is critical to discover associated, but often subtle, nondisplaced humeral neck fractures.

Special Studies

Posterior dislocations can be ruled out by a CT scan of the shoulder when reduction is difficult or unsuccessful and when associated tuberosity fractures exist. Arteriography or later EMG is required for associated arterial or neural injuries.

EMERGENT MANAGEMENT

In most cases, closed reduction is performed in the emergency department after the physical examination is completed. A surgical neck fracture should not be reduced closed without adequate anesthesia. Relaxation and analgesia are provided by 20 ml of intraarticular lidocaine (1% without epinephrine) injected inferiorly off the tip of the acromion. The extended arm is held in slight abduction and is pulled with linear traction and axillary bedsheet countertraction. Alternatively, the prone method of Stimson can be used. Posterior dislocations are reduced by application of gentle traction in abduction by an assistant while the surgeon lifts the humeral head back into the glenoid with thumb pressure. This maneuver consists of gentle anterior and lateral traction on the arm accompanied by manual medial rotation of the scapula.

DEFINITIVE MANAGEMENT

First-time shoulder dislocations occurring without associated tuberosity fractures are treated by closed reduction and shoulder rehabilitation. When the dislocation is associated with a surgical neck fracture, reduction is performed under general anesthesia. Operative management is reserved for significantly displaced anterior glenoid rim fractures. Open reduction of anterior glenoid rim fractures is done through a deltopectoral approach, with the patient in the beach-chair position. After closed reduction, a shoulder immobilizer is applied for comfort. Deltoid isometric exercises are begun immediately; strengthening exercises for internal and external rotation are begun between 2 and 3 postoperative weeks. Internal rotation exercises are vital to restore function after an anterior dislocation; external rotation exercises are important for posterior dislocations.

COMPLICATIONS

Recurrence of an anterior dislocation is the most common complication and is a significant problem when the initial dislocation occurs at an early age. Half of all initial anterior dislocations occuring in patients who are 18 years old or younger at the time of the first dislocation become recurrent. Posterior dislocations are often misdiagnosed; an impacted posterior shoulder dislocation must be suspected when the shoulder cannot be rotated externally to a neutral position. Recurrent dislocations are strongly suspected in patients with histories of seizure or alcohol withdrawal.

SKELETALLY IMMATURE PATIENTS

Shoulder dislocations are rare in children, but when they occur they are treated in the same way as dislocations in adults.

Proximal Humeral Fractures

MECHANISMS OF INJURY

Proximal humeral fractures can be caused by a fall onto an abducted arm or by high-energy trauma with the arm abducted or held to the side. Dislocations are common associated injuries, although fractures from falls often occur as isolated injuries in elderly patients. Neuropraxias involving the axillary, musculocutaneous, and radial nerves may occur. Axillary arterial injuries may occur with high-energy mechanisms.

ANATOMIC CONSIDERATIONS

The stability of the proximal humerus depends on capsular and muscular integrity. The tuberosities are the tendinous insertions. When these injuries are managed, the proximity of the axillary artery and the brachial plexus must be kept in mind. The blood supply to the humeral head has direct implications for treatment (Fig. 9).

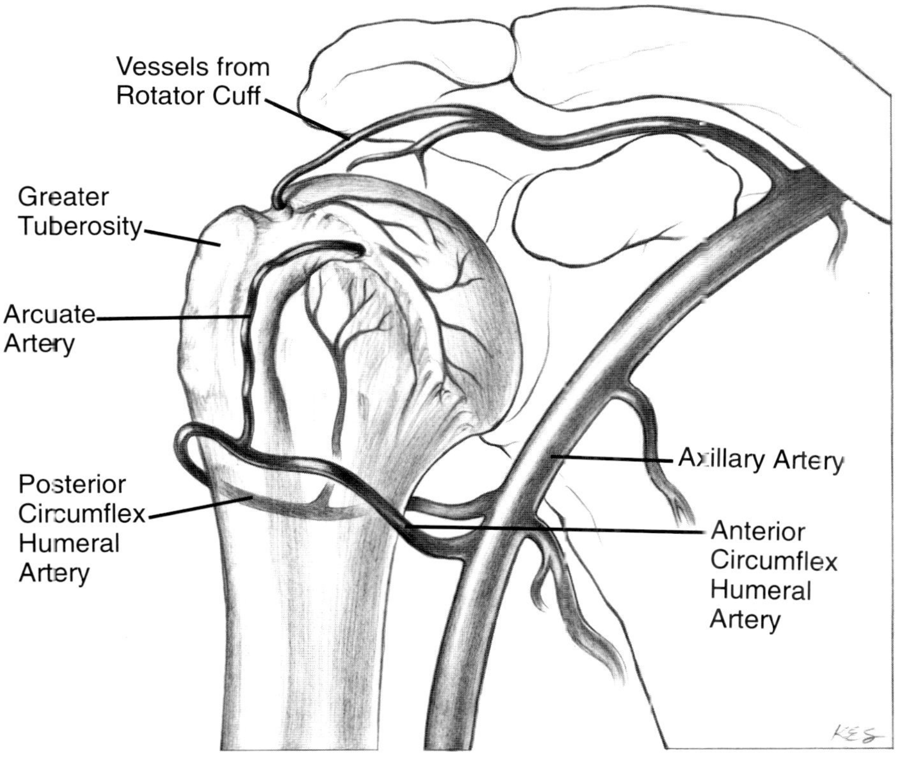

FIG. 9. Proximal humeral vascular anatomy. The anterior humeral circumflex artery supplies the majority of the humeral head.

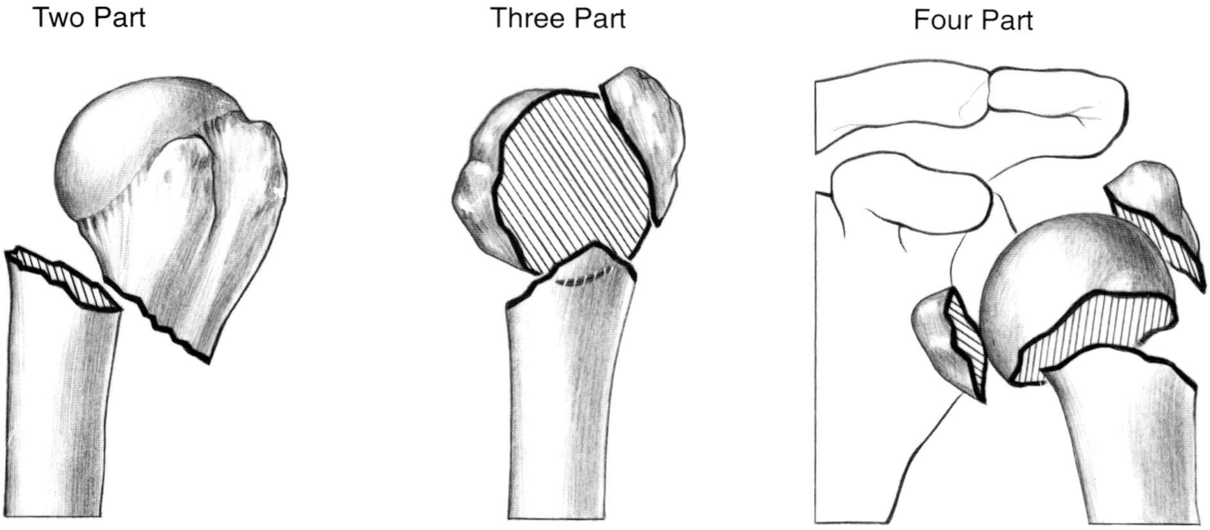

FIG. 10. Neer's proximal humerus fracture classification. Fragments are identified as the shaft, humeral head, and greater and lesser tuberosities. Displacement of greater than 1 cm must exist in this system.

CLASSIFICATION

The Neer classification is the most widely used, and despite its shortcomings, is useful in directing management (Fig. 10). This scheme is based on displacement of the four primary fragments: the greater and lesser tuberosities, the head, and the shaft.

ASSESSMENT

Physical Examination

Shoulder deformity, contusion, swelling, and tenderness occur to a variable degree. The circulatory status is carefully assessed by palpation of the distal pulses and by ultrasound Doppler. A sensory examination (light touch and pinprick) is used to test all peripheral distributions. Motor testing is limited by pain, but palpation of the muscle bellies can provide useful information.

Radiographic Evaluation

Anteroposterior, lateral, and axillary radiographic views of the scapula are obtained. An axillary view is taken with the patient's arm supported to ensure adequate abduction.

EMERGENT MANAGEMENT

Almost all proximal humeral fractures occur as closed injuries. Arteriography and emergent repair are essential after diagnosis of an axillary arterial injury.

DEFINITIVE MANAGEMENT

Isolated, minimally displaced (< 1 cm), or impacted fractures of the surgical neck or the greater tuberosity are treated nonoperatively. Anterior or posterior fracture–dislocations are treated by urgent closed reduction under general anesthesia.

The indications for operative management include unstable surgical neck fractures (no contact between the fracture fragments) and partially unstable fractures (partial contact) with associated ipsilateral upper-extremity injuries. Tuberosity fractures that remain displaced less than 5 mm after closed reduction should be carefully observed for secondary displacement. Anatomic restoration is most important in young patients who have sustained a traumatic injury to the ipsilateral limb. Displaced (>5 mm) three- and four-part fractures in young patients should be fixed percutaneously or internally. Widely displaced (>1 cm) three- and four-part fractures in elderly patients may warrant prosthetic hemiarthroplasty with wiring of the tuberosities.

Two- and Three-Part Fractures

Percutaneous pinning of two-part fractures and some three-part fractures is done with fluoroscopy, with the patient in the beach-chair position (2). After closed reduction and a fluoroscopic examination, the surgical neck fracture can be fixed with two or three 2.5-mm terminally threaded Schanz screws directed into the head fragment from an area 2 to 3 cm proximal to the deltoid tubercle (Fig. 11). In some cases percutaneous screw placement can add stability to this construct. A third or fourth pin is added anteriorly in a fan configuration to stabilize a lesser tuberosity fragment in four-part fractures. For greater tuberosity fractures, the final pin can be placed just lateral to the acromion process.

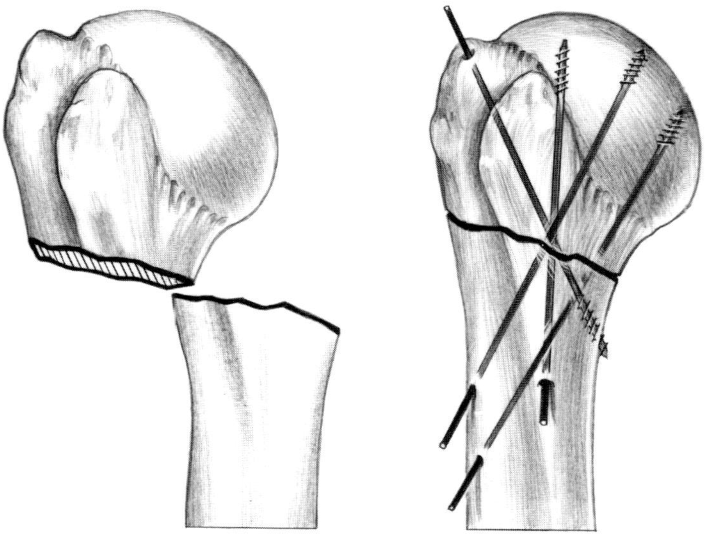

FIG. 11. Percutaneous fixation of a two-part proximal humeral fracture. Three planes receive 2.5-mm Schanz pins.

Three- and Four-Part Fractures

Open reduction of displaced three- and four-part fractures is also performed with the patient lying supine in the beach-chair position. A standard deltoid–pectoral incision is used and every effort is made to minimize soft-tissue stripping at the fracture sites. With this in mind, exposure can be minimized by use of percutaneous Schanz or standardcortical screws, particularly for tuberosity fractures (Fig. 12) Screws and washers are usually preferred for head and greater tuberosity fragments in young patients. In highly unstable fracture patterns, plates can be applied directly over the remaining soft tissues. Older patients with softer bone may require fixation with tension-band wiring techniques.

Anterior and Posterior Fracture–Dislocations

Anterior and posterior fracture–dislocations are managed whenever possible by closed reduction and pinning with the patient supine. In young patients, open reduction for common anterior fracture–dislocations is done through a deltopectoral incision with a tension-band wiring technique or screws and washers. A critical aspect of the operation is to move the greater tuberosity far enough laterally to allow external rotation. Patients over 60 years of age, especially those with compromised bone density, may require a hemiarthroplasty with wiring or suturing of the tuberosities.

Postoperative Care

Pendulum exercises are started with physical therapy supervision 2 to 3 days after injury whenever stability permits. Patients progress to assisted exercises after 3 weeks and gradually to strengthening exercises at 6 weeks. The percutaneous Schanz screws are removed from the greater tuberosity after 2 or 3 weeks pins that stabilize the surgical neck are removed at 4 to 6 weeks. After fixation with tension-band wires, screws, or small plates, a shoulder immobilizer is added for comfort. Pendulum exercises and deltoid isometric exercises are begun on the second or third postoperative day and assisted exercises are begun at 2 weeks. ROM exercises and a strengthening program are begun gradually at 6 postoperative weeks.

COMPLICATIONS

The incidence of pin-tract inflammation and entrance-point soft-tissue infection after percutaneous pinning is 20% to 30%. These infections can be treated successfully with oral antibiotics and local pin-tract care. The offending pin can be removed early at 3 weeks. Nonunion of a surgical neck fracture that was treated nonoperatively is rare but when it occurs can be salvaged by bone grafting and tension-band wiring. Malunion of the tuberosity is common after ORIF of three- and four-part fractures and results in limited ROM. In young patients this complication can be successfully managed by osteotomy and reapplication of the fixation device. In young adults, hemiarthroplasty is performed for degeneration of the joint surface of the humeral head. Symptomatic avascular necrosis can be managed by hemiarthroplasty.

SKELETALLY IMMATURE PATIENTS

Proximal humeral fractures in children usually occur in the surgical neck and rarely involve the tuberosities. Children's bones have a remarkable ability to remodel, and for this reason a significant amount of deformity is acceptable in pedi-

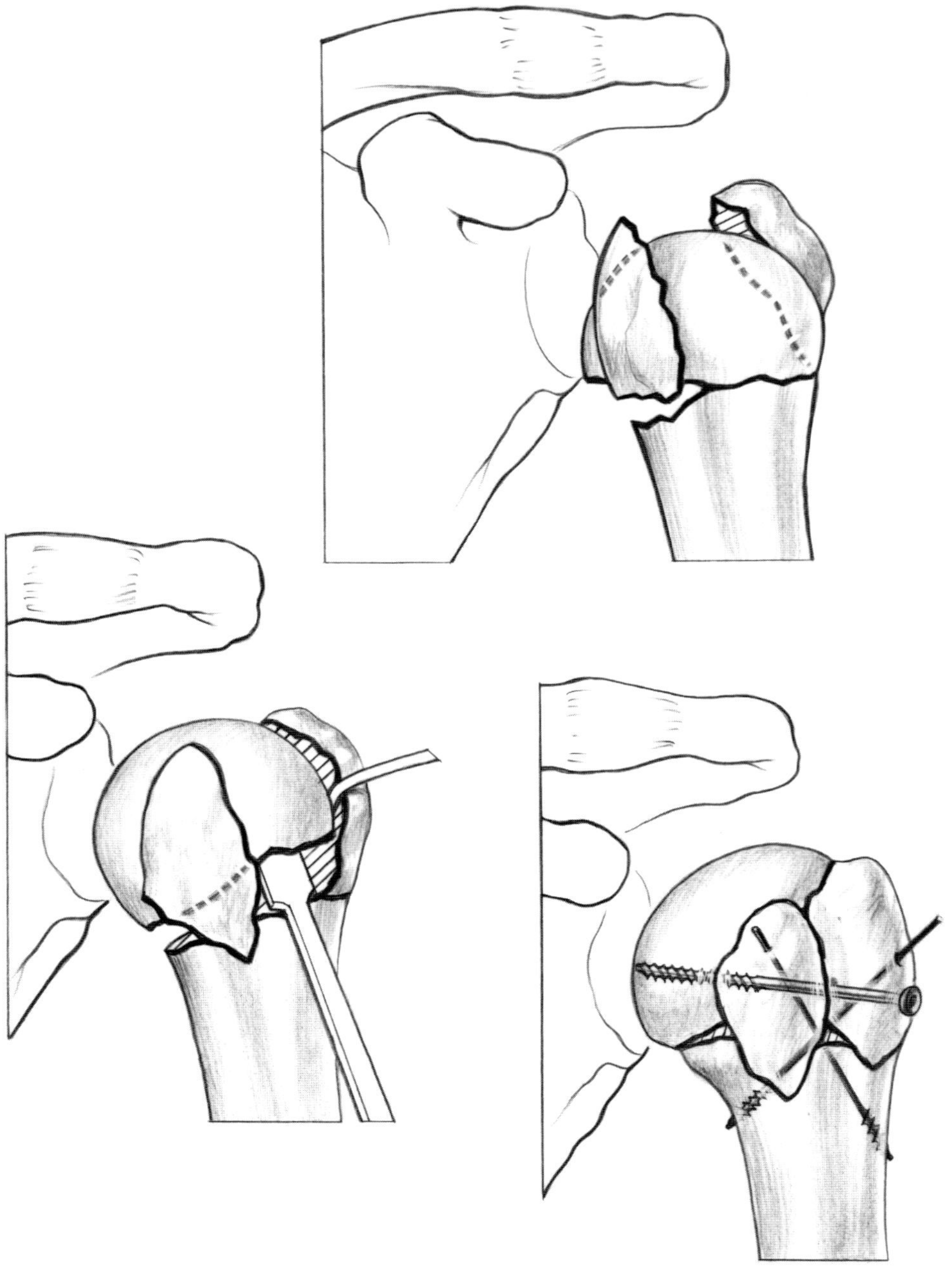

FIG. 12. Internal fixation of a four-part proximal humeral fracture. The emphasis must be placed on preserving soft-tissue attachments to all four fragments during the reduction. Minimal internal fixation with small fragment cancellous or cortical lag screws can be accompanied by percutaneous application of 2.5-mm Schanz pins.

atric fractures. Varus up to 45° is acceptable in children and can be treated without closed reduction. Fracture–dislocations with greater deformity warrant closed reduction and shoulder spica casting. Internal fixation is rarely indicated in children under the age of 10 years, but percutaneous fixation can be considered in children over the age of 10 years with significantly displaced fractures.

REFERENCES

1. Hardegger FH, Simpson LA, Weber BG. The operative treatment of scapular fractures. *J Bone Joint Surg* 1984;66B:725–31.
2. Jaberg H, Warner TJP, Jakob RP. Percutaneous stabilization of ustable fractures of the humerus. *J Bone Joint Surg* 1992;74A:508–15.

Orthopaedic Trauma Protocols, edited by
Sigvard T. Hansen, Jr., and Marc F. Swiontkowski,
Raven Press, Ltd., New York, ©1993.

CHAPTER 12

Humeral Shaft Fractures

M. Bradford Henley

MECHANISMS OF INJURY

Fractures of the humeral diaphysis commonly result from forces applied directly to the upper extremity. Although these fractures often occur as isolated injuries, sometimes they are a constituent element of multiple trauma. The mechanism of injury is usually a direct blow that fractures the humerus at the junction of its middle and distal thirds. The most common associated injury, radial nerve palsy, is seen in approximately 10% of patients with humeral shaft fractures.

ANATOMIC CONSIDERATIONS

The humeral shaft is surrounded by a thick, well-vascularized muscle cuff. The radial nerve and the deep brachial artery spiral around the middle and distal thirds of the humerus in the radial groove on the posterior side. The deltoid, coracobrachialis, brachialis, and triceps muscles attach into the humerus and help maintain fracture alignment during healing.

CLASSIFICATION

No universal classification system has been adopted for long-bone diaphyseal fractures, including humeral fractures. Humeral fractures are described as open or closed injuries and are further identified by the location and pattern of the fracture and by the degree of comminution (1). Alternatively, the AO classification for diaphyseal fractures can be used (Fig. 1) (2).

Department of Orthopaedics. Harborview Medical Center, University of Washington, Seattle, Washington 98104

ASSESSMENT

Physical Examination

A humeral fracture exhibits symptoms that are typical of all long-bone fractures. A thorough evaluation of radial, medial, musculocutaneous, and ulnar nerve functions must be performed on a patient who is awake and alert. The circulatory status is assessed by palpation or by Doppler examination.

Radiographic Evaluation

Anteroposterior and lateral radiographs of the humerus are obtained. These radiographs should visualize not only the humeral shaft but also the shoulder and the elbow joints. If open reduction and internal fixation (ORIF) is considered, the radiographs are scrutinized for nondisplaced fractures extending proximally or distally from the site of the injury.

Special Studies

No special studies are required.

EMERGENT MANAGEMENT

Closed reduction of a humeral shaft fracture is performed after adequate analgesia and relaxation have been obtained. After reduction, a U-shaped coaptation sugar-tong splint is applied to the humerus. The splint is applied from the axilla and is extended around the apex of the elbow and up the lateral aspect of the arm over the deltoid. A collar and cuff are applied to hold the elbow in a gravity-dependent position for maintenance of fracture alignment. Active motion is encouraged in the wrist and the hand during healing.

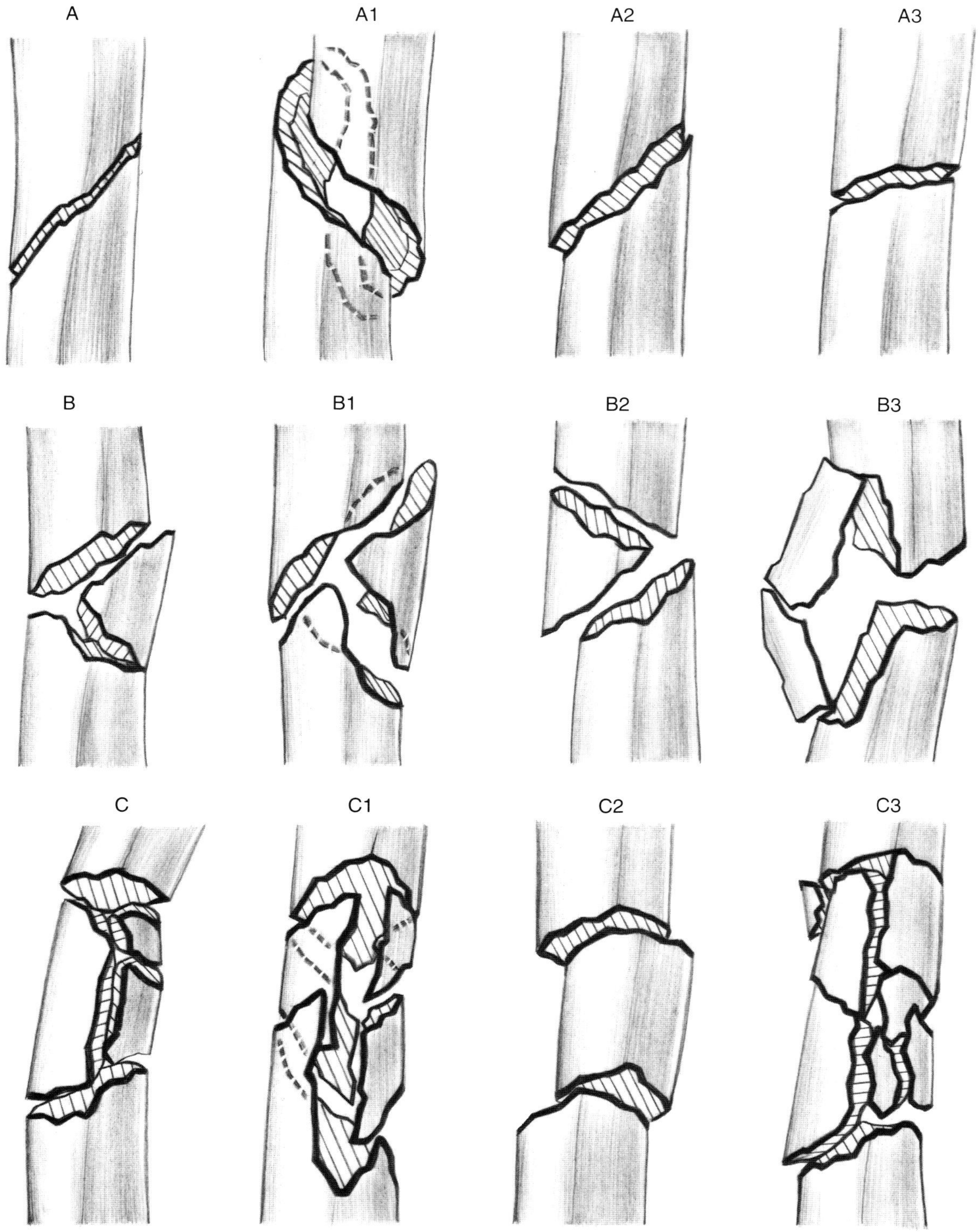

FIG. 1. The AO classification used for humeral shaft fractures. **A:** Simple fracture. A1—Spiral fracture. A2—Oblique fracture (≤30°). A3—Transverse fracture (≥30°). **B:** Wedge fracture. B1—Spiral wedge fracture. B2—Bending wedge fracture. B3—Fragmented wedge fracture. **C:** Complex fracture. C1—Spiral fracture with comminution. C2—Segmental fracture. C3—Irregular fracture with comminution.

A,B 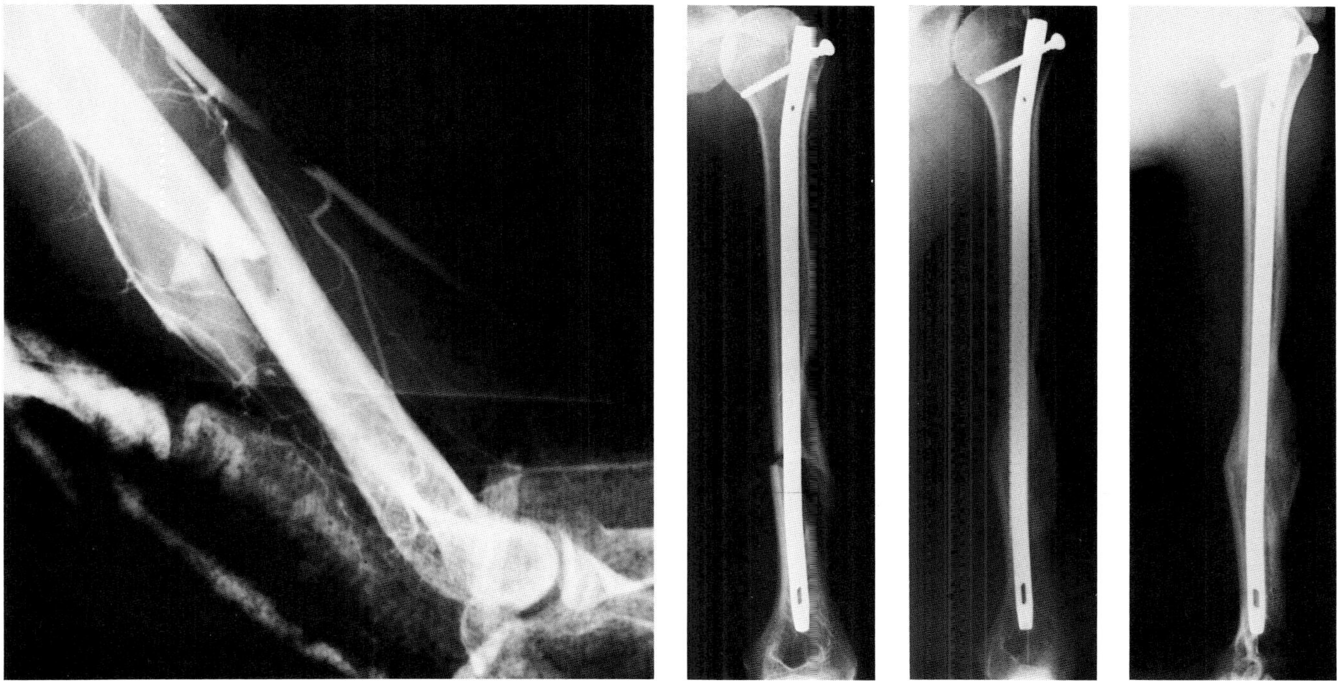 C,D

FIG. 2. A: Preoperative lateral angiographic film of a patient with a comminuted humeral shaft fracture and concomitant brachial artery laceration. **B:** Prior to stabilization of the humerus with an intramedullary nail, the arterial injury was bypassed with a shunt. Definitive arterial repair was performed after fracture fixation. **C,D:** AP lateral films of healed and remodeled fracture.

DEFINITIVE MANAGEMENT

Most humeral fractures are managed nonoperatively. The coaptation splint is removed 10 to 14 days postinjury, after acute pain and edema have subsided, and a humeral fracture orthosis is applied (3). An abduction pillow can be used to prevent varus angulation. Active and active-assisted range-of-motion exercises for the shoulder and elbow are added to the therapeutic regimen. An arm sling can be used intermittently for additional comfort.

Indications for osteosynthesis of humeral fractures are limited. They include open fractures, progressive neurologic deficits, multiple injuries, bilateral humeral fractures, floating elbow lesions, and failure of nonoperative methods to obtain or maintain satisfactory reduction. Initial exploration is not indicated for closed fractures with associated primary radial nerve lesions.

The choice of implant depends on the extent of soft-tissue injury, the fracture pattern, the location of the fracture, and bone quality. In general, all open fractures are treated by plating. Grade IIIB open injuries may warrant external fixation and autogenous bone grafting. Intramedullary fixation is an alternative when the patient must use the upper extremities for weight-bearing during ambulation and for patients with extensive segments of comminuted or osteoporotic bone. Until recently, the bundled nails of Hackethal (4) or small-diameter Enders nails were the best choices of intramedullary hardware for humeral fractures (5). At present, we are gaining experience with 6-mm, 7-mm, and 8-mm interlocking nails (Fig. 2).

An anterolateral approach is used for plating proximal and middle third diaphyseal humeral fractures. The patient is positioned supine on the operating table with a pad under the affected shoulder and the arm draped free. The fracture is exposed through a standard deltopectoral incision extending down the anterolateral aspect of the arm (6). The radial nerve must be identified and protected during all approaches by locating the nerve between the brachioradialis and brachialis muscles near the lateral intermuscular septum and tracing it in proximally. Fractures in the distal third of the humerus are stabilized through a posterior approach, with the patient lying prone or in a lateral decubitus position.

A diaphyseal fracture is stabilized with a broad 4.5-mm dynamic compression plate (DCP) or a limited contact–dynamic compression plate (LC-DCP) (Fig. 3). In a proximal or middle third fracture, the plate is applied to the anterolateral aspect of the humerus (Fig. 4); in a distal third fracture, it is applied directly to the posterior side (Fig. 5). Stacked intramedullary nails of Hackethal or Enders are inserted by a retrograde technique through a unicortical window above the olecranon fossa. Unreamed, locked intramedullary nails are inserted antegrade through the proximal humerus. Both nailing techniques are performed on a radiolucent table with fluoroscopy.

After stabilization, the arm is immobilized in a plaster splint with the elbow in approximately 90° of flexion. Active

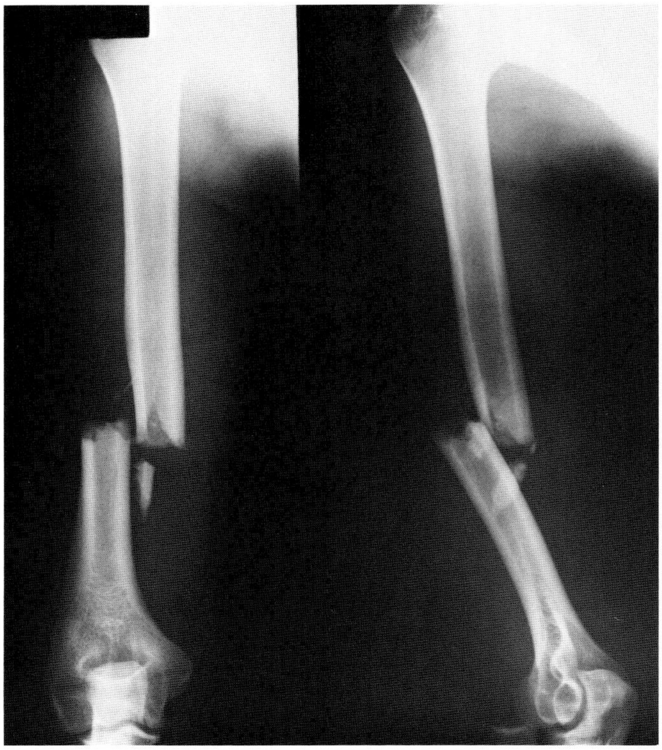

A

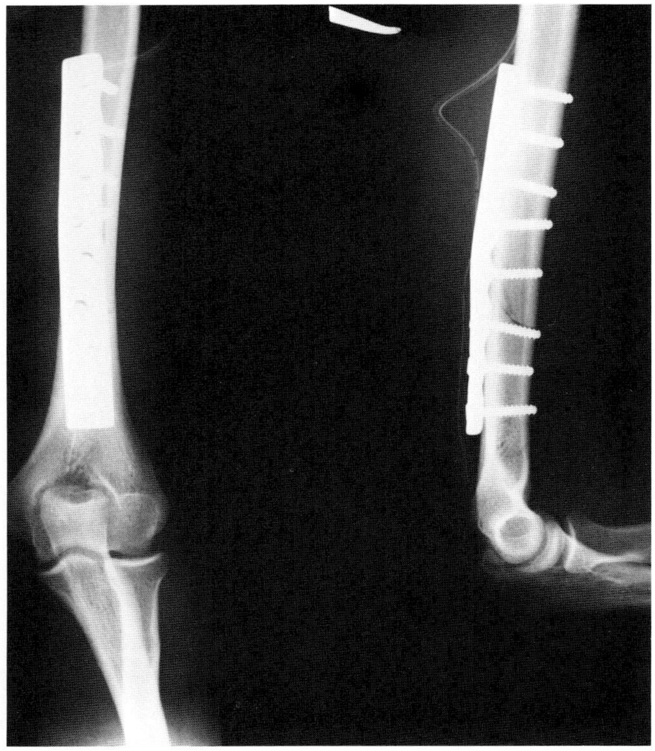

B

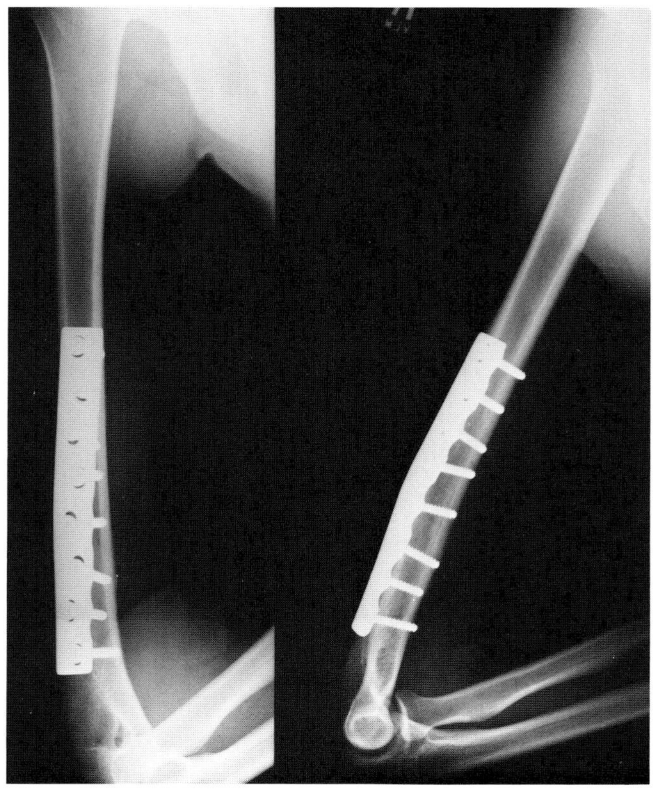

C

FIG. 3. AP (**A**) and lateral (**B**) radiographs of a transverse humeral diaphyseal fracture treated with a contoured 8-hole LC-DCP (intraoperative film). The fracture has completely united with restoration of full elbow flexion (**C**).

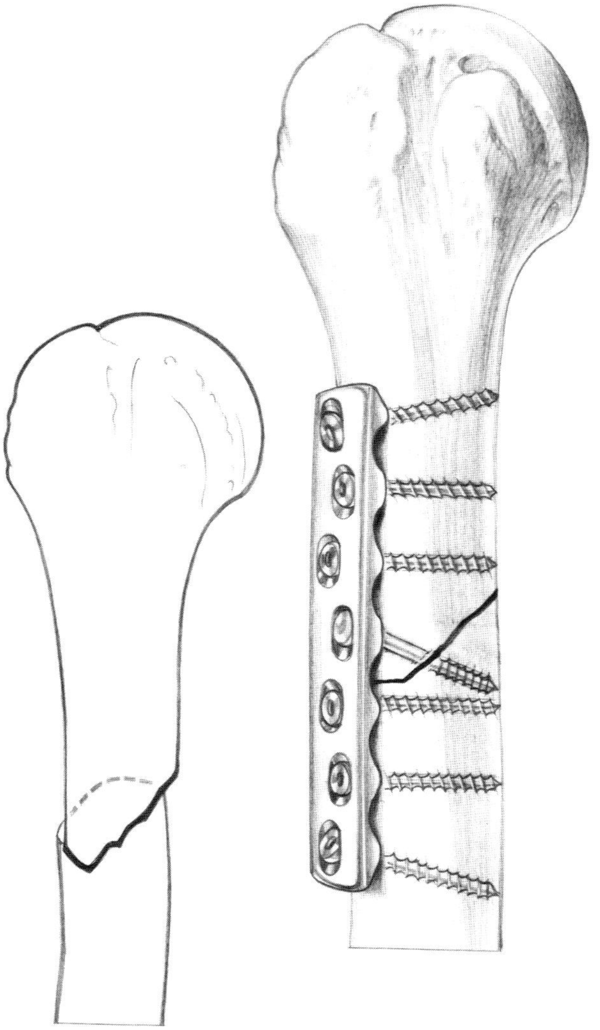

A,B

FIG. 4. A,B: Anterolateral plate placement for oblique fracture of the proximal middle third of the humerus.

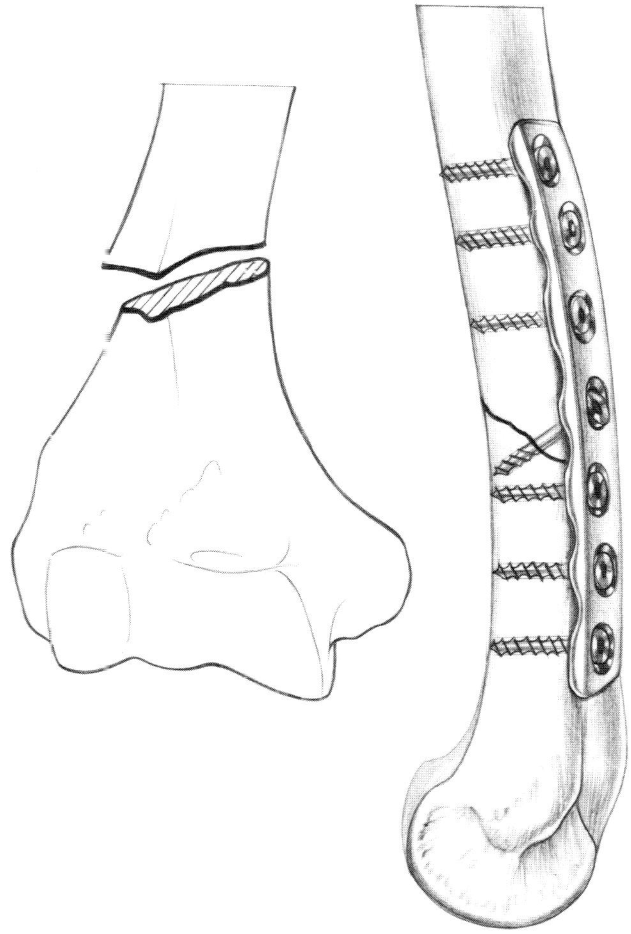

A,B

FIG. 5. A,B: Posterior LC-DCP application for a distal third fracture.

mobilization is begun after the suction drains have been removed and the wound is stable. In plated fractures, resitive exercises are not instituted until evidence of fracture union is seen radiographically, usually between 10 and 12 weeks posttrauma.

COMPLICATIONS

Delayed union or nonunion of a diaphyseal fracture can occur in transverse or short oblique fractures that have been distracted by dependent traction. Soft-tissue interposition may prevent healing of displaced long oblique or spiral fractures. In these instances, plating and autogenous bone grafting is indicated after the radial nerve has been identified. Primary radial nerve palsy is not an indication for surgical exploration. Progressive radial nerve palsy, especially palsy that develops after fracture manipulation, should be explored and the fracture should be stabilized.

SKELETALLY IMMATURE PATIENTS

Almost all humeral shaft fractures in children are treated nonoperatively unless the soft tissues have been severely injured. The treatment principles for severe open fractures in children are the same as those for adults.

REFERENCES

1. American Academy of Orthopaedic Surgeons. Trauma: femur. In: *Orthopaedic Knowledge Update 2 Home Study Syllabus.* Park Ridge, IL: 1987;370–1.
2. Müller ME, Allgöwer M, Schneider R, et al. *Manual of internal fixation: techniques recommendation by the AO Group.* 3rd ed. New York: Springer-Verlag; 1990: 126–7.
3. Sarmiento A, Kinman PB, Galvin EG, Schmitt RH, Phillips JG. Functional bracing of fractures of the shaft of the humerus. *J Bone Joint Surg* 1977;59A:596–601.
4. Chapman JR, Henley MB. Hackethal intramedullary nailing for the treatment of humeral fractures. *Techn Orthop* 1988;3:88–93.
5. Burmback RJ, Bosse MJ, Poka A, et al. Intramedullary stabilization of humeral shaft fractures in patients with multiple trauma. *J Bone Joint Surg* 1986;68A:960–70.
6. Rüedi T, von Hochstetter AHC, Schlumpf R. *Surgical approaches for internal fixation.* Berlin: Springer-Verlag; 1984:21–7.

Orthopaedic Trauma Protocols, edited by
Sigvard T. Hansen, Jr., and Marc F. Swiontkowski,
Raven Press, Ltd., New York, © 1993.

Chapter 13

Elbow

M. Bradford Henley

Elbow Dislocations

MECHANISMS OF INJURY

The most common mechanism of elbow dislocation is a fall on an outstretched hand with the elbow incompletely extended, the arm abducted, and the forearm supinated. Although elbow dislocation usually occurs as an isolated injury, associated injuries may include disruptions of the medial or lateral collateral ligaments and fractures of the coronoid process, the capitellum, the trochlea, or the radial head. The median and ulnar nerves and, rarely, the brachial artery may also be involved.

ANATOMIC CONSIDERATIONS

The elbow joint comprises three articulations: the humeroulnar, the humeroradial, and the radioulnar. The osseous contours of these articulations and their ligaments contribute to joint stability. The well-developed medial collateral ligament consists of anterior oblique, posterior oblique, and transverse oblique components. Of these three ligaments, the anterior oblique is the most important. On the lateral side, the lateral collateral complex ligament merges with the annular ligament and stabilizes varus stresses.

CLASSIFICATION

Stimson's directional classification is the most widely used grading system for elbow dislocations (Table 1) (1). Most elbow dislocations (80–90%) are posterior or posterolateral. Anterior, lateral, medial, and divergent dislocations are less common.

Department of Orthopaedics. Harborview Medical Center, University of Washington, Seattle, Washington 98104

Table 1. *Classification of adult elbow dislocations*

Both the radius and ulna	Posterior • Lateral • Medial Medial Lateral Divergent • Anteroposterior • Mediolateral
Ulna alone	Anterior Posterior
Radius alone	Anterior Posterior Lateral

(After Stimson LA. *A practical treatise on fractures and dislocations.* New York: Lea & Febiger; 1910:638. Used with permission.)

ASSESSMENT

Physical Examination

Simultaneous dislocations of the radius and the ulna are usually evident on clinical examination. A patient with this deformity typically exhibits a prominent olecranon, a shortened forearm, and a moderately extended elbow. A neurovascular examination must be performed before and after reduction.

Radiographic Evaluation

Anteroposterior and lateral radiographic views are obtained based on the position of the humerus and are scrutinized for associated fractures. Associated coronoid fractures have been classified by Regan and Morrey (Fig. 1) (2). Dis-

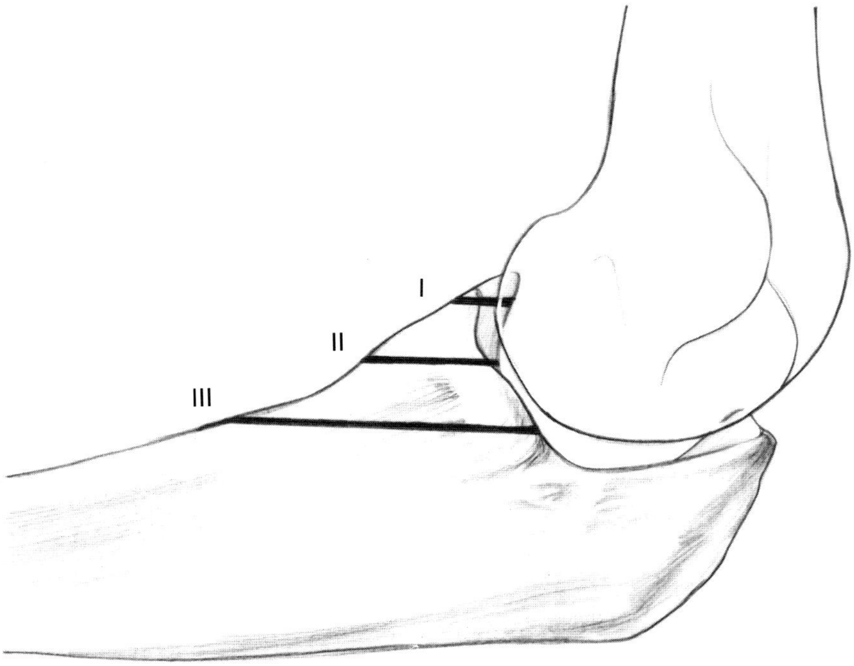

FIG. 1. In Morrey's classification, coronoid fractures are classified by the size of the fracture fragment.

locations with associated disruptions of the proximal radioulnar joint, as seen in divergent dislocations, are indicative of injury to the interosseous membrane. In this case, radiographs of the distal radioulnar joint should be made to identify a possible subluxation. Postreduction radiographs are taken to assess joint congruity and to detect osteochondral fractures and ligament avulsions. Stress radiographs taken with the elbow in approximately 30° of flexion are useful for assessing ligamentous disruptions and joint stability.

Special Studies

No special studies are required.

EMERGENT MANAGEMENT

An atraumatic closed reduction requires complete muscle relaxation. If complete relaxation cannot be achieved with sedation, a general anesthetic should be considered. Manual traction is applied in line with the supinated forearm while the upper arm is stabilized by an assistant. Hyperextension of the elbow must be avoided to prevent additional soft-tissue injury. Joint stability, absence of crepitus, and full range of motion are confirmed after reduction.

DEFINITIVE MANAGEMENT

The definitive treatment of an elbow dislocation is determined after the stability of the elbow and its range of motion are evaluated. When the elbow is stable in pronation and retains full range of motion, it is reduced closed and immobilized in a posterior splint in 90° of pronation (3). Early active flexion exercises are begun 3 to 5 days after reduction, using the splint to block extension. Range of motion is increased after 10 to 14 days. A flexion contracture of 5° to 15° is expected after healing.

Indications for arthrotomy include an unstable reduction, crepitus from interposition of cartilage or bone, any mechanical hindrance to full range of motion, an asymmetric joint space on postreduction radiographs, and associated osteochondral fractures. Simultaneous primary ligamentous repair is recommended for all these conditions. Before arthrotomy, varus and valgus stress tests are conducted under general anesthesia to reassess joint stability.

A lateral arthrotomy is performed through a Kocher incision. Irrigation and debridement and primary repairs of the lateral collateral, annular, and lateral humeroulnar ligaments, and the common origin of the forearm extensor muscle are performed through this incision. Nonabsorbable braided suture is passed through drill holes to secure the ends of the ligaments to bone at their epicondylar origins. A medial incision is indicated in addition to a lateral incision for correction of valgus instability. The ulnar nerve must be identified and protected. The flexor–pronator muscle group is usually avulsed from its origin or torn in the proximal portion of the muscle. Primary repair of the medial collateral ligament, especially the anterior oblique portion, is performed before reattachment or repair of the overlying flexor–pronator muscle group (Fig. 2) (4,5). Large coronoid fractures should be stabilized by lag screws (Fig. 3).

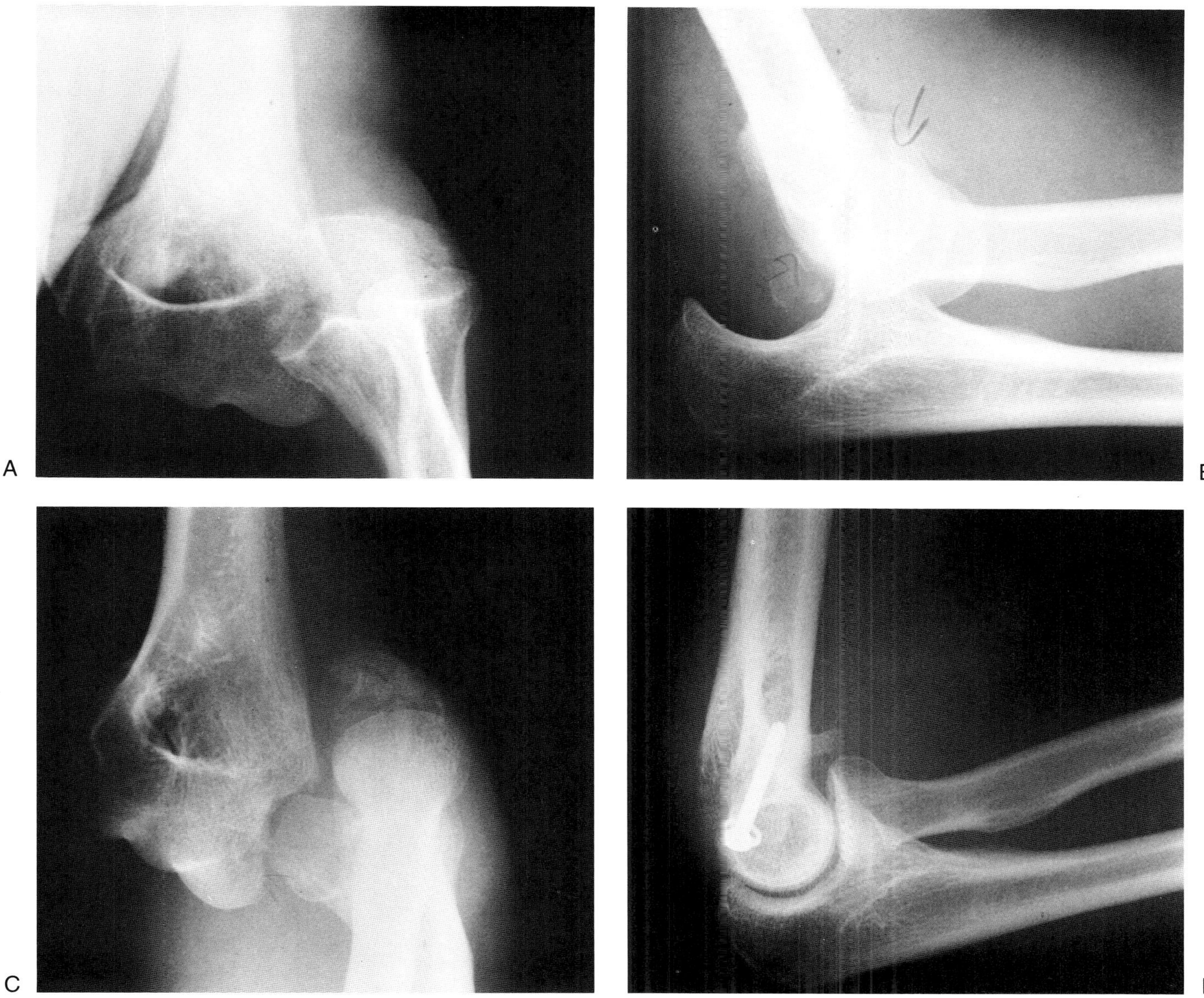

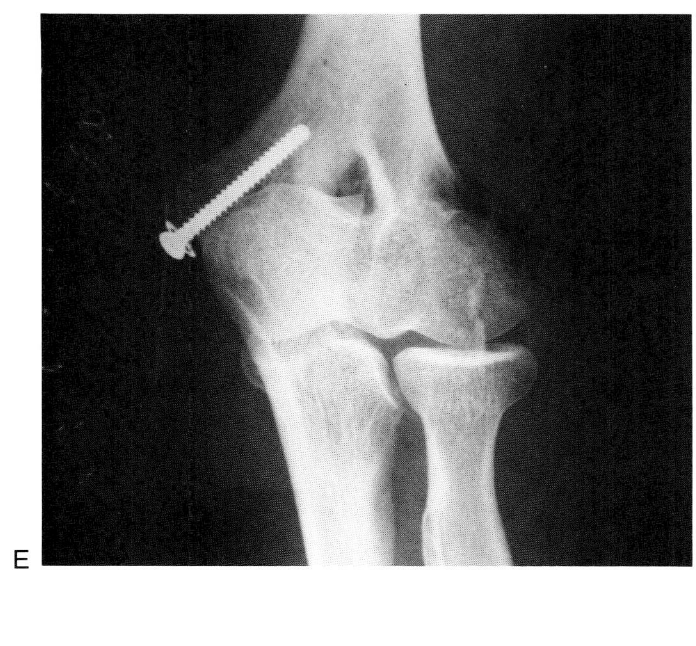

FIG. 2. A–C: Three radiographic views of a 50-year-old male's posterolateral elbow dislocation with associated medial epicondylar avulsion fracture and impaction fracture of lateral condyle. **D,E:** Medial and lateral arthrotomies were performed for debridement and ligament repairs. The avulsion fracture was reattached with a soft-tissue washer and 3.5 mm screw.

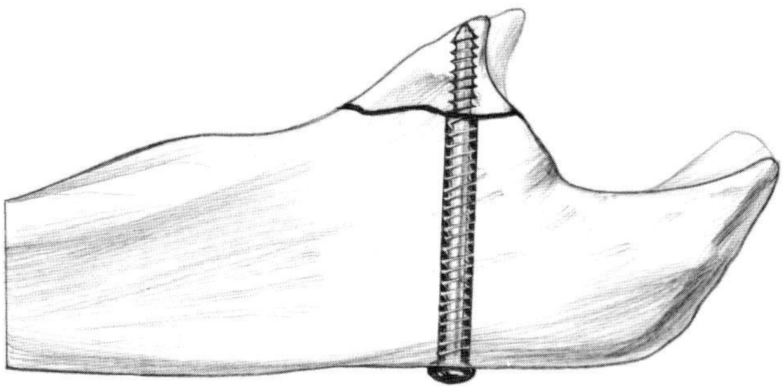

FIG. 3. A type II coronoid fracture is stabilized with a 3.5-mm lag screw.

In dislocations that require arthrotomy and ligament repair, active flexion is delayed until the suction drains are removed. Operative repair allows full unprotected motion in the elbow joint immediately after reduction. A sling can be used intermittently for comfort during the first 7 to 10 postoperative days.

COMPLICATIONS

Surgical repair of the collateral ligaments and closed management of stable elbow fractures have identical long-term outcomes (2). With either method, less than 20° of elbow extension can be expected to be lost when motion is begun early during rehabilitation. High-energy injuries that damage the anterior capsule and the brachialis muscle are associated with heterotopic bone formation. Entrapment of the brachial artery is rare. The presence of circulatory embarrassment mandates immediate arthrotomy, reestablishment of blood flow, and decompression fasciotomy distal to the elbow joint. Similarly, neurologic deficit resulting from reduction is an indication for exploration.

SKELETALLY IMMATURE PATIENTS

Elbow dislocations in children usually involve an avulsion fracture of the medial epicondyle and can easily be mistaken for a physeal injury of the distal humerus. Single- or double-contrast arthrography is useful for distinguishing these injuries. In young children, closed reduction of an elbow dislocation should be performed under general anesthesia. A stable congruent reduction with full range of motion should be confirmed both clinically and radiographically. Postoperative treatment consists of immobilization in a long-arm cast for 2 to 3 weeks.

REFERENCES

1. Stimson LA. *A practical treatise on fractures and dislocations.* NewYork: Lea & Febiger; 1910:638.
2. Regan W, Morrey B. Fractures of the coronoid process of the ulna. *J Bone Joint Surg* 1989;71A:1348–54.
3. Josefsson PO, Gentz C-F, Johnell O, Wendeberg B. Surgical versus nonsurgical treatment of ligamentous injuries following dislocations of the elbow joint. *Clin Orthop* 1987;214:165–9.
4. Osborne G, Cotterill P. Recurrent dislocation of the elbow. *J Bone Joint Surg* 1966;48B:340–6.
5. Dürig M, Müller W, Rüedi TP, Gauer EF. The operative treatment of elbow dislocation in the adult. *J Bone Joint Surg* 1979;61A:239–44.

Distal Humeral Fractures

MECHANISMS OF INJURY

Extraarticular supracondylar fractures are usually extension injuries caused by a fall onto an outstretched hand. In contrast, intercondylar fractures are usually caused by high-energy injuries and often include open soft-tissue injuries. In addition to transcondylar or supracondylar fracture components, T-shaped intercondylar fractures often include dissociated condylar fragments. Proximal displacement of the condyles occurs as the biceps and triceps muscles contract and the forearm muscle origins rotate the condylar fragments towards each other.

ANATOMIC CONSIDERATIONS

The cylindrical diaphysis flattens posteriorly in its distal third and then diverges into medial and lateral columns. The articular portions of both condyles project anteroinferiorly at 40° angles in relation to the midsagittal plane of the humerus. The distal articular surface of the trochlea inclines 10° to 15° radially in relation to the humeral shaft and contributes to the carrying angle. When they are unencumbered, the coronoid and olecranon fossae allow 150° of elbow rotation.

CLASSIFICATION

The AO classification for distal humeral fractures is the most comprehensive system available (Fig. 4) (1). T-shaped fractures in the Riseborough and Radin system correspond to AO type C fractures and are cited commonly in the literature (2). Unfortunately, this schema does not emphasize that fractures with supracondylar comminution are more severe injuries.

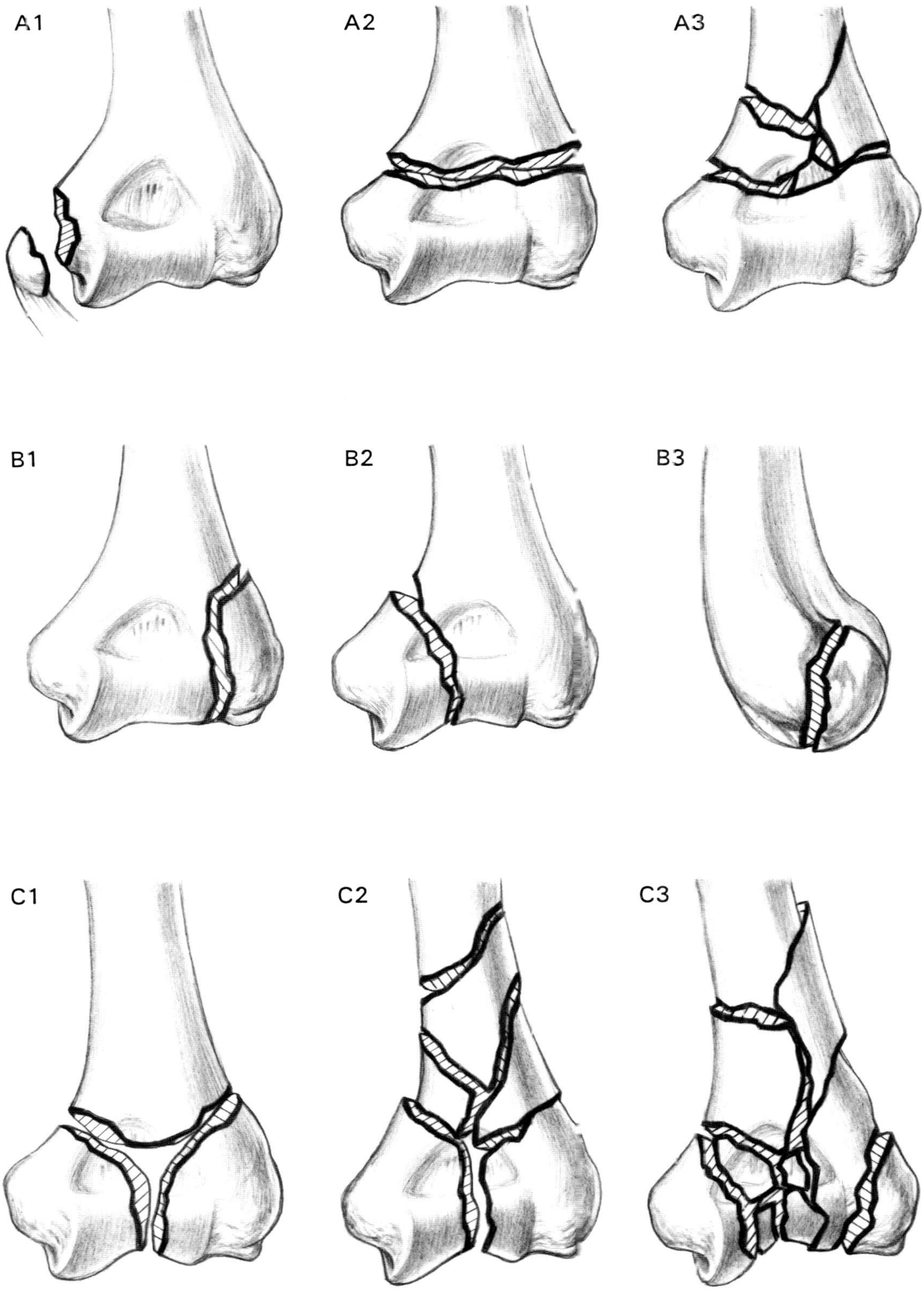

FIG. 4. The AO classification for distal humeral fractures.

A—Extraarticular fracture
  A1—Epicondylar avulsion fracture
  A2—Simple metaphyseal fracture
  A3—Comminuted fracture
B—Unicondylar fracture
  B1—Lateral condylar fracture (sagittal plane)
  B2—Medial condylar fracture (sagittal plane)
  B3—Medial or lateral condylar fracture (frontal plane)
C—T-intercondylar fracture
  C1—Simple articular, simple metaphyseal
  C2—Simple articular, comminuted metaphyseal
  C3—Comminuted articular

(Adapted from Müller ME, Algöwer M, Schneider R, Willenegger H. *Manual of Internal Fixation.* Berlin: Springer-Verlag, 1991. Müller ME, Nazarians, Koch P, Schatzker J. *Comprehensive Classification of Fractures of Long Bones.* Berlin: Springer-Verlag, 1990. Used with permission.)

ASSESSMENT

Physical Examination

In supracondylar fractures, deformities usually are evident on clinical examination. In an intercondylar fracture pattern, the width of the elbow is increased and the arm is slightly shortened. A careful neurovascular examination must be performed before reduction and splinting. The carrying angle of the contralateral arm is variable and should be noted.

Radiographic Evaluation

Anteroposterior and lateral radiographs are obtained to visualize the fracture. If the articular segment of the distal humerus cannot be visualized adequately, these radiographs should be repeated after moderate traction is applied and the elbow is partially extended. Optimal diagnostic radiographs can be obtained under general anesthesia before open reduction and internal fixation (ORIF).

Special Studies

Oblique radiographic views, CT scans, and hypocycloidal polytomograms are useful for evaluating intraarticular displacement and comminution. These tests are usually not required when high-quality radiographs are available.

EMERGENT MANAGEMENT

Open fractures require immediate irrigation, wound debridement and simultaneous definitive management. All other fractures are splinted, and patients with these injuries are admitted to the hospital for edema management and neurovascular observation.

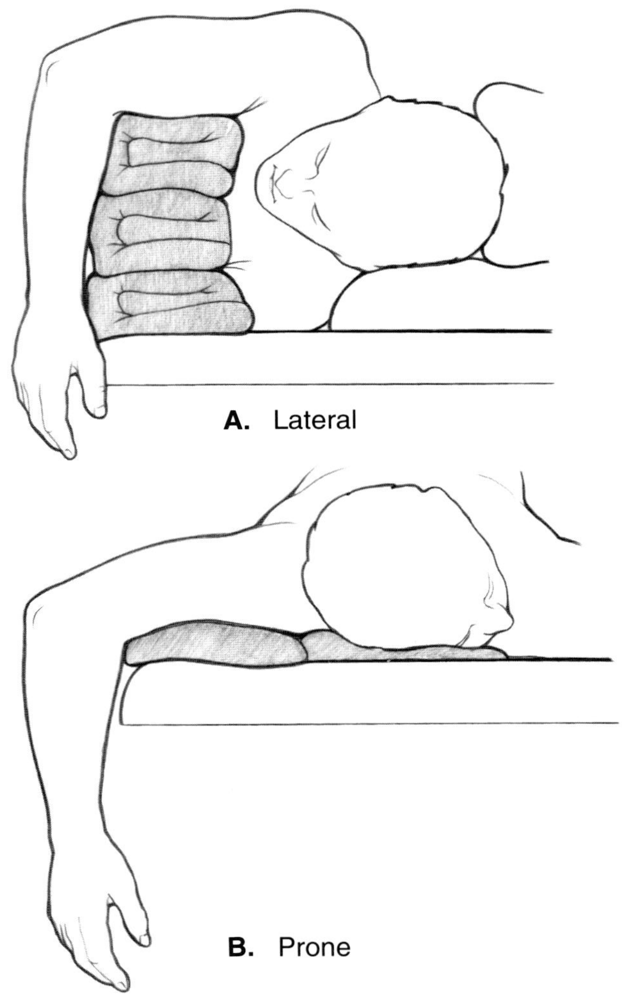

FIG. 5. The patient lies in a lateral decubitus position (**A**) or a prone position (**B**) for a posterior approach to a distal humeral fracture.

DEFINITIVE MANAGEMENT

The fracture pattern dictates the type of operative management and the surgical approach to be used. In general, all displaced fractures are reduced open and are stabilized with rigid internal fixation to allow immediate unrestricted range of motion.

Distal-Third Diaphyseal Supracondylar Fractures

A supracondylar fracture of the distal third of the humerus is approached through a posterior triceps-splitting incision with the patient positioned prone or straight lateral on the operating table (Fig. 5A,B). A broad 4.5-mm direct compression plate (DCP) or an LC-DCP is placed on the posterior cortex of the bone and screws are inserted to grasp 6 to 8 cortices of each major fragment. (see also Chapter 12).

Extraarticular Metaphyseal Supracondylar Fractures (A2 and A3)

Extraarticular metaphyseal supracondylar fractures that extend through or lie just proximal to the olecranon fossa require dual-plate fixation. Malleable reconstruction plates can be used, but in the presence of supracondylar comminution at least one of the plates should be a 3.5-mm DCP or LC-DCP. This type of fracture is approached through a posterior incision, with or without an olecranon osteotomy, or through separate medial and lateral incisions, depending on the location of the fracture and the degree of comminution.

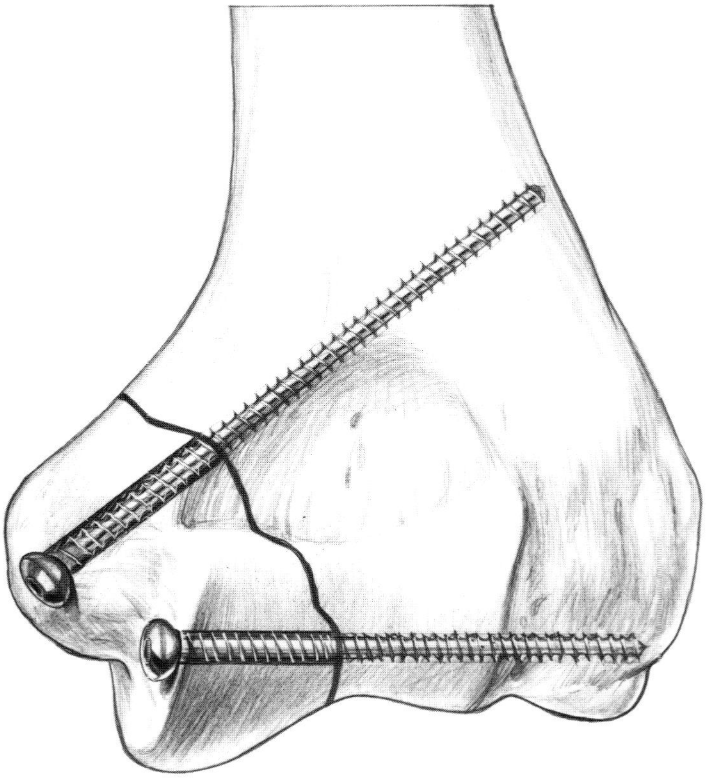

FIG. 6. A medial unicondylar fracture is stabilized with 3.5-mm and 4-mm lag screws, avoiding the olecranon fossa

Unicondylar Fractures of the Lateral Column (B1J)

This type of fracture is approached through a lateral arthrotomy with the patient lying supine or on one side. Fixation is provided by 3.5-mm lag screws or 4-mm cancellous screws. A small antiglide or buttress plate can be applied for additional stability. Anatomic reduction of the articular surface is visualized through the arthrotomy.

Unicondylar Fractures of the Medial Column (B2)

A unicondylar fracture of the medial column is approached through a medial incision after the ulnar nerve is identified. Fixation is similar to that for a lateral condylar fracture (Fig. 6).

Capitellar Fractures (B3.1)

The surgical approach to capitellar fractures is similar to that for lateral condylar fractures. At least two screws are required to provide stable fixation and to prevent rotation. Two 4-mm or 3.5-mm screws can be used for large fracture fragments, whereas 2.7-mm screws or minifragment screws are used for small fragments. The screws are usually inserted from posterior to anterior but can be inserted anterior to posterior if they are countersunk (Fig. 7).

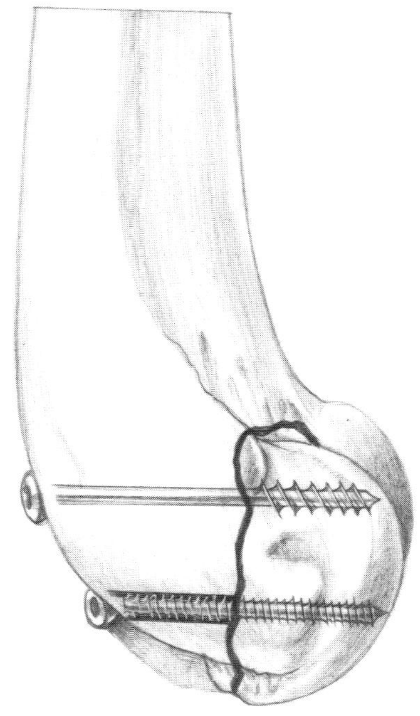

FIG. 7. A capitellar fracture stabilized with 2.7-mm and 4-mm lag screws.

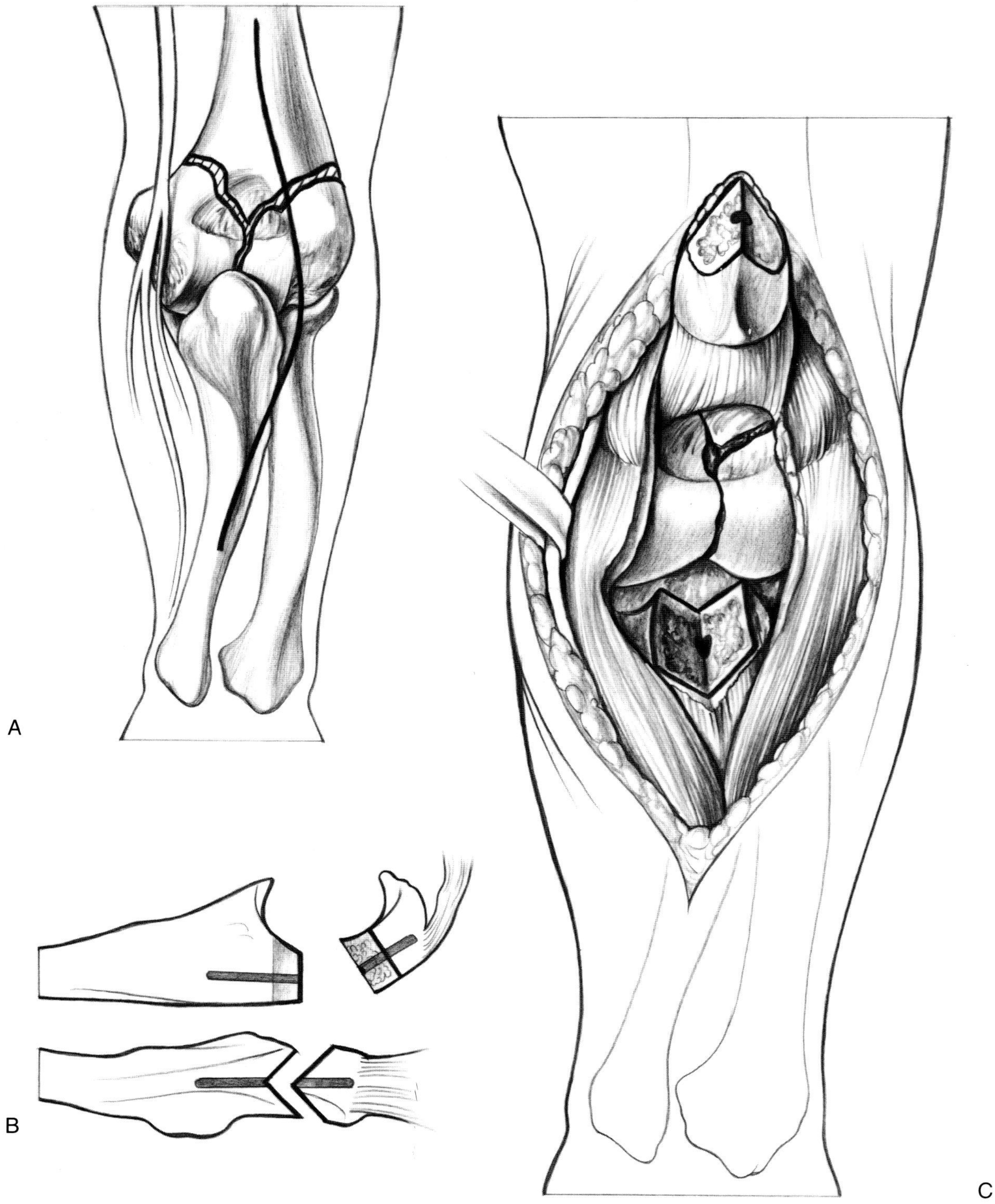

FIG. 8. The skin incision for a posterior approach (**A**). The chevron-shaped olecranon osteotomy is seen in lateral and dorsal views (**B**). The distal humerus is seen in a posterior intraarticular view after the proximal olecranon fragment and the triceps are elevated (**C**). The ulnar nerve is protected by a Penrose drain.

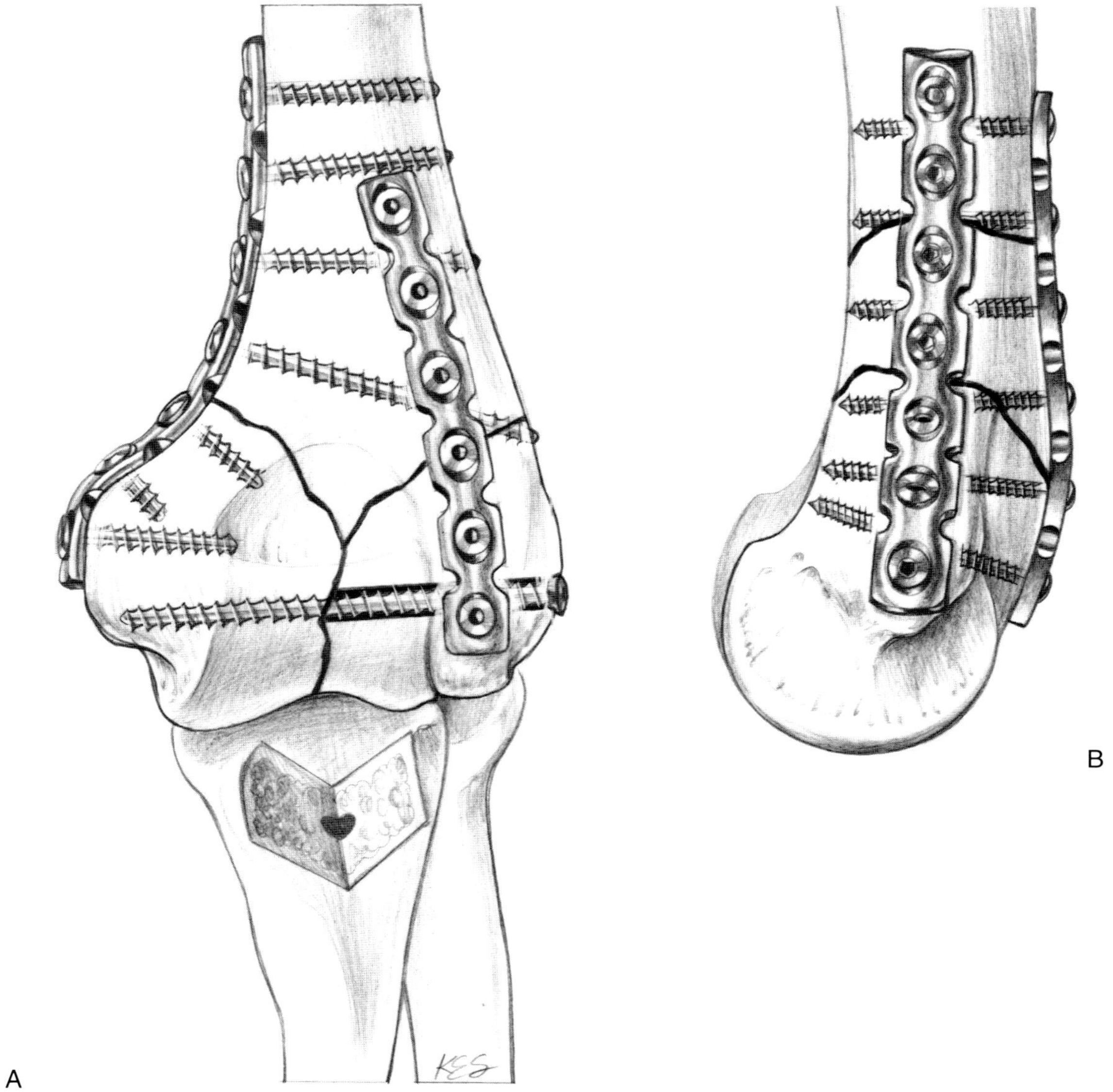

FIG. 9. Posterior view (**A**) and medial view (**B**) of a posterior T-intercondylar distal humeral fracture stabilized with two 3.5-mm reconstruction plates.

T-shaped Intercondylar Fractures (C1, C2, and C3)

A T-shaped intercondylar fracture is stabilized through a posterior approach (Fig. 8) and requires a transverse or chevron olecranon osteotomy (Fig. 8B,C). Before the osteotomy is performed, the ulnar nerve must be identified and protected. The nerve may be transposed anteriorly if it is to lie adjacent to internal hardware. Although a chevron osteotomy is technically more difficult to create, this procedure enhances reduction and fixation. The olecranon is stabilized later with a long (greater than 90 mm) 6.5-mm lag screw and a tension-band wire.

The humerus is stabilized with two 3.5-mm plates (reconstruction plates, DCP, or LC-DCP) placed at 90° angles to each other (3). The plate on the lateral column is placed directly on the posterior aspect of the humerus (Fig. 9A,B) (4). The medial plate is placed on the medial column in the sagittal plane (Fig. 10). Comminuted fractures above the olecranon fossa or fractures involving the cylindrical portion of the distal humerus require a stiffer plate (3.5-mm DCP or LC-DCP) applied on the lateral column. Bone graft may be added.

Postoperatively, the elbow is immobilized between 90° and 120° with a posterior splint and the arm is elevated for 24 to 48 hours. Active range-of-motion exercises are begun after the suction drain is removed and the wound is secure, usually between the third and fifth postoperative days.

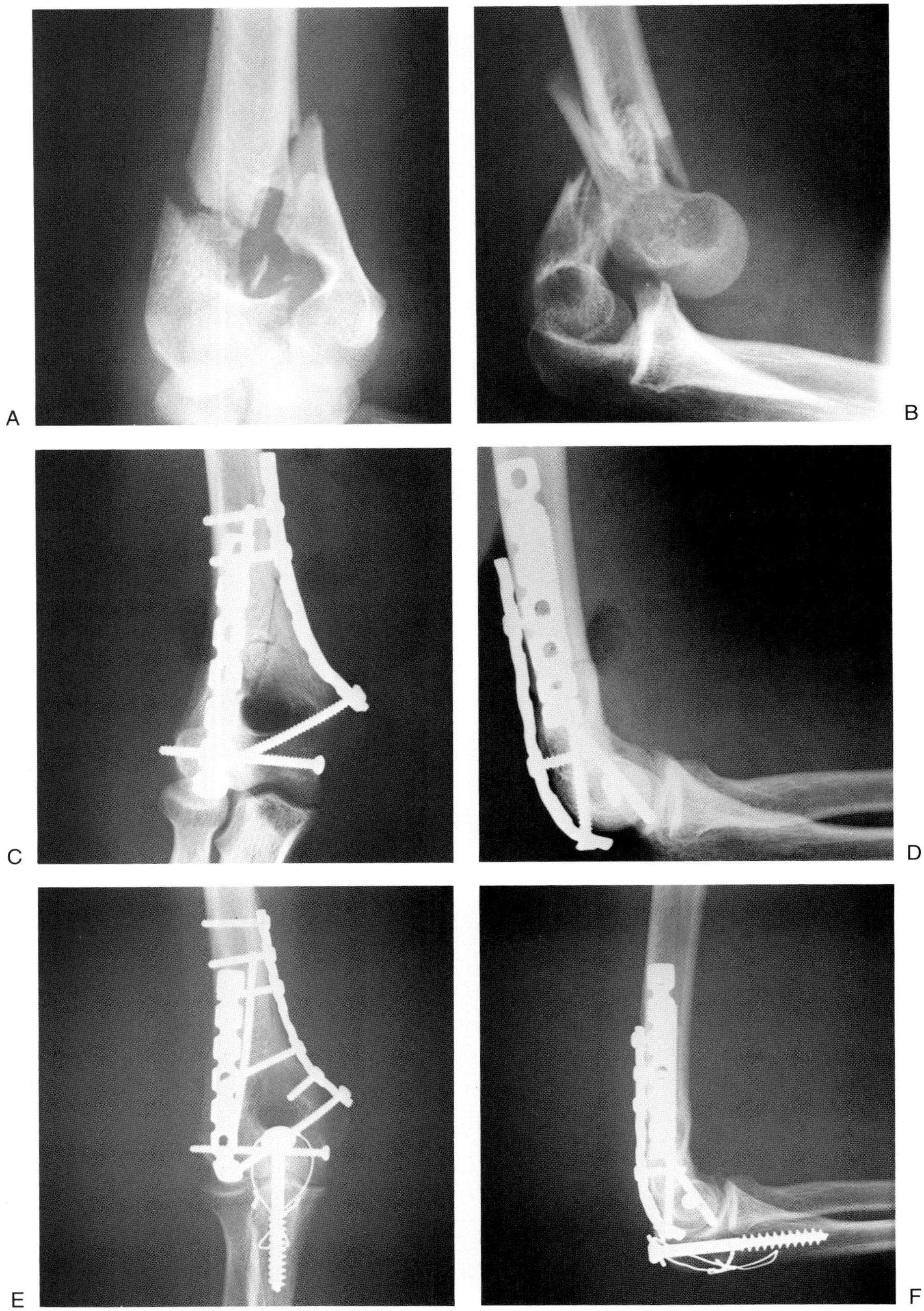

FIG. 10. Radiographs of a displaced T-intercondylar distal humeral fracture of a 17-year-old female. **A:** Anteroposterior view. **B:** Lateral view. **C,D:** Intraoperative films after provisional plate stabilization prior to fixation of the olecranon oteotomy. **E,F:** Four months postinjury, the fracture and osteotomy are healed.

COMPLICATIONS

Heterotopic bone formation is a common sequela of high-energy distal humeral fractures. Patients' functional outcomes can be favorably influenced by initiation of early range-of-motion exercises and a regimen of antiinflammatory medications. If motion is restricted, the ossification can be excised after the fracture has healed.

SKELETALLY IMMATURE PATIENTS

Supracondylar fractures in children are treated by closed reduction and percutaneous pin fixation performed under general anesthesia and fluoroscopy. Stable fixation allows elbow extension for intraoperative evaluation of Bauman's angle and the carrying angle. Postoperatively the elbow can be splinted in moderate extension, a position that allows edema to resolve and frequent vascular checks to be obtained. Before hospital discharge, the elbow is splinted in 90° of flexion. Immobilization is maintained for 3 weeks.

Displaced fractures of the lateral condyle are reduced open and stabilized internally with Kirschner wires. A fracture of the medial epicondyle may occur in association with an elbow dislocation. Open reduction and fixation with Kirschner wires is indicated when the epicondyle is displaced more than 2 mm.

REFERENCES

1. Müller ME, Allgöwer M, Schneider R, et al. *Manual of internal fixation: techniques recommended by the AO Group.* 3rd ed. New York: Springer-Verlag; 1990
2. Riseborough EJ, Radin EL. Intercondylar T fractures of the humerus in the adult. A comparison of operative and non-operative treatment in twenty-nine cases. *J Bone Joint Surg* 1969;51A:130–41.
3. Henley MB. Intra-articular distal humeral fractures in adults. *Orthop Clin North Am* 1987;18:11–23.
4. Helfet DL, Hotchkiss RN. Internal fixation of the distal humerus: a biomechanical comparison of methods. *J Orthop Trauma* 1990;4:260–4.

Radial Head and Neck Fractures

MECHANISMS OF INJURY

An isolated fracture of the radial head and neck is usually caused by a fall onto an outstretched hand. However, radial head and neck fractures can also be caused by directly applied forces. Associated injuries can include fractures of the capitellum or the proximal ulna. Radial head fractures often occur in conjunction with elbow dislocations and may result in disruption of the collateral ligaments, the interosseous membrane, or the distal radioulnar joint.

ANATOMIC CONSIDERATIONS

The intracapsular radial head articulates with the capitellum and the lesser sigmoid notch of the proximal ulna, and maintains articular contact with the ulna throughout forearm rotation. If stabilization is provided by a minifragment plate, its placement must not interfere with forearm rotation.

CLASSIFICATION

Mason's classification is used to provide treatment guidelines (Fig. 11) (1); type I, nondisplaced fractures; type II, marginally displaced fractures with depression, angulation, and impaction; type III, comminuted fractures, which usually involve the entire radial head; and type IV, fractures associated with a dislocation of the elbow.

ASSESSMENT

Physical Examination

Presenting symptoms include pain with passive and active rotation of the forearm. The radial head and neck are tender to palpation and a hemarthrosis is noted. Clinical examination should include assessment of the collateral ligaments, their insertions, and the stability of the elbow.

Radiograhic Evaluation

Anteroposterior, lateral, and oblique radiographs are obtained. A positive fat-pad sign is seen when the integrity of the joint capsule has not been disturbed. The radiographs are carefully examined for loose foreign bodies and a fracture of the capitellum.

Special Studies

The posterior portion of the radial head is best visualized on a radiocapitellar radiographic view, which clearly delineates the radiocapitellar and radioulnar joints (2).

Emergent Management

Nondisplaced fractures of the radial head and neck are treated nonoperatively. The hemarthrosis is aspirated and the

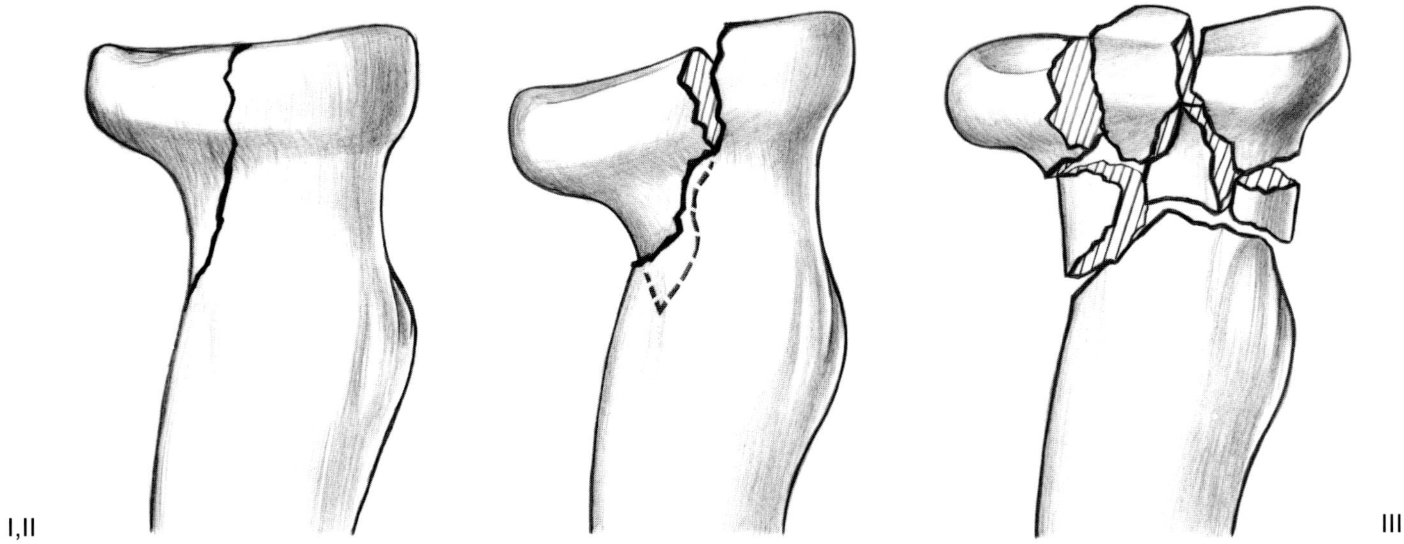

FIG. 11. Diagrammatic representations of Mason's type I, II, and III fractures.

joint is injected with approximately 3 ml to 5 ml of 0.5% or 1.0% lidocaine or bupivacaine without epinephrine. Full passive range of motion must be confirmed before splinting. The splint is removed after 2 or 3 days and early active range-of-motion exercises are initiated. Fractures requiring operative treatment are immobilized in a posterior splint for comfort.

DEFINITIVE MANAGEMENT

The goals of treatment of any intraarticular fracture are preservation of joint function and joint motion. Because loose bodies or displaced fractures can cause joint impingement, only nondisplaced Mason type I fractures and minimally dis-

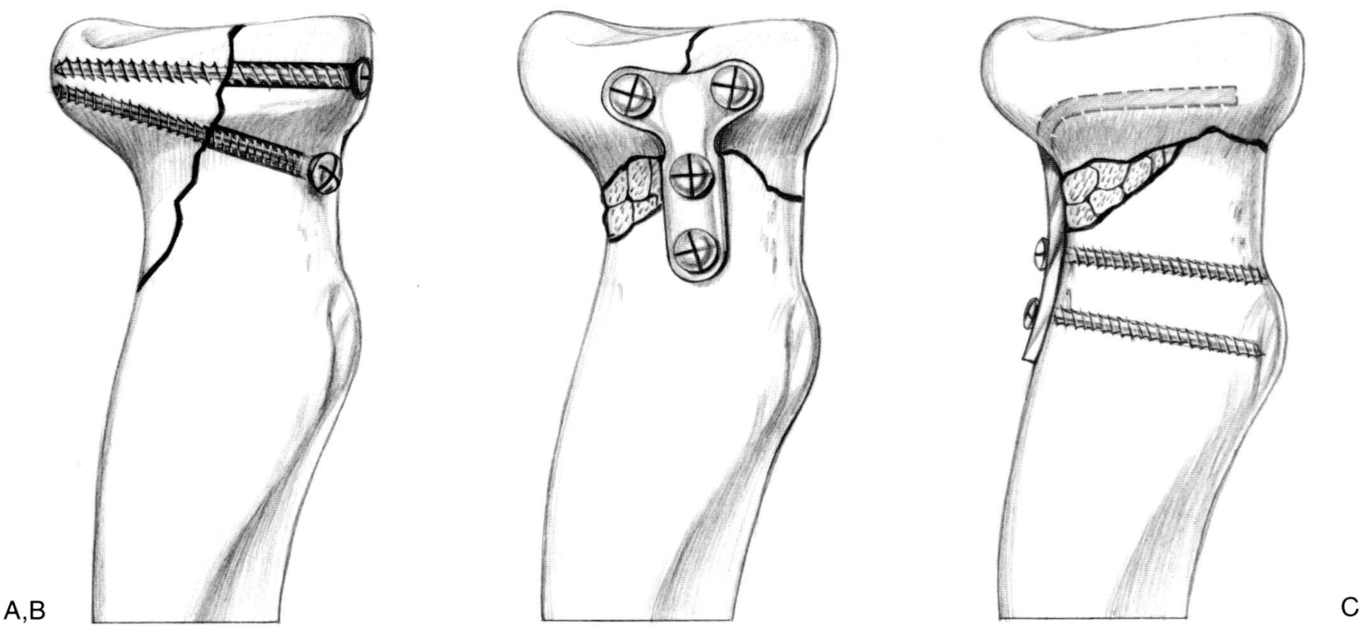

FIG. 12. Three methods of stabilization for radial head and neck fractures. **A:** Minifragment screws are used to stabilize wedge fractures. **B:** Mini-T-plates are used for transverse radial neck fractures and comminuted radial head fractures. **C:** Miniplates are used as buttress plates or as small blade plates.

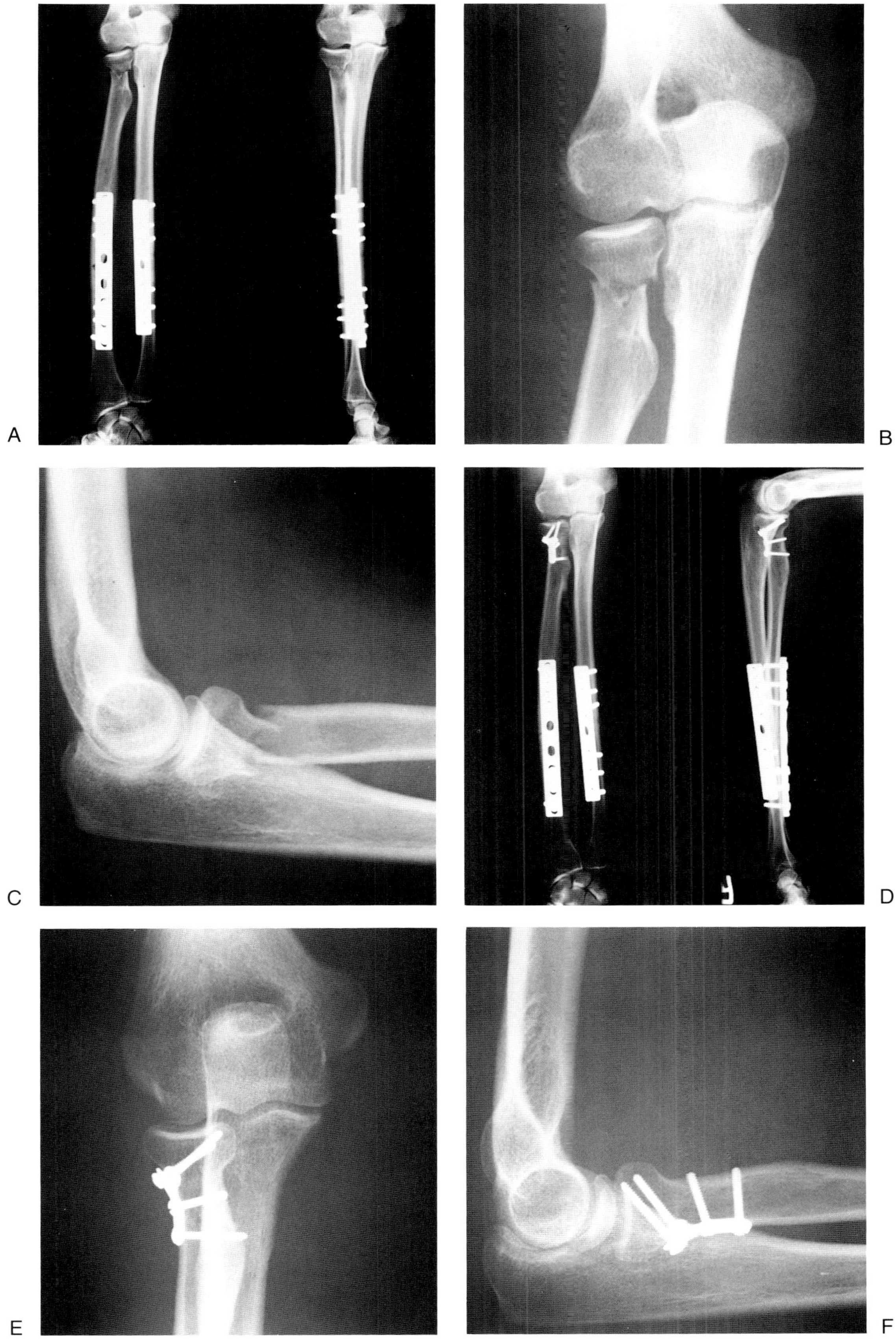

FIG. 13. A–C: A displaced radial neck fracure in a patient with ipsilateral radial and ulnar shaft fractures. **D–F:** The fracture has healed three months after mini T-plate stabilization.

placed Mason type II fractures are considered for nonoperative treatment. Unrestricted active or passive range of motion must be confirmed before splinting.

Because the results of late radial head excision are good, preservation of the head is recommended whenever feasible (3,4). Therefore, most type II and type III fractures are treated by open reduction and internal fixation ORIF. However, severely comminuted type III fractures that cannot be reconstructed and that interfere with normal range of motion are treated by excision of the radial head (5). Type IV fractures warrant immediate reduction of the elbow joint, and the treatment of the radial head depends on the fracture pattern. Use of a silastic radial head replacement is associated with a high incidence of prosthetic complications and is not recommended (6). Treatment of elbow instabilities is described above.

The patient is positioned supine on the operating table and a direct lateral Kocher incision is made to approach the radial head and neck. This approach spares the humeroulnar ligament. To safeguard the posterior interosseous nerve, the dissection is not extended distal to the annular ligament. Wedge fractures are reduced and stabilized with minifragment screws (1.5-mm, 2-mm, or 2.7-mm lag screws), and the screw heads are recessed below the articular surfaces (Fig. 12A). Transverse fractures of the radial neck and comminuted fractures of the radial head usually require plate fixation (Fig. 13). For these fractures, mini-T-plates are contoured and positioned so that they do not interfere with the radioulnar articulation (see Fig. 12B). Alternatively, miniplates are used as buttress plates or they are fashioned into small blade plates for fixation (see Fig. 12C) (7). Cancellous bone graft is used to fill any defect that remains after the impacted fragments are elevated.

An intraarticular suction drain is inserted postoperatively and is used for 24 to 48 h. After the drain is removed, flexion, extension, pronation, and supination exercises are begun. If a posterior splint was used for the first 2 days, it is discontinued at this time. Prolonged use of a sling is not recommended.

COMPLICATIONS

Pronation and supination deficits average 5° to 15° after rehabilitation. In addition, the last few degrees of elbow extension may be lost. Other complications include wrist pain (Essex–Lopresti injury), posterior interosseous nerve injury, elbow instability, heterotopic ossification, and degenerative arthritis.

SKELETALLY IMMATURE PATIENTS

Proximal radial fractures in children usually involve the radial neck or the proximal physis. Transarticular injuries are rare. A closed reduction is performed when angulation in a fracture exceeds 15° or 20°. Residual angulation greater than 30° is treated by open reduction and crossed Kirschner wire fixation (8). The radial head must never be excised in a child.

REFERENCES

1. Mason ML. Some observations on fractures of the head of the radius with a review of 100 cases. *Br J Surg* 1954;42:123–32.
2. Greenspan A, Norman A, Rosen H. Radial head-capitellum view in elbow trauma: clinical application and radiographic-anatomic correlation. *AJR* 1984;143:355–9.
3. Broberg MA, Morrey BF. Results of delayed excision of the radial head after fracture. *J Bone Joint Surg* 1986;68A:669–74
4. Goldberg I, Peylan J, Yosipovitch Z. Late results of excision of the radial head for an isolated closed fracture. *J Bone Joint Surg* 1986;68A:675–9.
5. Coleman DA, Blair WF, Shurr D. Resection of the radial head for fracture of the radial head. *J Bone Joint Surg* 1987;69A:385–92.
6. Carn RM, Medige J, Curtain D, Koenig A. Silicone rubber replacement of the severely fractured radial head. *Clin Orthop* 1986;209:259–69.
7. Geel CW, Palmer AK, Ruedi T, Leutenegger AF. Internal fixation of proximal radial head fractures. *J Orthop Trauma* 1990;4:270–4.
8. Steinberg EL, Golomb D, Salama R, Wientroub S. Radial head and neck fractures in children. *J Pediatr Orthop* 1988;8:35.

Olecranon Fractures and Comminuted Proximal Ulnar Fractures

MECHANISM OF INJURY

Olecranon fractures are usually caused by application of direct or indirect forces. When these forces occur simultaneously (for example, in a side-swipe injury) a severely comminuted fracture or a fracture–dislocation can result. Associated injuries may include elbow dislocations, radial head dislocations, radial head fractures, and coronoid fractures.

ANATOMIC CONSIDERATIONS

Important osseous landmarks in the proximal ulna include the insertion of the triceps tendon, the greater sigmoid notch of the olecranon, and the coronoid process. The greater sigmoid notch articulates congruently with the trochlea; the lesser sigmoid notch articulates with the radial head. An intact coronoid process can block dislocation.

CLASSIFICATION

The most useful classification system for selecting the optimal treatment for an olecranon fracture is a combination of the grading systems devised by Colton (1) and by Horne and Tanzer (2). Colton divides olecranon fractures into two major categories: nondisplaced and displaced. Fractures displaced less than 2 mm are considered nondisplaced if the amount of displacement does not increase with elbow flexion and if the elbow extensor mechanism remains intact.

Horne and Tanzer classify fractures on the basis of the lateral radiograph (Fig. 14): type I, either transverse intraarticular fractures originating on the proximal third of the articular surface of the olecranon or oblique extraarticular fractures involving the point of the olecranon; type II, oblique or transverse fractures involving the middle third of the greater sigmoid notch; and type III, fractures originating in the distal third of the greater sigmoid notch, which might involve the coronoid process.

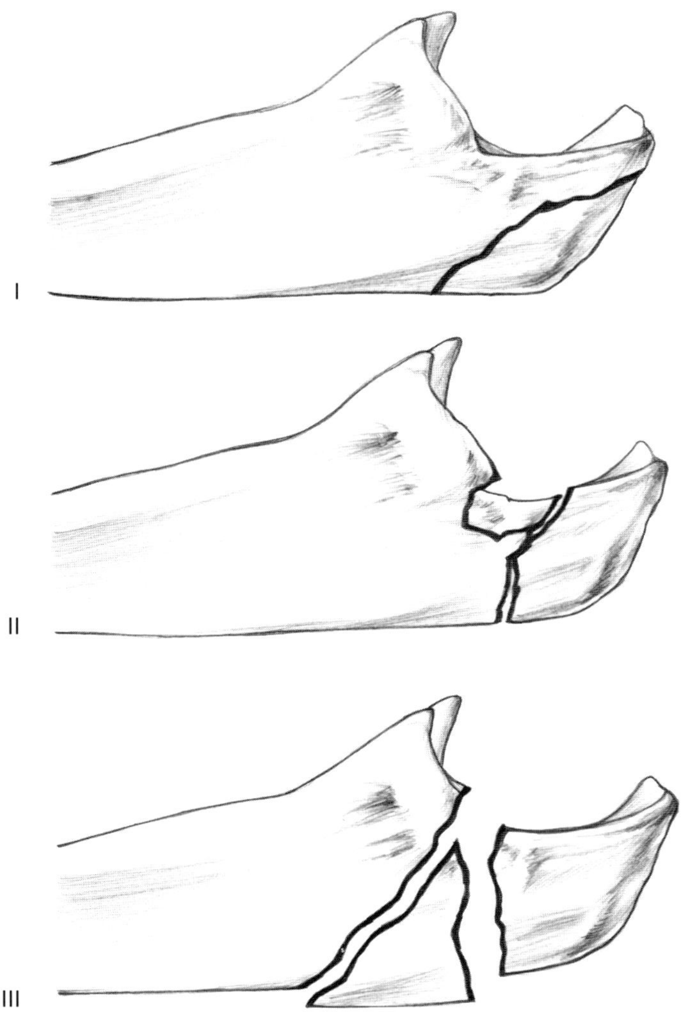

FIG. 14. Examples of types I, II, and III fractures according to Horne and Tanzer's classification.

ASSESSMENT

Physical Examination

Hemarthrosis, subcutaneous swelling, and ecchymosis are commonly seen after an olecranon fracture. A displaced fracture pattern permits communication between the olecranon bursa and the elbow joint. The integrity of the elbow extensor mechanism must be assessed in all olecranon fractures. In a stable fracture, the elbow can be extended against gravity without fracture displacement.

Radiographic Evaluation

Anteroposterior and true lateral radiographs are obtained of the elbow joint. On a true lateral radiograph, the trochlea and the capitellum are superimposed, their axes are coaxial, and the joint space is clearly visible. In addition to fracture displacement and comminution, radiographs are examined for a small osseous depression in the middle third of the greater semilunar notch.

Special Studies

Two oblique radiographs may provide additional information in comminuted fractures. Tomograms usually are not necessary.

EMERGENT MANAGEMENT

Nondisplaced fractures are treated by immobilization of the elbow in 45° to 90° of flexion. Stability is confirmed by observing range of motion under fluoroscopy. Displaced fractures are immobilized in a long-arm splint before ORIF. Comminuted fractures caused by high-energy injuries are often open injuries which demand emergent irrigation and debridement with concomitant fracture stabilization.

DEFINITIVE MANAGEMENT

Nondisplaced fractures with intact extensor mechanisms can be managed nonoperatively. Operative treatment is required for all fractures with disrupted extensor mechanisms and those that are displaced by more than 1.5 mm. A longitudinal posterior approach is made with the patient lying supine or in a lateral decubitus position on the operating table. The ulnar nerve is identified and protected during the approach and the joint surface is inspected. Impacted articular fragments are elevated and their corresponding deficits are grafted. Two parallel Kirschner wires and a tension-band wire are used to provide stable fixation for type I and type II fractures (3,4). The tension-band should be

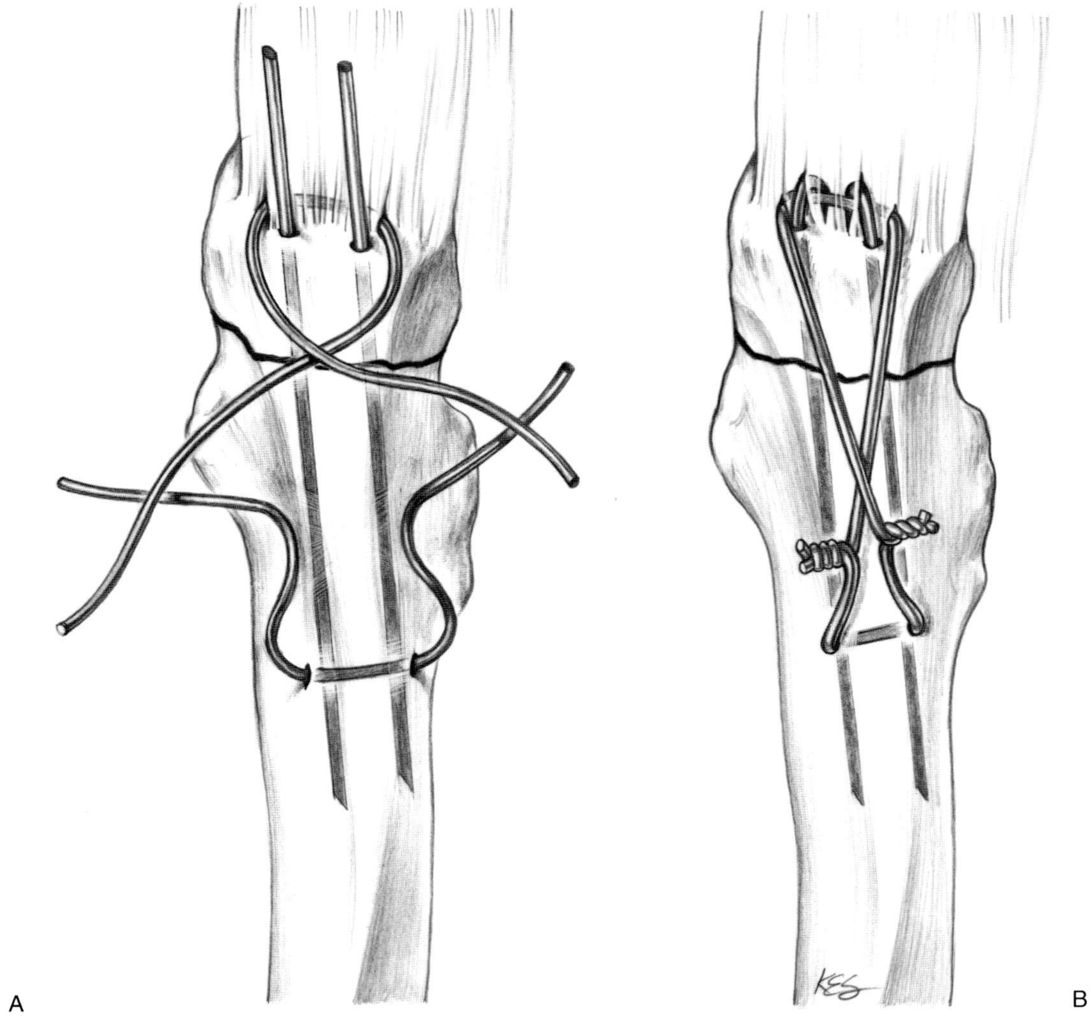

FIG. 15. The tension-band wiring technique. Two parallel Kirschner wires cross an olecranon fracture at right angles. One strand of 18-gauge wire has been inserted within the triceps tendon anterior to the Kirschner wires. The second wire is inserted through the dorsal ulnar cortex of the ulna (**A**). The fixation is secured (**B**).

placed within the triceps tendinous insertion (Fig. 15A). The proximal ends of the Kirschner wires are bent 180° and impacted deep into the tendon, flush with the cortex of the proximal fragment (Fig. 15B) (5). Sutures can be wrapped around the ends of the Kirschner wires and buried into the triceps fascia to prevent expulsion of the Kirschner wires (Fig. 16).

Type III fractures or comminuted proximal ulnar fractures are stabilized with interfragmentary compression and a 3.5-mm neutralization DCP or LC-DCP (Fig. 17). Concomitant fixation of the coronoid process is performed in fractures involving more than 50% of the process (see Fig. 2) (6). Occasionally, a tension-band one-third tubular hook plate applied with a tension-band technique or a 3.5-mm DCP is used to buttress a comminuted type II fracture. Excision of the olecranon process compromises joint stability and is not advisable (7). Similarly, lag screw fixation alone is not advocated. Unrestricted range of motion, stability of the fixation, and radiographic confirmation of screw placement are confirmed before wound closure.

A posterior splint is applied with the elbow in 90° of flexion and is worn for 36 to 48 h postoperatively. Active flexion and extension exercises are begun after the suction drains are removed. Comminuted fractures require a longer time to consolidate, and in these cases the use of continuous passive motion and assisted active range of motion should be considered.

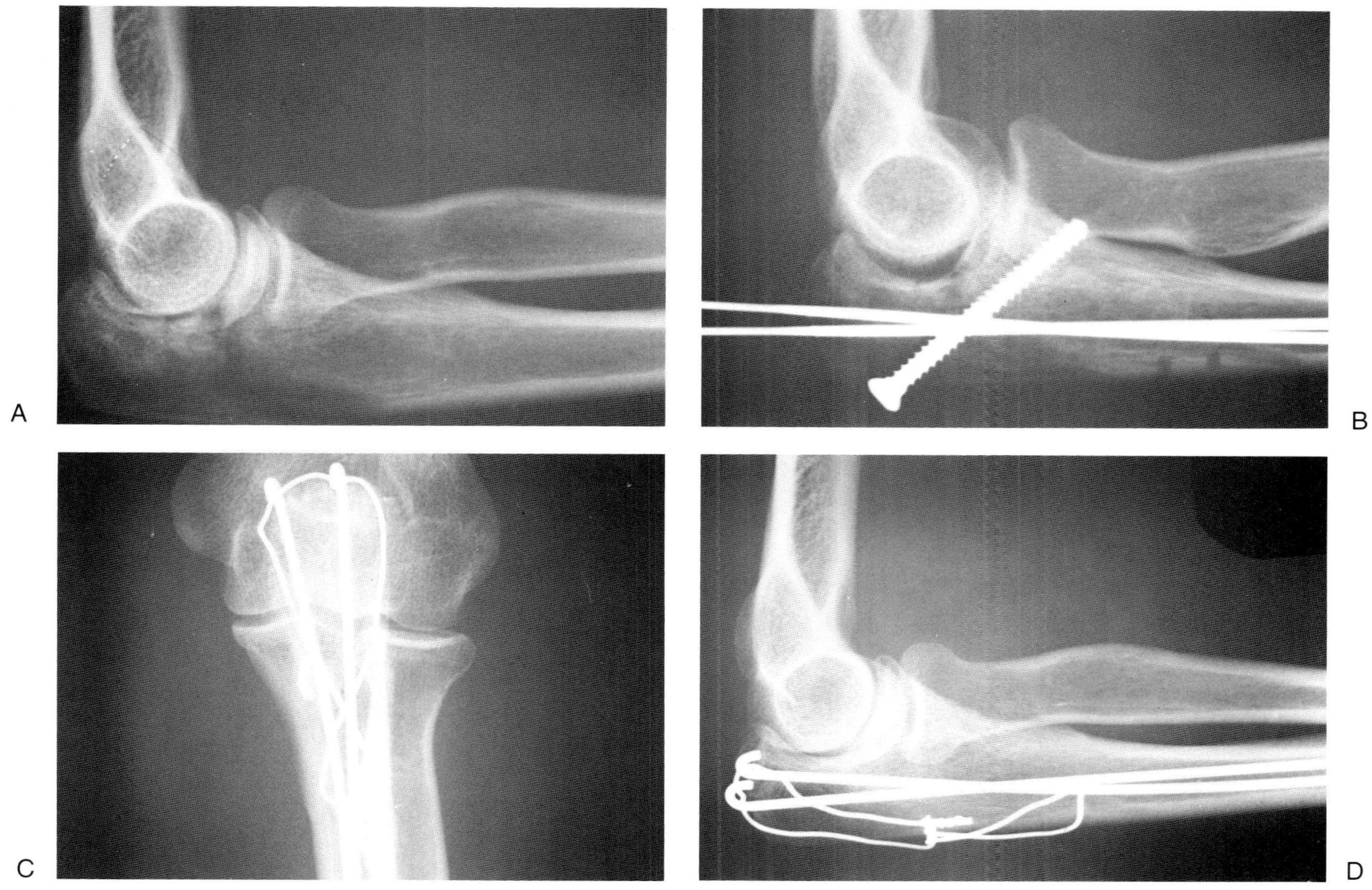

FIG. 16. An injury radiograph of an oblique olecranon fracture wth a small impacted intraarticular fragment. **B:** The intraoperative film demonstrating humeroulnar joint congruity after elevation of the impacted fragment and provisional stabilization. **C,D:** AP and lateral radiographs after screw removal and modified tension-band wire fixation.

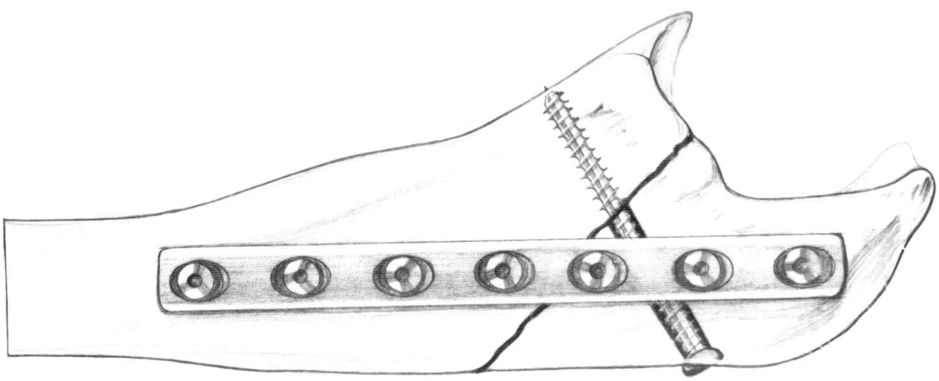

FIG. 17. Fixation for a type II olecranon fracture.

COMPLICATIONS

A slight loss of extension can be expected after any elbow injury. Posttraumatic arthritis might be prevented by anatomic reduction. Damage to the ulnar nerve is seen in less than 10% of patients. The most common complaint is a symptomatic prominence of the Kirschner wire ends or tension-band wire knots. To avoid these discomforts, the proximal ends of the Kirschner wires are bent 180° and are impacted securely into the olecranon. Similarly, tension-band wire knots are buried in soft tissues. Proximal migration of the Kirschner wires can sometimes be prevented by capturing the distal tips of the wires in the ulnar metadiaphysis.

SKELETALLY IMMATURE PATIENTS

Isolated olecranon fractures are rare in children. However, Monteggia fractures must not be overlooked.

REFERENCES

1. Colton CL. Fractures of the olecranon in adults: classification and management. *Injury* 1973;5:121–9.
2. Horn JG, Tanzer TL. Olecranon fractures: a review of 100 cases. *J Trauma* 1981;1:54–8.
3. Horne G. Olecranon fractures: classification and techniques of internal fixation. *Tech Orthop* 1986;1:54–8.
4. Fyfe IS, Mossad MM, Holdsworth BJ. Methods of fixation of olecranon fractures. An experimental mechanical study. *J Bone Joint Surg* 1985;67B:367–72.
5. Macko D, Szabo RM. Complications of tension-band wiring of olecranon fractures. *J Bone Joint Surg* 1985;67A:1396–1401.
6. Regan W, Morrey B. Fractures of the coronoid process of the ulna. *J Bone Joint Surg* 1989;71A:1348–54.
7. Kai-Nan A, Morrey BF, Chao EYS. The effect of partial removal of proximal ulna on elbow constraint. *Clin Orthop* 1986;209:270–9.

Orthopaedic Trauma Protocols, edited by
Sigvard T. Hansen, Jr., and Marc F. Swiontkowski,
Raven Press, Ltd., New York, © 1993.

CHAPTER 14

Forearm Fractures

M. L. Chip Routt, Jr.

Isolated Ulnar Fractures

MECHANISM OF INJURY

An isolated diaphyseal ulnar fracture is usually caused by a direct blow to the medial aspect of the ulna. Sometimes called a nightstick injury, an ulnar fracture often occurs when the arm is raised to assume a position of self-defense (Fig. 1). Because the ulna is subcutaneous in this region, the resulting fracture may be an open injury (Fig. 2).

ANATOMIC CONSIDERATIONS

The ulna is slightly bowed and is bordered by the volar and dorsal compartments. Implants in this area must be placed carefully because the articular surface of the proximal ulna constitutes a portion of the elbow joint.

CLASSIFICATION

Three criteria are used to classify isolated diaphyseal ulnar fractures: skin integrity, the fracture pattern, and the amount of displacement.

ASSESSMENT

Physical Examination

A patient with this injury usually presents with symptoms of localized swelling, pain, and diminished forearm function. The skin over the ulna is examined carefully to rule out an open injury. The elbow is palpated for tenderness around the radial head. Crepitus may not be manifested in a nondis-

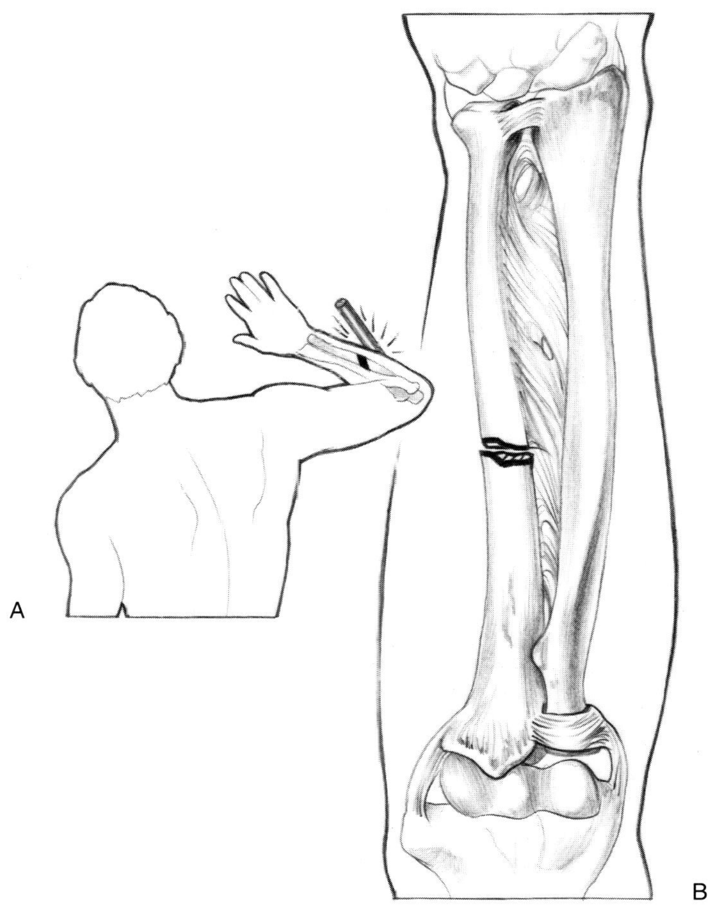

FIG. 1. A: Mechanism of injury producing an isolated ulnar shaft fracture. **B:** Representation of an isolated ulnar fracture.

Department of Orthopaedics. Harborview Medical Center, University of Washington, Seattle, Washington 98104

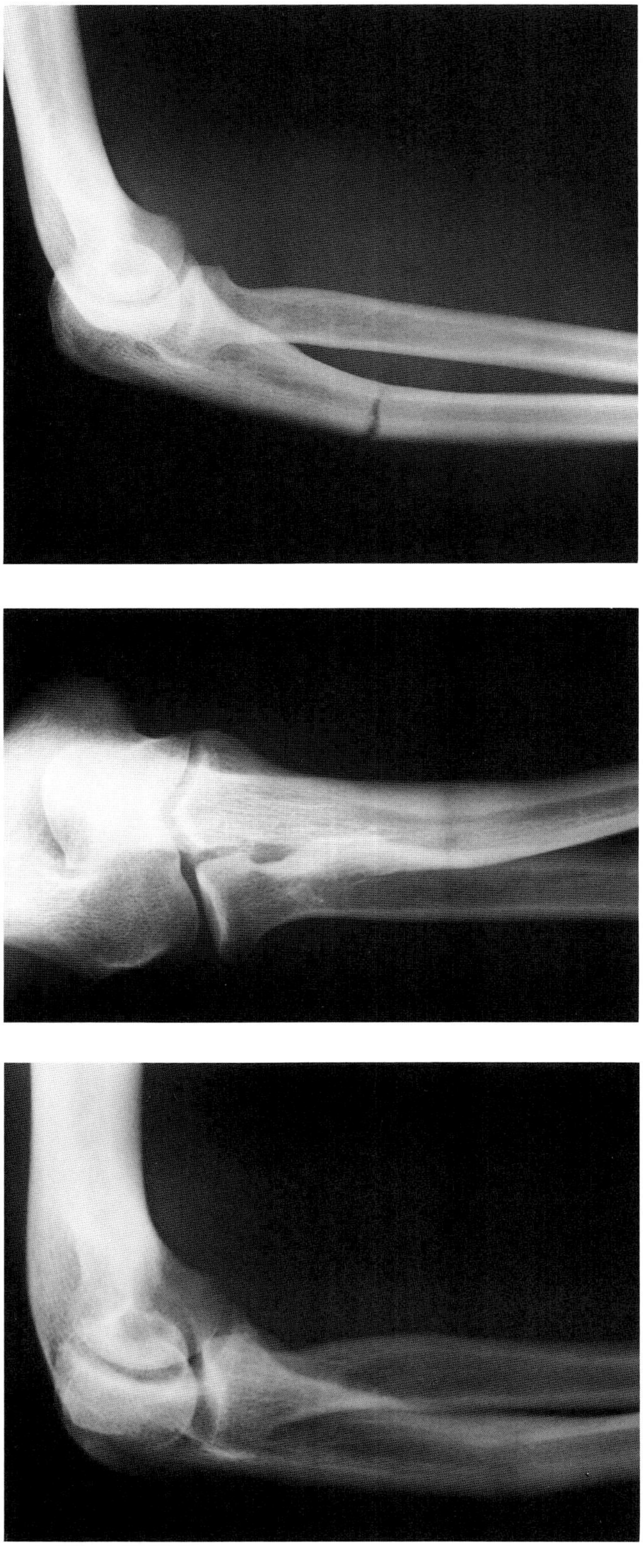

A

B

C

FIG. 2. A: This patient was assaulted with a lead pipe. Soft-tissue air densities surrounding the acute fracture reflect an open fracture. **B,C:** After operative debridement and irrigation, the surgeon chose conservative management with a cast. An angular malunion resulted, producing decreased rotation of the forearm.

placed fracture. The results of the neural and vascular examinations are documented and the presence of a compartmental syndrome is ruled out. Open fractures and those associated with compartmental syndromes require rapid evaluation to expedite treatment.

Radiographic Evaluation

Good quality plain AP and lateral radiographs of the elbow, the forearm, and the wrist should be obtained, with the radial head aligned with the humeral capitellum in all views. Fracture displacement and comminution are evident on radiographs.

Special Studies

Angiography may be indicated in the rare instance of a fracture with an associated vascular injury.

EMERGENT MANAGEMENT

Open wounds are assessed and aseptically dressed, a prophylactic tetanus immunization is administered, and the fracture is splinted. Compartmental pressures are measured and documented when a compartmental syndrome is suspected.

DEFINITIVE MANAGEMENT

Closed reduction and splinting are recommended for nondisplaced, closed, isolated ulnar shaft fractures and for fractures in noncompliant patients (1). Fractures that are treated closed must be followed radiographically during healing.

Operative treatment is recommended for displaced isolated diaphyseal ulnar shaft fractures, open isolated ulnar shaft fractures, and fractures associated with compartmental syndromes. After the open wound is irrigated and debrided and a fasciotomy has been performed as needed, the fracture is reduced anatomically and fixed rigidly with a 3.5-mm dynamic compression plate (DCP). Rarely is stabilization with an intramedullary nail or an external fixator recommended. Indirect reduction techniques are used, and narrow retractors are placed precisely to preserve vital soft-tissue attachments. Traumatic and fasciotomy wounds are left open for 5 to 7 postoperative days and are closed or skin grafted at that time. The arm is splinted before the patient is awakened from anesthesia.

Rehabilitation is begun as soon as the wound shows evidence of healing and proceeds according to the limitations imposed by the type of fracture and the rigidity of fixation. Ideally, active range-of-motion exercises are begun early.

COMPLICATIONS

The incidence of nonunion is higher with intramedullary nailing than with plating. Infection may occur in open injuries.

SKELETALLY IMMATURE PATIENTS

A child with an isolated ulnar shaft fracture frequently demonstrates plastic deformation of the ulna and often of the radius. Greenstick fractures are sometimes difficult to reduce and may require completion of the fracture before satisfactory closed alignment can be achieved. The elbow joint must be visualized radiographically with high-quality AP and lateral views to rule out a Monteggia lesion.

REFERENCE

1. Pollock FH, Pankovich AM, Prieto JJ, et al. The isolated fracture of the ulnar shaft. Treatment without immobilization. *J Bone Joint Surg* 1983; 65A:339–42.

Monteggia Fractures

MECHANISM OF INJURY

A fracture in the proximal third of the ulna with an associated radial head dislocation was first described by Monteggia in 1814 (1). This fracture can result from various mechanisms including falls, vehicular trauma, and direct blows. The history of injury usually involves an application of axial load combined with rotation.

ANATOMIC CONSIDERATIONS

Familiarity with forearm anatomy decreases the likelihood of injury to the important structures and vessels during examination and treatment in this area. The radial head, the capitellum, and the annular ligament are well-defined structures and are easily located. The posterior interosseous nerve is located near the proximal radius and the ulnar nerve is subcutaneous at the elbow. The integrity of the articulation between the radial head and the proximal ulna must be maintained when an associated radial head fracture requires fixation. The intraarticular chondral surface of the proximal ulna at the elbow joint should not be penetrated by implants of inappropriate length.

CLASSIFICATION

In 1967 Bado (2) classified Monteggia fractures into four categories (the incidence of each type of injury appears in parentheses):

Type I (60%): fracture of the ulna at any level with anterior angulation associated with anterior dislocation of the radial head;

Type II (15%): fracture of the ulna at any level with posterior angulation associated with a posterior or posterolateral dislocation of the radial head;

Type III (20%): ulnar metaphyseal fracture associated with a lateral or anterolateral dislocation of the radial head; and

Type IV (5%): fractures of the proximal third of the ulna and the proximal radius at the same level associated with an anterior dislocation of the radial head.

ASSESSMENT

Physical Examination

Early diagnosis of a Monteggia fracture is essential to a good prognosis. The wrist, the forearm, and the elbow are carefully assessed by palpation and a neurovascular examination. The region of the elbow and the forearm is painful, and the radial head is palpable in some types of injuries. The neurovascular status of the upper extremity is noted, especially that of the posterior interosseous nerve, which controls extension of the metacarpophalangeal joints.

Radiographic Evaluation

Anteroposterior and lateral radiographs of the wrist, the forearm, and the elbow are obtained for an accurate diagnosis of this injury. The radial head is examined carefully for the presence of an occult fracture. Normally the radial head and the capitellum are aligned on all radiographic projections, including the oblique views (Fig. 3).

Special Studies

Angiography is indicated in cases of vascular disturbance.

EMERGENT MANAGEMENT

Emergent management of a Monteggia fracture consists of splinting the injured limb.

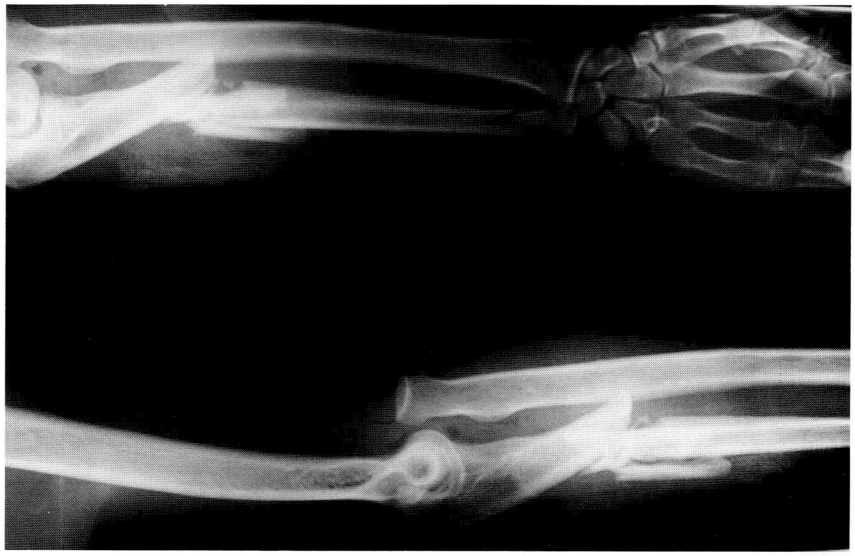

FIG. 3. Bado type I injury. The ulna is fractured segmentally, with extensive comminution and periosteal stripping of the proximal ulnar component.

DEFINITIVE MANAGEMENT

Closed reduction is rarely successful and should be attempted only when the posterior interosseous nerve is not damaged. Open reduction and internal fixation (ORIF) are needed to restore the normal anatomy of the forearm. The length of the ulna is vital to forearm stability and anatomic length is best maintained by plating. An unstable radial head fracture or dislocation, one that cannot be reduced closed, and a Bado type IV injury warrant open treatment. The ulnar fracture is approached along its subcutaneous border and a 3.5-mm DCP or LC-DCP is applied for stabilization. The radial head usually remains stable after the ulnar fracture is plated (Fig. 4).

Open reduction of a radial head fracture should include repair of the annular ligament at the same operation. The stability of the radial head is confirmed by fluoroscopy before the patient is awakened from anesthesia.

A

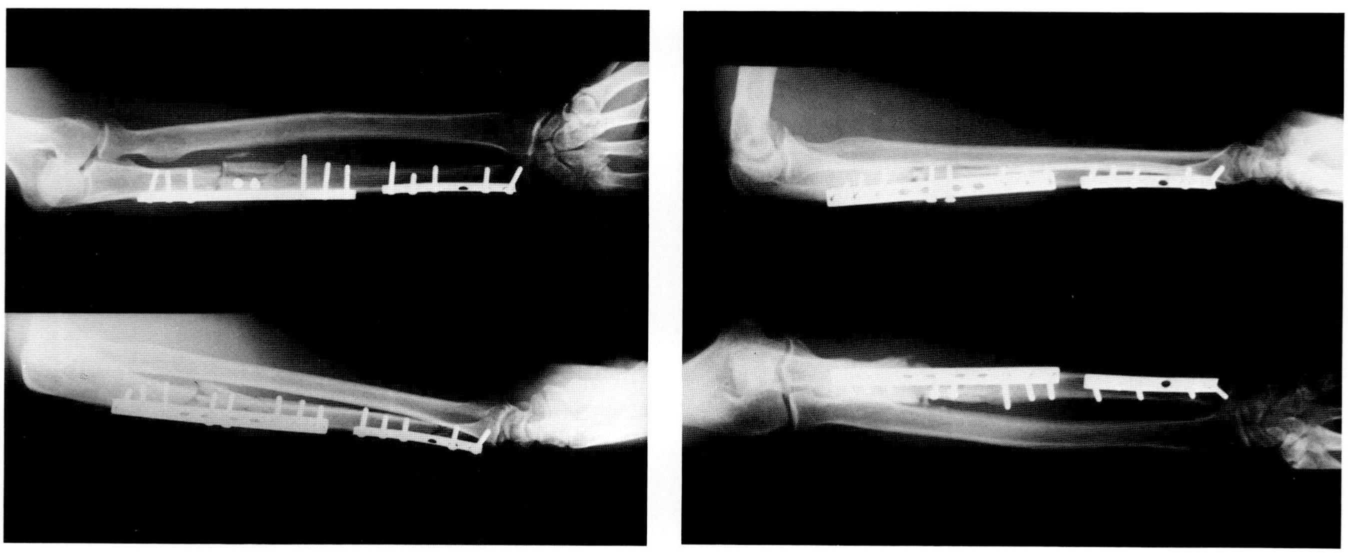

B

FIG. 4. Bado type I injury. **A:** The ulnar fractures have been reduced and stabilized with plates. The radial head dislocation has been closed reduced indirectly. **B:** A nonunion of the ulna resulted, despite attention to soft-tissue detail during fixation. Bone grafting was necessary.

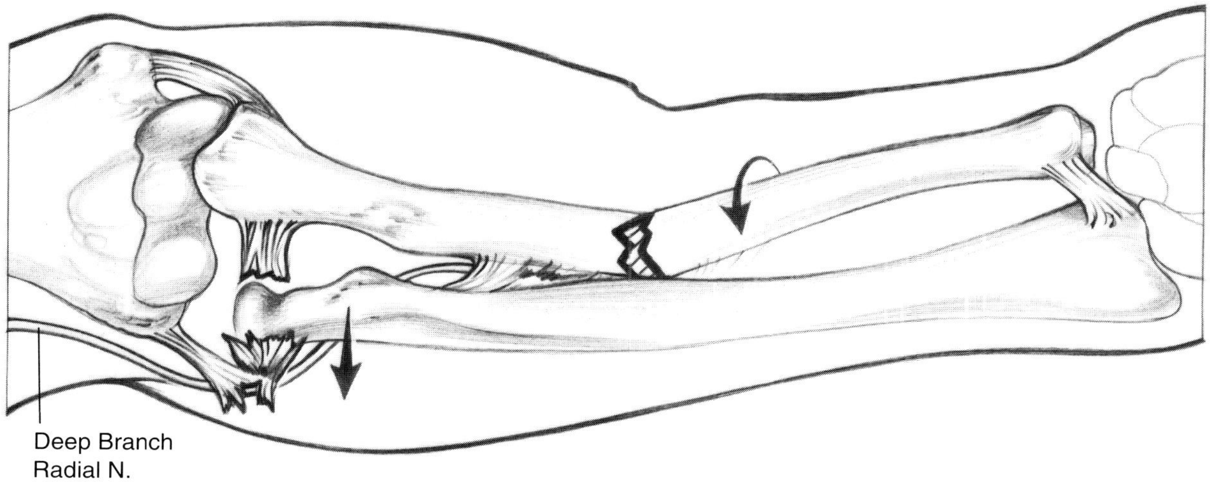

FIG. 5. Mechanism of associated neural injury in a Monteggia fracture.

Rehabilitation is guided by the rigidity of the ulnar fixation and by the stability of the radial head reduction. Casting the elbow past 90° of flexion may rarely be necessary to maintain reduction of the radial head. The elbow must remain in this position for 6 weeks to allow the soft tissues to heal. Close radiographic follow-up is necessary when the stability of the radial head is in question.

COMPLICATIONS

The deep branch of the radial nerve is often injured in a Monteggia fracture, and most complications are related to radial nerve injuries (Fig. 5). Other common neurologic complications include transient palsy from postoperative neuropraxia of the posterior interosseous nerve and posterior interosseous nerve entrapment after closed reduction. An entrapped nerve should be explored. Nonunion is rare with this injury.

SKELETALLY IMMATURE PATIENTS

The radial head and the capitellum of a very young child may not be ossified, and a Monteggia fracture might therefore be difficult to diagnose. Plastic deformation of the ulna may require completion of the fracture before successful reduction can be achieved.

REFERENCES

1. Monteggia GB. *Instituzioni chirurgiche* vol. 5. Milan: Maspero; 1814.
2. Bado JL. The Monteggia lesion. *Clin Orthop* 1967; 50:71–86.

Galeazzi Fracture–Dislocation

MECHANISM OF INJURY

Fracture of the distal radial diaphysis with associated disruptions of the capsule and ligaments of the distal radioulnar joint (DRUJ) was first described by Galeazzi in 1934 (1). Although the exact mechanism of injury is unknown, this fracture–dislocation is thought to be caused by a traumatic application of axial load to a hyperpronated forearm. The two most common causes of this injury are a vehicular accident and a twisting fall onto a pronated, outstretched arm. Galeazzi fracture–dislocations are relatively rare injuries, accounting for approximately 6% to 7% of all diaphyseal forearm fractures. Associated injuries are common, especially in cases of high-energy vehicular trauma.

ANATOMIC CONSIDERATIONS

The radius and the ulna lie almost parallel to each other and share a complex mechanical relationship. The radius is slightly curved and its concave surface faces the ulna. The medullary canal of the radius is funnel-shaped, wide at its distal end, and narrow in its midsection. The radial fracture component of a Galeazzi fracture–dislocation usually occurs at the junction of the middle and distal thirds of the bone. As a result, the triangular fibrocartilage complex (TFCC) is commonly disrupted, a condition that allows the distal radial fragment and the DRUJ to become unstable. Dislocation of the DRUJ cannot occur without rupture of the TFCC.

CLASSIFICATION

A Galeazzi fracture–dislocation has been called a Piedmont fracture, a reverse Monteggia fracture, and a fracture of necessity. No grading system exists for this injury, and classification is limited to the characteristics of the fracture (location, angulation, fracture pattern, displacement) and skin integrity.

ASSESSMENT

Physical Examination

Clinically, Galeazzi fracture–dislocations exhibit a typical appearance. A concave angular deformity is seen on the radial side of the forearm, and the forearm appears shortened. The DRUJ is deformed, swollen, and tender. A dorsal prominence over the ulnar head indicates a volar dislocation of the radiocarpus, but this deformity may be difficult to recognize in a swollen, tender wrist. Assessment of the DRUJ is an important element of the physical examination and must not be omitted. A neurovascular examination of the upper extremity is carefully documented and particular attention is paid to the integrity of the ulnar nerve, the dorsal interosseous nerve, and the extensor carpi ulnaris muscle.

Radiographic Evaluation

Shortening, rotatory, and angulation deformities of a radial fracture are evident on good-quality AP and lateral radiographs that include the forearm, the wrist, and the elbow (Fig. 6). Radiographic diagnosis of a DRUJ disruption is not always possible because the DRUJ appears normal when the ulnar head is subluxated. Disruption is evident on radiographs only when the dislocation is complete.

Obvious radiographic signs of DRUJ instability include: widening of the DRUJ articular interval on an AP view of the wrist; volar dislocation of the radiocarpus from the distal ulna on a true lateral view of the wrist; radial shortening greater than 5 mm; and an ulnar styloid fracture.

Special Studies

Comparison radiographs of the normal wrist are essential for making a diagnosis. The value of arthrography is limited for diagnosing a TFCC disruption.

EMERGENT MANAGEMENT

Emergent management consists of open wound care, prophylactic tetanus immunization and antibiotic administration, and a careful neurovascular examination conducted both before and after the initial splinting.

DEFINITIVE MANAGEMENT

Closed treatment of Galeazzi fracture–dislocations in adults rarely yields a good functional outcome. The definitive management of a Galeazzi fracture–dislocation begins with clinical and radiographic comparisons of the injured DRUJ and the normal DRUJ on the opposite side. The funnel-shaped anatomy of the medullary canal in the radius precludes the use of medullary fixation devices to stabilize this injury, and fixation must be accomplished by plating.

Both dorsal and volar surgical exposures have been advocated. Proponents of a dorsal incision maintain that malposition of the plate on the volar aspect of the radius limits rotation of the forearm in supination and pronation

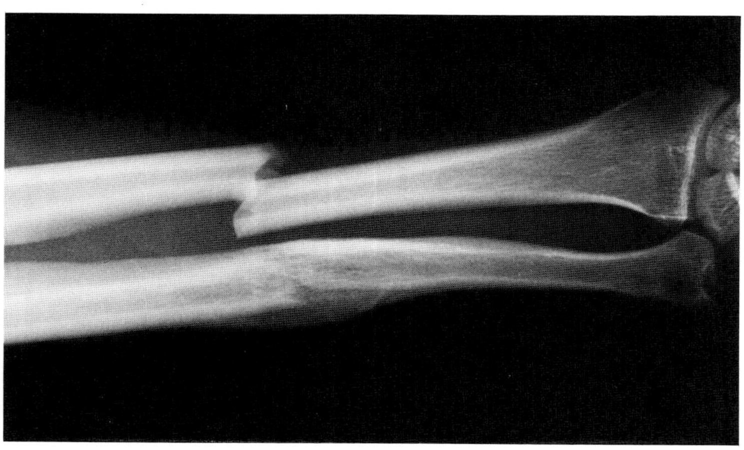

FIG. 6. This patient had a healed nightstick fracture of the ulna and an acute Galeazzi fracture–dislocation.

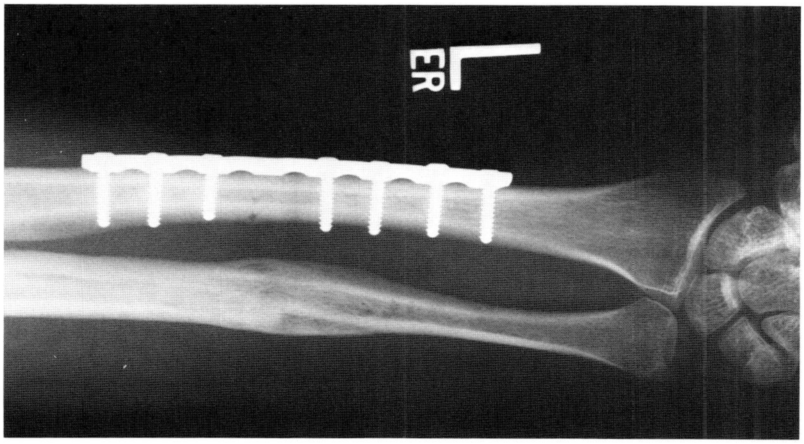

FIG. 7. Union after anatomic reduction and LC-DC plate fixation. No fixation of the DRUJ was needed in this case.

and that this incision is associated with a higher incidence of iatrogenic injury to the sensory branch of the radial nerve, especially when the nerve has not been identified and protected (2). Those who favor a volar approach postulate that the presence of a subcutaneous plate on the dorsal aspect of the radius can irritate the long thumb abductors (3).

We prefer to use the volar approach of Henry for a closed Galeazzi fracture–dislocation, but this standard approach can be altered when severe traumatic open wounds dictate a change (4). The sensory branch of the radial nerve must first be isolated and protected. Reduction can be hindered by entrapment of the extensor carpi ulnaris tendon within the DRUJ. Indirect reduction techniques are used to reduce comminuted fracture fragments (5). Intraoperative radiographs are taken after reduction and fixation with plates and screws (Fig. 7). Rigid anatomic fixation of the radius does not always guarantee DRUJ stability. When the DRUJ remains unstable after fixation of the radial fracture, stabilization of the DRUJ is indicated.

After reduction the upper extremity is immobilized in a long-arm cast in 90° of elbow flexion for approximately 4 weeks. The amount of forearm supination in cast is determined by the degree of DRUJ stability that was achieved intraoperatively. When screws or wires are used to secure an unstable DRUJ, they must be removed after 6 to 8 postoperative weeks. Adequate rehabilitation is vital for normal function because loss of motion at the wrist and the forearm greatly diminishes the limb's ultimate function. Early unrestricted motion is initiated only when the radius and the DRUJ are stable (see Fig. 7).

COMPLICATIONS

Nonunion can occur but is rare when good surgical techniques are used to apply appropriate 3.5-mm DC or LC-DC plates. A deficit in the sensory branch of the radial nerve may occur if the nerve is not identified and protected during the dorsal surgical exposure. Refracture after plate removal is discussed on page 126.

SKELETALLY IMMATURE PATIENTS

Closed manipulation of the radius with the forearm in supination is usually successful in a child who has been adequately sedated. Anatomic reduction is essential. Postoperatively, a long-arm cast is applied with the elbow flexed at 90° and with the forearm supinated. The cast is maintained for 6 weeks. After this time the cast can be replaced by a short-arm cast or left off, depending on the progress of healing and the comfort requirements of the patient.

REFERENCES

1. Galeazzi R. Über ein besonderes Syndrom bei Verletzungen im Bereich der Unterarmknochen. *Arch Orthop Unfallchir* 1934;35:557–62.
2. Moore TM, Klein JP, Patzakis MJ, Harvey JP. Results of compression-plating of closed Galeazzi fracture. *J Bone Joint Surg* 1985;67A:1015–21.
3. Hughston JC. Fracture of the distal radial shaft. Mistakes in management. *J Bone Joint Surg* 1957; 39–A:249–64.
4. Henry AK. *Extensile exposure*. Edinburgh: Livingstone; 1956.
5. Mast J, Jakob R, Ganz R. Reduction with plates. In: *Planning and reduction technique in fracture surgery*. Berlin: Springer-Verlag; 1989:48–51.

Fractures of Both Bones of the Forearm

MECHANISM OF INJURY

Diaphyseal radial and ulnar fractures usually result from moderate- to high-energy trauma. Motor vehicle accidents and falls produce most of these fractures, and direct blows, ballistic trauma, and pathologic lesions account for the rest. The neural injury most commonly associated with these injuries is neuropraxia due to contusion. Other neural or vascular injuries can occur from laceration by sharp bony fragments, compartmental syndrome, or disruption in the course of an open injury.

ANATOMIC CONSIDERATIONS

The radius lies almost parallel to the ulna and is curved in a unique lateral bow at the midshaft. The annular ligament connects the radius and the ulna proximally at the elbow capsule. Distally, the two bones are connected by the wrist capsule, the anterior and posterior radial and ulnar ligaments, and a fibrocartilaginous disk. An interosseous membrane tethers the two bones obliquely from the distal ulna to the proximal radius (Fig. 8).

Major neural, vascular, and muscle structures contribute to

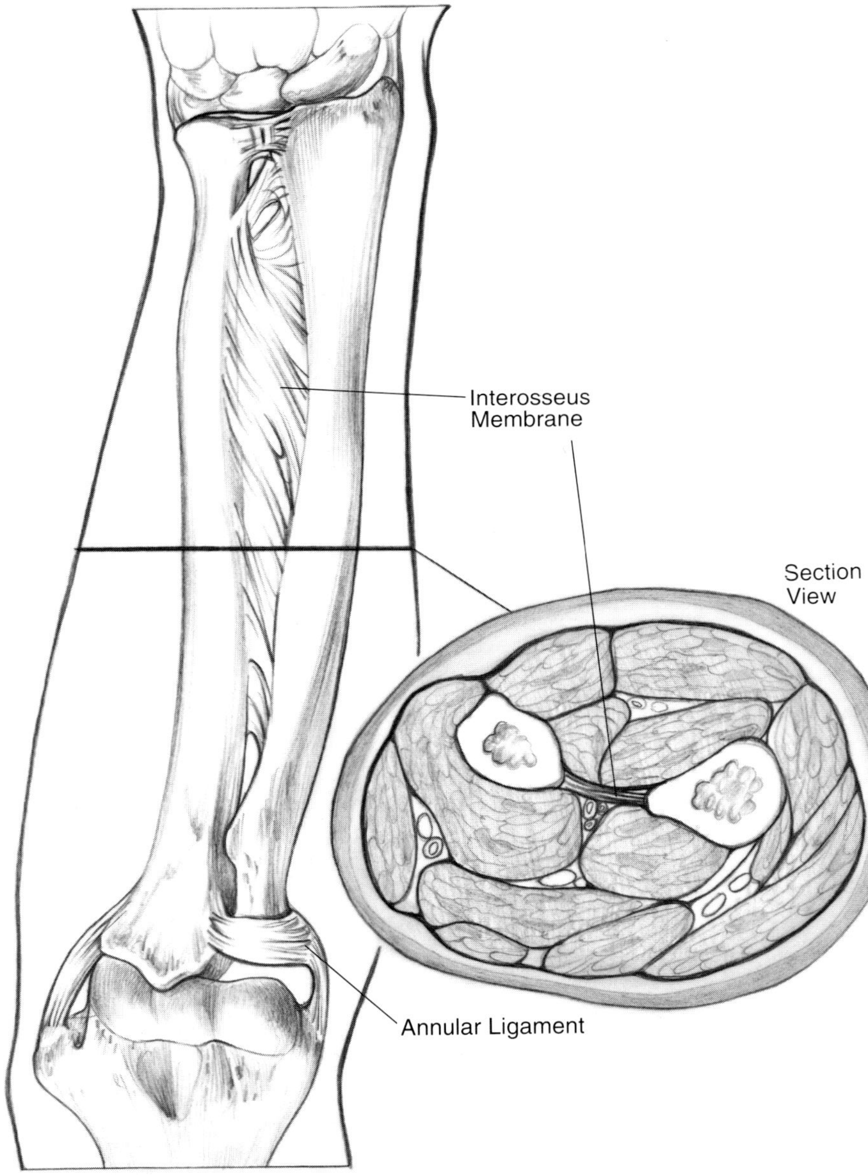

FIG. 8. Diagrammatic representation of forearm anatomy.

the complexity of the forearm's anatomy. The three compartments of the forearm are surrounded by dense fascia. The muscles within these compartments span the elbow, the forearm, and the wrist obliquely and allow flexion, extension, ulnar and radial deviation, supination, and pronation in these joints. Application of these forces to disrupted bone results in fracture deformity.

CLASSIFICATION

No widely used classification schema exists for diaphyseal fractures of the radius and the ulna. The AO classification of long bone fractures, as adapted by the OTA, is recommended for reporting purposes.These fractures are classified by description of skin integrity, the level of fracture and the fracture pattern, displacement, angulation, and rotatory malalignment.

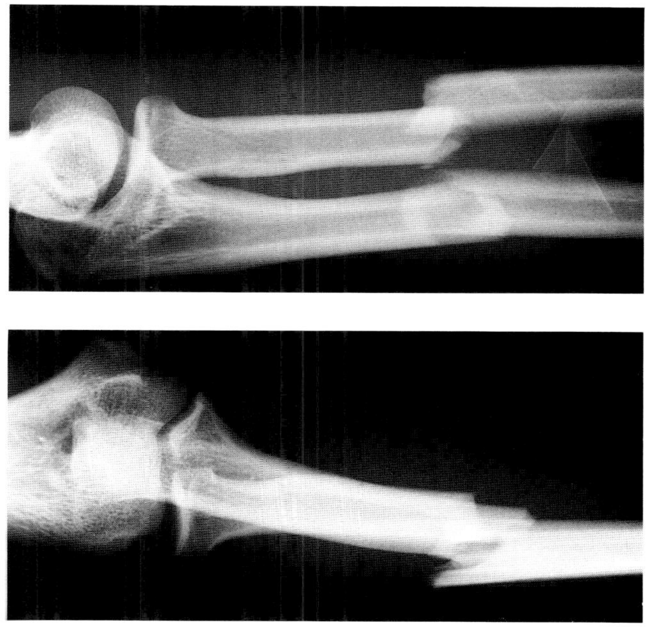

A

B

FIG. 9. A,B: This patient was involved in a high-speed auto accident. The fractures were associated with a forearm compartmental syndrome.

ASSESSMENT

Physical Examination

A patient with radial and ulnar fractures experiences pain and diminished function immediately after injury. Swelling, deformity, and crepitus are usually noted in the forearm. Before the extremity is manipulated, the results of complete neurologic and vascular assessments of the entire extremity must be documented. The skin is carefully inspected for open wounds.

Radiographic Evaluation

Good-quality AP and lateral radiographs must include the elbow, the forearm, and the wrist. Fracture characteristics, including comminution, shortening, angulation, and rotatory malalignment, are assessed (Fig. 9).

Special Studies

Compartmental pressure measurements are taken of the three forearm compartments when a compartmental syndrome exists or is suspected. Angiography is indicated when a vascular injury is likely to exist, particularly after high-energy ballistic trauma.

EMERGENT MANAGEMENT

Emergent intervention in open injuries usually consists of controlling hemorrhage by direct pressure. Open wounds are dressed aseptically and a prophylactic tetanus immunization is administered. Splinting is done carefully in situ or after gentle distal traction is applied. The neurovascular examination is repeated after the limb is splinted and the results are documented.

DEFINITIVE MANAGEMENT

Closed treatment of displaced fractures of both bones in the forearm is associated with a high incidence of unsatisfactory results and is not recommended. If closed management is performed follow-up must include radiographic evaluation of the fracture at regular intervals. A good functional outcome correlates directly with the maintenance of anatomic reduction. Accurate reduction is usually achieved and maintained by ORIF with rigid plate and interfragmentary screw fixation, used in conjunction with bone grafting (1,2).

A volar approach is usually recommended for a distal radial fracture and either a dorsal or a volar approach is used for middle and proximal radial fractures. The ulna is exposed along its subcutaneous border between the dorsal and the volar compartments. Open reduction and internal fixation do not increase the rate of infection of open forearm fractures. Open wounds, especially those caused by ballistic injuries, require immediate stabilization.

The extent of soft-tissue damage is reduced by using indirect reduction techniques. Periosteal stripping must be kept to a minimum. Narrow retractors are placed strategically to avoid penetration of the interosseous membrane. Butterfly fragments are manipulated carefully to protect the vital soft-tissue envelopes and are fixed with interfragmentary screws

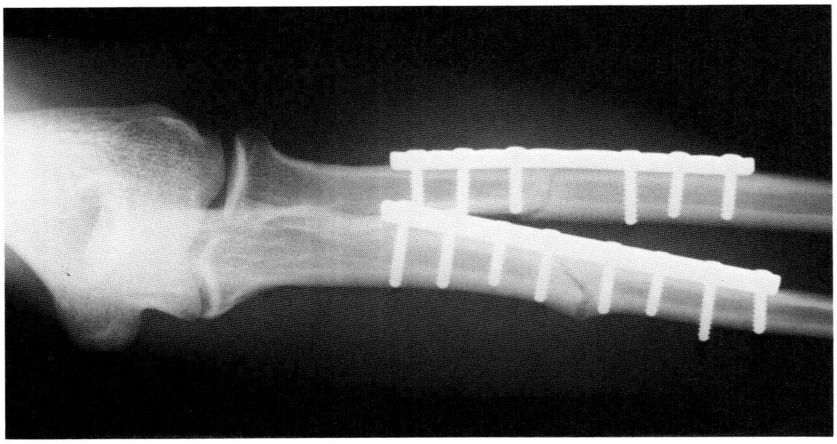

FIG. 10. Forearm fasciotomies followed by reduction and plate fixation. Both plates are poorly contoured, producing fracture gaps opposite the plate. Delayed union may result. Lag screws through the plates should have been used. Skin grafting was necessary.

or with small-diameter lag screws, depending on the sizes of the bony fragments. An appropriately contoured eight-hole, 3.5-mm DCP or LC-DCP is used to stabilize most adult fractures. Before the wound is closed, intraoperative radiographs are taken to verify the accuracy of the reduction and the placement of the implants. Screws of inappropriate length are replaced at that time. Autogenous bone grafting is recommended for significantly comminuted fractures and those with significant bone loss (1).

The functional results achieved by intramedullary nail fixation are less satisfactory than those after plating (3). External fixation of open fractures is reserved for fractures with massive bone and soft-tissue contamination and loss and is rarely used. When external fixation is planned it is usually temporary and the pins should be placed remotely. Provisions must be made for frequent surgical debridement and early skin-flap coverage. In the event of bone loss, treatment consists of delayed plate fixation with tricortical iliac bone grafting after soft-tissue coverage is achieved. A compartmental syndrome warrants immediate fasciotomies along with release of the carpal tunnel. The wounds are managed by delayed skin closure or by split-thickness skin grafting (Fig. 10).

The guidelines for rehabilitation depend on several factors, including the compliance of the patient, the stability of the fracture, and the number of associated injuries that were sustained. The time to union varies. Active range-of-motion exercises of the wrist and the elbow are begun as soon as the clinical situation permits.

COMPLICATIONS

Many complications can be avoided by the use of proper surgical techniques. Iatrogenic neural or vascular injuries can be prevented by a good understanding of forearm anatomy and the nature of the injury. Nonunion rates are low when compression plating techniques are followed and appropriate bone grafting techniques are used.

Plate removal is usually a safe procedure but is accompanied by some risk of refracture. Refracture after plate removal is usually related to an inappropriately large plate; a 4.5-mm plate is too large for most adult forearm fractures. Plate removal is not mandatory, but the long-term effects of retained plates are not known.

Crossunion of the radius to the ulna is a well-recognized yet poorly defined complication that results in diminished supination and pronation in the forearm. The risk of crossunion increases with delayed open reduction, the presence of bony fragments in the interosseous space, the protrusion of inappropriately long screws through the opposite cortex, fractures of both forearm bones at the same level, and associated closed head injuries. A diaphyseal crossunion is resected when it is metabolically inactive on a bone scan (4).

SKELETALLY IMMATURE PATIENTS

Fractures of both forearm bones in a child rarely require open treatment. Closed reduction and splinting are performed under anesthesia and a well-molded splint is applied. The arm must be monitored closely for compartmental syndrome.

REFERENCES

1. Chapman NW, Gordon JE, Zissimos AG. Compression-plate fixation of acute fracture of the diaphyses of the radius and ulna. *J Bone Joint Surg* 1989;71A:159–69.
2. Anderson LD, Sisk TD, Tooms RE, Park WI. Compression-plate fixation in acute diaphyseal fractures of the radius and ulna. *J Bone Joint Surg* 1975;57A:287–97.
3. Sage FP. Medullary fixation of fractures of the forearm. A study of the medullary canal of the radius and a report of fifty fractures of the radius treated with a prebent triangular nail. *J Bone Joint Surg* 1959;41A:1489–1516.
4. Vince KG, Miller JE. Cross-union complicating fracture of the forearm. Part I: adults. *J Bone Joint Surg* 1987;69A:640–53.

Orthopaedic Trauma Protocols, edited by
Sigvard T. Hansen Jr., and Marc F. Swiontkowski,
Raven Press, Ltd., New York, © 1993.

CHAPTER 15

Wrist

Allan W. Bach

Distal Radial Fractures

MECHANISMS OF INJURY

Next to phalangeal fractures, distal radial fractures are the most common injuries of the upper extremity in all age groups. Many fracture patterns can occur and the resulting pattern depends upon the age of the patient, the quality of the bone, the level at which energy was absorbed, and the mechanism of injury. Most distal radial fractures occur when axial load is applied with a rotatory component to an extended wrist. Rotation of the forearm into pronation on a fixed wrist can cause a dorsally angulated fracture or a dorsal lip fracture (Colles' fracture) (Fig. 1A); rotation of the forearm into supination on a fixed wrist results in volar angulation or an anterior lip fracture (Smith's fracture) (Fig. 1B). Forced hyperflexion is also a common mechanism. Distal radial fractures in children are often incomplete (torus or greenstick), owing to the plastic nature of their bones. Fractures in this age group often occur through the distal radial physis. In young adults, distal radial fractures typically are associated with high-energy trauma. Scaphoid fractures or ligamentous ruptures occur from the same mechanisms and forces that would cause distal radial fractures in older patients with osteopenic bone. A direct blow to the distal forearm may cause a fracture in addition to displacement or, if the force is very strong, a comminuted fracture. Associated injuries include distal radioulnar joint displacement, ulnar styloid fractures, carpal fractures, and ligamentous ruptures.

ANATOMIC CONSIDERATIONS

The two articular facets on the surface of the distal radius, the elliptical (scaphoid) and the spheroid (lunate), are separated by an anteroposterior ridge. The normal angulation of

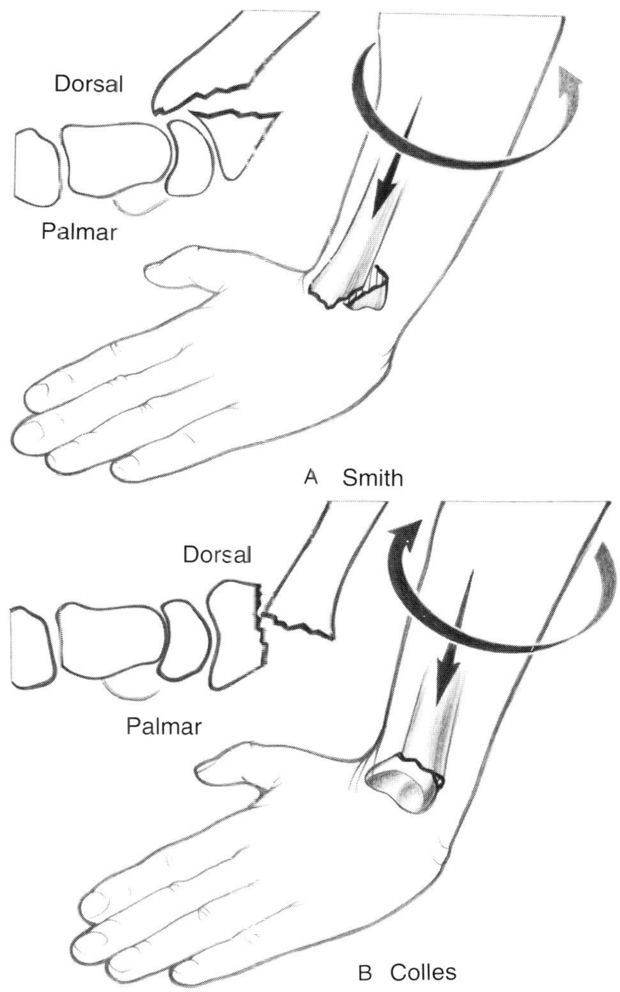

FIG. 1. A: A Smith's fracture, caused by forearm supination on a fixed wrist, results in volar angulation of the distal fragment. **B:** A Colles' fracture, caused by forearm pronation on a fixed wrist, is associated with dorsal angulation of the distal fragment.

Department of Orthopaedics, Harborview Medical Center, University of Washington, Seattle, Washington 98104

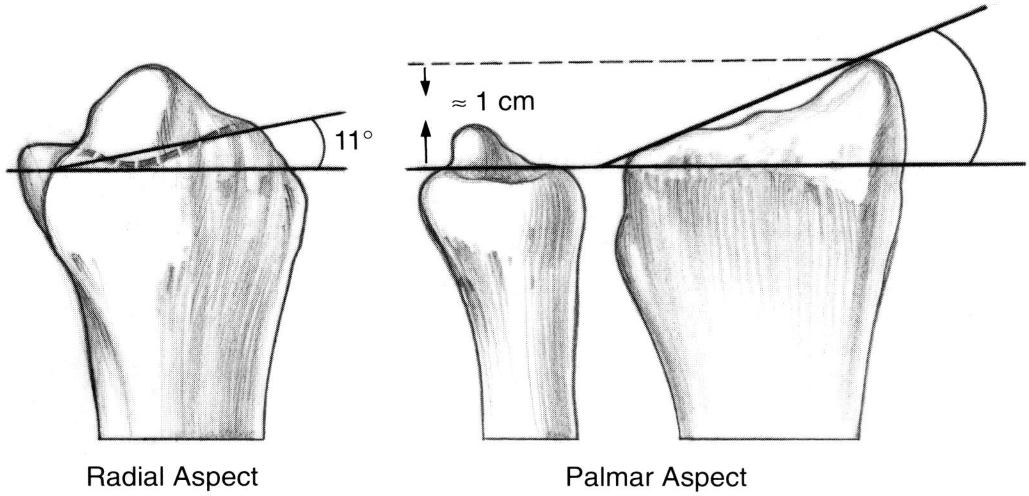

FIG. 2. These measurements represent the normal relationship of the distal radius and ulna in an average adult.

the articular surface of the distal radius is approximately 11° in volar tilt and 23° in the radioulnar plane (Fig. 2). The sigmoid notch of the distal radius articulates with the ulnar head in an arc of approximately 70°.

The ligamentous attachments on the volar aspect of the carpus form two triangular structures and are stronger than the more transverse dorsal radiocarpal ligaments. The triangular fibrocartilaginous complex (TFCC) connects the distal ulna to the radius.

CLASSIFICATION

Many eponyms are associated with the various classifications that exist for distal radial fractures. Although the names are historically significant, they can make classification confusing. Melone's classification (1) is useful for directing treatment of many distal radial fractures but it does not include all fracture types. The AO classification is preferred because it includes all types of distal radial and ulnar fractures (Fig. 3).

ASSESSMENT

Physical Examination

Swelling and deformity are typical presenting symptoms of a distal radial fracture. Dorsally angulated fractures demonstrate a characteristic silver-fork deformity. The initial examination must include an immediate evaluation of neurovascular function, particularly of the median nerve. Sudden loss of median nerve function usually indicates a direct injury to the nerve (neuropraxia); progressive loss of median nerve function indicates a carpal tunnel syndrome (compressive neuropathy) secondary to soft-tissue swelling or hematoma.

Radiographic Evaluation

Standard radiographic evaluation includes AP and lateral views of the entire forearm and hand. Oblique radiographic views of the distal forearm are obtained to assess the amount of fracture displacement and the fracture pattern. Traction views are useful for assessing severely displaced fractures but must be taken with the patient sedated.

Special Studies

Tomography is indicated to assess displacement of intraarticular fragments (e.g., die-punch injuries). Computerized tomography scans can be substituted for tomograms if the AP and lateral reconstructions are of good quality. Unresolved ulnar or median nerve dysfunction is evaluated by nerve conduction studies and electromyography (EMG) three weeks after injury.

EMERGENT MANAGEMENT

Many closed distal radial fractures can be treated definitively by closed reduction immediately after radiographic assessment. A hematoma block with 1% lidocaine or 0.5%

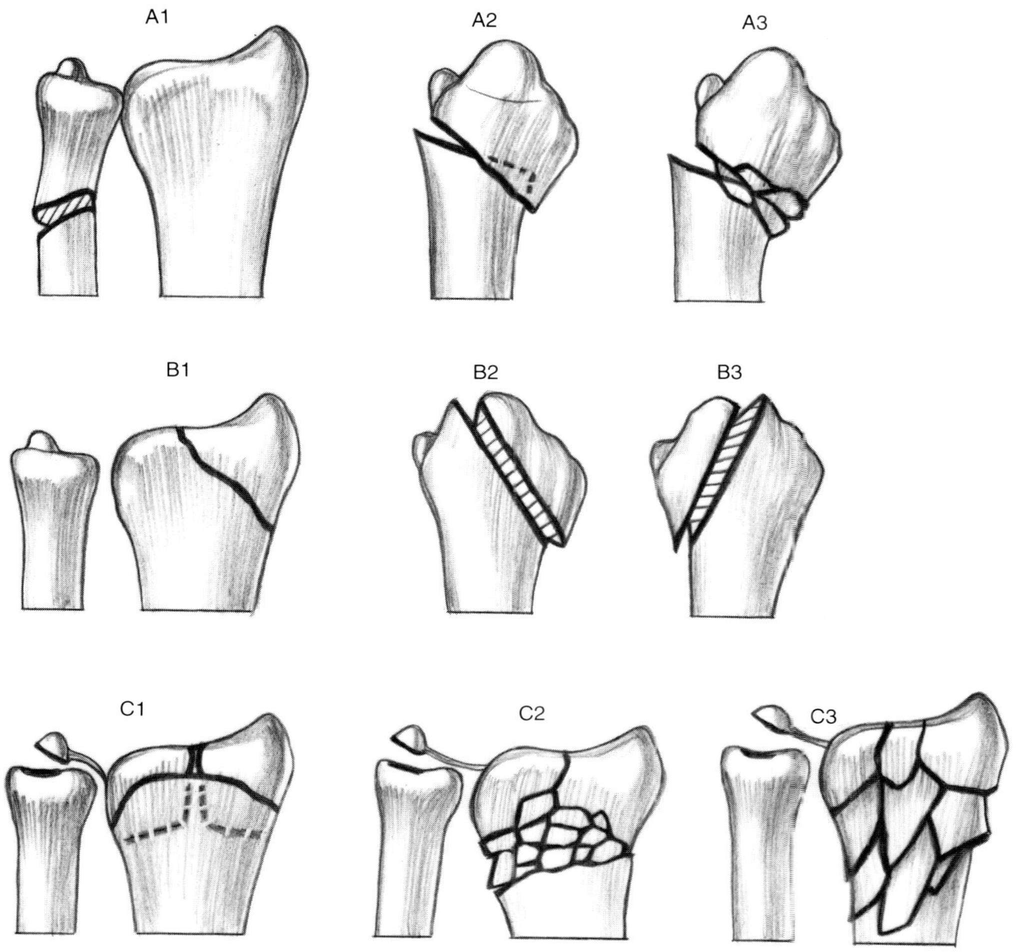

FIG. 3. The AO classification for distal radial fractures. (Adapted from Müller ME, Algöwer M, Schneider R, Willenegger H. *Manual of Internal Fixation,* 3rd ed. Berlin: Springer-Verlag, 1991. Müller ME, Nazarian S, Koch P, Schatzker J. *Comprehensive Classification of Fractures of Long Bones.* Berlin: Springer-Verlag, 1990. Used with permission.)

bupivacaine without epinephrine provides adequate anesthesia for closed reduction in children and elderly patients. Young adults may require a regional or a general anesthetic. All distal radial fractures are splinted after they are assessed, whether they were reduced or not.

DEFINITIVE MANAGEMENT

The optimal treatment for a distal radial fracture depends on several factors: the stability of the fracture, the amount of displacement, the quality of the bone, the age and functional requirements of the patient, the experience of the surgeon with the various treatment modalities, and the availability of equipment. The timing of definitive treatment depends on the characteristics of the fracture and the general condition of the patient. Distal radial fractures are treated by one of the following five procedures; two of these are accomplished by closed reduction and three require operative intervention.

Closed Reduction and Splinting

This method is appropriate for extraarticular fractures and for fractures with a nondisplaced intraarticular component. Manual traction or finger-trap distraction may have to be applied before reduction.

Closed Reduction and Percutaneous Pinning

Percutaneous pinning is indicated for unstable extraarticular fractures. This method is also used to treat intraarticular fractures with nondisplaced fragments and unstable fractures that were reduced closed (2).

External Fixation

External fixation is appropriate for axially unstable fractures that cannot be managed by closed methods (3) (Fig. 4). A small external fixator is applied to stabilize the distal radius with the wrist in a neutral position. Extreme positions are to be avoided. The pin sites for the fixator are predrilled and the pins are placed by hand. The length of time that the external fixator remains in place varies; the device should be left on for the shortest possible amount of time and should be removed as soon as fracture union is demonstrated radiographically.

Open Reduction and Internal Fixation

When wrist motion is of primary consideration and the patient's bone is of good quality, unstable distal radial fractures are treated by ORIF. However, ORIF offers no advantages over simpler methods of fixation unless it can provide adequate stability and near-anatomic realignment of the articular surfaces (<1.0 mm of displacement) (Figs. 5–7).

The incision and the hardware to be used are determined on an individual basis according to the pattern of the fracture and its location. A volar approach is preferred for extraarticular fractures. A dorsal approach is used to visualize intraarticular fractures and dorsally displaced fractures which might require a dorsal plate. Fractures with volar displacement are plated through an anterior Henry incision. Temporary external fixation can be used intraoperatively to facilitate reduction of articular fragments.

External Fixation and Internal Fixation

External and internal fixation can be combined when open reduction is necessary to restore anterior alignment, but internal fixation does not provide definitive stabilization. Bone graft is applied to the metaphysis to buttress the articular fragments, to maintain reduction, and to reduce the time spent in an external fixator. The postoperative treatment of distal radial fractures is individualized according to the characteristics of the fracture and the type of treatment that was performed. Standard postoperative treatment consists of early mobilization of the fingers and shoulder and application of loose dressings and splints to prevent edema caused by tight dressings or by holding the upper extremity in a dependent position. Altered sensation in two-point discrimination and loss of thenar muscle function suggest a severe carpal tunnel syndrome, which is treated by early carpal tunnel release.

COMPLICATIONS

Loss of initial reduction is commonly associated with closed treatment of distal radial fractures. For this reason,

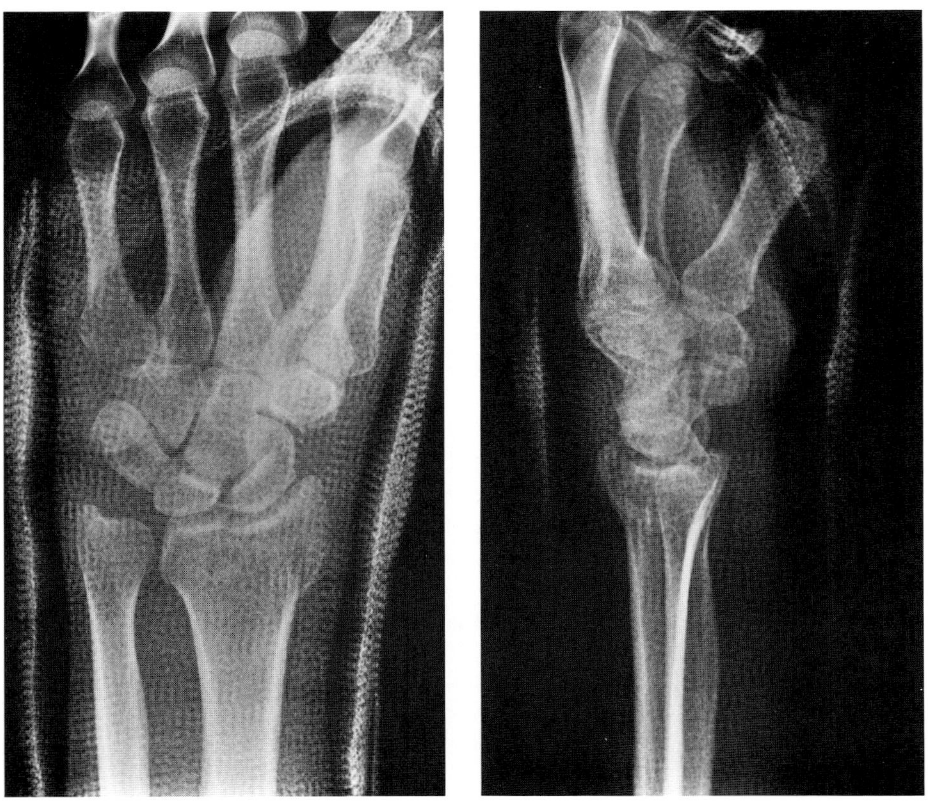

A,B

FIG. 4. A,B: Closed distal radius fracture in a young female with unacceptable position after closed reduction.

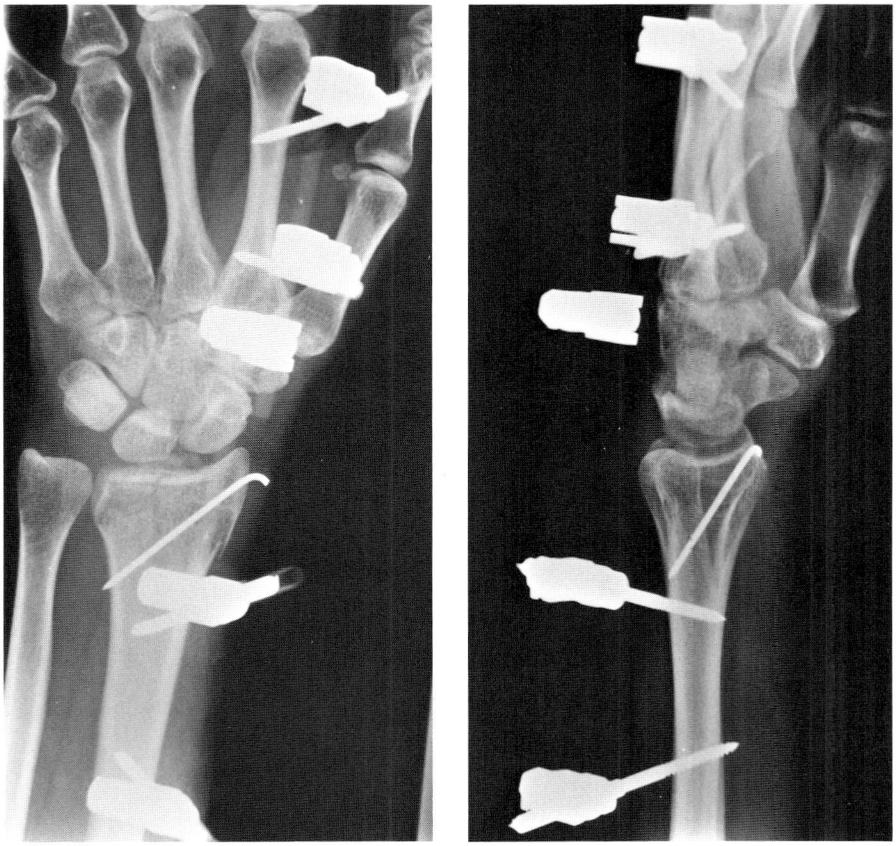

A,B

FIG. 5. A,B: After closed reduction and percutaneous pinning with external fixation, this combination of techniques allows maintenance of reduction without direct open treatment.

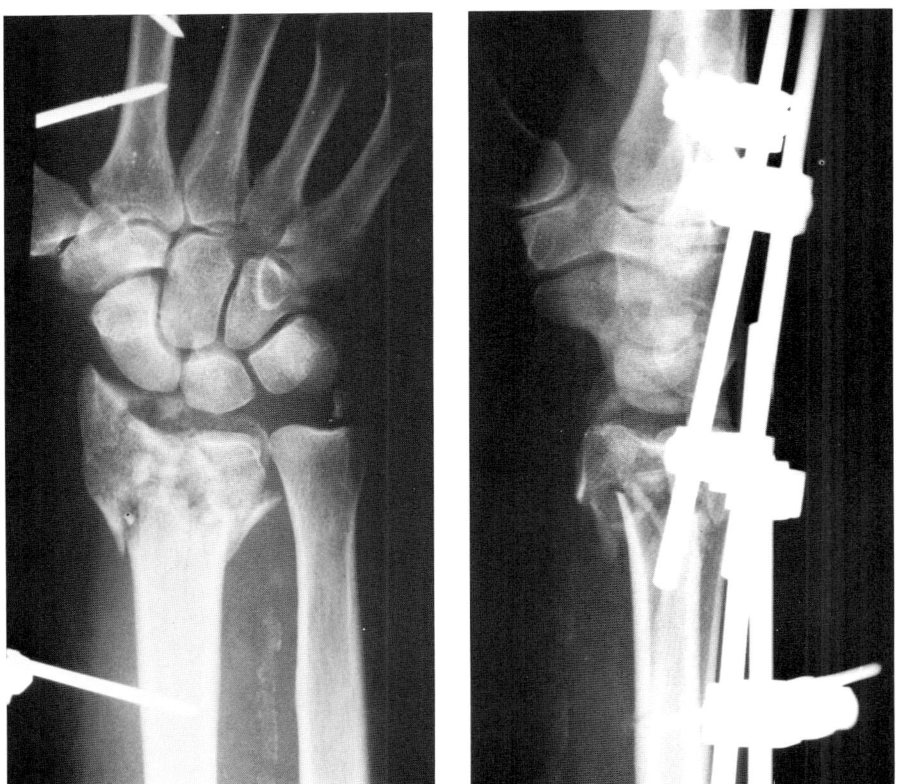

A,B

FIG. 6. A,B: Unacceptable position of a very comminuted distal radius fracture after external fixation. Note the incongruity of the distal radial surface.

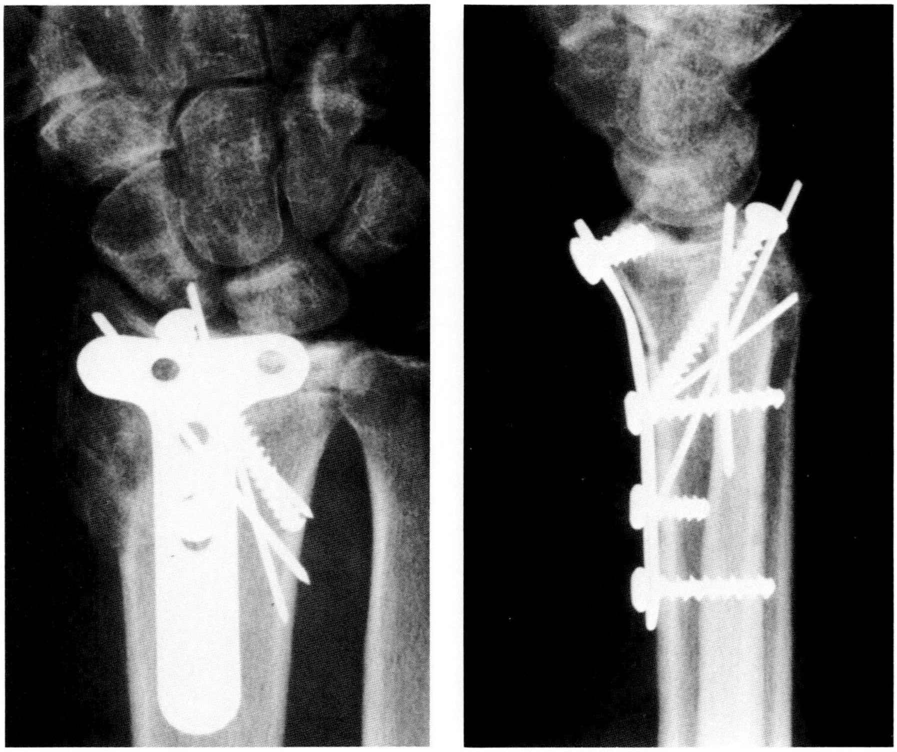

A,B

FIG. 7. A,B: Correction of the articular surface incongruity with open reduction and internal fixation with iliac crest bone graft.

radiographs are obtained at 3, 7, and 14 days after injury to verify continued reduction. Loss of reduction is an indication for repeat reduction, often with the addition of internal or external fixation. Malunion is common after a distal radial fracture and does not preclude a functional outcome if healing occurs without excessive malpositioning. Unacceptable malunions are those which have more than 5 mm shortening of the radius, loss of radial tilt, or more than 10° dorsiflexion of the articular surface on a lateral radiographic view.

Distal radioulnar joint instability is infrequently recognized but can occur with all types of distal radial fractures. Compression of the median nerve occurs in 10% to 20% of fractures secondary to neuropraxia from a direct blow or to a carpal tunnel syndrome from swelling or bone impingement. Injuries to the ulnar and radial nerves occur infrequently. Reflex sympathetic dystrophy can result from an excessively tight dressing or cast, an undiagnosed carpal tunnel syndrome, or other nerve lesions. The incidence of reflex sympathetic dystrophy is greatly decreased when early active finger and shoulder exercises are initiated early to prevent edema. Nonunion of a distal radial fracture is rare with appropriate treatment.

SKELETALLY IMMATURE PATIENTS

Most distal radial fractures in children and adolescents are treated by closed reduction with the same considerations that are applied to treating physeal fractures.

REFERENCES

1. Melone CP Jr. Articular fractures of the distal radius. *Orthop Clin North Am* 1984;15:217.
2. Clancey GJ. Percutaneous Kischner-wire fixation of Colles fractures. A prospective study of thirty cases. *J Bone Joint Surg* 1984;66A:1008–14.
3. Cooney WP III, Linscheid RL, Dobyns JH. External pin fixation for unstable Colles' fractures. *J Bone Joint Surg* 1979;61A:840–45.

Radiocarpal Dislocations

MECHANISMS OF INJURY

Radiocarpal dislocations are rare injuries that result from high-energy trauma. Dislocations can occur on the dorsal or the volar aspects of the wrist and are caused by compression and rotatory forces applied to a dorsiflexed or volar-flexed wrist. Dorsal dislocations are associated with dorsal lip or styloid process fractures of the radius. Rupture of the intercarpal ligaments is a common associated injury.

ANATOMIC CONSIDERATIONS

The proximal row of the carpus is supported by strong volar ligaments and the projecting dorsal lip of the radial articular surface blocks dorsal dislocation of the carpus. However, many wrist dislocations include gross ligamentous disruptions from high-energy forces and result in carpal drift, especially ulnar translation.

CLASSIFICATION

Dislocations on both the dorsal and the volar aspects of the wrist are classified into two types. Type I includes isolated radiocarpal joint injuries, and type II involves dislocations with associated intercarpal injuries.

ASSESSMENT

Physical Examination

The appearance of a dislocated wrist is similar to that of a severely displaced distal radial fracture. Both injuries demonstrate significant swelling and deformity. Physical examination includes an accurate neurovascular examination, with particular attention paid to median nerve function. Because a wrist dislocation is usually caused by high-energy trauma, the presence of associated injuries in the proximal upper extremity must be suspected and ruled out.

Radiographic Evaluation

Obvious deformities are evident on AP and lateral radiographs. However, fracture type and intercarpal alignment are more difficult to assess.

Special Studies

Tomograms or CT scans are occasionally necessary to assess the alignment of the carpus if anatomic relationships have been disrupted.

EMERGENT MANAGEMENT

Reduction of a dislocated wrist should be done as soon as possible after injury to relieve impingement on neurovascular structures. Reduction can be accomplished by applying traction along the axis of the deformity. Dorsal dislocations should be maintained in slight dorsiflexion and volar dislocations should be maintained in slight volar flexion.

DEFINITIVE MANAGEMENT

Correct classification of a wrist dislocation is an important element of planning the appropriate treatment. In type I injuries, the wrist is assessed for alignment and stability. If the alignment is satisfactory, the wrist is immobilized in the appropriate position in a long-arm cast for 8 weeks (Figs. 8 and 9). Open reduction and internal fixation are indicated if the alignment of a concomitant radial fracture is unsatisfactory. Most type II injuries are treated by open alignment of the carpus, Kirschner-wire fixation, and ligament repair. Stress radiographs with ulnar translation should be obtained to reveal ulnar translational instability in the carpus. Open repair of the radiocarpal ligaments is indicated in the presence of translational instability. Because ligament repair is difficult to accomplish through the volar incision of Henry, dorsal and volar incisions are used. The approach for ligament repair is made through the fourth dorsal compartment and through the extended carpal tunnel incision. The ligaments are repaired by ligament-to-bone fixation with nonabsorbable sutures. Traction radiographs and AP and lateral views are repeated after reduction. The wrist is immobilized in a cast for 8 weeks before active range-of-motion exercises are initiated. Full range of motion of the wrist is not permitted until 3 months postoperatively.

COMPLICATIONS

Loss of reduction can occur with any type of treatment, and therefore every patient with a radiocarpal dislocation,

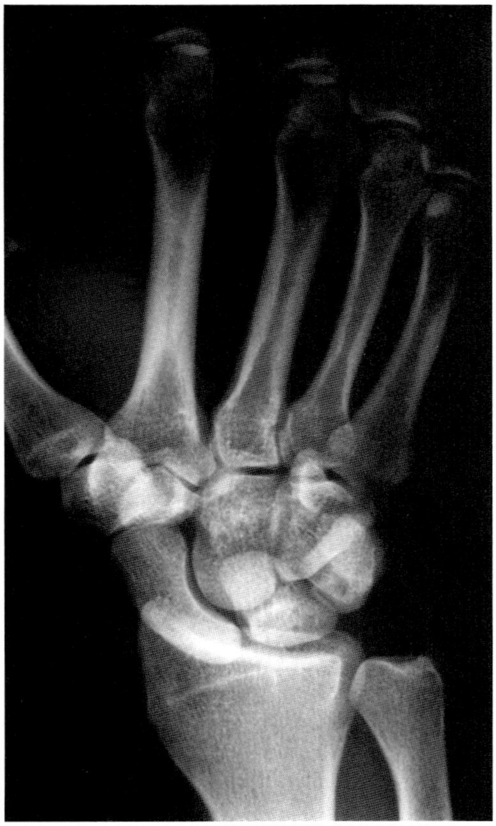

A

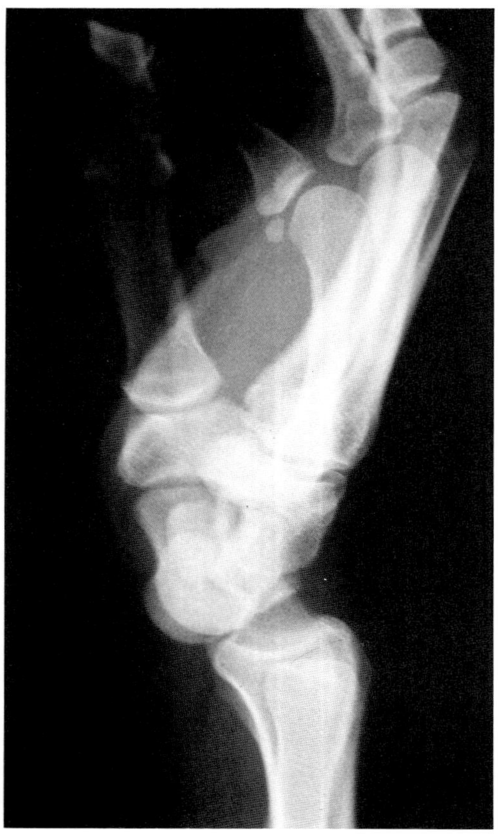

B

FIG. 8. A,B: Volar radial carpal dislocation type I.

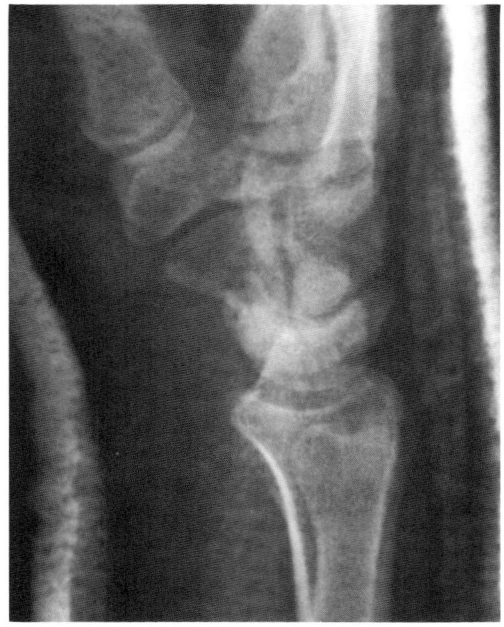

A

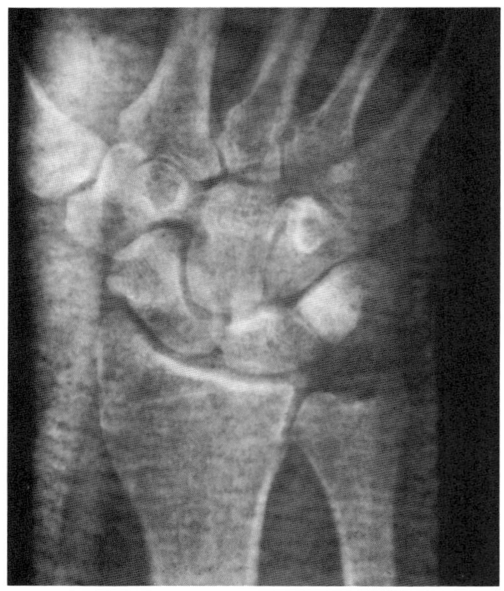

B

FIG. 9. A,B: After closed reduction of type I radial carpal dislocation, note the normal intercarpal relationships.

especially one treated by closed reduction, is followed up with serial radiographs. Commonly seen neurovascular complications include carpal tunnel syndrome and reflex sympathetic dystrophy. Significant joint stiffness is anticipated after a wrist dislocation.

SKELETALLY IMMATURE PATIENTS

Wrist dislocations occur rarely in children but are treated in the same manner as injuries in adults.

Carpal Instabilities

MECHANISMS OF INJURY

Like most wrist injuries, carpal instabilities can occur from excessive dorsiflexion of the wrist. However, carpal instabilities encompass many different injury patterns, depending on the position of the wrist and the amount of energy absorbed at the time of the injury. The severity of injuries can range from minor grade I sprains to major dislocations with complete ligamentous disruptions. Joint dislocations can cause significant traction injuries in the median or ulnar nerves. Open injuries are often associated with arterial, neural, or tendinous injuries.

Volar lunate and dorsal perilunate dislocations represent different stages of the same injury (1). Most injuries occur from excessive dorsiflexion during high-energy trauma. Dorsal lunate or volar perilunate dislocations are rare and occur from excessive volar flexion.

ANATOMIC CONSIDERATIONS

No universally recognized description of carpal functional anatomy exists, but the osseous anatomy of the wrist can be visualized by several concepts. Although contradictions exist among these theories, when considered together they help to explain the complex nature of carpal motion. In the traditional concept, the scaphoid acts as a link between the two carpal rows. Therefore, any break in the scaphoid may render the wrist unstable with compression forces.

The columnar carpal concept, introduced by Navarro in 1935 (2), was modified by Taleisnik (3). In this representation, the lunate, the capitate, the hamate, the trapezoid, and the trapezium form the stable central (flexion–extension) column; the scaphoid makes up the lateral (mobile) column; and the triquetrum, which is the pivotal point of the wrist, constitutes the medial (rotational) column. Lichtman et al. (4) presented the oval-ring concept, in which the carpus is attached to the rotatory triquetral–hamate articulation on the medial side and to the mobile scaphotrapezial articulation on the lateral side. The two carpal rows share reciprocal motion and become unstable when there is a break in the ring.

Mayfield (1) classified ligamentous injuries into stages of perilunate injuries (Fig. 10). Several aspects of the complex ligamentous anatomy of the wrist also should be noted. The small intrinsic ligaments are protected by a superficial joint capsule. The major stabilizing structures of the wrist are the

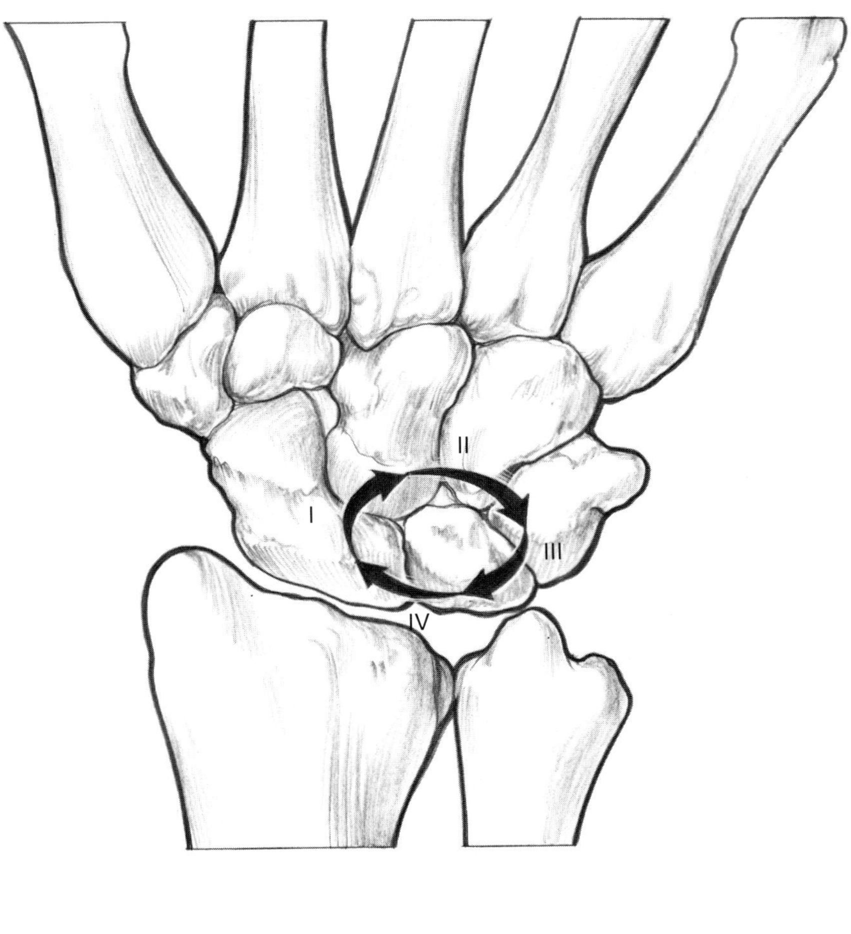

FIG. 10. The Mayfield classification of perilunate instability.

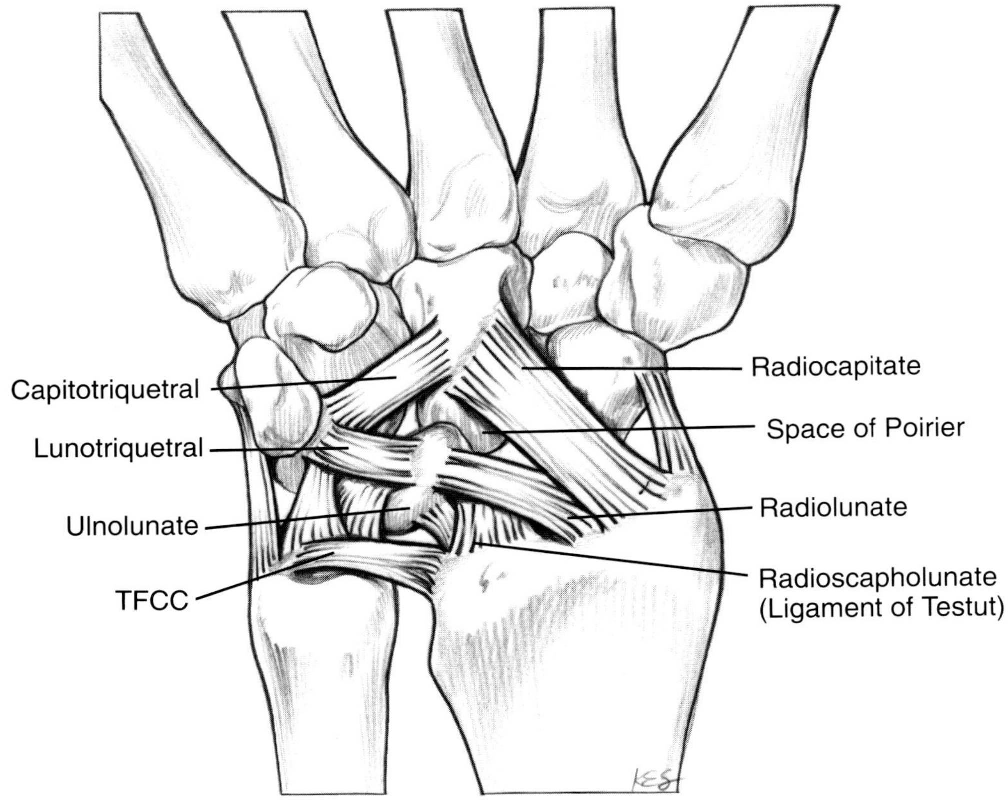

FIG. 11. The distal radial volar ligaments of the wrist.

volar ligaments, which are arranged in a double V-shaped structure. The weakest area is the space of Poirier, which is located over the volar capitate–lunate joint (Fig. 11).

Volar lunate and perilunate dislocations can involve ruptures of the scapholunate, the capitate–lunate, and the triquetral–lunate ligaments. Rupture of all three ligaments represents a stage IV injury of Mayfield. In a dorsal perilunate dislocation, the lunate remains fixed in the lunate fossa of the radius, whereas the carpus is displaced dorsally. Therefore, reduction of the carpus without traction forces the lunate through the volar capsular tear, displacing it from its normal position. As a result, the head of the capitate rests in the lunate fossa of the distal radius and the lunate is hinged on the volar radiolunate ligament.

CLASSIFICATION

Because the anatomic concepts of carpal instability are not in agreement, the classification of wrist instabilities remains descriptive. Green and O'Brien's classification (5) is most commonly used (Table 1).

Table 1. *Green and O'Brien's Classification*[a]

"Major" carpal dislocations
Dorsal perilunate/volar lunate dislocation[a]
Dorsal trans-scaphoid perilunate dislocations[a]
Transradial styloid perilunate dislocation
Scaphocapitate syndrome
Transtriquetral perilunate dislocation
Volar perilunate/dorsal lunate dislocation
Complete dislocation of the scaphoid
Capitate–hamate diastasis
Carpal instability, dissociative
Radial carpal instabilities
Scapholunate dissociation[a]
Dorsiflexion instability (DISI)[a]
Ulnar carpal instabilities
Triquetrohamate instability
Triquetrolunate instability
Volar flexion instability (VISI)
Central carpal instability
Carpal instability, nondissociative
Nondissociative instability of the proximal carpal row
Midcarpal joint
Radiocarpal joint

[a]Most common patterns of injury.

ASSESSMENT

Physical Examination

Most carpal injuries seen in the emergency department are caused by violent trauma. Patients with major carpal injuries present with significant swelling, ecchymosis, deformity, and possible neurovascular compromise. Those with minor instabilities usually attribute the injury to a sprain and might wait days, weeks, or even months before seeking treatment. Specific intercarpal instability or point tenderness may be the only presenting physical signs of an old "minor" instability.

Volar lunate and dorsal perilunate dislocations occur secondary to violent trauma and are accompanied by significant swelling, loss of motion, and pain. Acute compression of the median or ulnar nerves may occur.

Radiographic Evaluation

The key to radiographic examination of wrist instabilities is in recognizing the patterns of collapse or the zig-zag deformities that occur. Linscheid et al. (6) coined the acronyms for dorsal intercalated segment instability (DISI) and volar intercalated segment instability (VISI) to describe these patterns of collapse. These patterns are visible on lateral wrist radiographs taken with the wrist in a neutral position. The most important angles to note are the scapholunate, the capitate–lunate, and the radiolunate. Normally the range of the scapholunate angle is between 30° and 60° and the capitate–lunate and radiolunate angles are less than 15° (Fig. 12).

The standard radiographic evaluation of the wrist consists of AP, neutral–lateral, and oblique scaphoid views. A scapholunate dissociation is best seen on an AP radiograph of the supinated wrist. Normally, smooth arcs can be drawn along the proximal and distal surfaces of the proximal carpal row and the proximal capitate–hamate surface; an interrupted arc is indicative of an abnormality. Posteroanterior radiographs taken in radial and ulnar deviation may reveal other abnormalities. A scapholunate separation can be seen on an AP view with gripping. Lateral views taken with the wrist in flexion and extension can delineate instability patterns. Occasionally, many oblique radiographs must be taken before a nondisplaced fracture is seen. Comparison views are used to diagnose subtle carpal instabilities (Figs. 13–16).

Volar lunate and dorsal perilunate dislocations exhibit characteristic anatomic disruptions on AP and lateral radiographs. The lunate overlaps the capitate and the triquetrum on the AP view, resulting in a radiographic image in which the lunate appears triangular instead of trapezoidal and the volar process appears elongated. The rotation of the lunate appears as volar displacement on the lateral radiograph, which demonstrates a spilled-teacup sign.

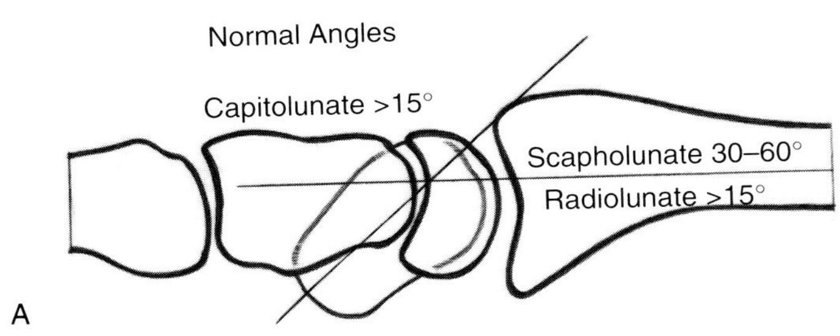

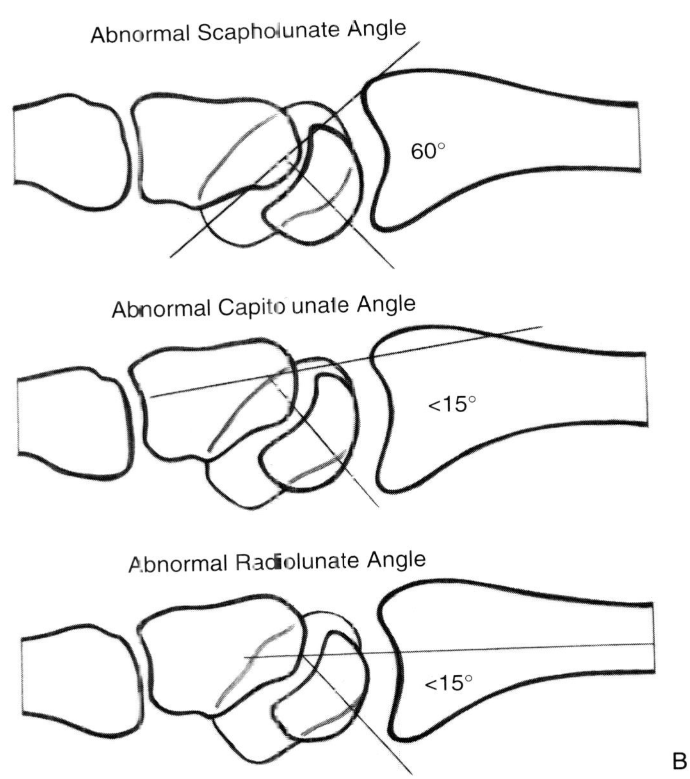

FIG. 12. Normal **(A)** and abnormal **(B)** carpal bone relationships seen from a lateral view.

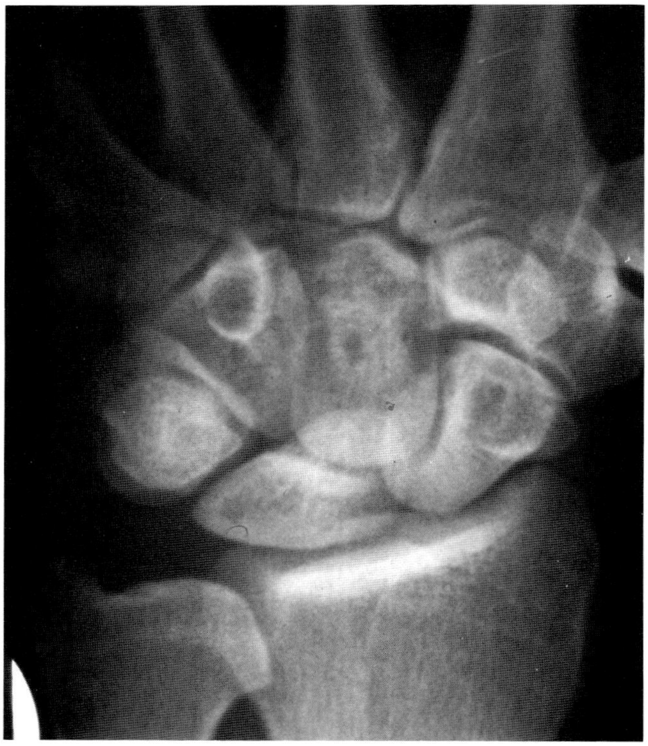

FIG. 13. AP view of wrist showing cortical ring sign.

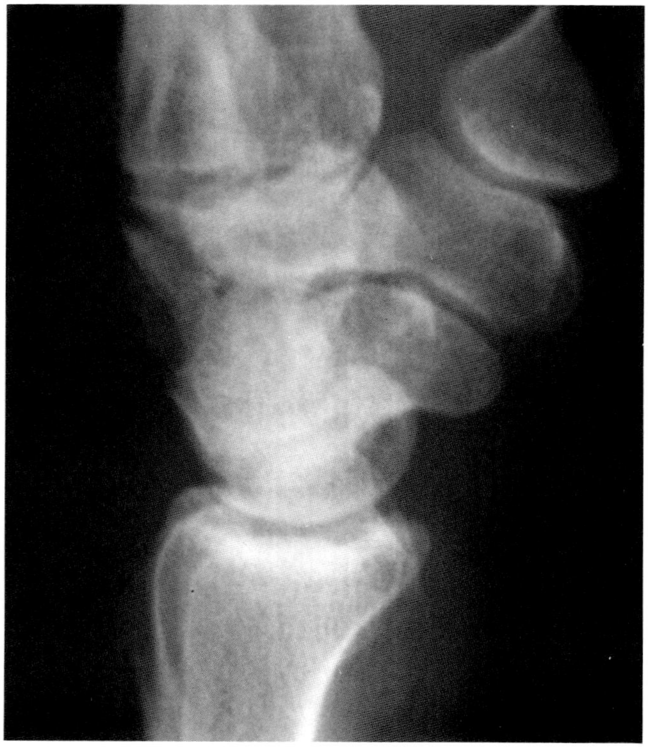

FIG. 14. Lateral view showing increased scapholunate angle and DISI collapse pattern of the wrist.

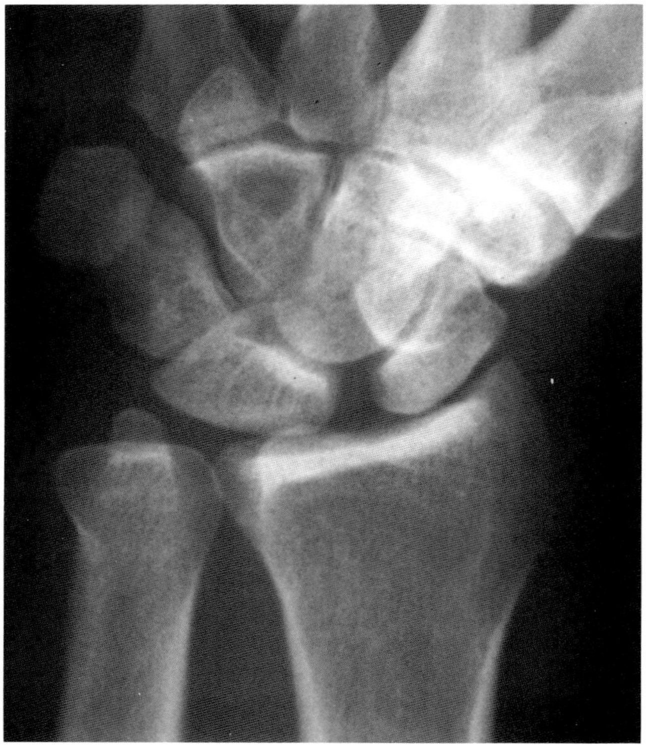

FIG. 15. Grip view showing increased scapholunate gap.

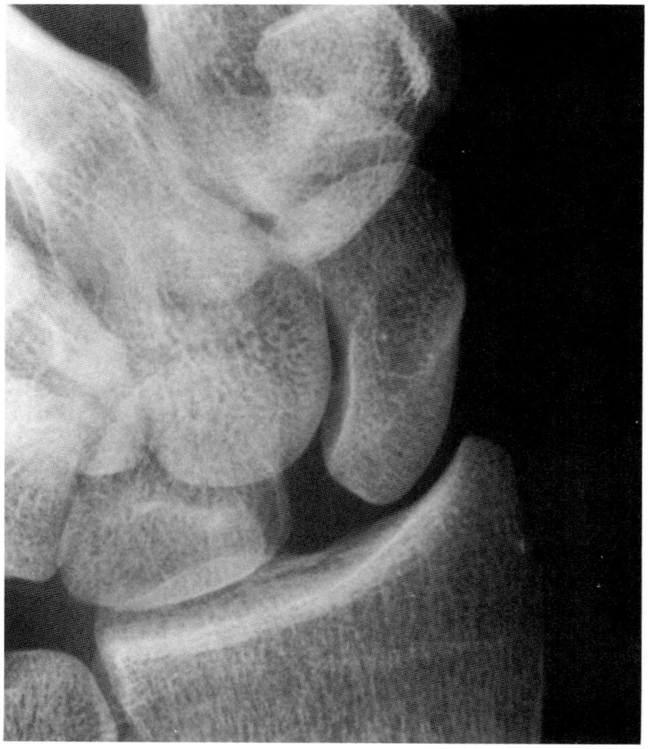

FIG. 16. Radial deviation view showing increased scapholunate gap.

Special Studies

Tomograms and CT scans are obtained to delineate subtle fractures in acute injuries. Videotaped arthrograms and bone scans are useful for identifying subacute or chronic injuries. Arthrography is used extensively in subacute situations. Magnetic resonance imaging is not widely used as a diagnostic tool for carpal instabilities.

EMERGENT MANAGEMENT

Acute ligamentous ruptures can be recognized easily and are treated initially by immobilization in a well-padded long-arm splint. Definitive operative care is recommended as soon as possible after injury.

DEFINITIVE MANAGEMENT

The appropriate treatment of a carpal instability depends on how recently the injury occurred: an instability less than 3 weeks old is considered acute, slightly older injuries are subacute, and those older than 4 months are considered chronic. Normal carpal anatomy must be restored in an acute carpal instability. However, this approach is usually not successful in subacute or chronic cases, and carpal instabilities in older injuries must be treated by ligamentous reconstruction or intercarpal fixation.

Scapholunate Instability

Acute scapholunate instabilities are treated by ligamentous repair and fixation of the scaphoid, the lunate, and the capitate in their anatomic positions with Kirschner wires. Two approaches are necessary for adequate visualization: a dorsal incision and an extended carpal tunnel incision (Fig. 17). The superficial wrist capsule is opened and the injury to the radioscaphoid ligament is identified. The dorsal incision is used to visualize the scapholunate joint. The carpus is then aligned and fixed anatomically with Kirschner wires and, if necessary, the ligaments are sutured through drill holes at

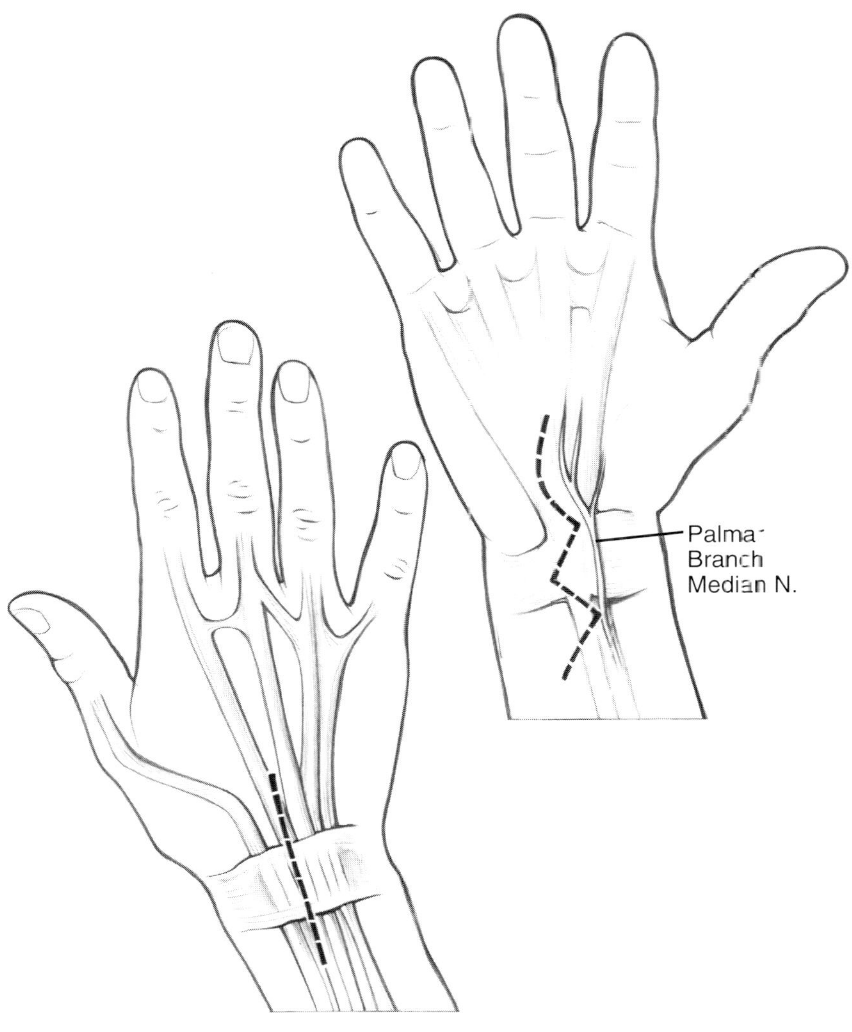

FIG. 17. The incisions used for acute and chronic carpal instabilities.

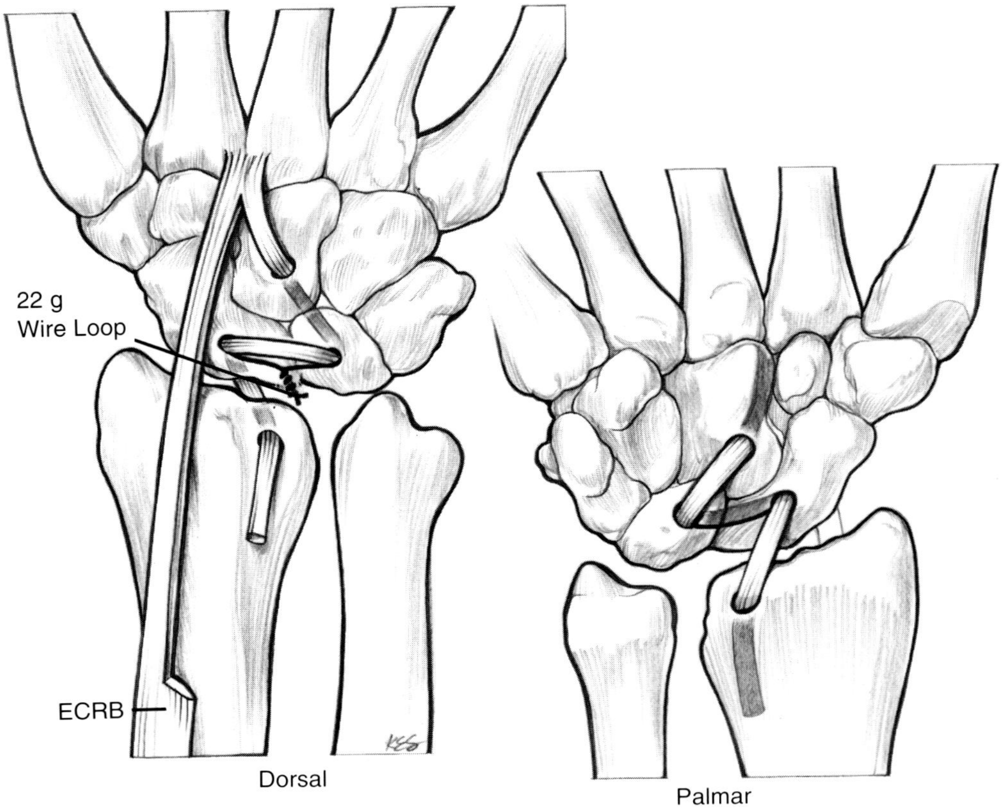

FIG. 18. Ligamentous reconstruction of a chronic complete scapholunate separation by the technique of Almquist, et al.

that time. Subacute or chronic scapholunate dissociations are treated by scaphoid–trapezium–trapezoid (S-T-T) fusion and ligamentous reconstruction (Fig. 18) (7).

Acute scapholunate repairs are immobilized for 8 weeks in a long-arm cast that includes the first metacarpal. After that time, the pins are removed and a short-arm cast is applied. Range-of-motion and light strengthening exercises are permitted in the cast between 8 and 16 weeks, followed by removal of the cast and unrestricted use of the limb. The same protocol is used in the postoperative management of chronic injuries.

Lunate–Triquetral Instability

Ligamentous ruptures on the ulnar side of the carpus can produce VISI deformities when the lunate–triquetral (L-T) ligament is unstable. Repair of the L-T ligament is very difficult, even in the acute stage, but is best accomplished by initial pinning in an anatomic position. Chronic L-T instabilities require fusion, which is associated with a high rate of nonunion. Many internal fixation techniques can be used to stabilize an L-T fusion, but fixation with Kirschner wires and a tension-band wiring technique is preferred to fixation with lag screws. A long-arm cast is applied to immobilize an L-T fusion or repair; the thumb is not included in the cast. An L-T fusion may require cast immobilization for as long as 4 months. If the fusion is not solid at the end of this time, reoperation might be indicated.

Volar Lunate and Dorsal Perilunate Dislocations

Closed reduction of a volar lunate or a dorsal perilunate dislocation should be attempted under anesthesia as soon as the patient's general condition allows reduction to be performed. The hand is suspended by Chinese fingertraps and 10–15 pounds of traction are applied. While the lunate is stabilized by the operator's thumb on the volar side of the wrist, closed reduction is performed by applying traction and maneuvering the wrist into dorsiflexion. Radiographs to reassess the injury are obtained after traction is applied. Reduction is complete when the hand is flexed. This technique is not difficult to perform in an acute situation but might no longer be possible a few days after injury. If normal carpal alignment is seen on radiographs, the wrist is immobilized in a long-arm–thumb spica cast. However, most cases reveal residual carpal instability and require open reduction. Percutaneous pinning is of doubtful value in this situation.

Operative fixation is accomplished through combined dorsal and volar incisions. If the initial attempt at closed reduction was unsuccessful, reduction can be accomplished under direct vision at this time. A volar approach is made through an extended carpal tunnel incision. Carpal collapse is corrected through a dorsal approach. The scaphoid, lunate, and capitate are held in anatomic alignment with .045-inch Kirschner wires. Radiocarpal fixation sometimes is necessary, and the Kirschner wires can be used as "joysticks" to control carpal position during hardware placement. Reduction is assessed intraoperatively by traction radiographs. Radiocarpal fixation is occasionally required to hold the carpals anatomically aligned. A volar ligament rupture is repaired with nonabsorbable suture and then immobilized in a long-arm–thumb spica cast.

Swelling can be expected after surgery and the splint must not be allowed to become too tight. A cast must remain in place for 12 weeks after either closed or open reduction. The Kirschner wires are removed after 8 weeks and the original long-arm cast is replaced with a short-arm cast for 4 weeks, or until fracture union is demonstrated radiographically. Recovery of full range of motion is a slow process and return to full activity takes at least 6 months.

COMPLICATIONS

Neurovascular injury, carpal tunnel syndrome, and reflex sympathetic dystrophy are common complications after treatment of wrist instabilities. After reduction, the ends of the Kirschner wires should be buried under the skin with the tips bent to prevent migration, breakage, and pin-tract infections. Patients should be informed that loss of some wrist motion is common after major ligamentous rupture. Despite advances in therapy, patients rarely regain more than 80% of normal wrist flexibility after a scapholunate dissociation. Loss of reduction is common when volar lunate and dorsal perilunate dislocations are managed without ORIF, and radiographs must be taken weekly for the first month to assess the position of the reduction. Other common complications include nerve compression, reflex sympathetic dystrophy, pin breakage, and pin-tract infection.

SKELETALLY IMMATURE PATIENTS

Because the carpus is still partially cartilaginous in children, documented cases of carpal instability are rare. Comparison radiographic views of the normal wrist and arthrograms should be obtained to rule out false-positive readings on plain radiographs in a child. Volar lunate and dorsal perilunate dislocations occur only in adults.

REFERENCES

1. Mayfield JK. Mechanism of carpal injuries. *Clin Orthop* 1980;149:50.
2. Navarro A. *Anales del Instituto de Clinica Quirurgica y Cirugia Experimental, Imprenta Artistica de Dornaleche.* Montevideo: 1935.
3. Taleisnik J. Wrist anatomy, function and injury. In: *AAOS Instructional Course Lectures.* St. Louis: CV Mosby; 1978.
4. Lichtman DM, Schneider JR, Wafford AR, et al. Ulnar midcarpal instability: clinical and laboratory analysis. *J Hand Surg* 1981;6:515–23.
5. Green DP, O'Brien ET. Classification and management of carpal dislocations. *Clin Orthop* 1980;149:55–72.
6. Linscheid RL, Dobyns JH, Beabout JW, Bryan RS. Traumatic instability of the wrist: diagnosis, classification, and pathomechanics. *J Bone Joint Surg* 1972;54A:1612–32.
7. Almquist EE, Bach AW, Sack JT, Fuhs SE, Newman DM. Four-bone ligament reconstruction for treatment of chronic complete scapholunate separation. *J Hand Surg* 1991;16:322–27.

Distal Radioulnar Joint Injuries

MECHANISMS OF INJURY

The most common mechanism of injury to the distal radioulnar joint is hyperrotation of the forearm in pronation or supination. This injury can occur in combination with other fractures, such Galeazzi's, Moore's, or Essex–Lopresti's lesions. Hyperrotation can also produce isolated ligamentous disruptions similar to TFCC tears. Most rotational injuries occur in conjunction with axial loading on the wrist, which causes a sudden change in the relative lengths of the radius and the ulna at the distal articulation.

ANATOMIC CONSIDERATIONS

The complex function of the distal radioulnar joint is not completely understood. The radioulnar joint is stabilized by several ligamentous structures: the TFCC, the ulnar meniscus homologue, the ulnar collateral ligament, the dorsal and volar radioulnar ligaments, the ulnolunate ligament, the ulnotriquetral ligaments, and the extensor carpi ulnaris tendon sheath. Other structures that help stabilize the distal radioulnar joint include the conformation of the radial sigmoid notch, the interosseous membrane, the extensor retinaculum, the extensor carpi ulnaris sheath, and the pronator quadratus muscle.

The dynamics of wrist motion help to show why hyperpronation results in radioulnar ligament tears and dorsal displacement of the distal ulna. The distal radioulnar joint rotates through an arc of approximately 150° from its stable axis at the base of the ulnar styloid. However, motion in this joint is not limited to rotation. A sliding movement occurs in two planes concurrently with wrist rotation. With pronation, the ulnar head moves dorsally and advances distally, forcing

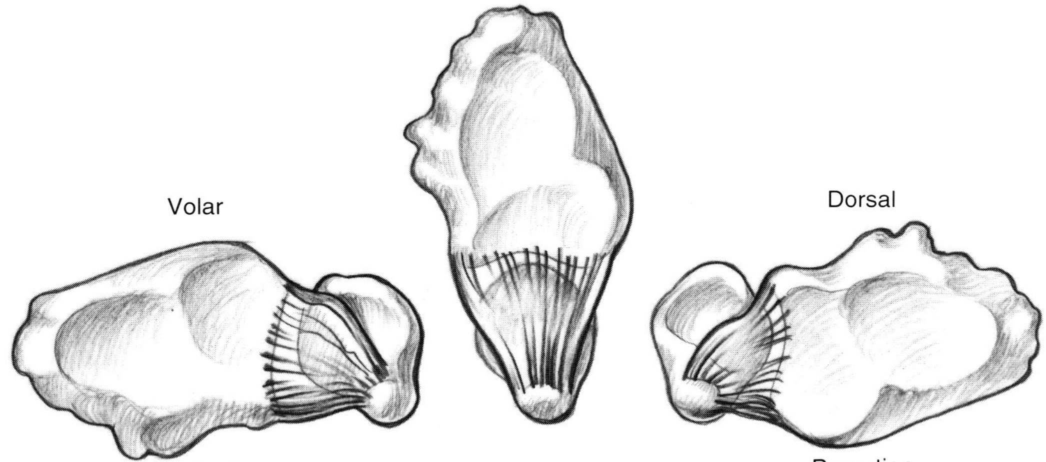

FIG. 19. Distal radioulnar joint stability with supination is dependent upon tension of the dorsal margin of the TFCC. The opposite is true for stability with pronation.

the distal ulna into abduction. With supination, the ulnar head moves in a volar direction and advances proximally, forcing the distal ulna into adduction. A portion of the important radioulnar ligaments remains taut during motion in any direction. During pronation, the volar segment is taut while the dorsal segment is lax. The opposite occurs with supination (Fig. 19).

CLASSIFICATION

No standard classification system exists for isolated instabilities of the distal radioulnar joint and these injuries are classified by association with other injuries. Bowers (1) grouped distal radioulnar joint injuries in the following manner:

I. Acute fractures
II. Acute joint injuries
III. Chronic or late-appearing joint disruptions
IV. Chronic joint disorders
V. Extensor carpi ulnaris tendon snapping
VI. Fixed rotational deformities

Palmer (2) classified TFCC tears by location and into acute and chronic injuries. Distal radioulnar joint stability in acute injuries is described by comparing the following characteristics to those on the opposite side:

1. Loss of motion
2. Deformity (ulnar, dorsal, volar)
3. Position of maximal instability
4. Position of maximal stability
5. Dorsal–volar translation of (3) and (4) in millimeters

ASSESSMENT

Physical Examination

Injury to the distal radioulnar joint is often a single component of multiple injuries in the forearm and the wrist, and the entire injured upper extremity must be examined. In an acute situation, a distal radioulnar joint injury usually is not the primary presenting complaint and diagnosis is made from the presence of localized tenderness, limited range of motion, and instability.

Radiographic Evaluation

Disruptions of the distal radioulnar joint (e.g., a Galeazzi's fracture) may be evident on plain radiographs (Fig. 20), but more subtle injuries may require further diagnostic efforts. Posteroanterior and lateral views must be taken with the forearm in neutral rotation and the x-ray beam centered over the joint. The normal anterior–posterior and proximal–distal translations of the joint that occur with rotation of the forearm can be eliminated only in this position. Oblique views are useful to delineate undisplaced or chip fractures.

Special Studies

Tomography is useful for detecting small fractures and defining the displacement of large fracture fragments. Comparison CT scans of the uninjured wrist are obtained to define displacement of the distal radioulnar joint in the transverse plane and to document abnormalities. Arthrography of the radiocarpal joint can help to identify TFCC tears, but this modality is associated with a 10% rate of false-negative results and is usually reserved for diagnosing chronic conditions (Fig. 21). Because asymptomatic age-related ruptures

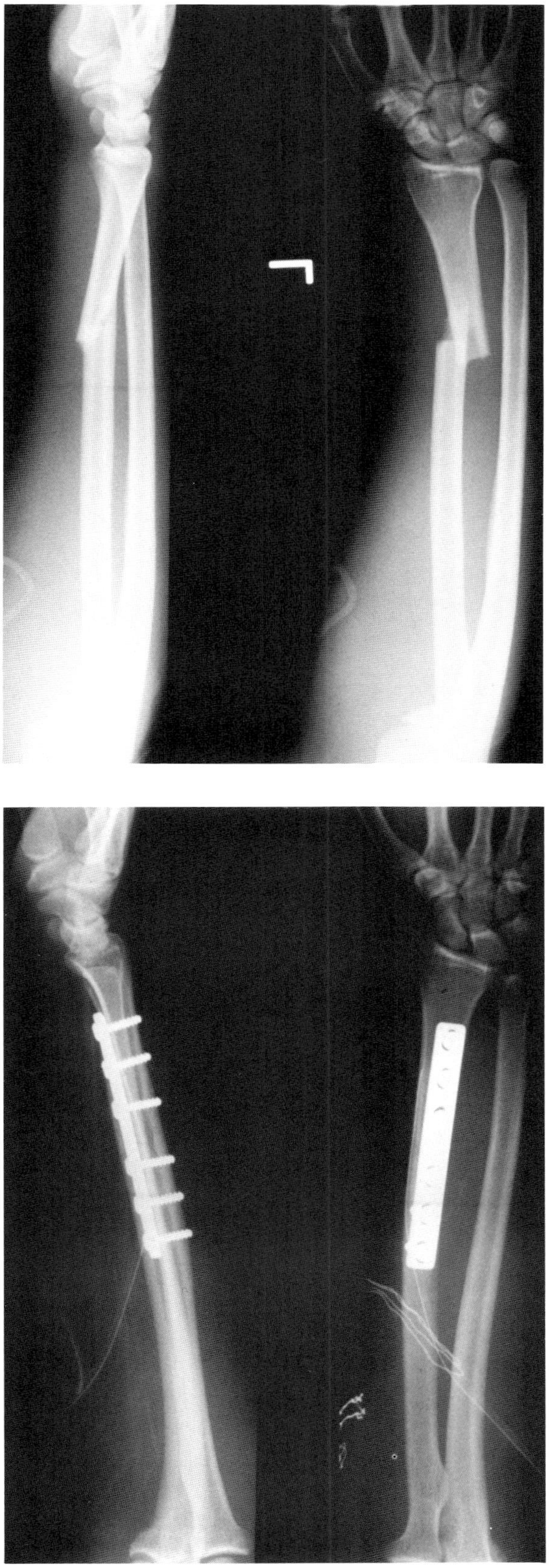

A

B

FIG. 20. A,B: Closed Galeazzi's fracture in an adult male. Note the correction of the distal radial ulnar joint relationships with anatomic fixation of the radius.

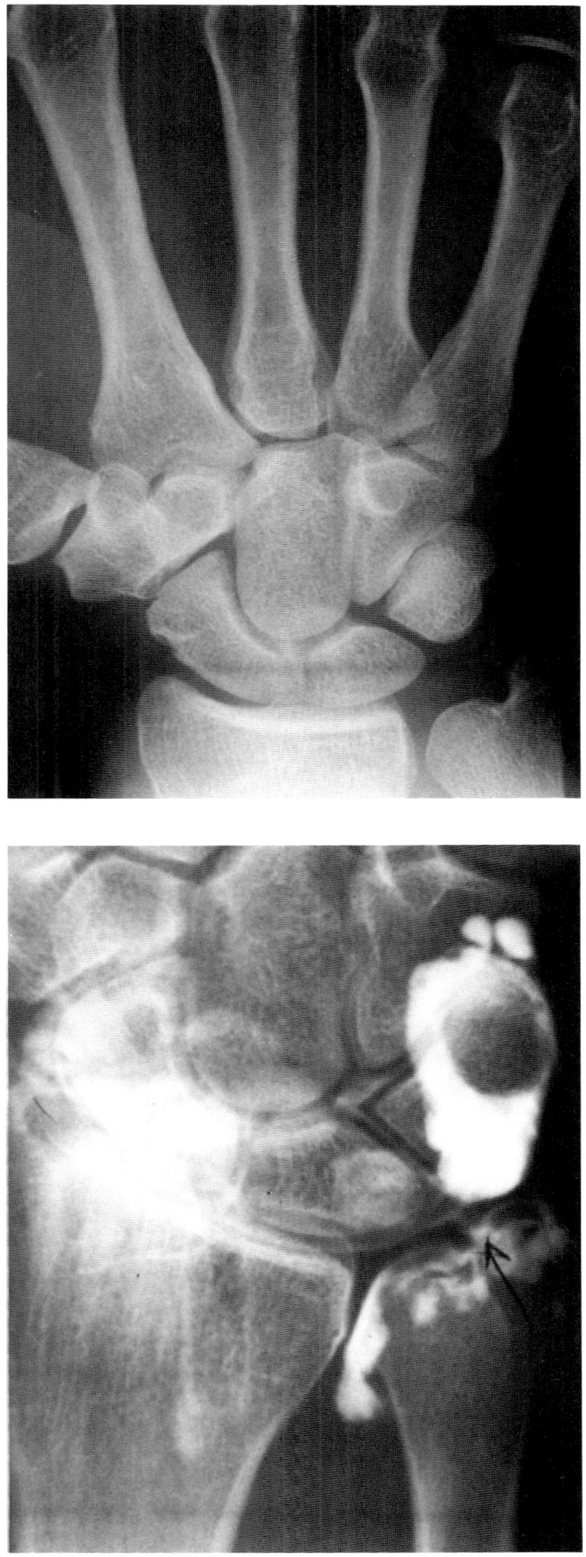

A

B

FIG. 21. A: An adult male with chronic wrist pain following a twisting injury. The standard radiographs of the wrist are normal. **B**: An arthrogram shows a large dye leak into the distal radial ulnar joint consistent with a tear of the triangular fibrocartilage complex which explains the patient's distal radial ulnar joint instability.

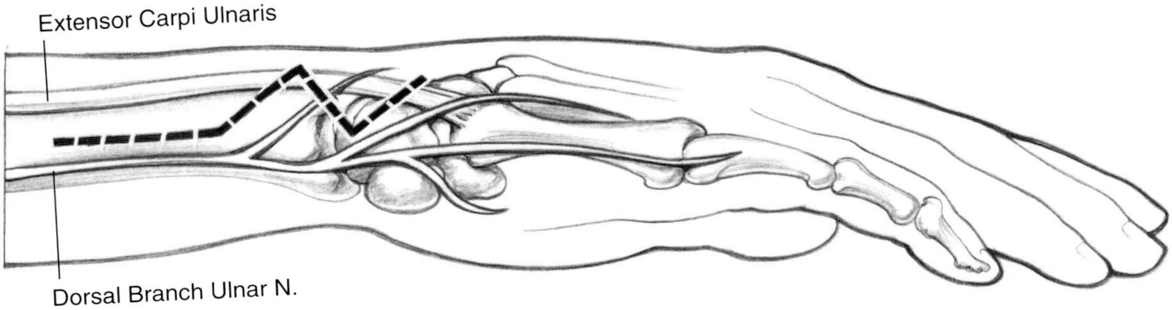

FIG. 22. The skin incision for an approach to the distal radioulnar joint.

are common, isolated arthrographic findings must be relevant to clinical findings to be considered meaningful. Technetium bone scanning is used to define chronic pain problems but has little place in the evaluation of an acute injury.

EMERGENT MANAGEMENT

An isolated distal radioulnar instability in which the ulna has been displaced dorsally is treated by splinting the arm in supination; volar displacement of the ulna is splinted in pronation. Rarely, the ulna may be locked on the volar aspect of the radius and an anesthetic will be required for reduction.

DEFINITIVE MANAGEMENT

An isolated distal radioulnar injury warrants a trial of cast treatment with the forearm immobilized in the appropriate rotation for 6 weeks. At the end of this time, range-of-motion exercises are initiated and stability is reassessed. If the joint remains unstable despite appropriate casting, operative treatment is indicated.

The distal radioulnar joint is visualized through an incision extending through the fifth and sixth dorsal compartments (Fig. 22). If the styloid has been fractured, it is repaired with a tension-band wiring technique to restore adequate stability to the distal radioulnar joint. If the injury is caused by ligamentous avulsion, the TFCC and the ulnar collateral ligament are sutured to the ulnar hilum through drill holes in the distal ulna. Pinning the distal radioulnar joint is not recommended to hold the reduction. Postoperatively, the wrist is immobilized in a long-arm cast for 6 weeks, at which time the joint should be stable in midrotation and the cast can be removed. Range-of-motion and strengthening exercises are initiated and a splint is used for protection until 3 months postoperatively.

COMPLICATIONS

Posttraumatic arthritis is a common complication of severe distal radioulnar joint injuries. Ulnar neuritis can occur secondary to local synovitis and may lead to chronic compression of the ulnar nerve. Tendinous adhesions and stiffness are commonplace after operative repair. Severe limitation of motion sometimes warrants tenolysis of the extensor carpi ulnaris tendon.

SKELETALLY IMMATURE PATIENTS

Few cases of distal radioulnar joint instability have been reported in children, but this injury must be suspected and ruled out in isolated radial fractures. Injuries occurring through the distal ulnar growth plate are treated according to guidelines for the type of injury sustained by the growth plate.

REFERENCES

1. Bowers WH. The distal radioulnar joint. In: Green DO, ed. *Operative hand surgery,* Vol II. New York: Churchill–Livingstone; 1988:939.
2. Palmer AK, Werner FW. The triangular fibrocartilage cmplex of the wrist: anatomy and function. *J Hand Surg* 1981;6:153–61.

Scaphoid Fractures

MECHANISMS OF INJURY

Fractures of the scaphoid commonly occur in young adults and make up approximately 60% of all carpal bone fractures. The usual mechanism of injury is compression of the wrist in approximately 95° of dorsiflexion (1). Scaphoid fractures usually occur as isolated injuries but may have associated distal radial fractures with ligamentous ruptures (trans-scaphoid perilunate dislocations). A direct blow to the radial side of the wrist can result in fracture of the scaphoid tubercle.

ANATOMIC CONSIDERATIONS

The scaphoid is a mobile bone that bridges the midcarpal joint. It is subjected to high stresses with extremes of carpal motion but is stabilized in its proximal pole by the radioscaphoid ligament. The radiocapitate ligament crosses the waist of the scaphoid and may contribute to the force of the bending moment on the scaphoid with dorsiflexion. When the scaphoid is fractured, the proximal fragment usually remains attached to the proximal carpal row, whereas the distal fragment is displaced. The amount of displacement depends on the position of the distal carpal row. The apex of the fracture is usually displaced dorsally if the scaphoid is angulated.

Over 80% of the surface of the scaphoid is covered by articular cartilage, resulting in a tenuous blood supply to the scaphoid. Dorsal vessels entering the dorsal ridge of the scaphoid from the radial artery supply blood to 70% to 80% of the bone, including the proximal pole (Fig. 23) (2). The time required for healing depends on the location of the fracture. Fractures of the scaphoid tubercle and those in the distal pole tend to heal quickly. Middle-third fractures are the most common. Proximal pole fractures are associated with slow healing and a high (30%) incidence of avascular necrosis.

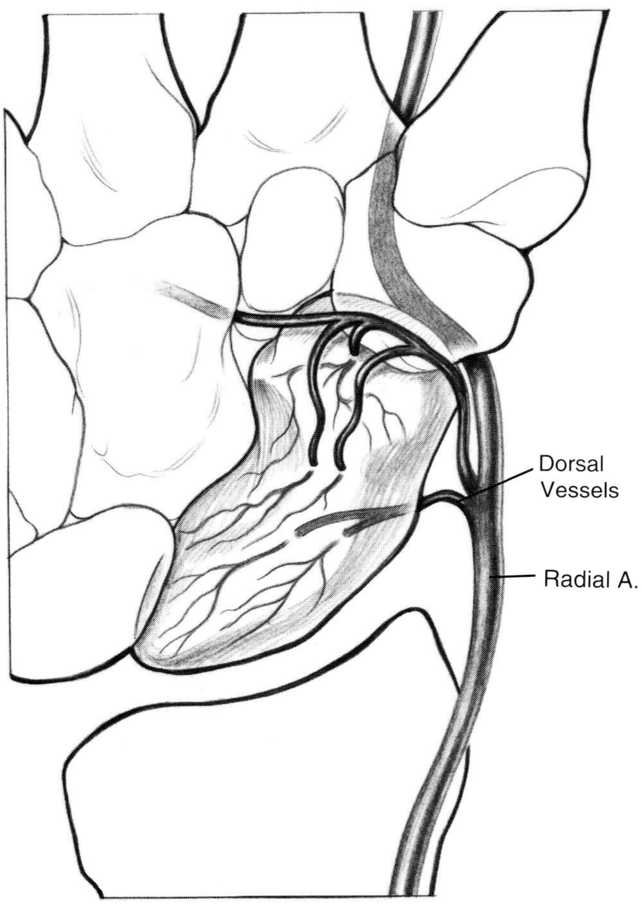

FIG. 23. Diagrammatic representation of the scaphoid blood supply.

CLASSIFICATION

A universal classification system does not exist for scaphoid fractures, and several factors must be considered to help direct treatment and to predict outcome. Russe (3) classified fractures as horizontal (90° to the long axis of the radius), transverse (in the plane of the scaphoid axis), and vertical (parallel to the long axis of the radius). Vertical fractures tend to be the most unstable. Fractures are also described as displaced or nondisplaced. Translation greater than 1 mm and angulation greater than 10° are considered excessive.

ASSESSMENT

Physical Examination

The presenting symptoms of a patient with a scaphoid fracture are usually swelling, decreased range of motion in the wrist, pain with compression of the anatomic snuff-box, and decreased grip strength. Some nondisplaced scaphoid fractures exhibit few physical findings.

Radiographic Evaluation

Standard radiographic evaluation of a painful wrist includes AP and lateral views taken with the wrist in a neutral position and ulnar deviation, and oblique views taken with the wrist in pronation. Most scaphoid fractures can be seen on these two radiographic projections. If the initial films are unremarkable but a scaphoid fracture is suspected, the wrist is immobilized in a thumb spica cast for 2 weeks and radiographs are repeated at that time.

Special Studies

If the second set of radiographs does not reveal a scaphoid fracture but a fracture is still suspected, special studies are indicated. Technetium bone scanning is the most sensitive technology for diagnosing a scaphoid fracture when a lesion is not evident on radiographs. The prevalence of false-positive results associated with bone scanning is approximately 10%; false-negative results have not been reported.

AP and lateral tomograms can detect nondisplaced scaphoid fractures not seen on plain radiographs (Fig. 24). However, because of the scaphoid's unique shape and oblique position, tomograms in the plane of the scaphoid axis are more helpful. Displaced fracture fragments are accurately assessed with tomograms or CT scans taken in the plane of the scaphoid axis. Blood flow to the proximal pole can be assessed accurately by MRI. Plain radiographs are not reliable for detecting the presence of osteonecrosis in the proximal pole.

EMERGENT MANAGEMENT

Scaphoid fractures are treated initially in a long-arm–thumb spica cast.

DEFINITIVE MANAGEMENT

Nondisplaced fractures demonstrate a high rate of healing and are managed by immobilization in a long-arm–thumb spica cast or a Muenster-type thumb spica cast for six weeks. The wrist is casted in neutral flexion and mild radial deviation with the thumb remaining in a functional position. Fractures displaced more than 1 mm are associated with perilunate dislocations and are treated operatively. Other fractures that require operative intervention are those with a radiolunate angle greater than 15° and those with a scapholunate angle greater than 60° (Figs. 25 and 26).

A volar approach poses a smaller risk of disrupting the important dorsal blood supply to the scaphoid than a dorsal approach. Reduction of a trans-scaphoid perilunate dislocation is accomplished through a volar approach. Restoring anatomic alignment to the scaphoid often produces gaps in the fracture and the need for access to a bone-graft donor

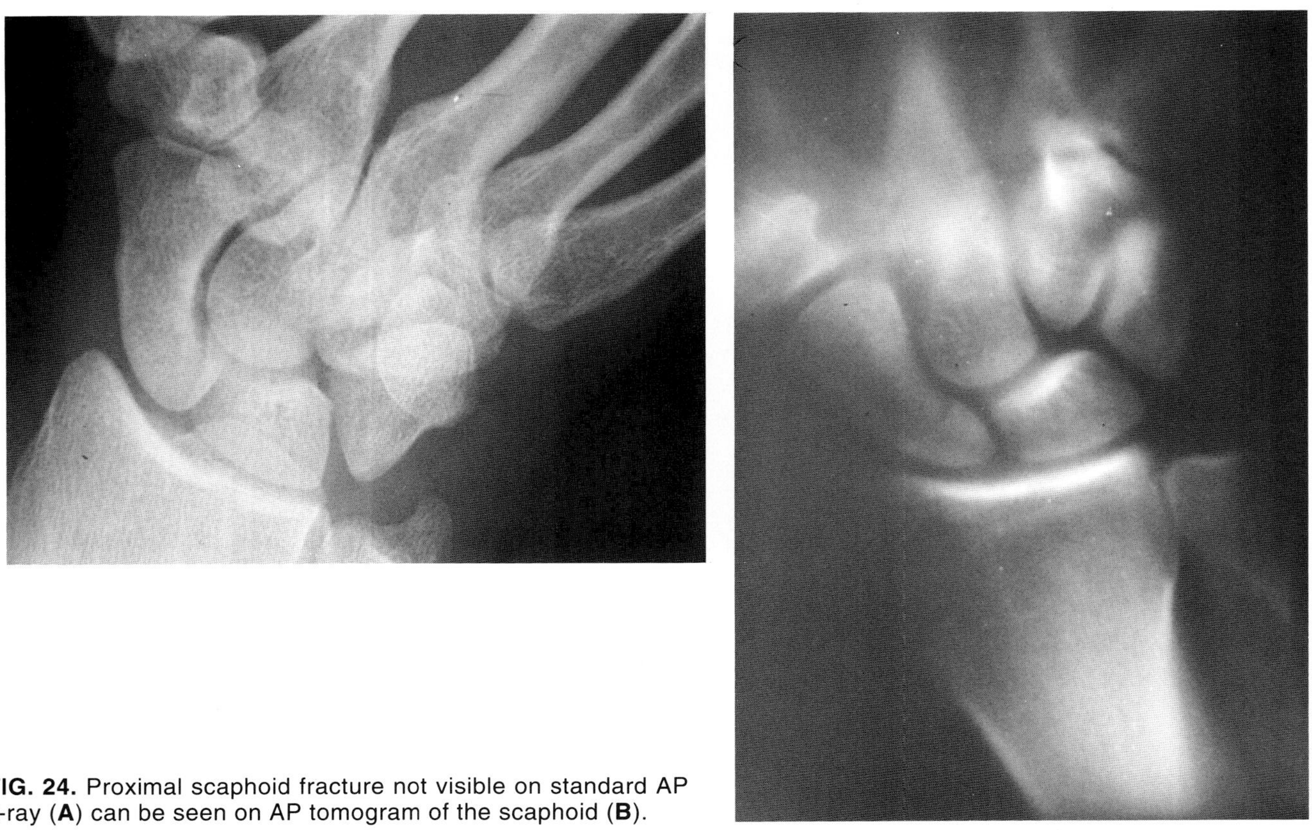

A

B

FIG. 24. Proximal scaphoid fracture not visible on standard AP x-ray (**A**) can be seen on AP tomogram of the scaphoid (**B**).

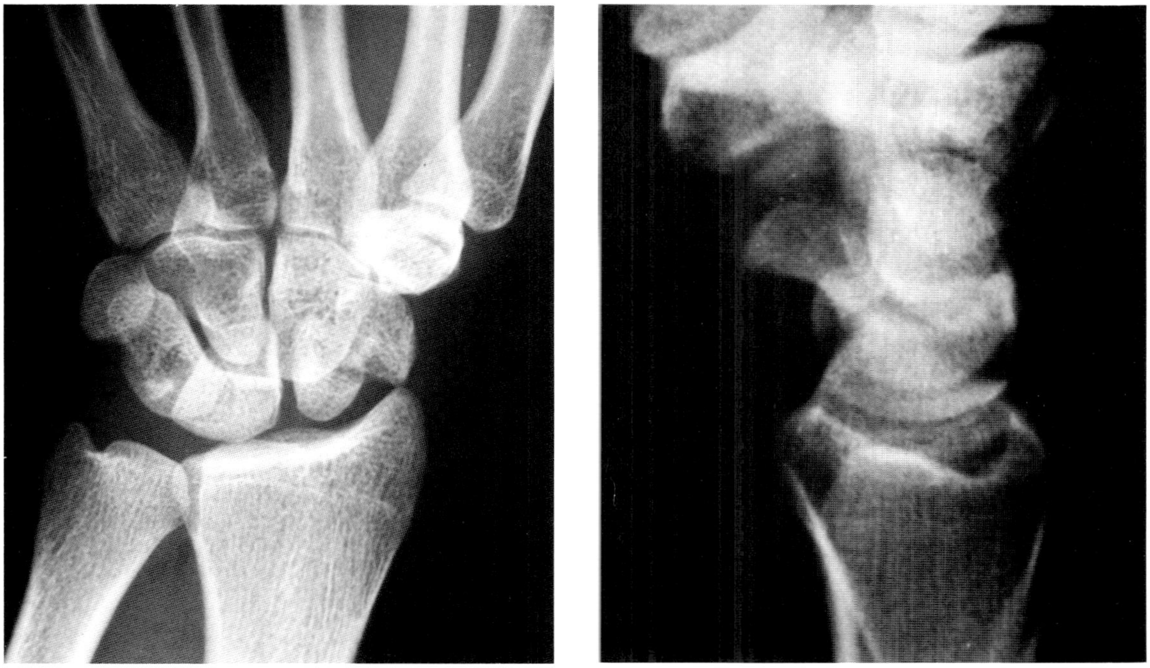

A B

FIG. 25. A,B: AP and lateral views of trans-scaphoid perilunate dislocation. The displacement of the scaphoid requires anatomic reduction.

site, usually the iliac crest or the distal radius, should be anticipated. Stable fixation can be accomplished with cancellous screws, Herbert screws (4), or Kirschner wires. After operative repair, the wrist is immobilized in a thumb spica cast and rehabilitated in the same manner as fractures that are reduced closed. A cast is kept in place until the fracture demonstrates radiographic and clinical signs of healing, regardless of the type of fixation that was used.

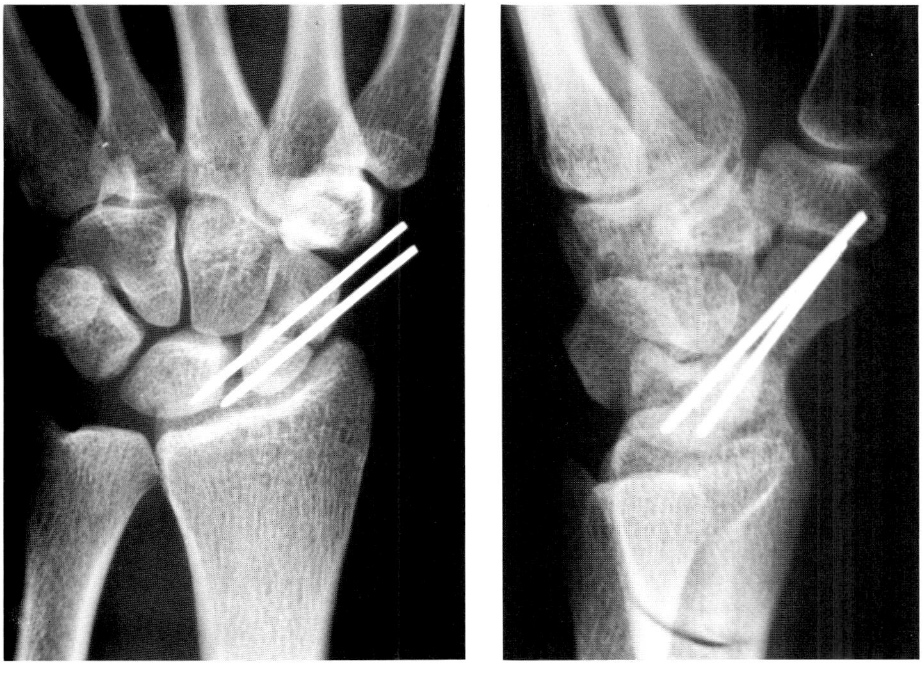

A,B

FIG. 26. A,B: Postoperative views after correction of trans-scaphoid perilunate dislocation through a volar approach. The volar ligaments were repaired and anatomic position of the scaphoid is maintained with two Kirschner wires (K-wires).

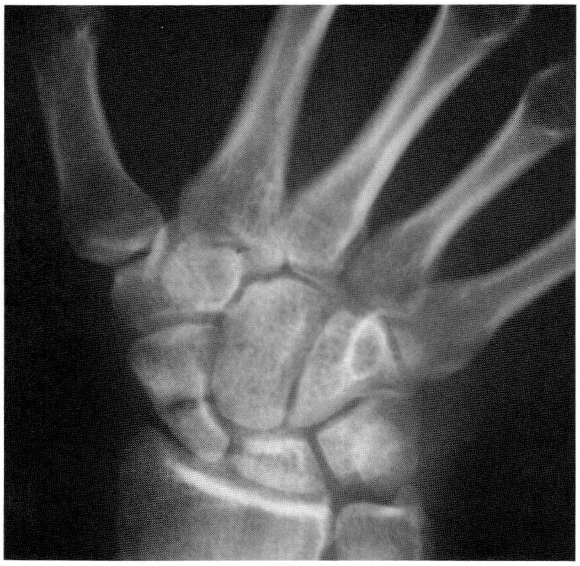

FIG. 27. AP view showing nonunion of a nondisplaced scaphoid fracture after cast immobilization. Note the cyst at the level of the fracture.

COMPLICATIONS

Nonunions are common in untreated scaphoid fractures but the incidence of nonunion in nondisplaced fractures decreases to less than 10% with adequate immobilization (Fig. 27). Nonunions are treated by bone grafting. Treatment with a pulsed electromagnetic field has demonstrated a success rate of 80%, but this treatment modality is not indicated for synovial nonunions, carpal collapse with nonunion, or displaced fractures. Malunion may result in functional limitations. As little as 5° angulation in the scaphoid can decrease wrist extension by as much as 20°. Severe cases of scaphoid malunion are treated by osteotomy.

SKELETALLY IMMATURE PATIENTS

Scaphoid fractures are rare in children and can be difficult to diagnose. Magnetic resonance imaging provides a noninvasive means of diagnosis in a child. All displaced fractures should be treated by ORIF using Kirschner wires.

REFERENCES

1. Weber ER, Chao EY. An experimental approach to the mechanism of scaphoid wrist fractures. *J Hand Surg* 1972;3:142–153.
2. Gelberman RH, Manon J. The vascularity of the scaphoid bone. *J Hand Surg* 1980;5:508.
3. Russe O. Fracture of the carpal navicular: diagnosis, non-operative treatment, and operative treatment. *J Bone Joint Surg* 1960;42A:759–768.
4. Herbert TJ, Fisher WE. Management of the fractured scaphoid using a new bone screw. *J Bone Joint Surg* 1984;66B:114–123.

Lesser Carpal Fractures: Trapezial Fractures

MECHANISMS OF INJURY

The lesser carpals include the trapezium, the triquetrum, and the capitate. The trapezial body is commonly fractured when it is compressed with radial deviation between the first metacarpal and the radial styloid. Trapezial ridge fractures are caused by direct blows or by avulsions of the volar ligaments. Isolated injuries are rare, and trapezial injuries are often associated with fractures of the first metacarpal or the distal radius.

ANATOMIC CONSIDERATIONS

A fracture in the trapezial body often involves a portion of the extensive articular surface. The trapeziometacarpal joint, which is susceptible to arthritic changes without acute injury, is often involved. The volar process of the trapezium serves as a radial attachment for the flexor retinaculum and comes into direct contact with the flexor carpi radialis tendon.

CLASSIFICATION

Trapezial body fractures are described as nondisplaced, displaced, or comminuted fractures. Fractures that involve ligamentous disruption of the first carpometacarpal (CMC) or the scaphotrapezial joints may appear as small flecks of bone and are not associated with the hyaline cartilage surface. All other fractures are considered intraarticular (1).

Trapezial ridge fractures are classified into two types: Type I includes fractures of the base of the volar process. Type II involves fractures of the tip of the volar process.

Physical Examination

Fractures or fracture–dislocations of the trapezial body are accompanied by pain, swelling, and loss of thumb function. Because trapezial fractures are often associated with ulnar carpal injuries, the entire carpus should be carefully examined. All carpal injuries should be examined for damage to

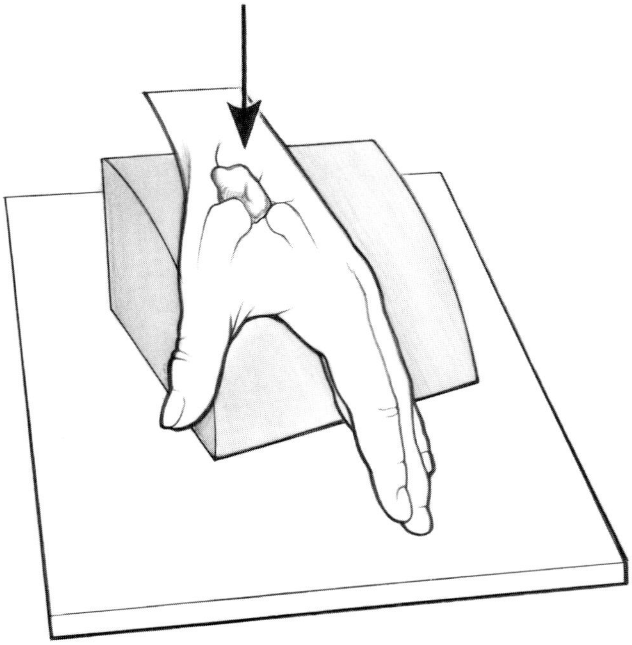

FIG. 28. Bett's view for visualizing the trapezium.

the median nerve. Trapezial ridge fractures demonstrate more subtle physical symptoms. After injury, the volar aspect of the trapezium is painful to palpation and the wrist is painful with resisted flexion because this motion forces the flexor carpi radialis tendon against the trapezial ridge.

Radiographic Evaluation

Anteroposterior, lateral, and navicular radiographic views of the carpus should be obtained. In addition to these standard radiographic views, Bett's view is obtained to define the outline of the trapezium without overlapping of the other carpals (Fig. 28). Trapezial ridge fractures are best seen on a carpal tunnel view.

Special Studies

Tomography may be useful to assess comminution and joint congruity.

EMERGENT MANAGEMENT

Emergent management of lesser carpal fractures consists of splinting, gentle compression, elevation, and icing, the same treatment that is appropriate for most minor fractures. If radiographic evaluation reveals a trapezial fracture with an associated dislocation, reduction should be performed immediately under a hematoma block.

DEFINITIVE MANAGEMENT

Operative management is indicated for displaced fractures of the trapezial body and for unreduced or incompletely reduced fracture–dislocations (2). Trapezial ridge fractures are treated in a thumb spica cast for 6 weeks. Type I fractures usually heal without complications, but type II fractures often fail to unite. Excision of the volar fragment is the preferred treatment for trapezial nonunions. To perform an open reduction, the trapezial body is exposed through a dorsoradial approach (Fig. 29). Care must be taken to protect the branches of the superficial radial nerve and the radial artery. The fracture is stabilized with a Kirschner wire, with or without a tension-band wiring technique, or with miniscrews (Fig. 30). If the fracture is associated with an unstable first CMC joint, careful capsular repair can be augmented with a

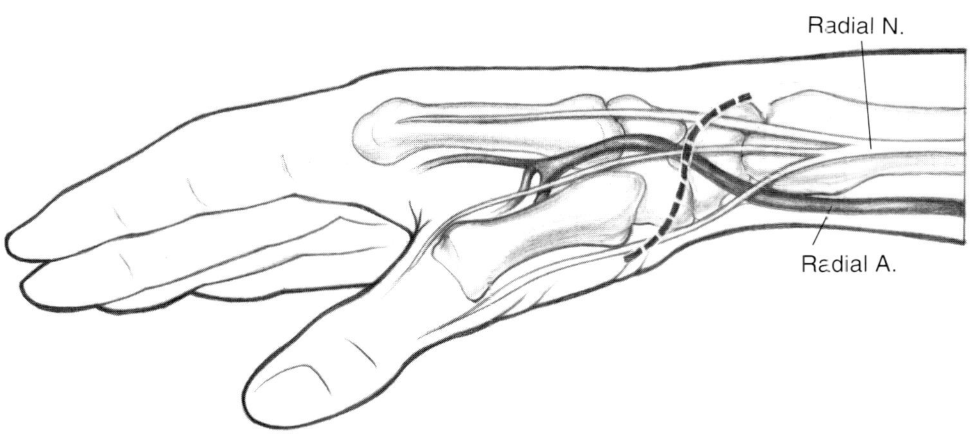

FIG. 29. The dorsoradial approach for a trapezial fracture.

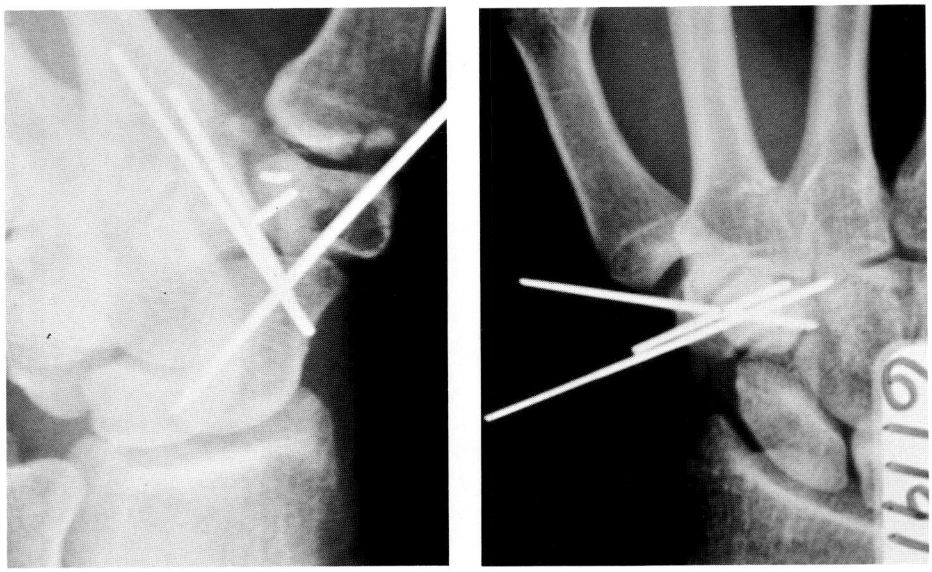

A,B

FIG. 30. A,B: Postoperative fixation of a comminuted trapezial fracture. Inaccurate reduction leads to arthritic changes of the first CMC joint.

slip of abductor pollicis longus tendon or a portion of the flexor carpi radialis tendon.

The trapezial ridge is approached by a direct volar incision, avoiding the volar branch of the median nerve. Treatment can be delayed up to 6 weeks without negative sequelae when the wrist is splinted in a thumb spica cast. In fractures stabilized with rigid fixation, early active range of motion can be started in a removable splint.

COMPLICATIONS

Radial nerve and arterial injuries are avoided by meticulous operative technique. Nonanatomic joint restoration results in posttraumatic degenerative arthritis and a weak pinch.

SKELETALLY IMMATURE PATIENTS

The trapezium begins to ossify in girls at age 4 years and in boys at age 6 years. Trapezial fractures are rare in children.

REFERENCES

1. Palmer A. Trapezial ridge fractures. *J Hand Surg* 1981;6:561–65.
2. Foster RJ, Hastings H. Treatment of Bennett, Rolando, and vertical intraarticular trapezial fractures. *Clin Orthop* 1987;214:121–29.

Lesser Carpal Fractures: Triquetral Fractures

MECHANISMS OF INJURY

Fractures of the triquetrum usually occur by one of two mechanisms. The first is a shear fracture of the dorsoulnar aspect of the bone. This occurs from wrist extension and ulnar deviation and fracture follows from avulsion by the triquetral–hamate ligament or by compression of the triquetrum against the ulnar styloid process (Fig. 31). The second mechanism involves fractures associated with perilunate or carpal dislocation. Acute wrist flexion can avulse the dorsal radiotriquetral ligament with a bone fragment.

ANATOMIC CONSIDERATIONS

The triquetrum is attached to the lunate by a short, strong ligament that allows 10° to 15° of rotation (Fig. 32). Its intercarpal connection to the hamate consists of a complex helicoidal joint, which allows rotation and angulation in two planes. In the columnar concept of the carpus that was described above, the triquetrum is the rotational column. The strong dorsal radiotriquetral ligament controls flexion and ulnar deviation and the meniscus homologue connects the triquetrum to the TFCC.

CLASSIFICATION

Fractures of the triquetrum are classified by their location and the mechanism of injury. Associated perilunate instability must be noted.

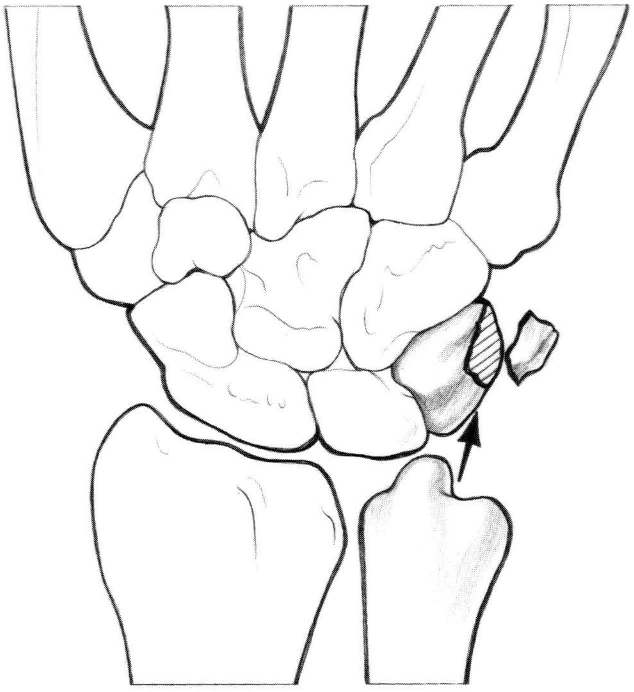

FIG. 31. Triquetral fracture, secondary to ulnar deviation shear from the ulnar styloid. This fracture is usually treated by immobilization.

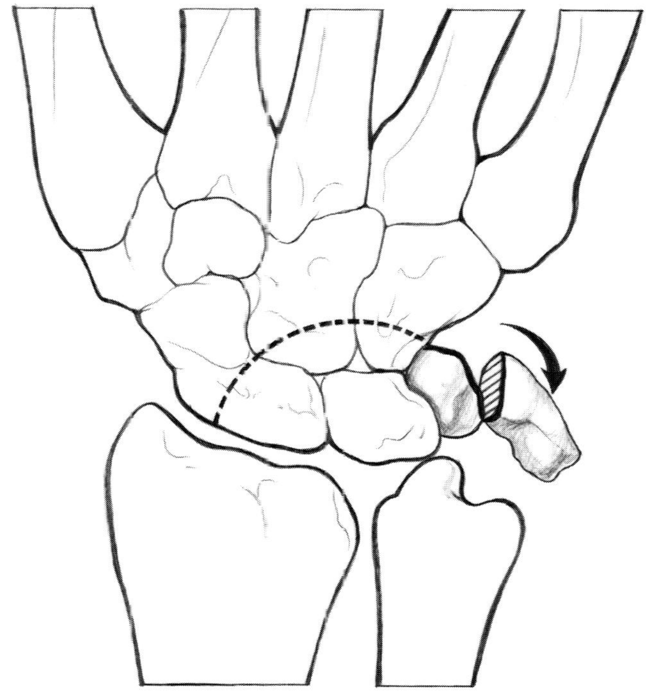

FIG. 32. Triquetral body fracture, often associated with midcarpal ligament injury or greater arc fracture. ORIF is indicated for a displaced fracture.

ASSESSMENT

Physical Examination

Local swelling and tenderness are characteristic of most triquetral fractures. Fractures with associated perilunate instability demonstrate a greater amount of swelling and, possibly, greater radial wrist pain.

Radiographic Evaluation

Standard radiographic projections may not reveal small triquetral fractures. An oblique view is often necessary to reveal a dorsal avulsion fracture. Dorsal fractures can be mistaken for lunate injuries on lateral views.

Special Studies

Tomograms or triphasic bone scans are needed to visualize occult triquetral injuries.

EMERGENT MANAGEMENT

A triquetral fracture is managed initially by splinting, gentle compression, elevation, and icing.

DEFINITIVE MANAGEMENT

Operative treatment of triquetral fractures is rarely necessary (1,2). Cortical fractures usually resolve after 3 to 6 weeks of immobilization; body fractures usually heal in 6 weeks. Nonunions may occur but are rarely symptomatic.

COMPLICATIONS

A symptomatic nonunion of a triquetral body fracture is treated by ORIF and bone grafting, but nonunion of a triquetral cortical fracture may require excision of the displaced fragment. Excision of the fragment is reserved for exceptionally severe cases of associated posttraumatic degenerative joint disease.

SKELETALLY IMMATURE PATIENTS

Few cases of triquetral fractures in children have been reported.

REFERENCES

1. Bartone NF, Grieco V. Fractures of the triquetrum. *J Bone Joint Surg* 1956;38A:353.
2. Taleisnik J. Fractures of the triquetrum. In: The Wrist, New York: Churchill–Livingstone; 1985.

Lesser Carpal Fractures: Capitate Fractures

MECHANISMS OF INJURY

Fractures of the capitate, or the "os magnum," make up only 1% of all carpal fractures. Capitate fractures have been produced experimentally by applying extreme flexion or extension forces combined with axial loading to the wrist. Application of direct load on the third metacarpal can produce an isolated oblique capitate fracture which involves the third CMC joint. This injury is commonly associated with carpal fractures or fracture–dislocations occurring through a greater arc and the proximal pole of the capitate can be rotated as much as 180° (Fig. 33). A displaced scaphoid fracture occurring in association with a capitate neck fracture can result in a scaphocapitate syndrome.

ANATOMIC CONSIDERATIONS

The proximal pole of the capitate has weak ligamentous attachments. Consequently, all the soft-tissue attachments of the proximal pole are disrupted by excessive rotation when the capitate neck is fractured. Disruption of the soft-tissue attachment makes the capitate highly susceptible to avascular necrosis, much like a displaced talar neck or talar fractures (1,2).

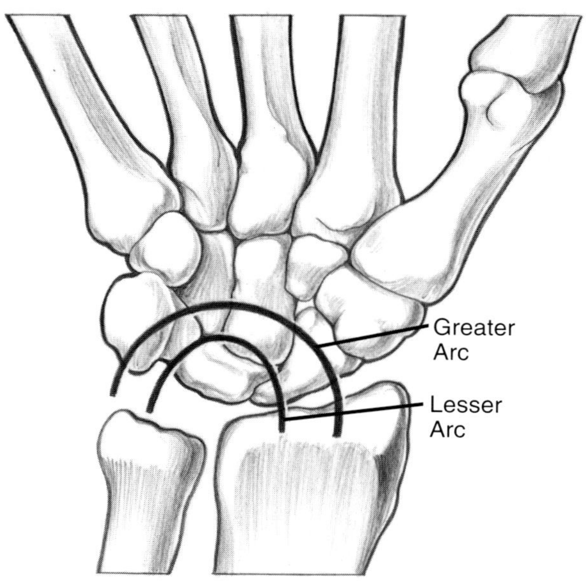

FIG. 33. Capitate fractures can be associated with other lesser arc or greater arc fractures.

CLASSIFICATION

No formal classification system exists for capitate fractures, which are described in terms of fracture characteristics.

ASSESSMENT

Physical Examination

Swelling, pain, and loss of motion are typical presenting symptoms of a capitate neck fracture. Like any severe carpal injury, a capitate fracture can compromise median nerve function.

Radiographic Evaluation

A capitate fracture is usually evident on standard radiographic projections, but oblique views are useful to define the plane of the fracture and traction views are useful to identify cases of carpal collapse.

Special Studies

Tomograms and CT scans can be obtained to define the fracture pattern further, but are usually not necessary for making treatment decisions.

EMERGENT MANAGEMENT

Adequate treatment of a capitate fracture is dependent upon an accurate early diagnosis. A fracture with a rotated proximal pole warrants immediate operative intervention, the same as a femoral neck fracture in a young patient. Other displaced fractures can be splinted while the patient awaits definitive treatment.

DEFINITIVE MANAGEMENT

Nondisplaced fractures of the capitate are uncommon and can be treated by cast immobilization. The preoperative planning of displaced capitate fractures includes diagnosis and treatment of all other carpal fractures and dislocations. Concurrent scaphoid and capitate fractures usually require internal fixation of both bones (Fig. 34). If traction radiographs were not taken during the initial examination, they should be obtained after anesthesia has been induced. Operative stabi-

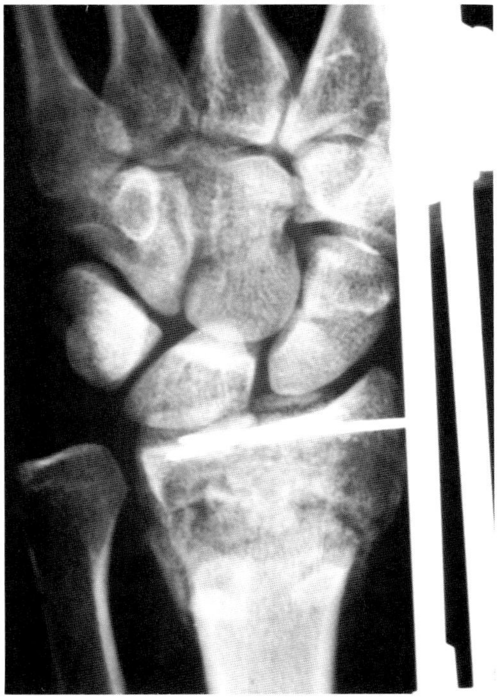

FIG. 34. Nondisplaced fracture through the capitate and scaphoid accompanying a distal radius fracture.

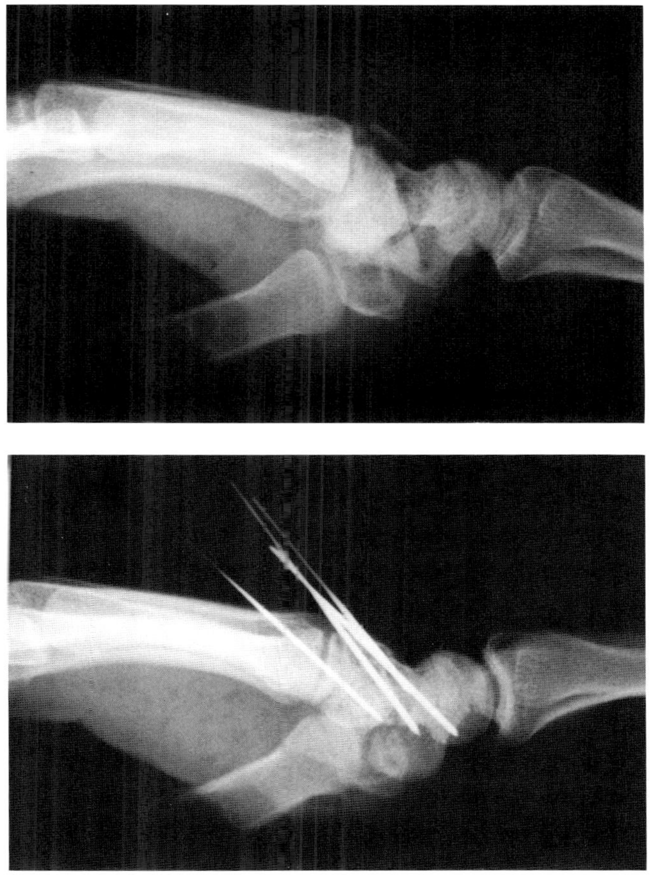

A

B

FIG. 35. Open capitate fracture involving the second and third CMC joints and neck of the capitate (**A**). Fracture fixation is obtained by K-wire reduction in this comminuted fracture. Note the transarticular wire holding reduction of the CMC joint in the lateral x-ray (**B**).

lization of a capitate fracture is performed through a dorsal approach but the incision varies according to the type of fracture. Carpometacarpal joint injuries can be approached through a longitudinal incision unless multiple CMC joints are involved, in which case a transverse incision is required. A capitate neck fracture is approached through a longitudinal incision.

The CMC joint is examined and debrided before reduction. Provisional Kirschner-wire fixation is followed by rigid fixation with lag screws. If the fixation is not absolutely rigid, a .045-inch or .054-inch transarticular wire is inserted across the CMC joint to prevent displacement. Capitate neck fractures require accurate reduction for a functional prognosis (Fig. 35). Insertion of lag screws or Herbert screws from the proximal to the digital pole is not recommended because these screws damage a large portion of the cartilage surface during insertion. Adequate fixation is provided by Kirschner wires placed across the lunocapitate joint for increased stability. A scaphoid fracture associated with a scaphocapitate syndrome is reduced through a dorsal approach. Excision of the proximal pole of the capitate may be necessary if the pole is fragmented. The definitive treatment for this injury is a midcarpal fusion. Fractures of the capitate are immobilized in cast until union is demonstrated on radiographs. The transarticular wires are removed and range-of-motion exercises are instituted at that time. Capitate neck fractures usually heal in 12 to 16 weeks.

COMPLICATIONS

Inadequate reduction of a capitate fracture can result in posttraumatic arthritis and subsequent functional limitations. Avascular necrosis of the proximal pole is common and may warrant a midcarpal fusion.

SKELETALLY IMMATURE PATIENTS

This injury is rare in children.

REFERENCES

1. Fenton RL. The naviculo-capitate syndrome. *J Bone Joint Surg* 1956;38A:681–84.
2. Vance RM, Gelberman RH, Evans EF. Scaphocapitate fractures. Patterns of injury, and preliminary results of treatment. *J Bone Joint Surg* 1980;62A:271–76.

Orthopaedic Trauma Protocols, edited by
Sigvard T. Hansen, Jr., and Marc F. Swiontkowski,
Raven Press, Ltd., New York, © 1993.

CHAPTER 16

Hand

Thomas E. Trumble and John T. Sack

Metacarpal Fractures of the Thumb

MECHANISMS OF INJURY

Two types of fracture occur in the proximal articular surface of the first carpometacarpal (CMC) joint: Bennett's and Rolando's. A Bennett's fracture is an avulsion that occurs in conjunction with a fracture–dislocation of the CMC joint. The usual mechanism of this injury is forced abduction and proximal displacement of the thumb metacarpal with radial subluxation of the metacarpal base (Fig. 1). Rolando's fractures generally occur due to axial loading that shatters the articular surface at the base of the first metacarpal. The resulting fracture patterns are T- or Y-shaped and consist of three or more fragments (Fig. 2) (1). Shaft fractures usually result from crushing or torsional forces. Crushing usually produces comminuted transverse fractures in the proximal third of the metacarpal; torsional forces produce spiral midshaft fractures.

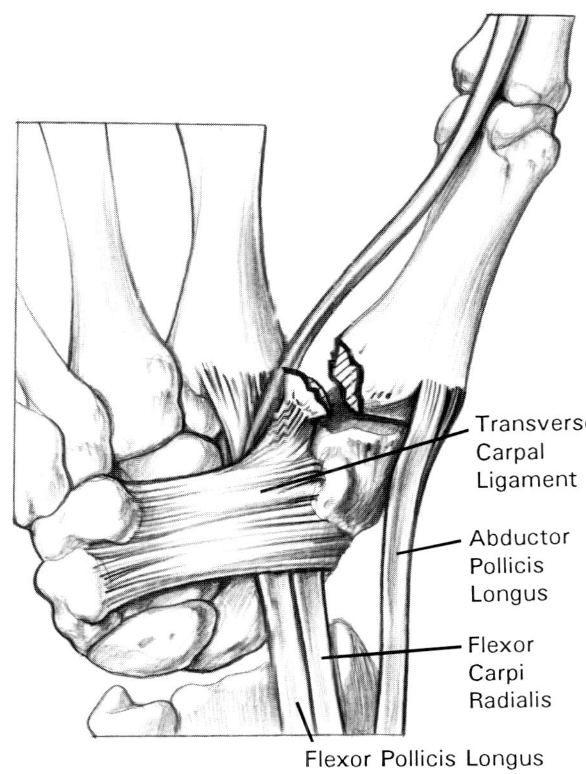

FIG. 1. Mechanism of injury of a Bennett's fracture.

ANATOMIC CONSIDERATIONS

The first CMC joint of the thumb is an intrinsically unstable structure that is supported by the volar oblique ligament, the wide insertion of the abductor pollicis longus, and the joint capsule (2). The contracting force of the surrounding intrinsic muscles can shorten the metacarpal when fracture occurs.

CLASSIFICATION

Intraarticular Bennett's and Rolando's fractures are identified by name. Extraarticular injuries are classified as transverse, oblique, comminuted, or avulsion fractures.

Department of Orthopaedics. Harborview Medical Center, University of Washington, Seattle, Washington 98104

ASSESSMENT

Physical Examination

The typical symptoms of a first metacarpal fracture include swelling and tenderness near the thenar eminence. Because these symptoms are also common to other injuries,

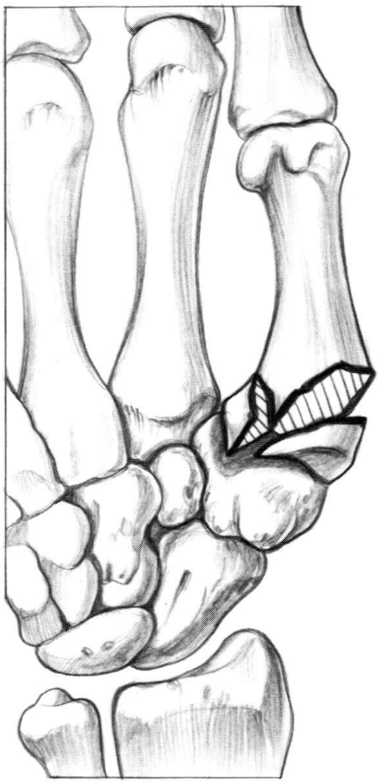

FIG. 2. Fracture pattern described by Rolando.

an accurate diagnosis is needed to differentiate thumb metacarpal fractures from trapezial or scaphoid fractures and from first CMC joint dislocations. Concomitant ligamentous injuries are ruled out by stability testing.

Radiographic Evaluation

Anteroposterior, lateral, and oblique radiographs are essential for making a diagnosis. An additional radiographic view taken with the hand fully pronated and the x-ray beam angled 15° from distal to proximal is useful for diagnosing intraarticular fractures (3).

Special Studies

Trispiral tomograms can be obtained to evaluate the amount of comminution in a Rolando's fracture.

EMERGENT MANAGEMENT

Bennett's and Rolando's fractures are splinted to reduce swelling and discomfort. Closed reduction of a displaced metacarpal shaft fracture can be attempted within 24 to 48 h of injury under a wrist nerve block in the emergency department. The alignment of a transverse shaft fracture displaced in adduction and supination can be markedly improved by applying forces in abduction and pronation. Stable oblique fractures occasionally lock in place after this manipulation and are immobilized in a thumb spica splint.

DEFINITIVE MANAGEMENT

Bennett's Fractures

Failure to reduce a fracture anatomically by closed reduction is an indication for open reduction and internal fixation (ORIF). The CMC joint is approached through a curvilinear incision running along the radial border of the thenar muscles and centered over the joint (Fig. 3). The origins of the abductor pollicis brevis and the opponens pollicis muscles are reflected proximally off the first metacarpal and the trapezium. The CMC joint capsule is incised longitudinally, the flaps are elevated by sharp dissection, leaving the abductor pollicus longus attached to the capsule. Any granulation tissue is removed from the fracture site. The fracture is reduced

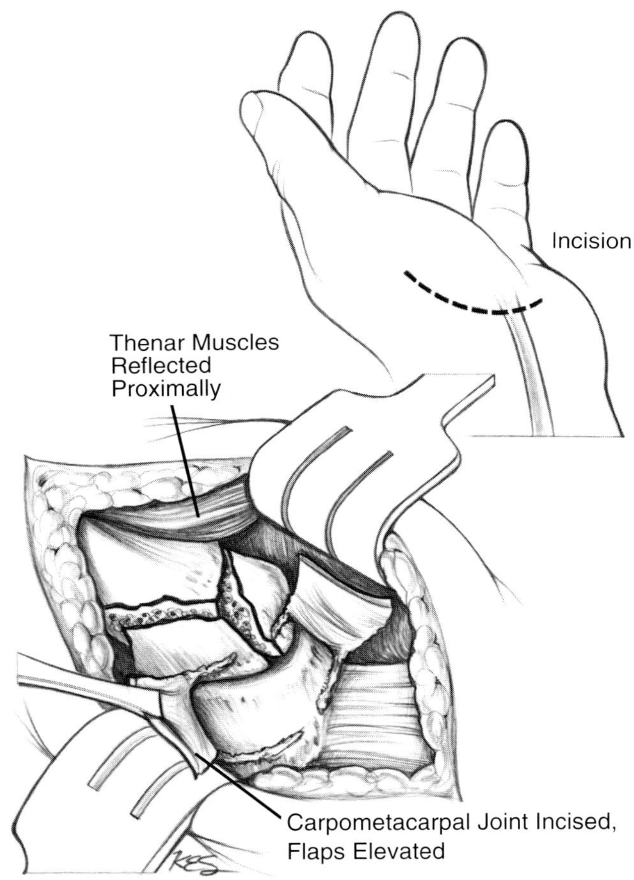

FIG. 3. Surgical approach for a Bennett's fracture.

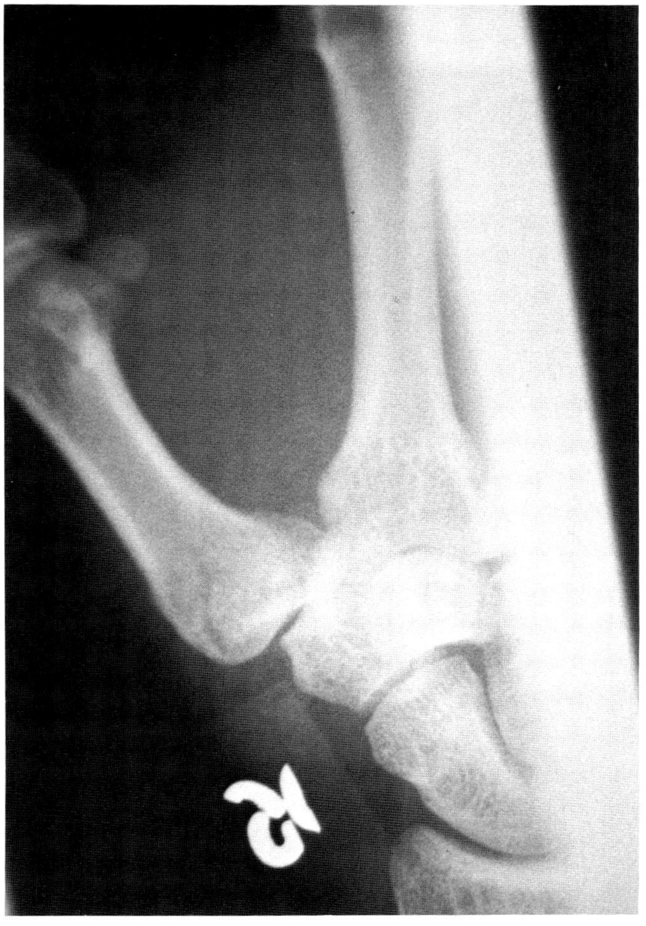

FIG. 4. Radiograph of a Bennett's fracture.

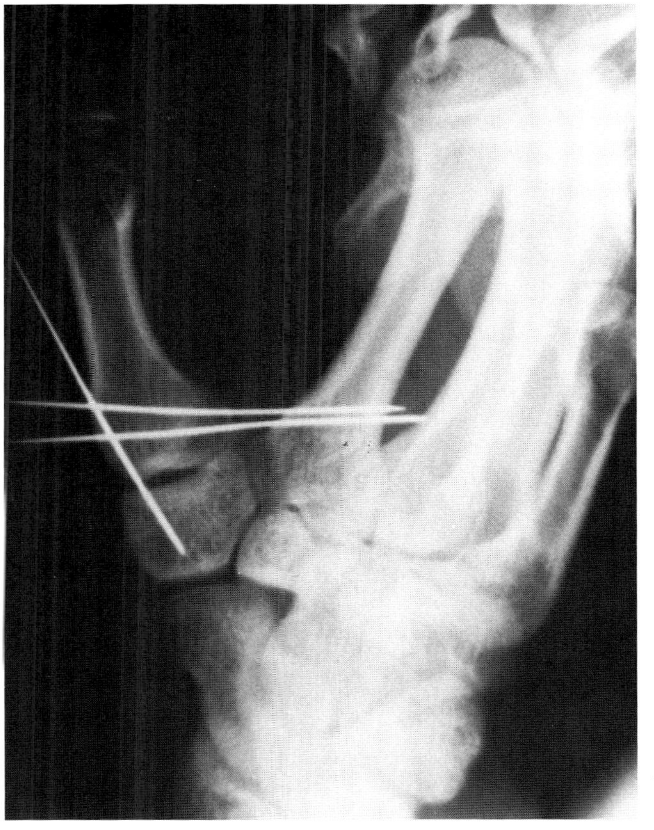

FIG. 5. Kirschner-wire fixation of a Bennett's fracture.

under direct vision and stabilized with Kirschner wires driven across the fracture site and into the base of the second metacarpal (Figs. 4 and 5) (4). The ends of the pins are buried beneath the skin. Screw fixation is reserved for large fracture fragments (5).

Rolando's Fractures

Rolando's fractures are visualized through the same surgical approach that is used for Bennett's fractures. Fractures consisting of two or three large proximal fragments are stabilized with Kirschner wires or screws. External fixation, such as the Hoffmann external minifixator or a frame improvised from Kirschner wires and methylmethacrylate, may be indicated for patients with extremely osteoporotic bone or comminuted fractures. In extremely comminuted fractures, an external fixation device that spans the joint can be made from pins placed in the trapezium and the metacarpal shaft. This device may be used in combination with percutaneous or open pinning to align the articular surfaces.

Postoperatively, both types of fractures are immobilized in a thumb spica splint for 7 to 14 days. The splint is then replaced with a thumb spica cast. Because motion in the first interphalangeal (IP) joint is not restricted in the cast, active range-of-motion exercises can be initiated early. Transarticular Kirschner wires are removed between 6 and 7 weeks after surgery. In uncomminuted fractures the Kirschner wires can be removed 8 to 10 weeks after surgery and a hand-based opponens splint, fabricated by a physical therapist, is used as a protective device during strenuous activities. External fixation devices are removed after 6 postoperative weeks.

Shaft Fractures

Significant displacement, translation greater than 75% of the diameter of the metacarpal, or angulation greater than 30° to 40° may warrant ORIF with small plates or Kirschner wires. Oblique fractures that cannot be stabilized by closed reduction and percutaneous Kirschner-wire fixation, particularly comminuted fractures or those with a butterfly fragment on the ulnar border of the first metacarpal, also require ORIF.

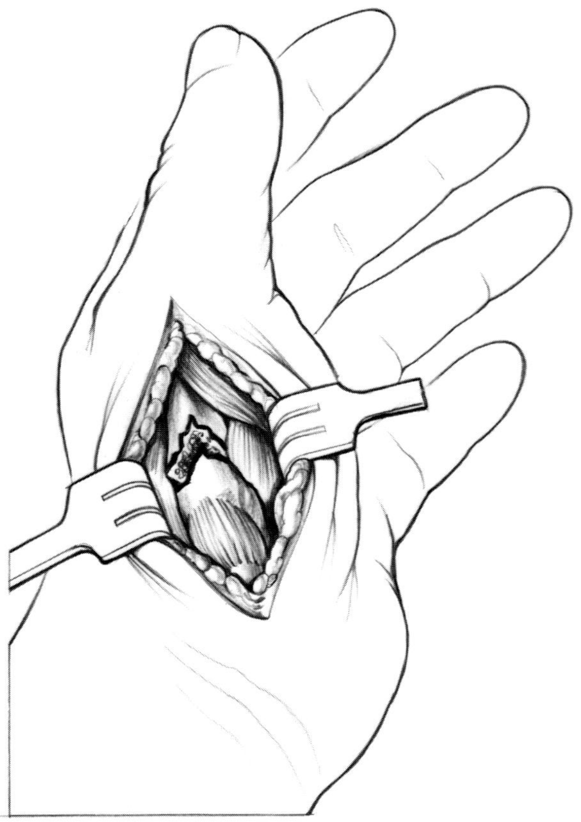

FIG. 6. Surgical approach for a metacarpal shaft fracture. The radial sensory nerve is protected during the exposure.

The surgical incision is made along the border of glabrous skin while protecting the small branches of the radial sensory nerve (Fig. 6). The origins of the abductor pollicis brevis and the periosteum are reflected sharply off the metacarpal with a longitudinal incision and the fracture site is exposed. Proximal fractures are stabilized with small T-plates; longer, oblique fractures require combination fixation with interfragmentary screws and 2.0 or 2.7-mm neutralization plates or Kirschner wires. The postoperative management of shaft fractures is similar to that of intraarticular fractures.

COMPLICATIONS

Pin-tract infection is the most common complication associated with first metacarpal fractures and is managed by local wound care and early pin removal. Burying the Kirschner wires beneath the skin greatly decreases the incidence of pin-tract infection. Rigid cast protection is needed to prevent breakage of transarticular Kirschner wires. Patients with Rolando's fractures may experience functional limitations from degenerative arthritis.

SKELETALLY IMMATURE PATIENTS

Salter-II fractures of the base of the first metacarpal are common in children. These fractures are treated by closed reduction and occasionally require percutaneous Kirschner-wire fixation.

REFERENCES

1. Rolando S. Fracture de la base du premier métacarpien: et principalement sur une variété non encore décrité. *Presse Med* 1910;33:303.
2. Pellegrini VD. Fractures of the base of the thumb. *Hand Clin* 1988;4:87–102.
3. Billing L, Gedda KO. Roentgen examination of Bennett's fracture. *Acta Radiol* 1952;38:471–476.
4. Gedda KO, Moberg E. Open reduction and osteosynthesis of the so-called Bennett's fracture in the carpometarcapal joint of the thumb. *Acta Orthop Scand* 1953;22:249–257.
5. Rüedi TP, Burri C, Pfeiffer KM. Stable internal fixation of fractures of the hand. *J Trauma* 1971;11:381–389.

Metacarpal Fractures of the Fingers

MECHANISMS OF INJURY

Metacarpal neck fractures usually result from striking a blow with a closed fist. Shaft fractures are caused by applying torsional or bending forces to the hand. Multiple metacarpal fractures are usually caused by industrial injuries that damage the intrinsic musculature of the hand.

ANATOMIC CONSIDERATIONS

The finger metacarpals form the distal arch of the hand (Fig. 7). Flexibility in the ulnar border of this arch is attributed to 30° of mobility in the little finger CMC joint and 20° of mobility in the ring finger CMC joint. The metacarpals articulate with several structures. The V-shaped surface of the index finger metacarpal joint articulates with the trapezoid and the capitate. The middle finger metacarpal, the central axis of the hand, articulates with the capitate. The ring finger metacarpal articulates with both the hamate and the capitate, and the little finger metacarpal articulates proximally exclusively with the hamate. The deforming force of the extensor carpi ulnaris muscle and the oblique slope on the distal surface of the hamate contribute to the inability of the little finger CMC joint to resist shear forces, which can produce avulsion type fracture–dislocations similar to a Bennett's fracture of the

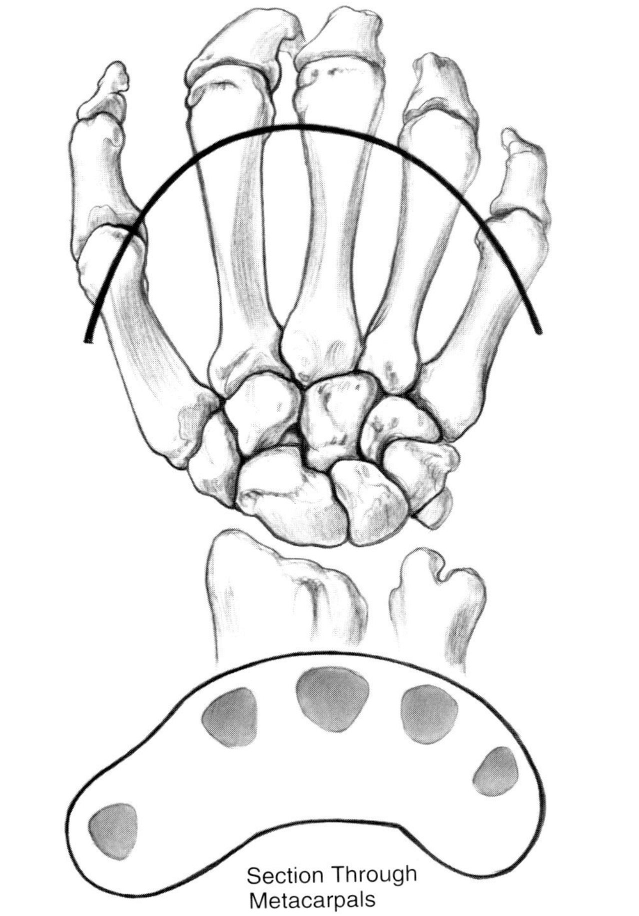

FIG. 7. Diagrammatic representation of the metacarpal and carpal arches of the hand.

thumb (1). The length of the collateral ligaments of the MCP joints and the tension placed on them is greatest in 70° of flexion (Fig. 8). Intraarticular fluid produced by an injury forces the joint into extension and decreases tension in the collateral ligaments. Loss of MCP joint flexion is a major obstacle in the rehabilitation of patients with metacarpal fractures.

CLASSIFICATION

Fractures are classified by the type and location of the injury (Table 1).

ASSESSMENT

Physical Examination

Compartmental pressures must be measured whenever severe swelling is noted after crushing injuries. An unusual prominence, particularly over a CMC joint, may be indicative of a fracture–dislocation that was not visualized on radiographs.

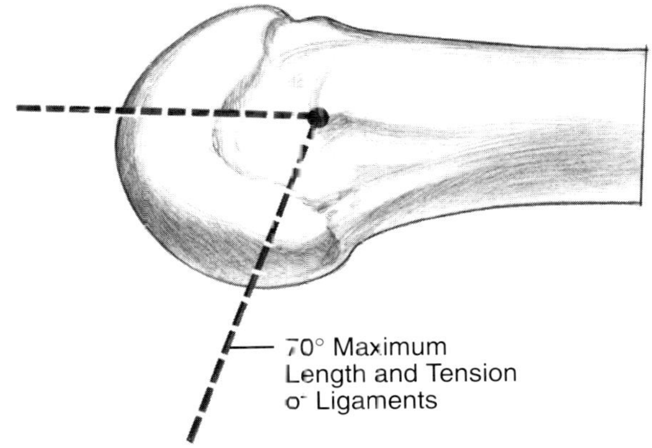

FIG. 8. The cam effect of the metacarpal head on ligamentous tension.

Radiographic Evaluation

Carpometacarpal dislocations are easily missed on routine radiographs and a high degree of suspicion must be maintained to make an accurate diagnosis. In addition to standard AP, lateral, and oblique radiographs, oblique films are taken in supination (for index and middle fingers) and pronation (for ring and little fingers) to evaluate CMC joint dislocations. Occasionally, the only sign of dislocation is a small gap between two metacarpal bases on an AP radiograph.

Special Studies

The positioning required for some radiographic views may be painful or inconclusive. Therefore, dislocations and intraarticular fractures at the bases of the CMC joints can be diagnosed by trispiral tomograms or by CT scans taken in the sagittal and coronal planes.

EMERGENT MANAGEMENT

Elevated compartmental pressures warrant immediate fasciotomy through two longitudinal incisions. The first is made over the second metacarpal to decompress the first and second web spaces, and the second is made over the third metacarpal to decompress the third and fourth web spaces. Open wounds require immediate irrigation and debridement.

Table 1. *Classification of metacarpal fractures*

Base fractures
Extraarticular
Intraarticular
Impaction fractures
Avulsion fractures
Fracture-dislocations
Shaft fractures (oblique and transverse)
Neck fractures
Head fractures

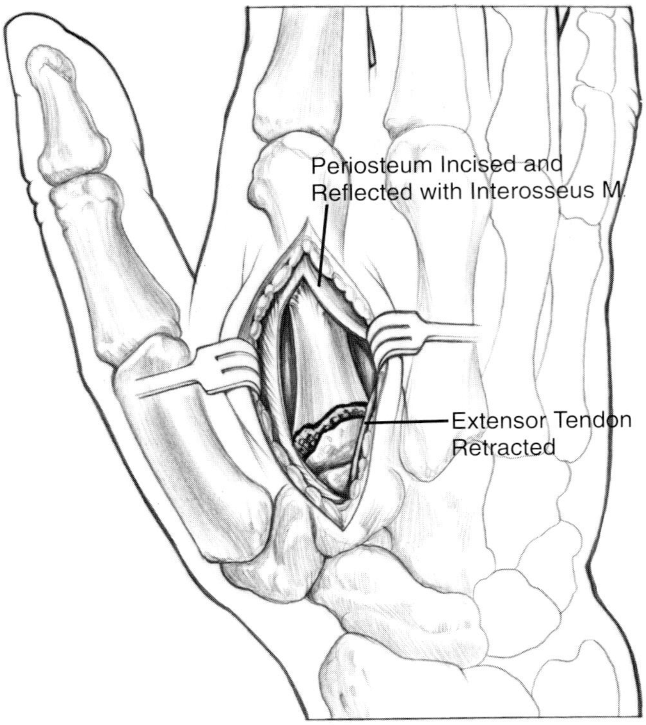

FIG. 9. Surgical approach for an extraarticular base fracture.

DEFINITIVE MANAGEMENT

Extraarticular Base Fractures

Angulation of 10° to 15° and shortening up to 2 mm are acceptable in the ring and little fingers after closed reduction because compensatory motion is provided by the CMC joints. The same amount of deformity is unacceptable and painful in the index and middle finger CMC joints, which form the stable strut of the hand. Realignment of the metacarpals should be attempted by closed reduction under a wrist nerve block. Closed reduction is achieved by distracting the fingers and applying pressure over the apex of the fracture, which is normally angulated dorsally. If satisfactory reduction is achieved, a splint is applied from the PIP joints to the forearm, immobilizing the MCP joints in 70° of flexion. The splint is replaced with a cast after 10 to 14 days.

Fractures that cannot be aligned in a satisfactory position by closed reduction are approached through a longitudinal incision centered over the proximal half of the metacarpal (Fig. 9). The extensor tendons are retracted to either side and the bridging juncturae tendinum might have to be divided, although efforts should be made to keep this structure intact to minimize the formation of postoperative adhesions. The periosteum on the dorsal surface of the metacarpal is incised longitudinally and the origins of the interosseous muscles are reflected slightly to expose the fracture site. Although crossed Kirschner wires can be used for fixation, a mini-T-plate and 2.7-mm cortical screws are preferred.

Intraarticular Base Fractures

Minimally displaced fractures resulting from impaction or avulsion can be treated by cast immobilization by the same protocols that were described for extraarticular base fractures.

Impaction Fractures

Impaction fractures are caused by significant axial loading on the CMC joint. The fracture pattern is usually T- or Y-shaped, and comminution is common. Open reduction and internal fixation is usually necessary to anatomically realign displaced fractures. A longitudinal incision is centered over the injured CMC joint and the extensor tendons are retracted to either side. The capsule is incised longitudinally and the flaps are elevated by sharp dissection to expose the joint. Length is restored by traction, and the fracture fragments are reduced by manipulation with a dental pick. The joint surface is restored by pinning together the two largest articular fragments (Fig. 10). After this, the shaft is fixed to the reconstructed articular surface with crossed Kirschner wires or a mini-T-plate. In very comminuted fractures, the shaft can be fixed to the adjacent metacarpal with transverse Kirschner wires to prevent shortening.

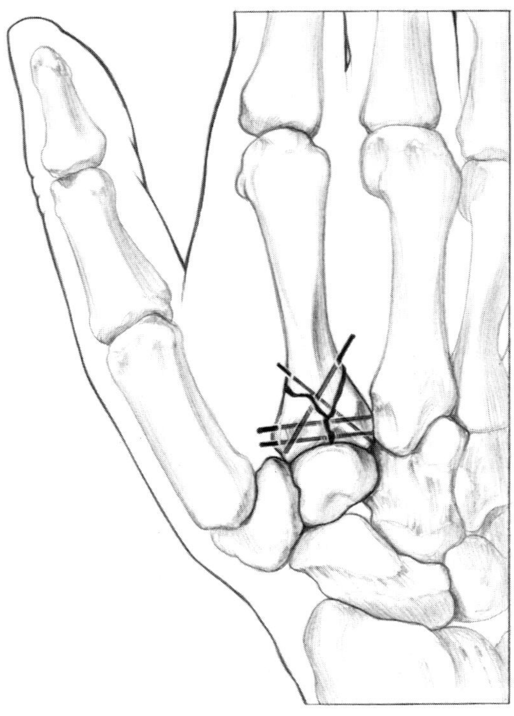

FIG. 10. Internal fixation of an intraarticular impaction fracture.

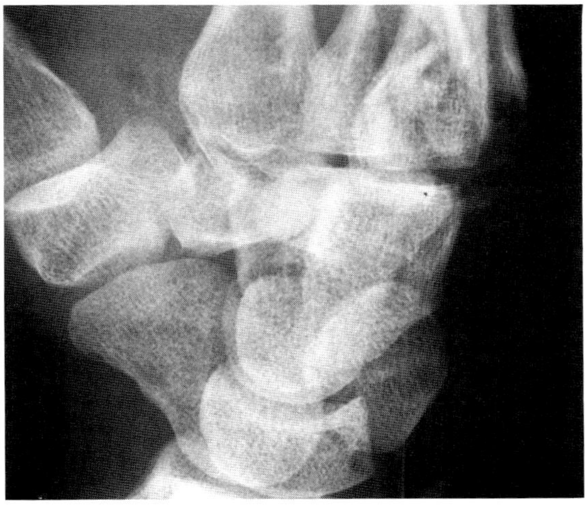

FIG. 11. Radiograph of an intraarticular avulsion fracture of the middle finger metacarpal.

Avulsion Fractures

Avulsion fractures are caused by forced palmar flexion of the wrist. They are traction injuries involving the insertion sites of the extensor carpi radialis brevis on the second metacarpal and the extensor carpi radialis longus and extensor carpi radialis brevis on the third metacarpal (Fig. 11). Small avulsion fractures can be managed by splinting the wrist in extension for 3 weeks. Fractures involving 15% to 20% of the articular surface require open reduction. The surgical approach for avulsion fractures is the same as for impaction fractures. Fractures are stabilized with 2-mm or 2.7-mm cortical lag screws or by a tension-band wiring technique (Fig. 12). If the fixation is stable, wrist range-of-motion exercises, except palmar flexion, can be started after 2 to 3 postoperative weeks. Palmar flexion can be started after 4 to 6 weeks.

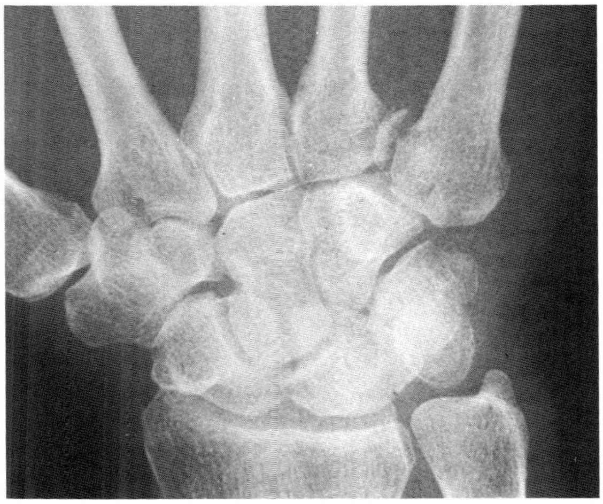

FIG. 13. Radiograph of an intraarticular fracture–dislocation of the little finger CMC joint.

Fracture–Dislocations

Intraarticular fracture–dislocations are often difficult to diagnose and consequently may be recognized late (2). Closed reduction and fixation with percutaneous Kirschner wires may be possible within a few days of injury, but older or markedly displaced fractures require ORIF. Stabilization may be provided by crossed Kirschner wires or Kirschner wires fashioned as staples, without tethering the extensor tendons. The surgical approach and immobilization times are the same as for intraarticular impaction injuries. Degenerative changes and pain result when chronic fracture–dislocations are left untreated (3). Fracture–dislocations of the little finger CMC joint are unstable injuries and require internal fixation in almost all cases to avoid degenerative changes in unstable joints (reverse Bennett pattern) (Figs. 13 and 14).

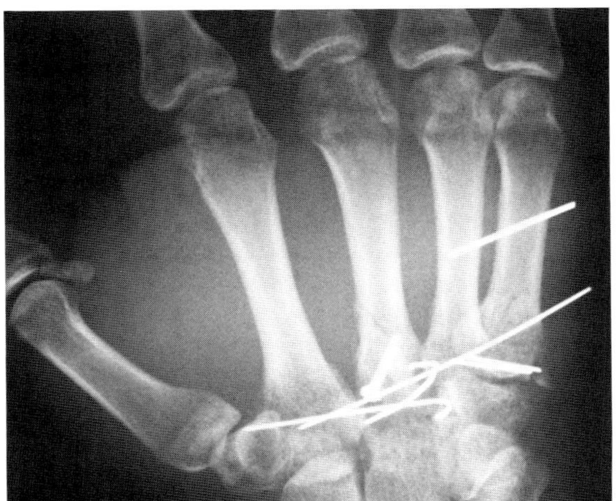

FIG. 12. Radiograph of internal fixation of an intraarticular avulsion fracture of the middle finger metacarpal.

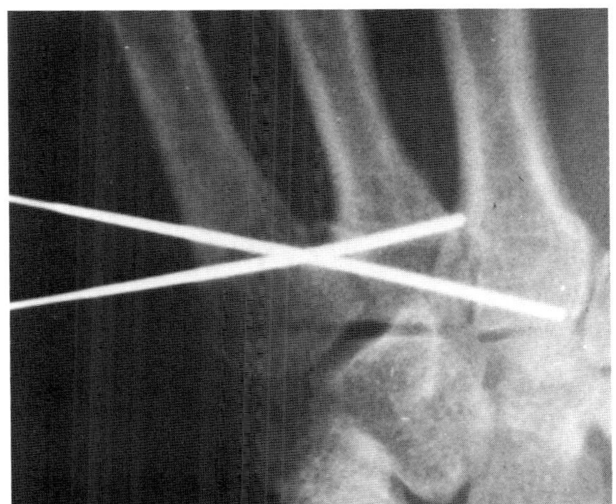

FIG. 14. Postoperative radiograph after open internal fixation of the little finger CMC joint.

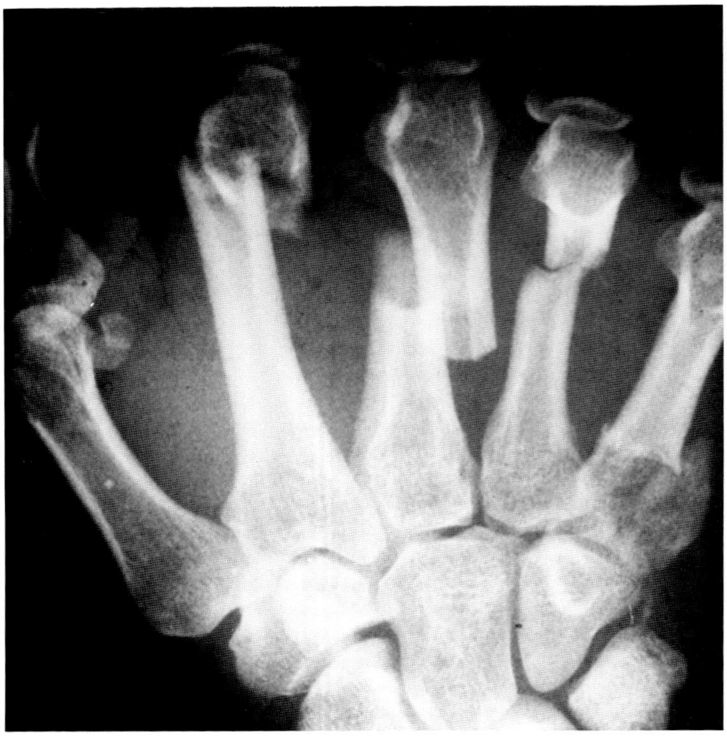

FIG. 15. A crushing injury resulted in metacarpal fractures of all four fingers.

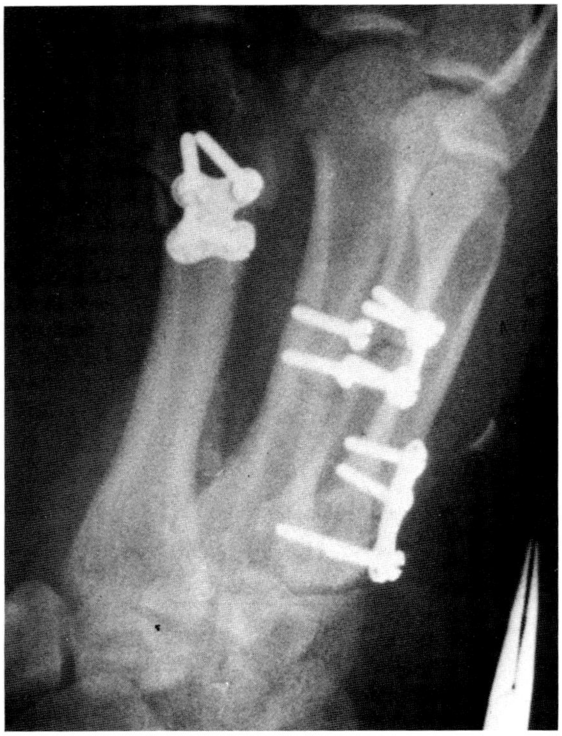

FIG. 16. Postoperative radiograph after internal fixation of multiple metacarpal shaft fractures.

Metacarpal Shaft Fractures (Oblique and Transverse)

Like base fractures, shaft fractures in the ring and little finger metacarpals can tolerate 10° to 15° of angulation and 2 mm of shortening. The technique for closed reduction is the same as the protocols described for extraarticular base fractures. Fracture displacement tends to occur as swelling decreases and the initial tight fit of the splint loosens. Follow-up radiographs are necessary at 1, 3, and 6 weeks after injury.

Multiple metacarpal fractures require rigid internal fixation for early motion and to prevent joint stiffness due to swelling (Figs. 15 and 16). The surgical approach for multiple fractures is similar to that for extraarticular base fractures, except that the incision is extended farther distally. Oblique fractures can be stabilized with lag screws and neutralization plates. Transverse fractures are stabilized with semitubular plates or H-plates. After surgery, a gutter splint is applied to the radial or the ulnar side of the hand as dictated by the fracture site. The splint should extend over the MCP joint and hold it in 70° of flexion to prevent extension contractures. The PIP joints are left free to prevent flexion contractures. A removable splint is prescribed for 3 to 4 weeks to facilitate hand therapy. Noncompliant patients are treated for 5 to 6 weeks in a short-arm cast that extends over the MCP joints.

Metacarpal Neck Fractures

The most common metacarpal neck fracture is a fighter's fracture of the fifth metacarpal. Evaluation of this injury must include a careful examination of the skin for small puncture wounds or lacerations that might have penetrated the MCP joints. Lacerations that penetrate the joint are treated by emergent surgical incision, drainage, and irrigation. Intravenous antibiotics and tetanus immunizations (or immunoglobulin) are administered prophylactically. Angulation with flexion at the neck of the fourth and fifth metacarpals almost always occurs in the plane of MCP and CMC joint motion and rarely causes functional limitations.

The force of the impact that produces a fighter's fracture usually tilts the distal metacarpal fragment in a volar direction. The angulated fragment can be reduced by flexing the MCP and PIP joints and applying upward pressure on the metacarpal head, using the shaft of the proximal phalanx as a lever (Fig. 17). A splint is applied from the ring and little finger PIP joints to the forearm, leaving PIP joint motion unhindered and the metacarpal joints immobilized in 70° of flexion to prevent extension contractures of the MCP joints (Fig. 18). These fractures usually heal after 5 to 6 weeks of immobilization in cast. Range-of-motion exercises for the PIP joint should be encouraged during this time. Flexion deformities of 50° to 70° in the little finger and 40° to 50° in the ring finger

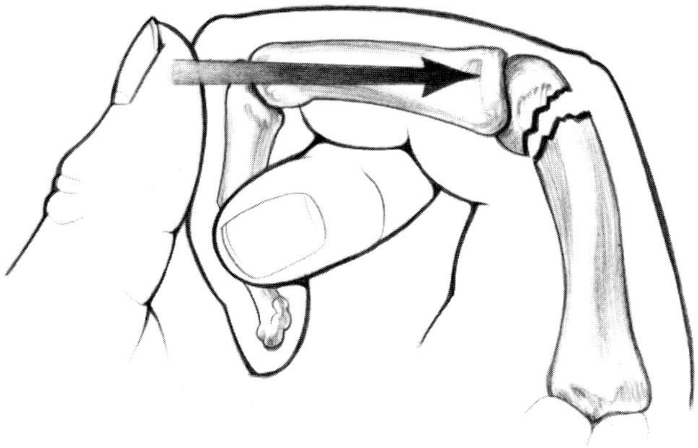

FIG. 17. Reduction of a metacarpal neck fracture.

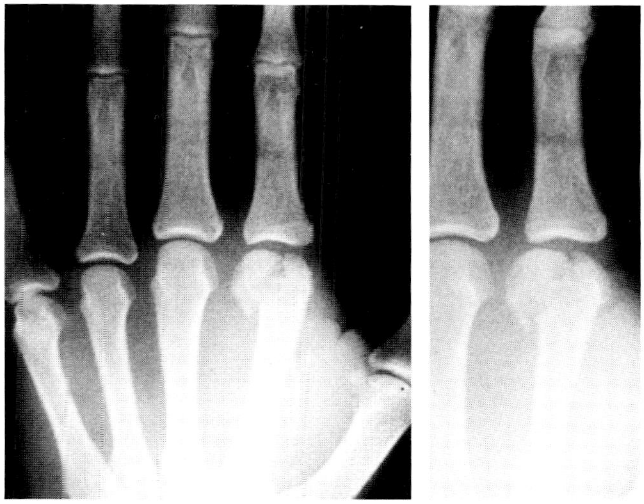

FIG. 19. Metacarpal head fracture.

metacarpals do not cause significant functional problems in most cases. Closed reductions of more severe deformities are stabilized with crossed percutaneous Kirschner wires placed along the mid-lateral axis of the metacarpal to avoid tethering the extensor hood mechanism. Angular deformities greater than 10° to 15° in the index and middle fingers require repeat reduction, possibly with percutaneous pinning. Many patients delay seeking treatment for this injury. Fractures seen 2 or 3 weeks after injury are allowed to heal, and late osteotomies are planned if function is limited after fracture union.

Metacarpal Head Fractures

Most intraarticular fractures of the metacarpal head occur in conjunction with open injuries. Late traumatic arthrosis is unavoidable when a portion of the articular head is destroyed or when a congruent articular surface cannot be restored. When the articular surface is displaced by more than 1 mm, ORIF is necessary to reestablish joint congruency and decrease the risk of joint arthrosis (Figs. 19 and 20).

A longitudinal incision is made 2 mm to 3 mm lateral to the border of the central tendon in the extensor hood mechanism and the extensor tendon is reflected to the side. The joint is exposed through a curvilinear incision centered over the MCP joint. The sagittal band is divided on the ulnar side and a longitudinal incision is made in the joint capsule by sharp dissection and the capsular flaps are reflected to either side. The fracture fragments are reduced with a dental pick, and the articular surface is reconstructed and stabilized with Kirschner wires or small 1.5-mm or 2-mm cortical lag screws. The heads of the screws are countersunk to prevent a

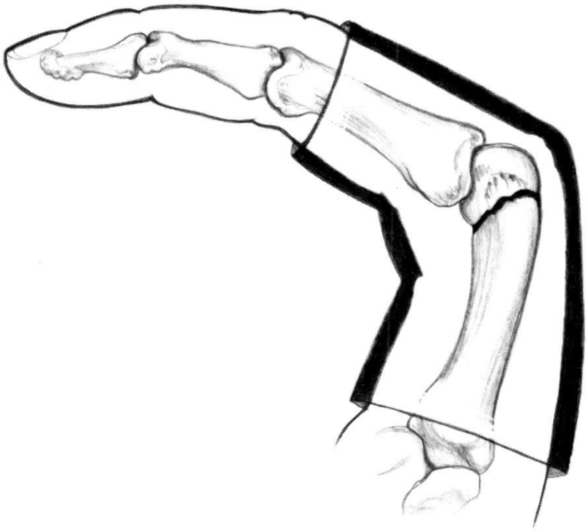

FIG. 18. Casting technique for a metacarpal neck fracture.

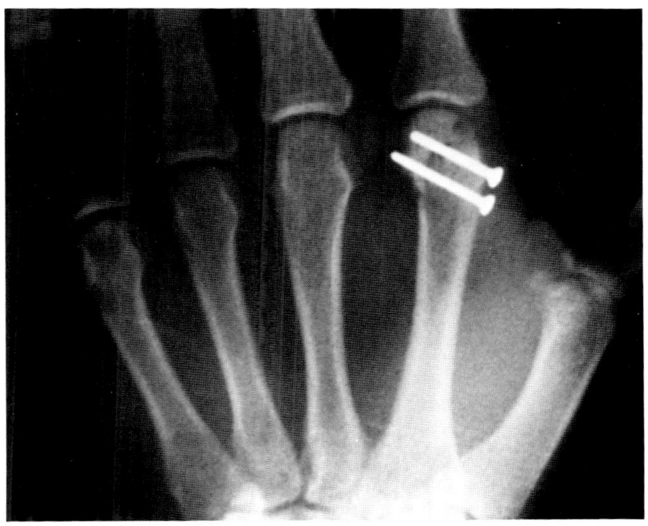

FIG. 20. Internal fixation for a metacarpal head fracture.

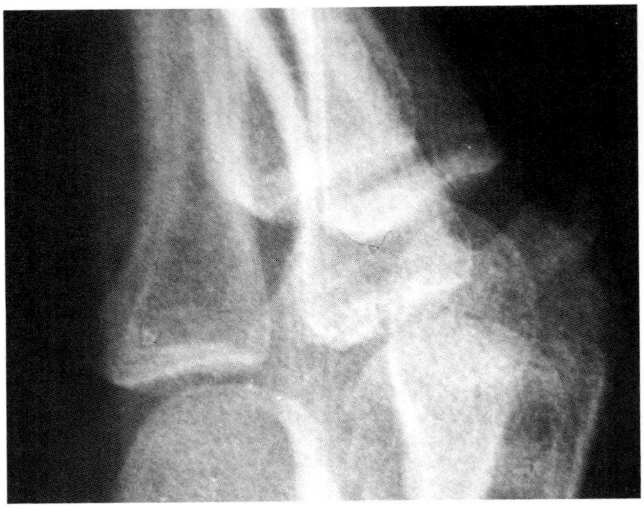

FIG. 21. Displaced segment of metacarpal head.

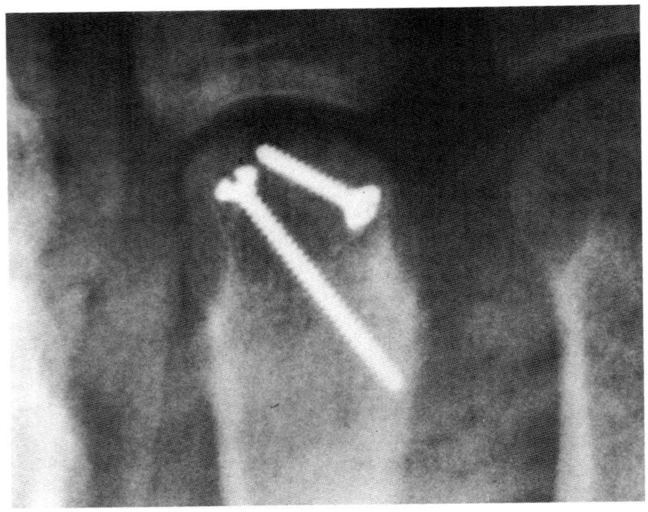

FIG. 22. Lag screws are countersunk to avoid injury to articular surfaces.

prominence over the joint when intraarticular lag screws are required (Figs. 21 and 22). Alternatively, large fracture fragments may be stabilized with a small Herbert screw. The wound is closed in two layers using fine absorbable sutures. Joint range-of-motion exercises are supervised by a hand therapist after swelling has subsided.

COMPLICATIONS

Joint stiffness is a serious problem after hand fractures. To minimize this complication, the MCP joint must be splinted in 70° of flexion and the IP joint must be splinted in extension. The incidence of adhesion formation between the extensor tendons and the metacarpals or interosseous muscles decreases when hand therapy is initiated early. Tenolysis may be necessary if adhesions continue to limit joint flexion.

SKELETALLY IMMATURE PATIENTS

Almost all metacarpal fractures in children can be treated by closed manipulation within the first week of injury. Exceptions include Salter-III and -IV fractures involving the MCP joint, which require ORIF to reestablish joint congruency. Patients with physeal injuries must be followed longitudinally for early identification of bony bridges across the physis.

REFERENCES

1. Bora FW, Didizian NH. The treatment of injuries to the carpometacarpal joint of the little finger. *J Bone Joint Surg* 1974;56A:1459–1463.
2. Joseph RB, Linsheid RL, Dobyns JH, et al. Chronic sprains of the carpometacarpal joints. *J Hand Surg* 1981;6:172–180.
3. Clendenin MB, Smith RJ. Fifth metacarpal/hamate arthrodesis for posttraumatic osteoarthritis. *J Hand Surg* 1984;9A:374–378.

Metacarpophalangeal Joint Subluxations and Dislocations

MECHANISMS OF INJURY

Thumb

Most MCP joint subluxations and dislocations are caused by hyperextension combined with rotation or lateral deviation. The most common acute injury, skier's thumb, occurs when the thumb is caught in a device such as the strap of a ski pole and the ulnar collateral ligament is torn. A gamekeeper's thumb is usually attributed to chronic stretching of the ulnar collateral ligament even though it is probably caused by an earlier acute injury. A dorsal dislocation involving the volar plate is caused by a hyperextension injury. When ulnar deviation is a component of the injury the radial collateral ligament also may be damaged. The severity of these injuries ranges from mild ligamentous tears to complete MCP joint disruptions and displaced avulsion fractures (1–5).

Fingers

Digital MCP injuries occur by similar mechanisms. However, the fingers are less susceptible to collateral ligament injuries because they are protected by adjacent digits.

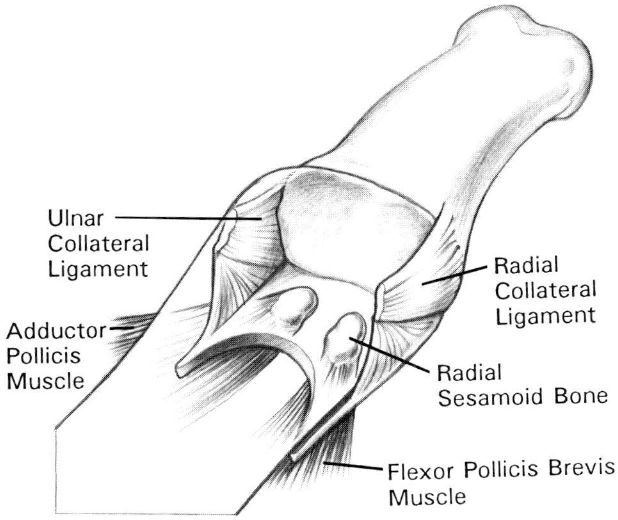

FIG. 23. Anatomy of the thumb MCP joint.

ANATOMIC CONSIDERATIONS

Thumb

The volar plate of the thumb MCP joint contains two sesamoids (Fig. 23). The adductor pollicis muscle inserts onto the ulnar sesamoid and the flexor pollicis brevis inserts onto the radial sesamoid. The collateral ligaments are located on both sides of the volar plate. Unlike the radial collateral ligament, the ulnar collateral ligament is covered by the broad expanse of the adductor aponeurosis. When it is severely avulsed, the ulnar collateral ligament can retract and turn back on itself, interposing the adductor aponeurosis between the end of the ligament and the base of the proximal phalanx. This injury is called a Stener lesion. Continuity of the ligament cannot be reestablished without operative repair (Fig. 24) (6).

Fingers

The anatomy of the finger MCP joints is similar to that of the thumb except for the location of the extensor hood mechanism, which makes interposition of the extensor hood between the torn collateral ligaments impossible in the fingers. Two sesamoids are found in the fingers, one in the volar plate of the index finger and one in the volar plate of the little finger.

CLASSIFICATION

Thumb

Classifications of thumb subluxations and dislocations correspond to the injured structures (Table 2).

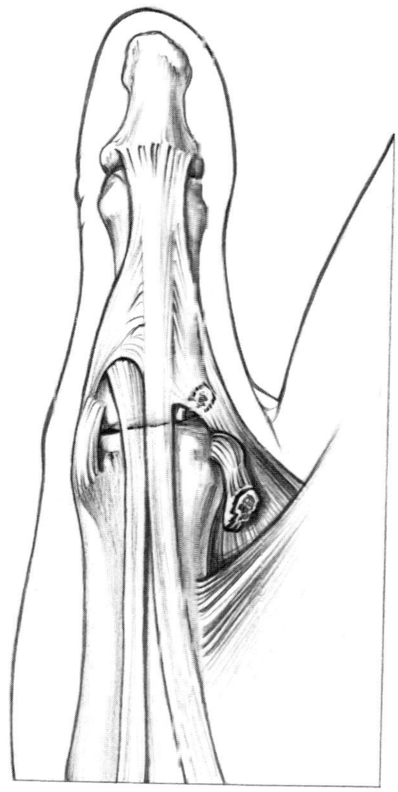

FIG. 24. A Stener lesion with an avulsion fracture.

Table 2. *Thumb MCP joint subluxations and dislocations*

Ulnar collateral ligament injuries secondary to *radial* subluxation and hyperextension
Radial collateral ligament injuries secondary to *ulnar* subluxation and hyperextension
MCP joint subluxations and dislocations with *dorsal* displacement and avulsion of the volar plate secondary to hyperextension
Simple dislocations
Complex dislocations

Fingers

The injured structure is also the key to classifying subluxations and dislocations in the fingers (Table 3).

Table 3. *Finger MCP joint subluxations and dislocations*

Collateral ligament injuries secondary to radial or ulnar deviation
Dorsal MCP joint dislocations with avulsion of the volar plate
Simple dislocations
Complex dislocations

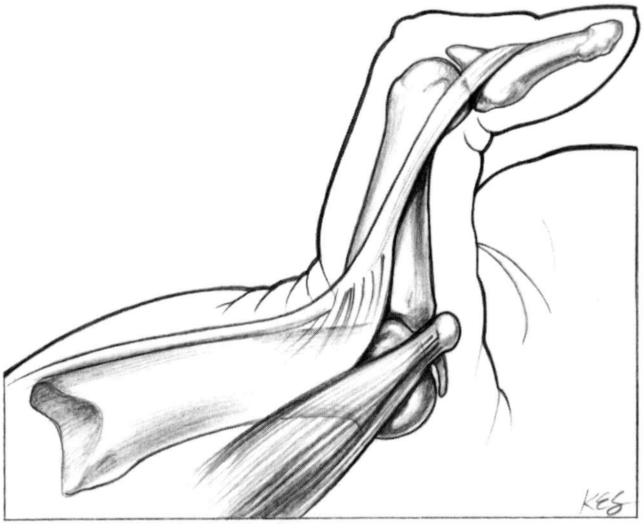

FIG. 25. Simple dislocation of the thumb MCP joint.

ASSESSMENT

Physical Examination

Thumb

Subluxations or dislocations may consist of soft-tissue injuries that are not apparent on radiographs. Swelling and ecchymosis are usually suggestive of severe ligamentous disruptions that require operative repair. A painful thumb may be indicative of a nondisplaced avulsion fracture. Stress testing is contraindicated in this case and radiographs should be obtained before the physical examination is conducted.

A simple thumb subluxation or dislocation presents as a hyperextended MCP joint (Fig. 25). In contrast, a completely dislocated MCP joint demonstrates dorsal displacement of the proximal phalanx but less overall deformity (Fig. 26). Ulnar and radial collateral ligament injuries are evaluated by positioning the thumb MCP joint in 30° of flexion to eliminate the stabilizing effect of the articular structures and by stressing the joint in radial or ulnar deviation, respectively.

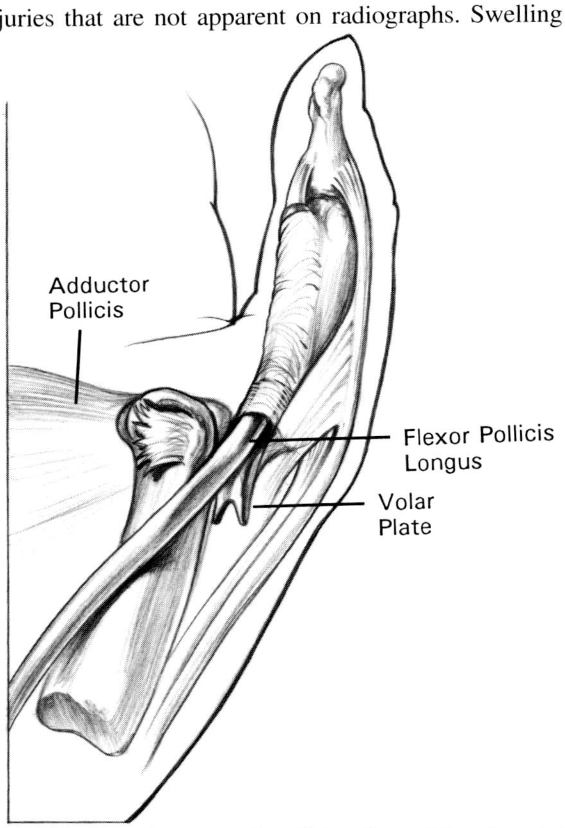

FIG. 26. Complete complex dislocation of the thumb MCP joint.

Fingers

Metacarpophalangeal dislocations and collateral ligament instability in the fingers are diagnosed in a similar manner after the radiographic evaluation is completed.

Radiographic Evaluation

Anteroposterior, lateral, and oblique radiographs are obtained to evaluate all MCP joint injuries before reduction. The appearance of a sesamoid in the MCP joint on an AP radiograph is indicative of a complex dislocation and interposition of the volar plate into the joint. Avulsed fragments that were not seen on the original radiographs can sometimes be identified on postreduction films.

Special Studies

An arthrogram can be taken with contrast dye injected into the MCP joint to diagnose a ligamentous injury that might otherwise be camouflaged by diffuse swelling and tenderness. Rapid leakage of dye from the joint is consistent with a large collateral ligament tear.

EMERGENT MANAGEMENT

Tenting of the neurovascular bundles over the metacarpal head occurs with complex MCP joint dislocations and warrants immediate joint reduction. Open injuries require immediate irrigation and debridement in addition to reduction.

DEFINITIVE MANAGEMENT

Thumb

Ulnar Collateral Ligament Injuries

When stress testing confirms an incomplete ligamentous

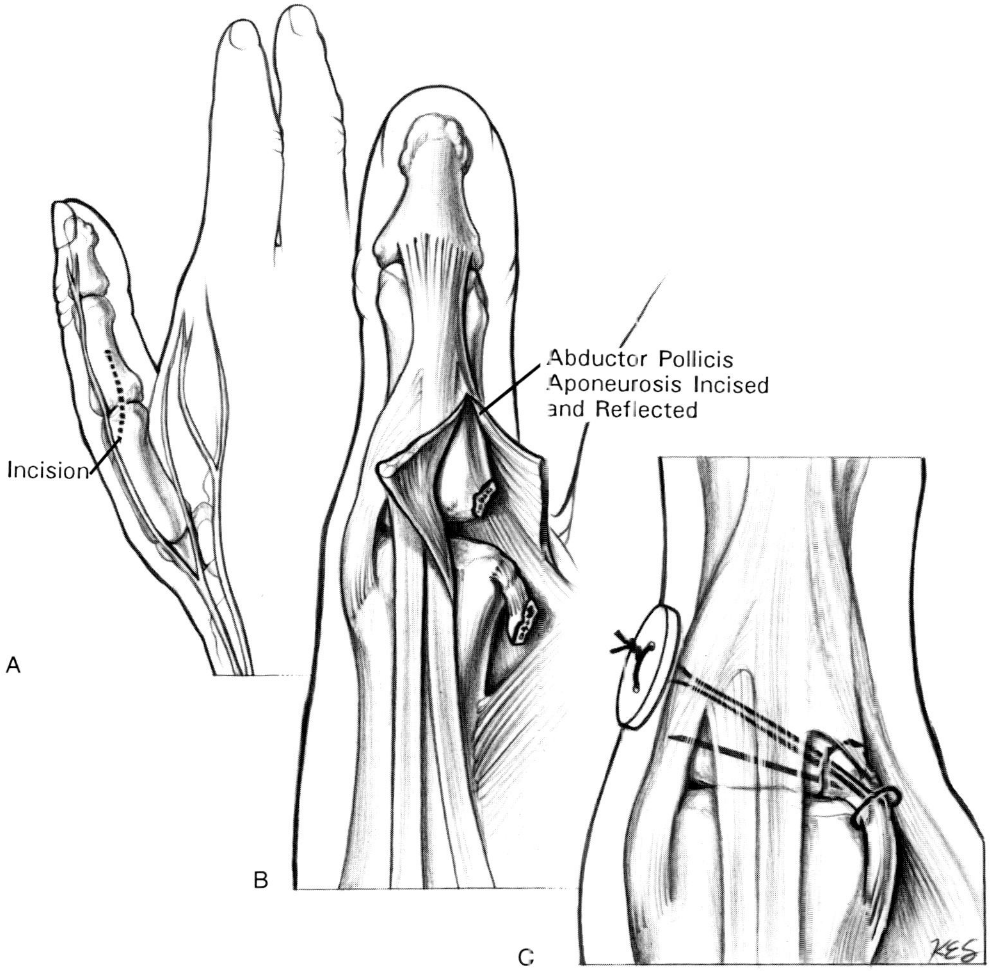

FIG. 27. A,B: Surgical approach for a thumb ulnar collateral ligament injury. **C:** Surgical repair of a thumb ulnar collateral ligament rupture.

injury, treatment consists of immobilization in a thumb spica cast for 5 to 6 weeks. After the cast is removed, a hand-based opponens splint is worn part-time for 3 weeks to protect the joint during exercise of the MCP and IP joints. Operative repair is indicated when radial deviation in the injured thumb exceeds 10° of radial deviation on the contralateral side, when total ulnar deviation is between 30° to 45°, or when an avulsion fracture is displaced by more than 1 mm (5).

The joint is approached through a longitudinal incision centered over the ulnar surface of the thumb MCP joint. A branch of the radial sensory nerve lies just dorsal to the margin of this exposure and must be identified and retracted. The proximal margin of the adductor aponeurosis is inspected for the presence of a Stener lesion (Fig. 27). The aponeurosis is divided several millimeters from the ulnar margin of the central tendon in the extensor hood. A suture is passed through the distal end of the ligament in a Kessler fashion.

The attachment site of the ligament on the base of the proximal phalanx is freshened with a rongeur to expose cancellous bone. A hole is made through the bone with a power drill and the suture is passed to the radial side of the thumb with a Keefe needle. The suture is tied over a button while the thumb is held in the reduced position (see Fig. 27C). Bone fragments attached to the distal end of the ligament are reduced and pinned to the fracture site with a .028-inch Kirschner wire or a 2-mm cortical screw. A combination of fixation using suture and internal fixation provides a "belt-and-suspenders" repair. The collateral ligament must be re-attached to the correct insertion site to avoid imposing a flexion or extension moment on the MCP joint. Because the volar plate is frequently detached, the distal end of the volar plate should be sutured to the periosteum on the volar aspect of the proximal phalanx if an injury is present. A splint is applied immedi-ately after surgery and is replaced with a thumb spica cast 2 weeks postoperatively. Flexion exercises for the thumb IP joint are started to prevent loss of motion secondary to the formation of adhesions around the adductor aponeurosis. The pull-out button and the cast are removed after 5 weeks and a hand-based opponens splint is worn part-time for 3 weeks to protect the repair without inhibiting motion in the MCP and IP joints. If an acute-on-chronic injury has destroyed all but a small remnant of the ulnar collateral ligament, reconstruction can be accomplished by tendon grafting (5).

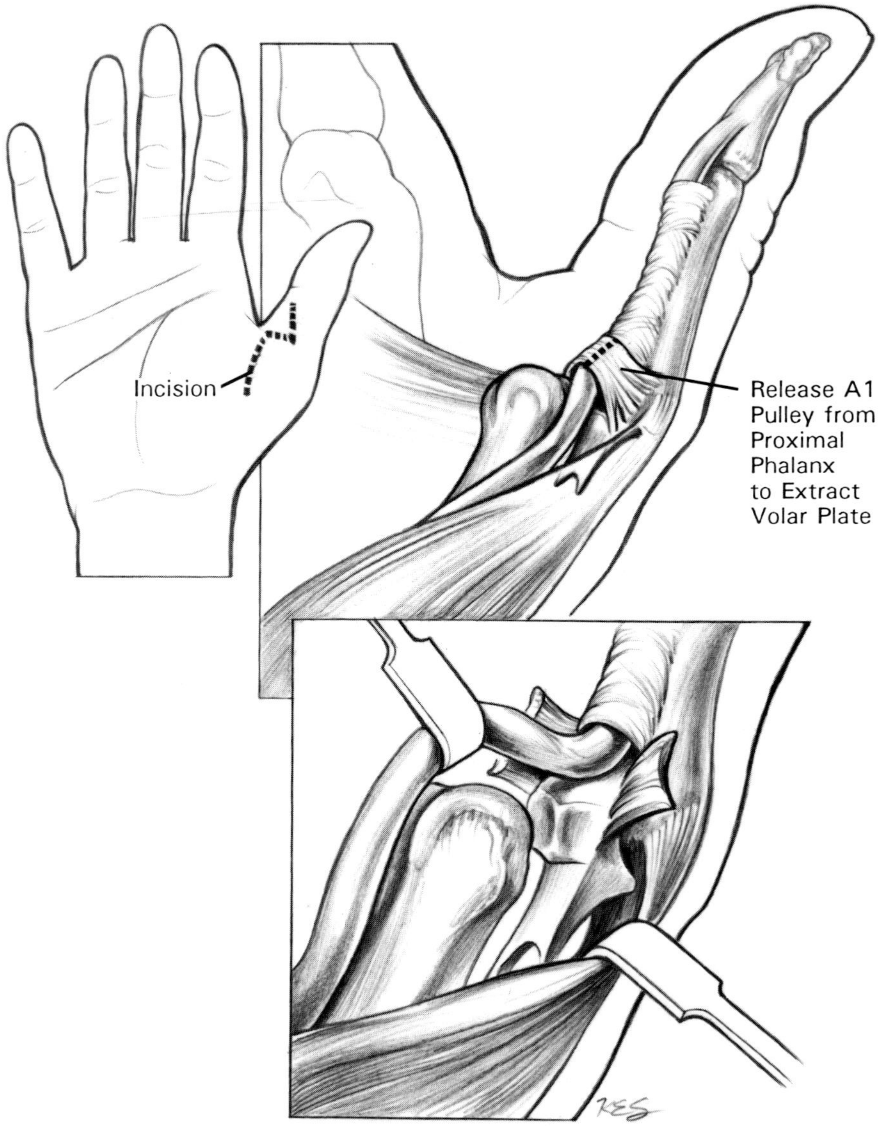

FIG. 28. Surgical exposure of a complex thumb MCP dislocation.

Radial Collateral Ligament Injuries

Most radial collateral injuries can be managed in a thumb spica cast for 6 weeks. Fractures with articular surface involvement, those with more than 1 mm of displacement, and joints that dislocate or luxate with stress testing require operative repair. The surgical approach for a radial collateral ligament repair is made through a longitudinal incision on the radial side of the MCP joint. A portion of the adductor pollicis brevis insertion is reflected from the base of the proximal phalanx to expose the radial collateral ligament. The ligamentous injury or the avulsion fracture is repaired in a manner similar to an ulnar collateral ligament repair, but in this case the pull-out suture is brought out the ulnar aspect of the thumb and tied over a button. The postoperative course is the same as that for an ulnar collateral ligament injury.

Dorsal Dislocations and Subluxations

Simple dislocations can be reduced easily because the joint surfaces maintain contact. To reduce simple dislocations, dorsal pressure is applied to the base of the proximal phalanx and the thumb is immobilized in a dorsal block splint that prevents the last 30° of motion. The splint is worn for 3 weeks while active and passive flexion exercises are carried out.

Complex dislocations often exhibit a bayonet deformity on radiographs. Closed reduction is often unsuccessful for complex dislocations because the soft tissues surrounding the metacarpal head tighten like a Chinese fingertrap with any type of manipulation. The main structure blocking reduction is the volar plate, which is displaced dorsally over the metacarpal head. Although a dorsal approach can be used, a palmar approach using a Bruner zig-zag incision over the distal palmar crease is preferred. The neurovascular bundles, which might be tented over the metacarpal head, are protected. Releasing the A1 annular pulley of the thumb facilitates retraction of the flexor tendon and extraction of the volar plate and reduction of the MCP joint (Fig. 28).

Fingers

MCP Collateral Ligament Injuries

Collateral ligament injuries are treated by buddy-taping the injured finger to an adjacent digit. Active and passive motion are initiated to prevent joint stiffness. In spite of this, patients occasionally experience chronic discomfort around the MCP joint, especially when the joint was not protected during the acute phase.

MCP Dorsal Dislocations

Simple dorsal dislocations in the fingers are usually reduced and splinted in the same way as thumb injuries. Complex dislocations generally occur in combinations that involve the index finger or the little finger, with or without involvement of the adjacent digits (Figs. 29 and 30). In complex dislocations of the index finger, the flexor tendons are wrapped tightly around the ulnar aspect of the metacarpal head and the lumbrical muscle is wrapped around the radial aspect. In the little finger, the flexor tendons are usually displaced to the radial side and the abductor digiti quinti muscle is displaced to the ulnar side of the metacarpal head. A dorsally displaced volar plate is the key structure preventing joint reduction.

To reduce a complex dislocation, the injury that caused the MCP joint dislocation is reproduced by hyperextending the MCP joint with the wrist in flexion, lessening the Chinese finger-trap effect and placing the joint surfaces in contact. Dorsal pressure is then applied to the base of the proximal phalanx to reduce the joint (Fig. 31). Open reduction can be done through dorsal or volar approaches, the same as for the thumb MCP joint. The postoperative regimen for simple and complex dislocations consists of a dorsal block splint that prevents the last 30° of extension for 3 weeks.

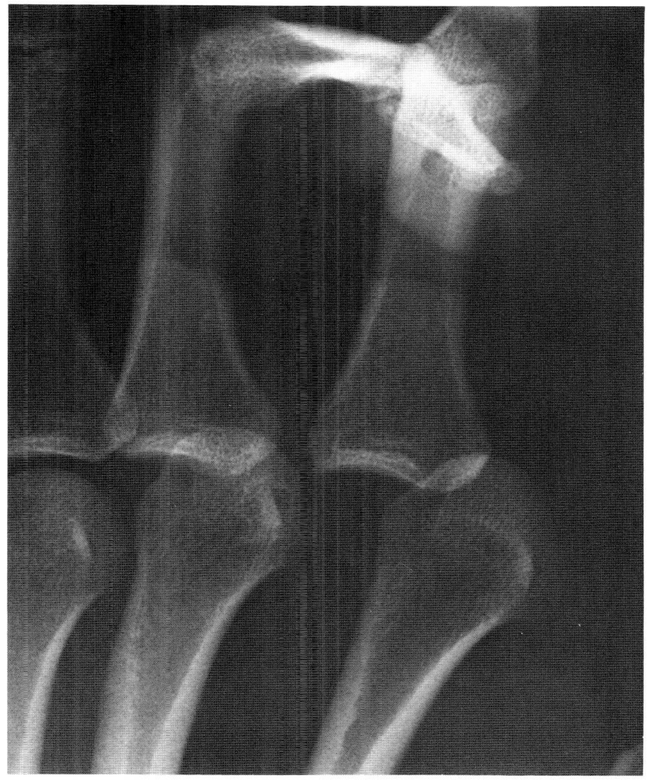

FIG. 29. Anteroposterior radiograph of complex dislocations of the index and middle fingers.

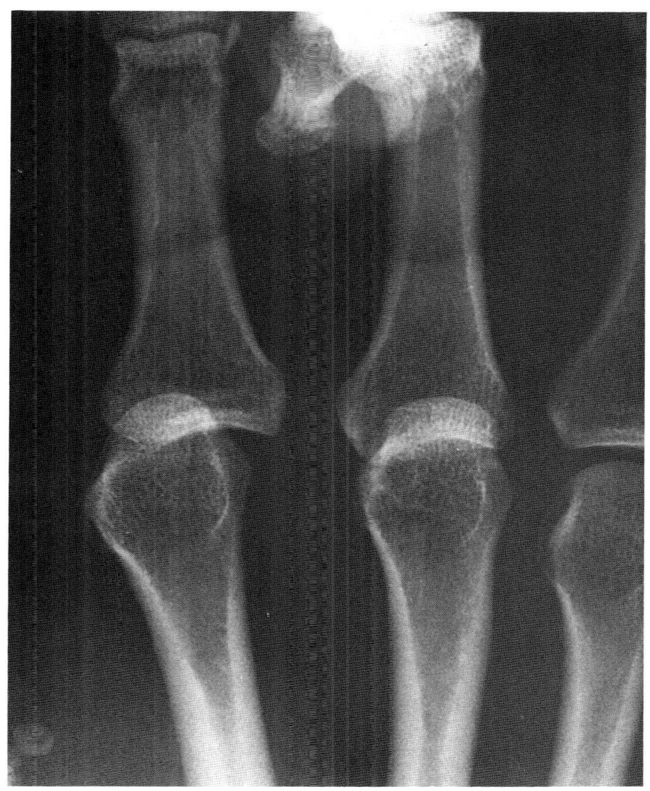

FIG. 30. Overlapping of the bones at the MCP joint is an indication of a complex dislocation.

COMPLICATIONS

Digital nerve injuries can be prevented by identifying the nerves proximally during the volar approach.

SKELETALLY IMMATURE PATIENTS

Metacarpophalangeal joint dislocations are rare in children. A high degree of suspicion must be maintained when

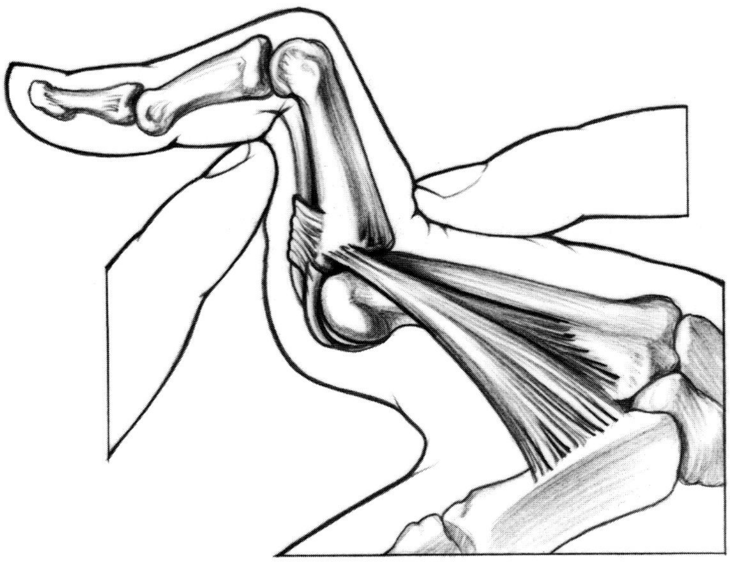

FIG. 31. Reduction of a complex dislocation.

evaluating these injuries in children because incomplete ossification of the phalanges and metacarpals makes radiographic interpretation of dislocations difficult. Salter II or III fracture–dislocations are common and should be ruled out.

REFERENCES

1. Browne EZ, Dunn HK, Snyder CC. Ski pole thumb injury. *Plast Reconstruct Surg* 1976;58:19–23.
2. Coonrad R, Golner J. A study of the pathologic findings and treatment in soft-tissue injury of the thumb metacarphophalangeal joint. *J Bone Joint Surg* 1968;50A:439–451.
3. Kaplan EB. The pathology and treatment of radial subluxation of the thumb with ulnar displacement of the head of the first metacarpal. *J Bone Joint Surg* 1961;43A:541–544.
4. Kessler I. Complete avulsion of the ulnar collateral ligament of the metacarpopohalangeal joint of the thumb. *Clin Orthop* 1961;29:196–200.
5. Smith RJ. Post-traumatic instability of the metacarpophalangeal joint of the thumb. *J Bone Joint Surg* 1977;59A:14–21.
6. Stener B. Displacement of the ruptured ulnar collateral ligament of the metacarpophalangeal joint of the thumb. *J Bone Joint Surg* 1962;44B:869–879.

Proximal and Middle Phalangeal Fractures

MECHANISMS OF INJURY

The fracture patterns of all phalangeal fractures are related to the mechanisms of injury. Torsional forces produce oblique fractures, bending moments produce transverse fractures, and crushing injuries produce comminuted fractures.

ANATOMIC CONSIDERATIONS

Proximal Phalangeal Fractures

Full digital range of motion is dependent on the smooth gliding motion of the extensor hood over the proximal phalanx. Loss of 2 to 3 mm of motion at this site can result in loss of 20° to 30° of arc motion. The entire circumference of the proximal phalanx is surrounded by tendons, making all surgical approaches difficult. Because the base of the middle phalanx must fit into the concavity on the volar side of the proximal phalanx as the volar plate shifts proximally as a unit (unlike the accordion action of the collapsible volar plate of the MCP joint), application of an internal fixation device or the presence of fracture fragments in this area will mechanically block PIP joint flexion (Fig. 32).

Middle Phalangeal Fractures

The central slip attaches to the base of the middle phalanx. The lateral bands cross both sides of the middle phalanx and

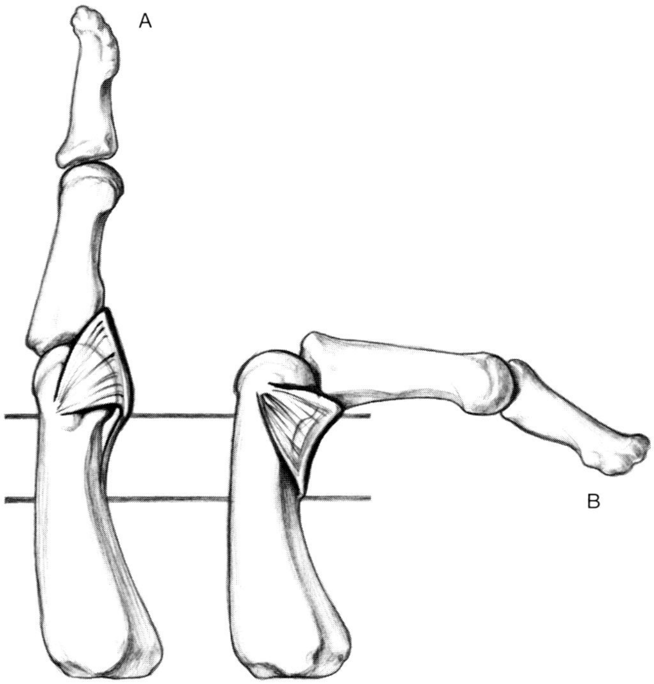

FIG. 32. The movement of PIP joint volar plate during finger flexion.

merge on the dorsal side to form the terminal branch of the flexor tendon, which inserts into the distal phalanx. The flexor tendon sheath adheres to the volar side of the middle phalanx.

CLASSIFICATION

Proximal and middle phalangeal fractures are classified by location and fracture pattern (Table 4).

ASSESSMENT

Physical Examination

Severe soft-tissue injuries are common in both proximal and middle phalangeal fractures. The soft-tissue cover in this area is meager and a seemingly minor laceration might in fact have communicated with the fracture site, producing a compound fracture or even an incomplete amputation. Malrotation is diagnosed by aligning all the fingers in the same degree of flexion. Normally, the tilt of the nail beds decreases from the index to the little fingers, the nail bed of the little finger being the most transverse. Loss of nail bed alignment or failure of a finger to remain parallel when it is flexed is indicative of malrotation that should be corrected with manipulation and pin fixation (Fig. 33). Care must be taken not to rotate the joint during attempt to correct the alignment of the fracture.

Table 4. *Classifying proximal and middle phalangeal fractures*

Base fractures
Extraarticular
Intraarticular
Shaft fractures
Oblique
Transverse
Comminuted fractures with extensive bone loss
Condylar fractures
Unicondylar
T- and Y-shaped bicondylar

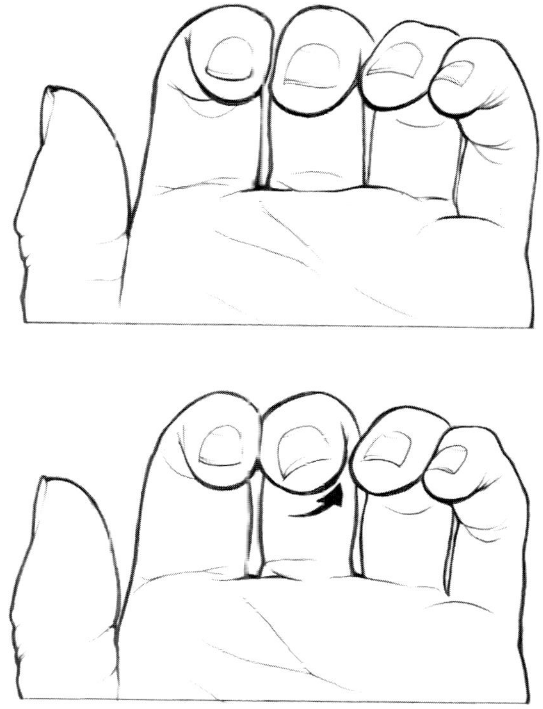

FIG. 33. Change in nail bed orientation signals a problem with malrotation of the long finger.

Radiographic Evaluation

Standard AP, lateral, and oblique radiographs are obtained. A digital nerve block with lidocaine is administered before positioning the hand for a true lateral radiograph.

Special Studies

Depressed areas on the articular surface are visualized best on traction radiographs and trispiral tomograms.

Emergent Management

Open wounds are treated immediately with irrigation and debridement. Reduction and splinting performed under a digital nerve block might be sufficient treatment for a closed injury. The finger must be splinted in a safe position, with the MCP joint in 70° of flexion and the PIP joint nearly neutral to avoid MCP joint extension contractures and PIP joint flexion contractures (see Fig. 8).

DEFINITIVE MANAGEMENT

Nondisplaced or minimally displaced fractures are routinely splinted in a safe position for 4 to 6 weeks, depending on the extent of comminution. Radial gutter splints are used for the index and middle fingers and ulnar gutter splints for the ring and little fingers. The fracture is assessed weekly for late displacement during the first 3 weeks. Active range-of-motion exercises must be delayed for at least 4 weeks in proximal phalangeal fractures. Indications for internal fixation include fractures with 5° of radial or ulnar angulation, 5° of rotation, or 10° to 20° of residual flexion or extension angulation after closed reduction. The digits are flexed after reduction to ensure that they do not overlap or diverge in flexion.

Proximal Phalangeal Fractures

Extraarticular Base Fractures

Extraarticular base fractures (especially short oblique fractures) usually redisplace almost immediately after manipulation (Fig. 34). A fracture near the web spaces is often difficult to stabilize with percutaneous Kirschner wires. These cases require fixation with 1.5- or 2-mm lag screws and a plate through a dorsal incision. A skin flap is reflected to expose the extensor hood mechanism and a longitudinal incision is made in the sagittal band to displace the extensor aponeurosis to one side (Fig. 35). The capsule is incised longitudinally to expose the joint. In this case, however, the incision is located slightly more distally and the joint capsule is not incised. The risk of adhesions forming between the extensor tendon and the proximal phalanx is greatly increased by the exposure and by internal fixation (Fig. 36). Therefore, a thin (0.05 mm) Silastic sheet is placed between the extensor tendon and the plate. Hand therapy that includes active flexion exercises in a dynamic extension splint must be initiated early.

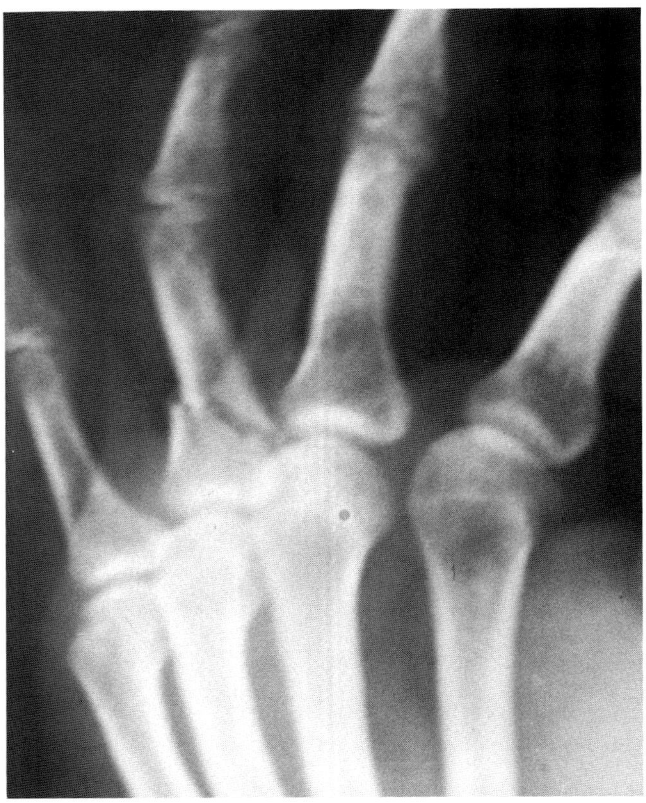

FIG. 34. Radiograph of a displaced oblique fracture at the base of the ring finger proximal phalanx.

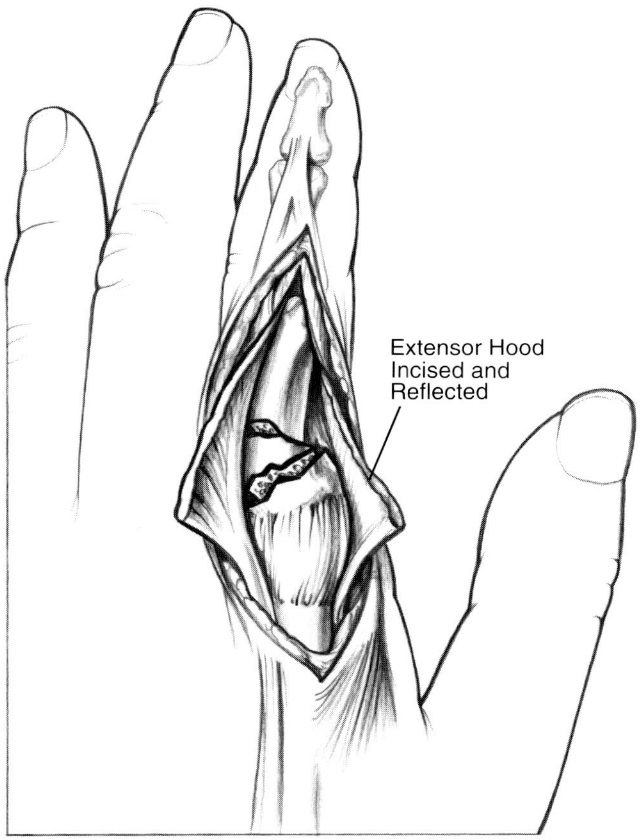

FIG. 35. Radiograph of the surgical exposure for a proximal extraarticular base fracture.

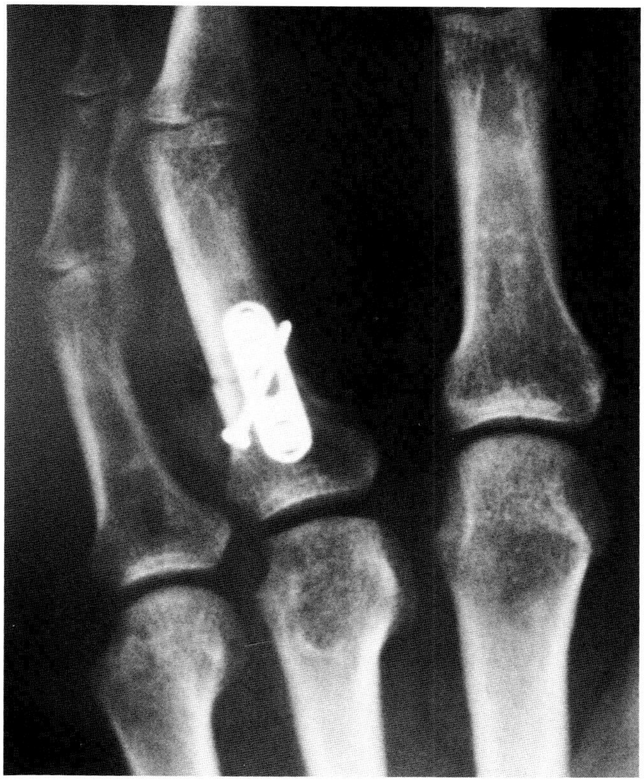

FIG. 36. Internal fixation for a proximal extraarticular base fracture.

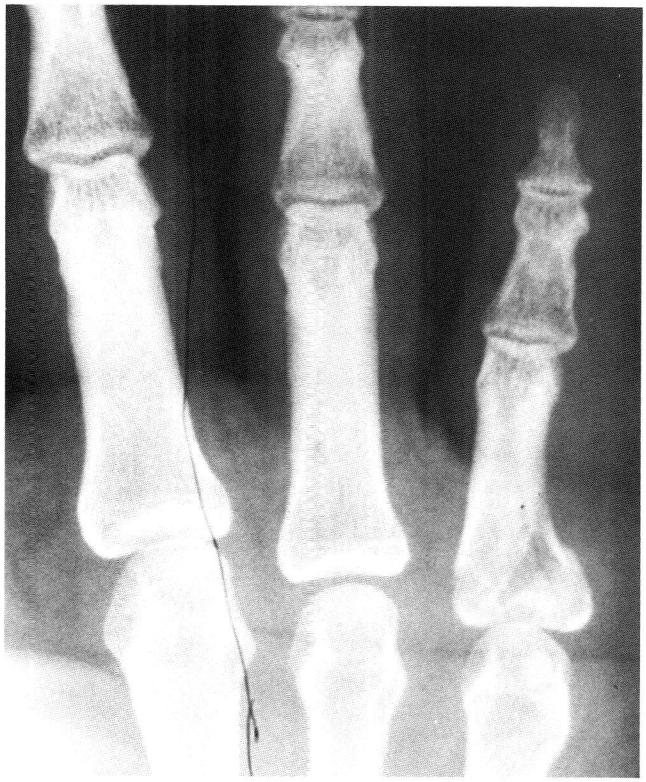

FIG. 37. Comminuted intraarticular base fracture of the little finger.

Intraarticular Base Fractures

Displaced proximal phalangeal fractures can be stabilized with Kirschner wires, small screws, or minifragment plates. Many fractures can be treated by closed reduction and percutaneous pinning if enough cortical contact exists at the fracture site to provide additional stability. When closed reduction is unsuccessful, the fracture is approached through a dorsal curvilinear incision made over the MCP joint as described for extraarticular fractures (Fig. 37). The fracture fragments are manipulated gently and fixed with small Kirschner wires. Large fracture fragments can be stabilized with a screw after initial temporary stabilization with Kirschner wires (Fig. 38). The ends of the pins are cut flush with the bone surface and are left in place permanently unless migration occurs after fracture union. The wound is closed in two layers to minimize extensor tendon adhesions. Unstable fractures and minimally displaced fractures treated without internal fixation are casted in a forearm-based volar splint with the MCP joints in only 30° of flexion to avoid an extensor lag, and the PIP joints in extension. Active PIP exercises are started at 3 weeks. In fractures that are stable after internal fixation, early active flexion is started in a dynamic extension splint for the first 3 weeks to prevent an extensor tendon lag from stretching out the repaired extensor aponeurosis. Active extension exercises are then initiated.

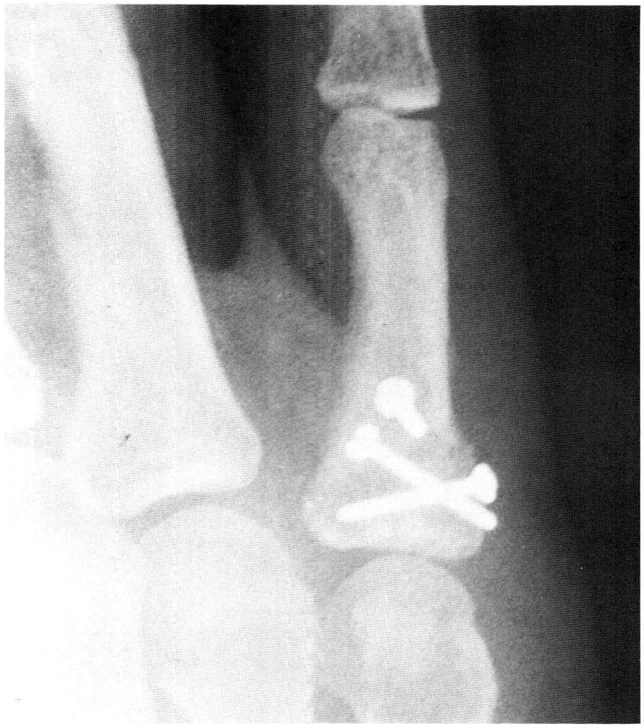

FIG. 38. Internal fixation of a comminuted intraarticular base fracture of the little finger.

Oblique Shaft Fractures

Fixation with percutaneous Kirschner wires does not compress the fracture site adequately and is associated with a high incidence of late fracture displacement except in minimally displaced fractures that are treated prophylactically with pins placed perpendicular to the fracture line. The optimal fixation for oblique fractures is provided by 1.5-mm or 2-mm screws. The screws are placed through a dorsolateral approach, similar to the incision for base fractures, except that in this case the extensor aponeurosis is retracted dorsally for a lateral exposure.

Transverse Shaft Fractures

Transverse fractures are usually stable after reduction and can tolerate approximately 10° to 15° of dorsal or volar angulation. No more than 5° of radial or ulnar deviation is considered acceptable. Malrotation can cause significant disability and is prevented by stabilizing the fracture with small-diameter Kirschner wires. Accurately placing more than two pins is difficult without tethering the extensor tendon at several sites and must be done extremely carefully (1–4). The distal ends of the pins are buried in the soft tissues.

Comminuted transverse fractures can redisplace after percutaneous pinning, and fixation is occasionally supplemented with a small plate applied through a dorsolateral approach. The presence of an open wound frequently dictates the surgical approach for internal fixation. For example, a laceration on the volar aspect suggests using a volar approach, which can be enlarged into a Bruner zig-zag incision. If the flexor tendons are not injured, the tendon sheath is reflected from the proximal phalanx by sharp dissection after the neurovascular bundles have been identified and protected. Although this approach is difficult and increases the risk of adhesion formation at the flexon tendons, it allows placement of a plate on the volar aspect of the phalanx and facilitates rehabilitation of the extensor tendons. Hand therapy is started immediately. A dynamic extension splint is used following a dorsal approach; early active and passive exercises are started following a palmar exposure.

Comminuted Shaft Fractures with Extensive Bone Loss

Extensive comminution may preclude stabilization with internal fixation devices. In this case, external fixation is used initially to maintain length until some of the comminuted fragments heal and definitive care can be undertaken. An external fixation device can be constructed by placing trans-

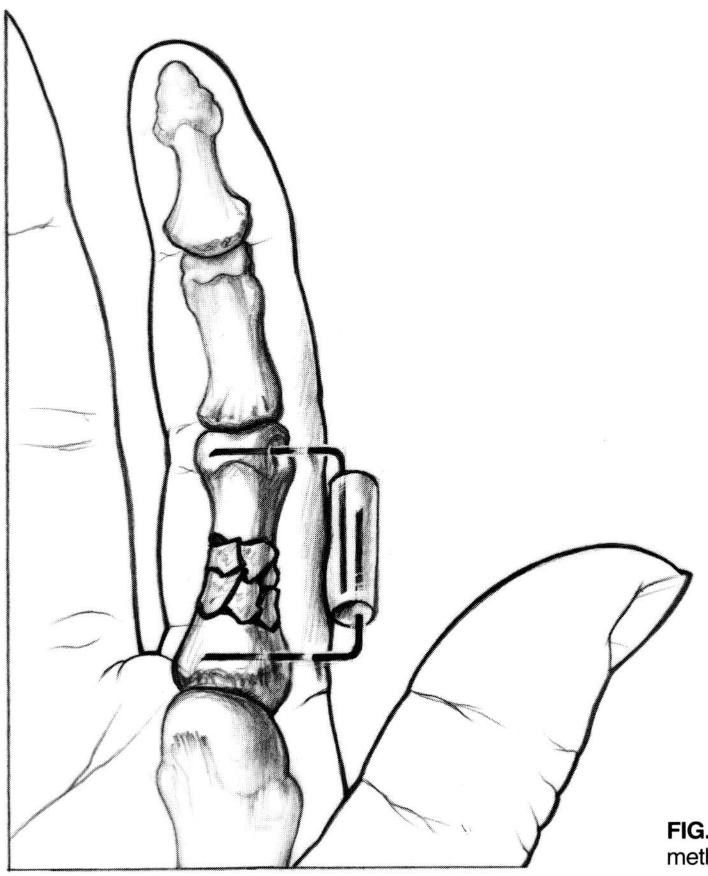

FIG. 39. Diagram of an external fixation device fashioned from methylmethacrylate.

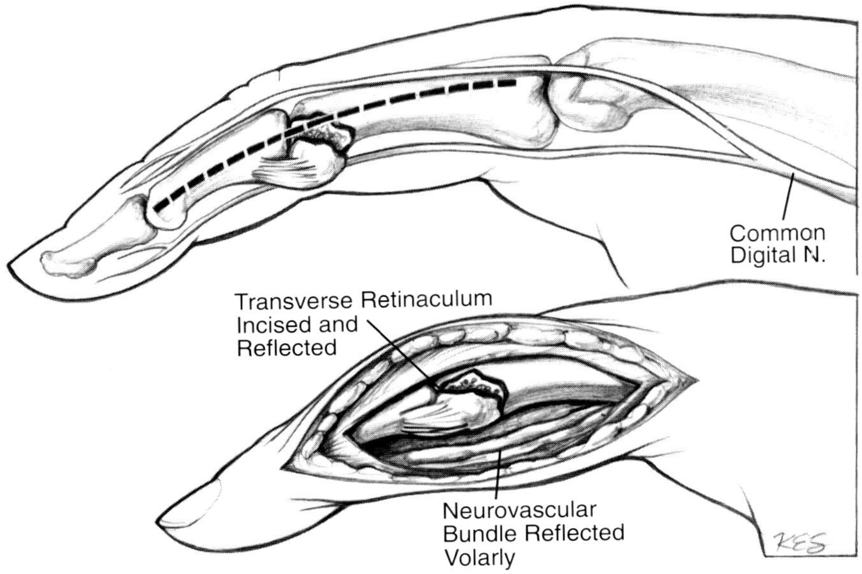

FIG. 40. Surgical approach for unicondylar fracture of PIP joint and Kirschner wires to stabilize the proximal phalanx.

verse Kirschner wires near the proximal and distal articular surfaces, bending them into an overlapping L-shaped configuration and cementing them together with methylmethacrylate (Fig. 39). This device allows some joint motion and facilitates wound care.

Condylar Fractures

Although they are uncommon, unicondylar and bicondylar (T- or Y-shaped) fractures may occur in the proximal phalanx. Nondisplaced fractures are immobilized in an extension splint. Fractures displaced more than 1 mm require closed reduction and percutaneous pin fixation or ORIF. Unicondylar fractures are approached through a mid-axial incision made between the extensor hood and the flexor tendon sheath (Fig. 40). The transverse retinaculum that stabilizes the lateral bands to the flexor tendon sheath is divided and the neurovascular bundles are reflected in a volar direction. The capsule is incised and the articular fragments are aligned and stabilized with small Kirschner wires or, occasionally, 1.5-mm screws (Figs. 41 and 42).

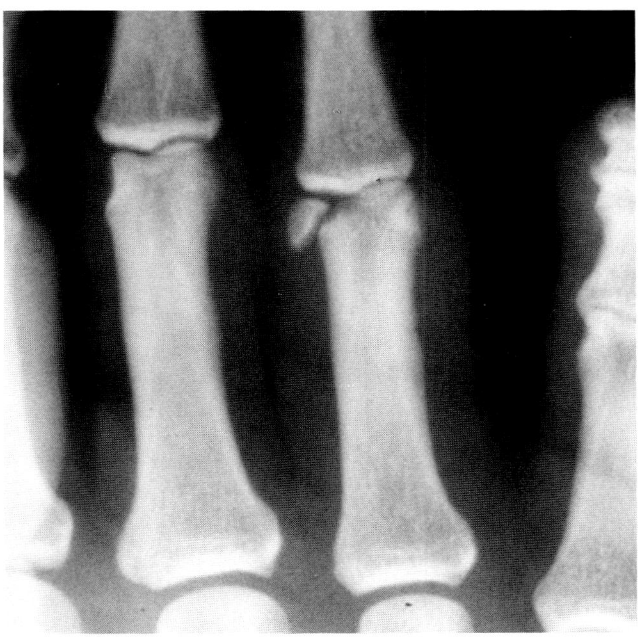

FIG. 41. Unicondylar fracture of the proximal phalanx.

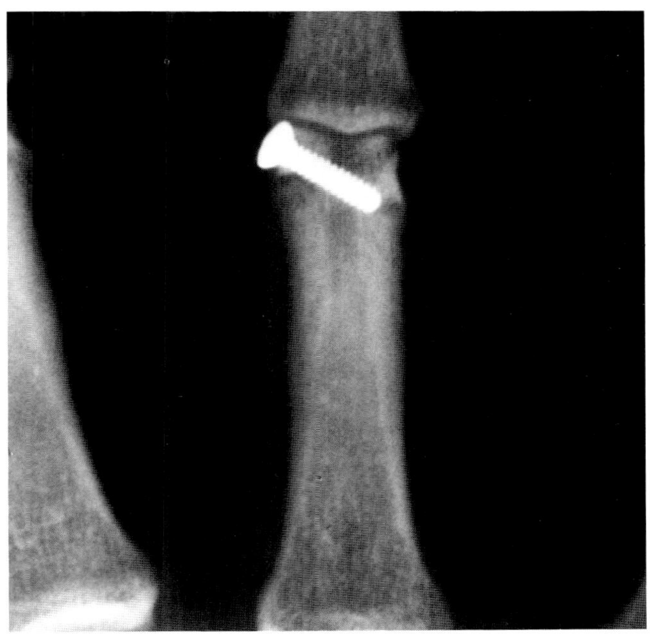

FIG. 42. Internal fixation of a unicondylar fracture of the proximal phalanx.

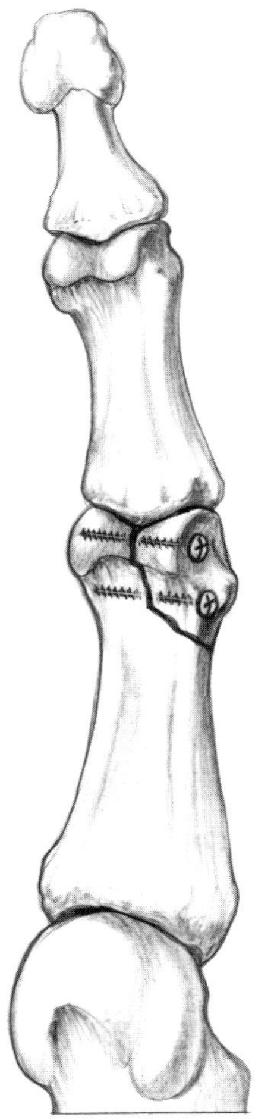

FIG. 43. Diagram of internal fixation of a bicondylar fracture of the proximal phalanx.

T- and Y-Shaped Bicondylar Fractures

In T- or Y-shaped fracture patterns, both sides of the joint are exposed through a dorsal incision made over the PIP joint. The skin flap is reflected and the joint is exposed through longitudinal incisions made on either side of the central slip, between the central slip and the lateral bands. The central slip must not be detached from the base of the middle phalanx. A congruent joint surface is restored by reducing and pinning together both condylar fragments with one or two small-diameter Kirschner wires (Fig. 43) (3). The reestablished condylar surface is then pinned to the shaft fragment with oblique Kirschner wires. The ends of the pins are cut flush with the bone and buried in the soft tissues. Active exercises in a removable protective splint are started immediately after stable fixation, with the MCP joint positioned in hyperextension.

Middle Phalangeal Fractures

Extraarticular Base Fractures

Extraarticular middle phalangeal fractures are treated the same as extraarticular proximal phalangeal fractures.

Intraarticular Base Fractures

Reduction of T- or Y-shaped fractures by traction and percutaneous pinning soon after the injury prevents scarring of the delicate extensor tendon mechanism. If the articular surface cannot be aligned by traction, the joint can be approached surgically in a manner similar to a condylar fracture of the proximal phalanx. Care is taken not to detach the central slip from its bony fragment. The articular surface is stabilized with transverse 0.028-inch Kirschner wires. Fracture alignment is confirmed by direct vision as the pins are passed percutaneously from the mid-axial region of the digits. Additional oblique wires are used to stabilize the articular surface to the shaft. The ends of the pins are cut and buried beneath the skin. Rehabilitation is similar to that for condylar fractures of the proximal phalanges.

Oblique Shaft Fractures

Displaced oblique shaft fractures require supplemental internal fixation for adequate stabilization. Within the first week after injury, the fracture frequently can be reduced by traction and stabilized with percutaneous Kirschner wires. When closed reduction is not possible, open reduction is performed through a dorsal approach. The skin flaps are elevated through a dorsal incision and the shaft of the middle phalanx is exposed through the space between the lateral bands. The central slip and the terminal extensor tendon must not be detached during this procedure (Fig. 44). In most cases, adequate stabilization is provided by .028-inch transverse Kirschner wires or 1.5-mm cortical lag screws. After internal fixation, the extensor tendon mechanism connecting the two lateral bands is repaired with closely spaced sutures without shortening the overall length of the tendon. Early active range-of-motion exercises are started several days after surgery, using a removable volar splint. A small aluminum splint is used to prevent extensor lag at the DIP joint, while allowing PIP joint rotation.

Transverse Shaft Fractures

Transverse shaft fractures in the middle phalanges are treated similar to oblique fractures, except that the preferred fixation in this case consists of crossed Kirschner wires or a plate and 1.5-mm screws.

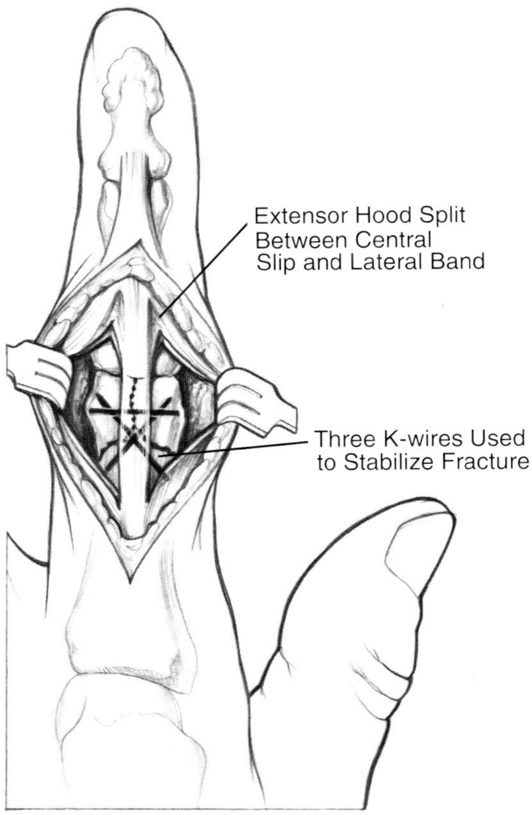

FIG. 44. Diagram of internal fixation of a bicondylar fracture of the middle phalanx.

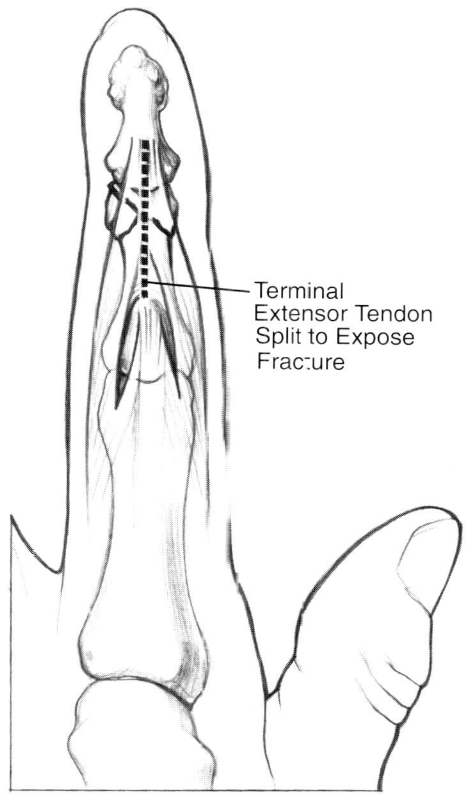

FIG. 45. Surgical exposure of middle phalanx condylar fracture via an extensor tendon splitting approach.

Comminuted Shaft Fractures

The guidelines for treating comminuted middle phalangeal shaft fractures are the same as those for comminuted proximal phalangeal fractures.

Condylar Fractures

Condylar fractures in the middle phalanges are treated the same as condylar fractures in the proximal phalanges, except that the terminal extensor tendon is split down the middle to expose the fracture (Fig. 45). Active PIP exercises are encouraged with the DIP joint splinted in extension.

COMPLICATIONS

Extensive soft-tissue injury can limit digital motion. The extensor tendon is very susceptible to the formation of adhesions after a proximal phalangeal fracture, and secondary surgery for tenolysis of extensor or flexor tendons is often necessary after these injuries. Reflex sympathetic dystrophy can occur after a crushing injury. The risk of pin-tract infections is minimized when the ends of the pins are buried in soft tissues. Loss of fixation may be a problem in noncompliant patients. These fractures are immobilized in cast until the fracture heals and a secondary capsulotomy with tenolysis is performed later to restore motion.

SKELETALLY IMMATURE PATIENTS

Salter-II fractures of the base of the proximal phalanx are common in children. Unlike proximal phalangeal fractures in adults, many of these fractures can be stabilized by closed reduction. Fractures that occur just proximal to the condyles are uncommon but when they do occur they require percutaneous pinning because the deforming force of the flexor tendon can overpower the limited stability provided by splinting. Middle phalangeal fractures are rare in pediatric patients, but when they occur they are usually minimally displaced.

REFERENCES

1. Clinkscales GS. Complications in the management of fractures in hand injuries. *South Med J* 1970;63:704–707.
2. Widgerow AD, Edinburg M, Biddulph SL. An analysis of proximal phalangeal fractures. *J Hand Surg* 1987;12A:134–139.
3. Belsky MR, Eaton RG, Lane LB. Closed reduction and internal fixation of proximal phalangeal fractures. *J Hand Surg* 1984;9A:725–729.
4. Viegas SF, Ferren EL, Self J, et al. Comparative mechanical properties of various Kirschner wire configuration in transverse and oblique phalangeal fractures. *J Hand Surg* 1988;13A:246–253.

Distal Phalangeal Fractures

MECHANISMS OF INJURY

Most distal phalangeal fractures are caused by crushing injuries and include associated comminution of the distal tuft or shaft. Open fractures are common, even in seemingly mild injuries. Two injuries, avulsion fractures and mallet deformities, are associated with injury to the tendinous insertions. Avulsion of the flexor digitorum profundus usually occurs in the ring and middle fingers when a flexed digit is forcefully hyperextended, for example, when a finger is caught in a football jersey during a tackle. A mallet injury occurs in an extended digit when the extensor tendon insertion is avulsed by forced flexion.

ANATOMIC CONSIDERATIONS

The volar plate and the flexor digitorum profundus insert onto the volar base of the distal phalanx, whereas the terminal portion of the extensor tendon attaches onto the dorsal surface. The extremely thin skin on the dorsum of the finger makes surgical approaches in that area susceptible to wound-healing problems. Fibrous septa attach from the skin surface to the distal phalanx on the volar side of the finger. Hypersensitivity of scars on the fingertip is common from arborization of digital nerves in this area.

CLASSIFICATION

Distal phalangeal fractures are described by fracture type and location (Table 5).

Table 5. *Distal phalangeal fractures*

Avulsion fractures from the base of the distal phalanx
Avulsions of the flexor digitorum profundus insertion
Avulsions of the extensor tendon insertion
Shaft Fractures
Closed
Open
Tuft Fractures

ASSESSMENT

Physical Examination

An open fracture is not always evident when the nail fold is disrupted, particularly when the fracture has been reduced emergently in the field (Fig. 46). Undiagnosed open fractures can lead to deep infections with related osteomyelitis and nail bed deformities. A neurovascular examination is performed and painful subungual hematomas are drained. When a hematoma involves more than 50% of the nail, the nail should be removed to inspect and repair any nail-bed lacerations.

Active DIP flexion is lost after avulsion of the flexor digitorum profundus tendon. Even a partially amputated digit can demonstrate some active movement under a digital nerve block when this tendon is intact. When the ability to flex the DIP is absent, the finger should be palpated for tenderness in case the tendon was avulsed and had retracted into the sheath or the palm.

Radiographic Evaluation

Distal phalangeal fractures are evaluated from standard AP, lateral, and oblique radiographs. A postreduction radiograph of the entire digit should be obtained.

Special Studies

No special studies are required.

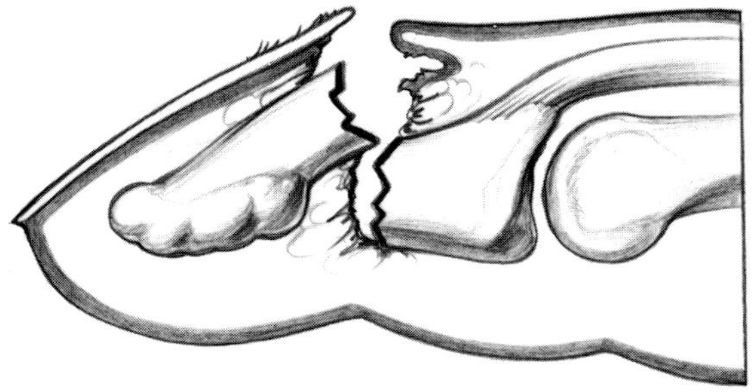

FIG. 46. Open fracture of the distal phalanx.

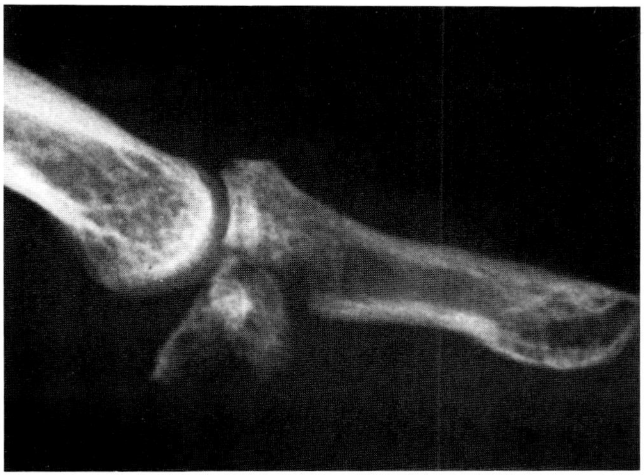

FIG. 47. Radiograph of the profundus tendon avulsion from the distal phalanx.

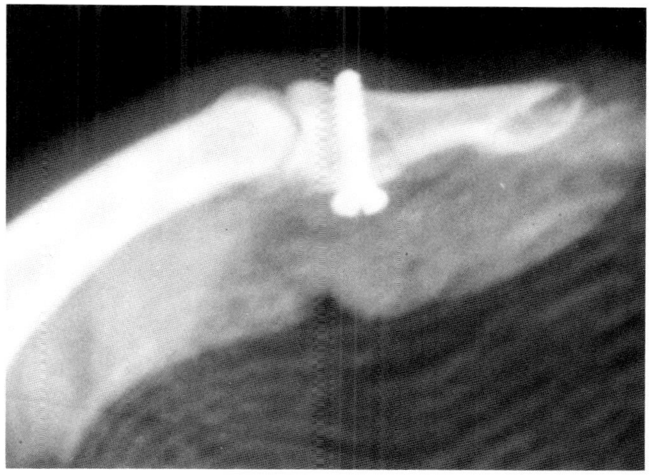

FIG. 49. Internal fixation of a distal phalangeal avulsion fracture.

EMERGENT MANAGEMENT

Open wounds are debrided to prevent infection. Subungual hematomas are drained by spinning the tip of a #11 blade on the nail and carefully boring several holes into the nail. The finger is immobilized in a splint that does not include the PIP joint.

DEFINITIVE MANAGEMENT

Avulsion Fractures

Avulsions of the profundus tendon frequently include fragments of the volar articular surface and extend into the intraarticular surface of the distal phalanx (Fig. 47) (1). The earliest possible repair usually provides the best functional results. Repair of a tendon that has retracted into the palm must be done within 10 days of injury (2). In contrast, repair of an avulsed tendon that has not retracted into the palm can be performed as late as 6 weeks after injury. However, a fracture fragment is not always present to predict the level of retraction, and early repair is indicated in all cases (3).

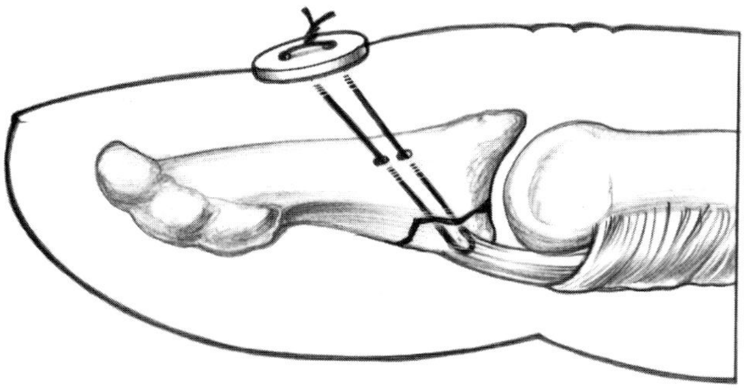

FIG. 48. Repair with a pull-out button.

The operative approach is made through a Bruner zig-zag incision centered over the distal phalanx. This incision can be enlarged proximally as far as necessary to identify the proximal extent of the flexor tendon. The site of avulsion is usually seen within the tendon sheath as an area of hemorrhage. The flexor tendon sheath is incised at the retraction site of the profundus tendon. A suture is placed into the tendon and passed to the distal end of the sheath to advance the tendon distally. A hole is drilled through the distal phalanx and a suture is passed with a Keefe needle to the dorsum of the finger and secured there with a pull-out suture tied over a button (Fig. 48). In large avulsed fragments, a Kirschner wire or a screw is added for extra stability before tying the tendon suture over the button (Fig. 49).

Shaft Fractures

A closed shaft fracture is usually reduced and immobilized in a splint. When swelling precludes application of a splint, immobilization is accomplished by a Kirschner wire placed percutaneously through the fingertip. Accurate positioning must be maintained and angulation must be avoided (Figs. 50 and 51). Displaced open fractures (apex dorsal) are reduced by retracting the nail fold and extending the distal fragment, a maneuver similar to closing a shotgun. Stabilization is provided by a Kirschner wire inserted in a retrograde fashion—first through the distal phalanx before reduction and then across the DIP joint after reduction.

Tuft Fractures

Tuft fractures are treated by draining the subungual hematomas and applying a splint for comfort.

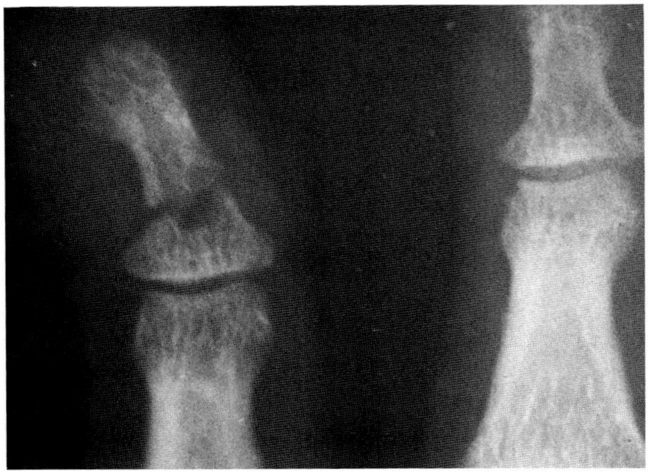

FIG. 50. Unstable distal phalangeal shaft fracture.

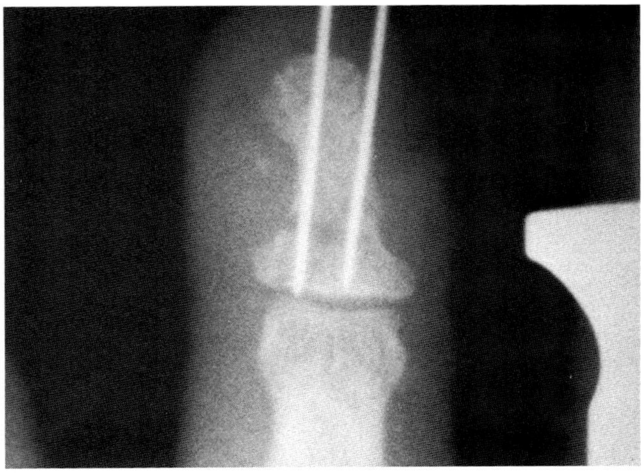

FIG. 51. Internal fixation of an unstable distal phalangeal shaft fracture.

COMPLICATIONS

Late infections can occur in open fracture–dislocations if debridement is not performed at the time of reduction. Some shaft fractures are very unstable and inadequate treatment can lead to unusual and painful deformities. Untreated nail bed lacerations result in nail bed deformities with grooved or split nails.

SKELETALLY IMMATURE PATIENTS

Displaced open fractures may occur in children as Salter-II fracture–dislocations at the base of the distal phalanx. Fractures in children are usually stable and are managed by splinting after irrigation and debridement. Incomplete ossification may complicate the diagnosis of avulsion fractures in children, which require ORIF to reestablish normal growth and tendon function.

REFERENCES

1. Smith JH. Avulsion of a profundus tendon wtih simultaneous intraarticular fracture of the distal phalanx. Case report. *J Hand Surg* 1981;6:600–601.
2. Leddy JP, Parker JW. Avulsion of the profundus insertion in athletes. *J Hand Surg* 1977;2:66–68.
3. Trumble T, Vedder NB, Benirsche SK. Misleading fractures following profundus tendon avulsions. *J Hand Surg (In press).*

Proximal Interphalangeal Joint Subluxations and Dislocations

MECHANISM OF INJURY

Proximal interphalangeal (PIP) joint dislocations include a wide spectrum of injuries. Hyperextension of the PIP joint produces injuries ranging from partial tears of the volar plate to complex dorsal dislocations; hyperflexion injuries range from partial or complete disruptions of the central slip to volar dislocations. Injuries from lateral ulnar or radial deviation usually occur with the digit extended and result in damage to the collateral ligaments. Most torsional injuries affect two adjacent structures, e.g., the volar plate and the collateral ligament, or the central slip and the collateral ligament.

ANATOMIC CONSIDERATIONS

The soft-tissue structures surrounding the PIP joint are vulnerable to injury. Deeper structures, which include the volar plate, both collateral ligaments, and their accessory collateral ligaments form a strong structure, analogous to three sides of a box, that supports the volar and lateral aspects of the PIP joint. Dorsally, the central slip controls joint extension. At the PIP level, the lateral bands cross the joint slightly dorsal to the central axis and merge with the triangular ligament to form the terminal branch of the extensor tendon. Unlike the MCP joint, which is susceptible to extension contractures, the PIP joint is vulnerable to flexion contractures because the volar plate glides like a piece of armor into the recess of the neck of the proximal phalanx during PIP joint flexion (see Fig. 33). Adhesions can form between the volar plate and the proximal phalanx if the joint is immobilized in flexion.

CLASSIFICATION

Proximal interphalangeal subluxations and dislocations are classified by description and by the mechanism of injury (Table 6).

ASSESSMENT

Physical Examination

Flexion injuries can be differentiated from extension injuries by the mechanism of injury. However, patients with PIP injuries typically do not recall how they were injured. When the history of injury is unavailable, point tenderness is used to reveal the area of maximal pathology.

In the absence of dislocation, a central slip injury must be ruled out by one of three diagnostic findings: (i) the absence of active extension of the PIP joint from a position of 90° of flexion under a digital nerve block (inability of the middle phalanx to provide resistance against the examiner's finger correlates with a central slip injury); (ii) loss of the tenodesis effect (the PIP joint should straighten to within 15° of neutral when the joint is blocked into full MCP flexion); and (iii) the absence of active DIP joint flexion with the PIP joint fully extended (this maneuver is not possible when the central slip has been disrupted and the lateral bands have been retracted proximally).

Table 6. *Classification of PIP subluxations and dislocations*

- Dorsal subluxations and dislocations
  - Hyperextension injuries of the volar plate without dislocation
  - Simple dislocations with volar plate disruption but with the articular surface maintaining contact
  - Complex dislocations with overriding articular surfaces and a bayonet deformity
- Volar subluxations and dislocations
  - Avulsions of the central slip
    - Without fracture
    - With a displaced or nondisplaced fracture
  - Volar dislocations
- Collateral ligament injuries
  - Without an avulsion fracture
  - With an avulsion fracture
    - Less than 25% articular surface involvement
    - More than 25% articular surface involvement

Radiographic Evaluation

Standard AP, lateral, and oblique radiographs are obtained for PIP joint injuries. Reduction and traction radiographs provide additional information.

Special Studies

Tomograms can be obtained to confirm the presence of a depressed fracture fragment at the base of the middle phalanx.

EMERGENT MANAGEMENT

Injuries to the PIP joint require immediate irrigation and debridement. Because an open injury might be a partial amputation, a complete neurovascular examination must be conducted.

DEFINITIVE MANAGEMENT

Dorsal Subluxations and Dislocations

Hyperextension Injuries

Hyperextension injuries of the volar plate without dislocations are managed by buddy-taping the injured finger to an adjacent digit for 3 weeks if it is stable with active and passive motion. When the finger is stable with active motion but not with passive motion, a hand-based dorsal block splint preventing the last 30° of extension is applied. Motion is begun early to prevent loss of finger flexion.

Simple Dislocations

Simple dislocations without fracture can be managed by closed reduction and a dorsal block splint for 3 weeks. The same treatment is used for simple dislocations with fracture unless more than 25% of the articular surface is involved. The fracture is exposed through a palmar approach using a Bruner zig-zag incision centered over the PIP joint. The skin flaps are elevated and the neurovascular bundles are identified. The flexor tendons are exposed and retracted through an incision made at the level of the C1 and A3 pulleys (Fig. 52A). The presence of an avulsed fragment is revealed as an area of hemorrhage after the volar plate is exposed. A pull-out suture is inserted into the distal end of the volar plate and attached to the base of the middle phalanx. The suture is brought out through the dorsal aspect of the finger and tied to a pull-out button (Fig. 52B). Occasionally a 1.5-mm screw is used to stabilize the fracture. Rehabilitation is the same as for a fracture treated by closed reduction.

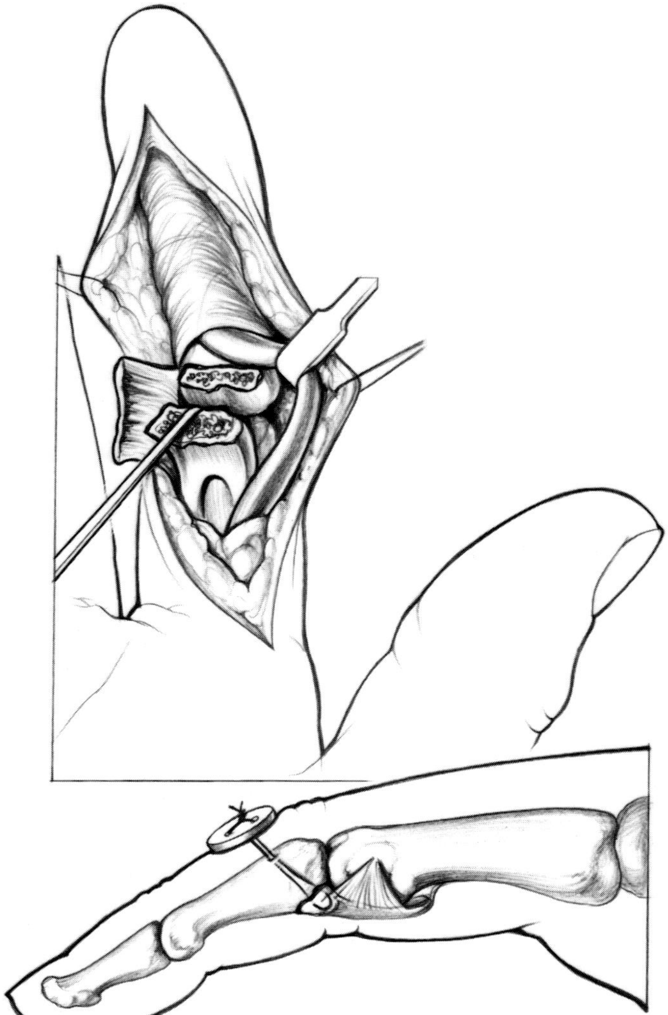

A

B

FIG. 52. A: Surgical approach for an unstable rupture of the volar plate. **B:** Repair of a volar plate avulsion fracture.

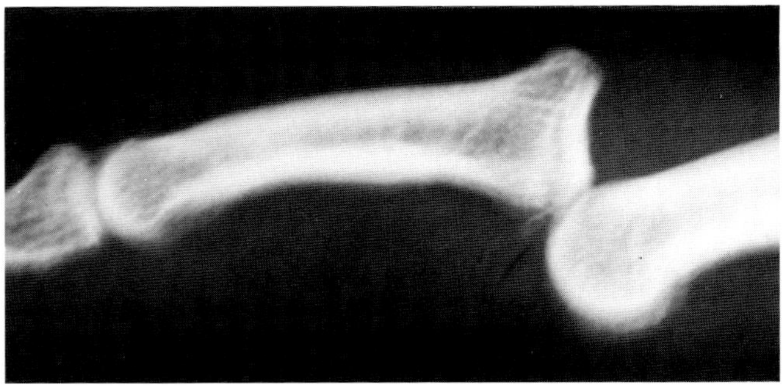

FIG. 53. Lateral radiograph of a complex PIP joint dislocation.

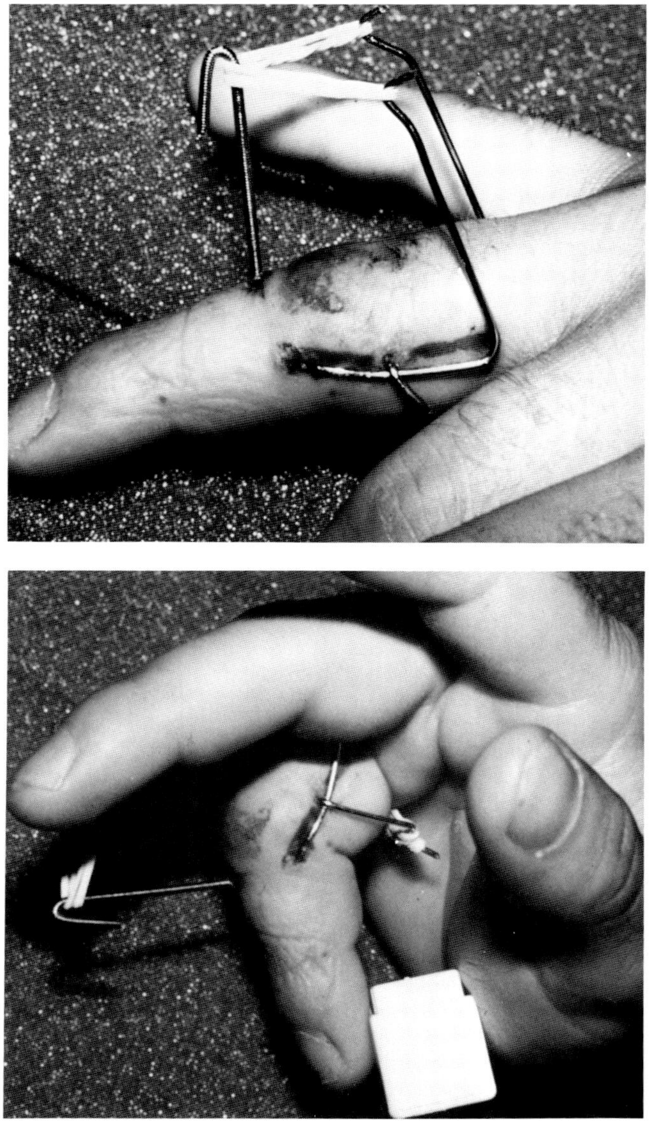

A

B

FIG. 54. A: An Agee dynamic extension splint reduces an unstable PIP joint after a dorsal dislocation. **B:** Early flexion exercises are allowed in the splint.

Complex Dislocations

A proximal condyle entrapped between the volar plate and the flexor tendon sheath can usually be released by closed methods but occasionally requires open reduction following complex dislocations (Fig. 53). A dorsal incision is made, the skin flaps are elevated, and the joint is exposed through an incision made between the central slip and the lateral bands, similar to the procedure for bicondylar fractures of the proximal phalanx. The volar plate is displaced and the joint is reduced. After reduction, the stability of the joint is assessed to determine the type of splinting that is required. If the joint is stable to active range of motion, a dorsal block splint is used.

Open repair is necessary when the joint is unstable to active range of motion or when more than 25% of the articular surface is disrupted (1,2). The technique used in this situation is the same as that described for hyperextension injuries. When the fracture is extremely comminuted, the fragments are excised and the volar plate is sutured to the

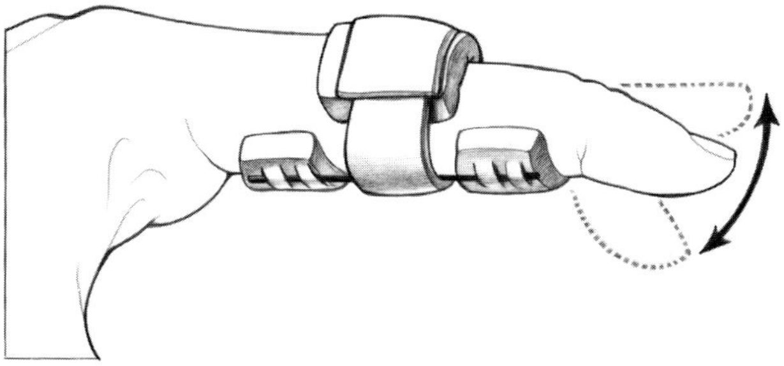

FIG. 55. A closed central slip injury treated with a Bunnell splint.

remaining portion of the middle phalanx (see Fig. 52B). This technique produces an obligatory flexion contracture. If the injury is first seen several days after it has occurred, immediate surgery is contraindicated by swelling and the joint is treated in an Agee dynamic-extension splint (Fig. 54) (3).

Volar Subluxations and Dislocations

Avulsions of the Central Slip Without Fracture

A central slip injury without dislocation is immobilized in a safety-pin or Bunnell splint with the PIP joint extended for 5 to 6 weeks. Active DIP joint flexion exercises are begun immediately to draw the lateral bands distally and to prevent proximal migration of the central slip (Fig. 55). Active flexion exercises with dynamic extension are begun in a Capener splint after 6 weeks (Fig. 56). Night splinting is continued for an additional 6 weeks to prevent formation of a late boutonniere deformity.

Avulsions of the Central Slip with Fracture

Avulsion fractures displaced less than 1 mm are treated like avulsions without fracture; those displaced more than 1 mm

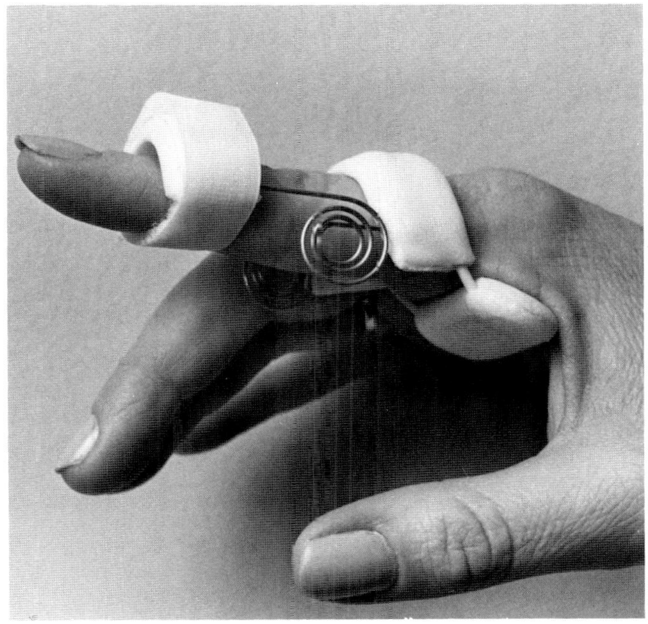

FIG. 56. A Capener splint is used to prevent extensor lag during mobilization of a central slip injury.

require surgical stabilization (Fig. 57). The surgical approach is made through a curvilinear incision on the dorsal aspect of the PIP joint. The skin flaps are elevated and the avulsed portion of the central slip is identified. Large bony fragments are fixed with screws to avoid tethering the extensor tendon with sutures or Kirschner wires (see Fig. 57B). Small fragments can be stabilized by a tension-band suture technique.

Volar Dislocations

Dislocations without fracture are rare. Closed reduction is accomplished by flexion of the CMP and PIP joints to

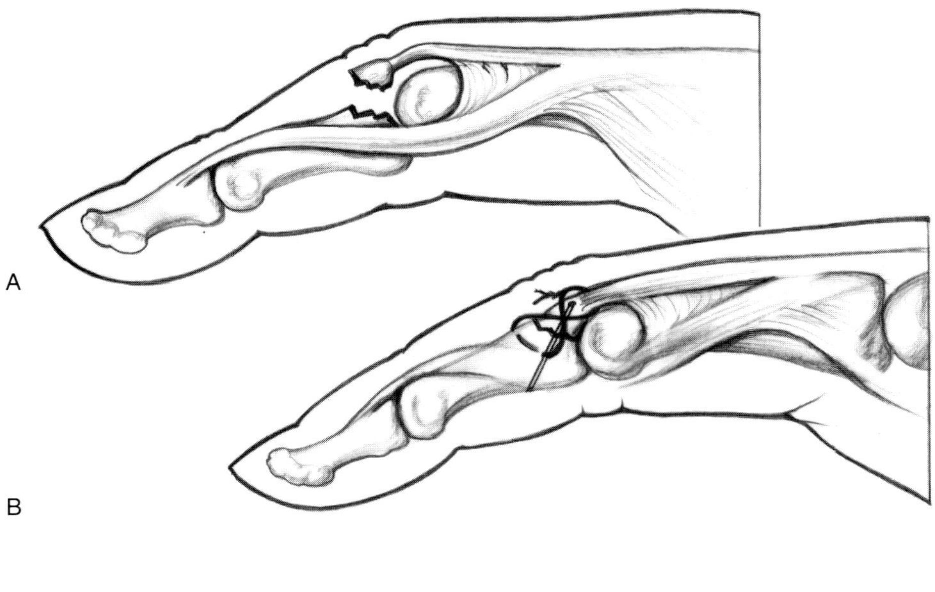

FIG. 57. **A:** Avulsion of a central slip attachment to the middle phalanx. **B:** Repair of a central slip avulsion fracture

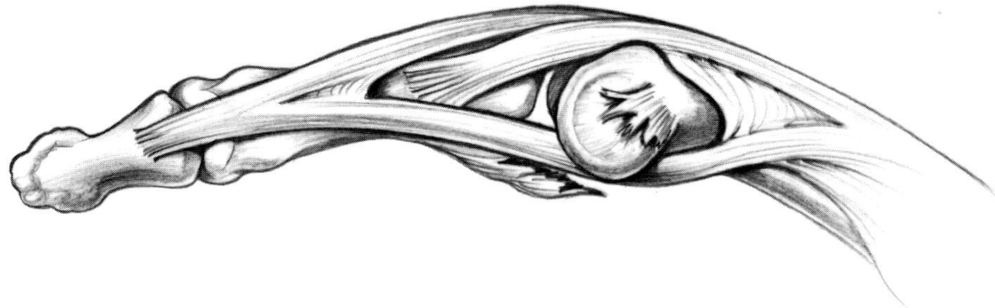

FIG. 58. Illustration of a volar PIP dislocation. (Adapted from Peimer CA, Sullivan DJ, Wild DR. Palmar dislocation of the proximal interphalangeal joint. *J Hand Surg* 1984; 9A: 39–40. Used with permission.)

decrease tension in the lateral bands and by extension and derotation of the middle phalanx. However, a condyle entrapped between the central slip and the lateral bands (Fig. 58) may be freed by using a dorsal approach similar to the technique described for condylar fractures of the proximal phalanx (4,5). The continuity of the central slip is confirmed after reduction and, if it is injured, is repaired in the same manner as a volar subluxation (Figs. 59 and 60).

Collateral Ligament Injuries

Ligamentous Injuries Without Avulsion Fractures

Buddy-taping is usually sufficient treatment for ligamentous injuries without fractures in the middle and ring fingers, even when the PIP joint is unstable with gentle radial or ulnar deviational stresses. Operative repair is indicated when the radial collateral ligament of the index finger is unstable with gentle passive stresses or active motion. The transverse retinaculum is divided through a mid-axial incision and the lateral bands are reflected dorsally, taking care to protect the neurovascular bundles on the volar side. The collateral ligament is repaired with a pull-out suture that is brought out of the opposite side of the middle phalanx and tied over a pull-out button (Fig. 61). Postoperatively, the finger is treated by buddy-taping and early active motion.

Ligamentous Injuries With Avulsion Fractures

Avulsion fractures involving less than 25% of the joint surface are treated the same as ligamentous injuries without fracture. Fractures involving more than 25% of the articular surface warrant internal fixation even when the joint is stable to lateral stress. The operative approach used is the same as that for unstable collateral ligament injuries, but in this case a Kirschner wire is inserted as supplemental fixation to the pull-out button to correct rotation. A screw can be used to stabilize large uncomminuted fracture fragments.

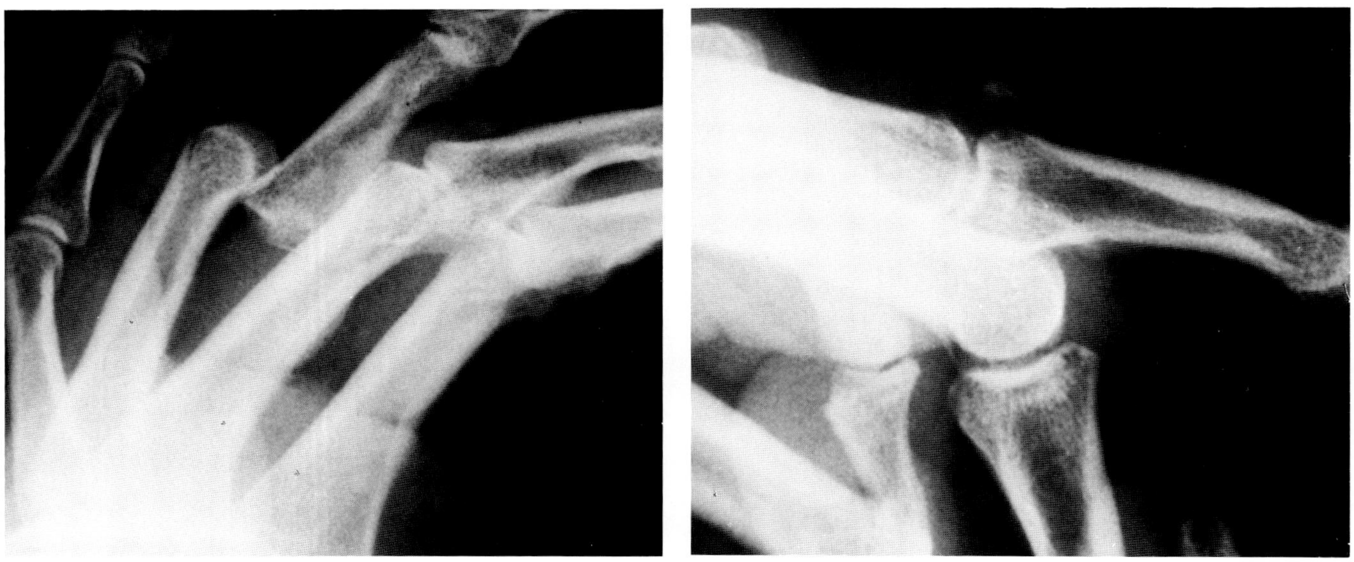

A B

FIG. 59. **A:** Radiograph of a volar subluxation with an avulsion fracture of the central slip. **B:** Despite closed reduction of the volar PIP joint dislocation, the fragment containing the central slip is still displaced.

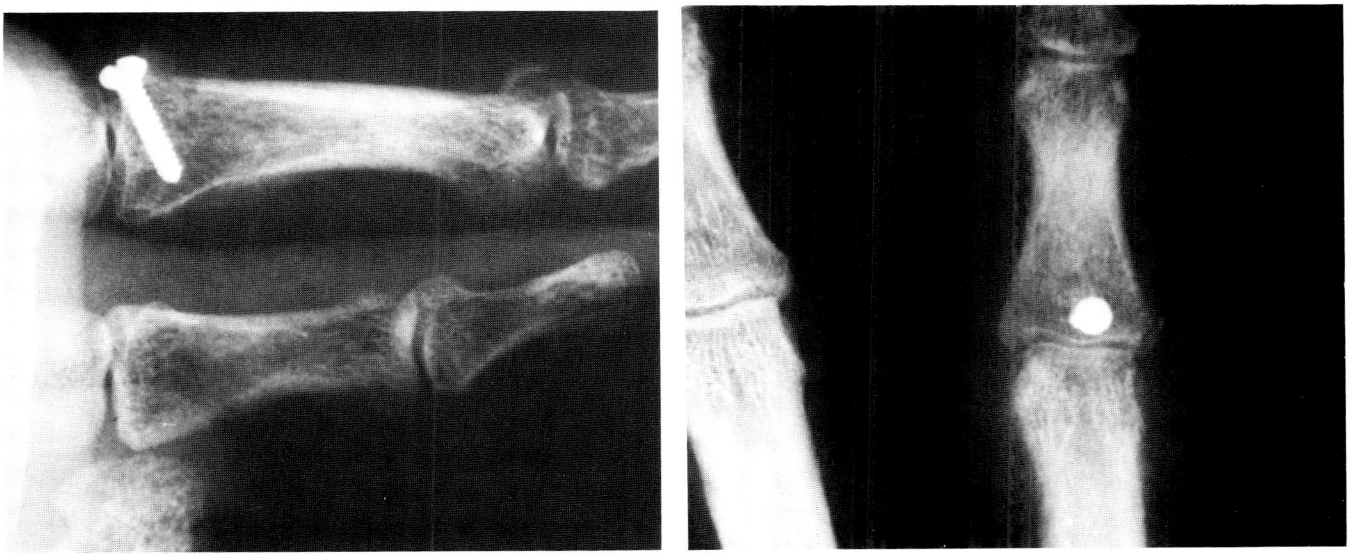

FIG. 60. Lateral (**A**) and anteroposterior (**B**) radiographs of a reduced volar subluxation and internally fixed avulsion fracture.

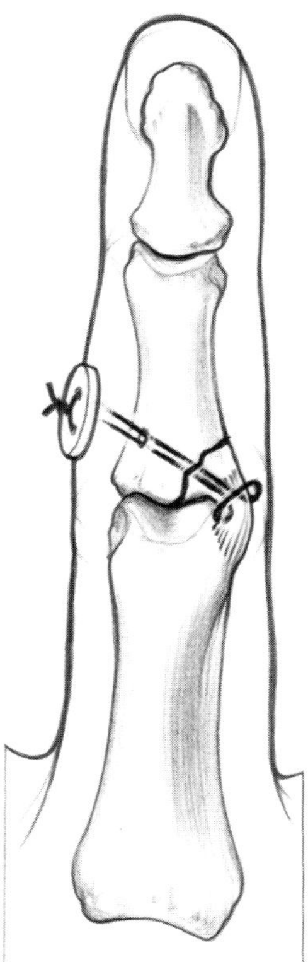

FIG. 61. Repair of a collateral ligament injury and an avulsion fracture using a pull-out button.

COMPLICATIONS

Loss of as little as 10° to 20° of PIP motion results in diminished hand function. Hyperextension injuries that are splinted for too long in extension lead to loss of finger flexion, and those immobilized in flexion for a prolonged period of time lead to flexion contractures. A late boutonniere deformity with volar subluxation of the lateral bands is a consequence of an unrecognized injury to the central slip that was treated in a Bunnell splint.

SKELETALLY IMMATURE PATIENTS

Although dislocations in this joint are rare in children, thorough radiographic evaluations should be done to rule out displaced Salter II or III fracture–dislocations, which require closed or open reduction and percutaneous pinning or open reduction to reestablish proper skeletal alignment and the orientation of the physis.

REFERENCES

1. Lee MLH. Intra-articular and peri-articular fractures of the phalanges. *J Bone Joint Surg* 1963;45B:103–109.
2. Wilson JN, Rowland SA. Fracture–dislocation of the proximal interphalangeal joint of the finger. Treatment by open reduction and internal fixation. *J Bone Joint Surg* 1966;48A:493–502.
3. Agee JM. Unstable fracture dislocations of the proximal interphalangeal joint of the fingers: a preliminary report of a new treatment technique. *J Hand Surg* 1978;3:386–389.
4. Murakami Y. Irreducible volar dislocation of the proximal interphalangeal joint of the finger. *Hand* 1974;6:87–90.
5. Peimer CA, Sullivan DJ, Wild DR. Palmar dislocation of the proximal interphalangeal joint. *J Hand Surg* 1984; 9A: 39–40.

Distal Interphalangeal Joint Subluxations and Dislocations

MECHANISM OF INJURY

The most common mechanisms of distal interphalangeal (DIP) joint injuries are usually volar subluxation and flexion. These injuries commonly occur in sports such as softball and basketball when an object strikes an outstretched finger and forces the DIP joint into flexion. The resulting injury avulses the terminal insertion of the extensor tendon from the dorsum of the distal phalanx and produces a mallet-finger deformity. Rarely, a dorsal dislocation can occur in association with an open injury and an incomplete amputation.

ANATOMIC CONSIDERATIONS

Anatomic considerations for the DIP joint are similar to those described for distal phalangeal fractures.

CLASSIFICATION

The classification of DIP injuries attempts to separate soft-tissue injuries from those with articular surface involvement (Table 7).

ASSESSMENT

Physical Examination

Typical symptoms of a DIP injury include swelling of the fingertip and sagging of the DIP joint into flexion. The joint cannot be extended actively to a neutral position and sometimes cannot be extended passively because of excessive swelling.

Radiographic Evaluation

The standard radiographic views used to diagnose PIP injuries are also required for DIP injuries.

Table 7. *Classification of DIP injuries*

Rupture of the terminal extensor tendon without an avulsion fracture
Disruption of the terminal extensor tendon with an avulsion fracture
Without joint subluxation
With joint subluxation

Special Studies

Tomography is useful in special circumstances.

EMERGENT MANAGEMENT

The DIP joint is splinted to avoid further fracture displacement. The splint should not block motion at the PIP joint.

DEFINITIVE MANAGEMENT

Extensor Tendon Rupture Without Avulsion Fracture

Fractures involving less than 40% of the articular surface and those without volar subluxation are immobilized in a neutral position in a dorsal splint (Fig. 62). The skin on the dorsal side of the finger must be monitored during joint extension to avoid hyperextension and blanching, which can lead to skin necrosis. Excessive swelling may prevent full extension of the DIP joint for up to a week. The splint should not immoblize the PIP joint (Fig. 63).

Extensor Tendon Rupture with Avulsion Fracture

Fractures with displaced fragments involving more than 40% of the articular surface usually involve the insertion of the collateral ligaments and cause volar subluxation of the DIP joint (1). These injuries require operative repair. The joint is approached through an H-incision on the dorsum of the finger (Fig. 64). Severely comminuted fractures are repaired with a tension-band wiring technique that is supplemented with a retrograde Kirschner wire (Fig. 65). Exercises

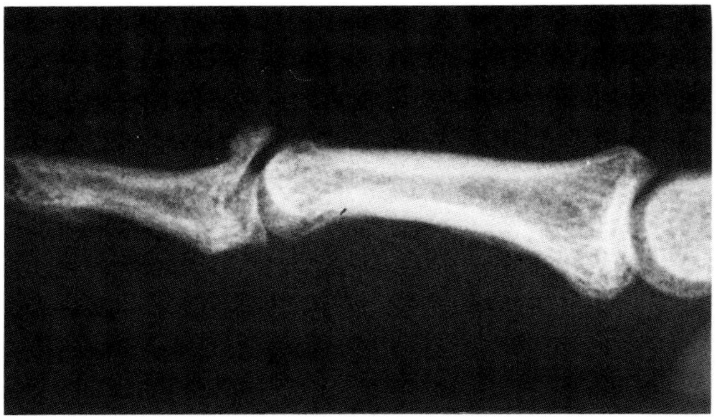

FIG. 62. Mallet finger with an avulsed terminal extensor tendon.

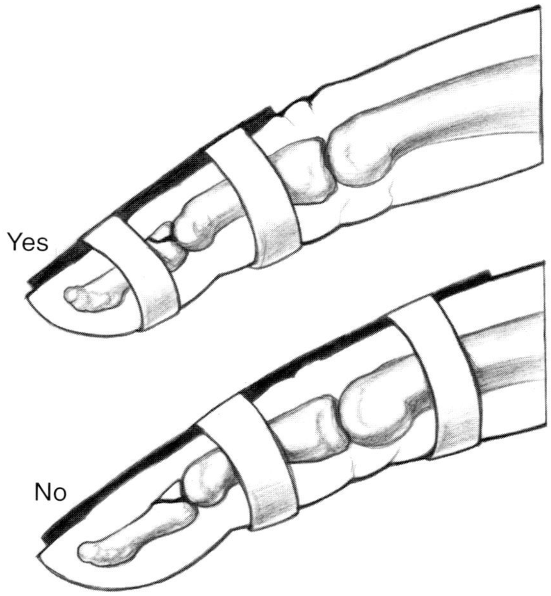

FIG. 63. Immobilization of a mallet finger should not block PIP joint flexion.

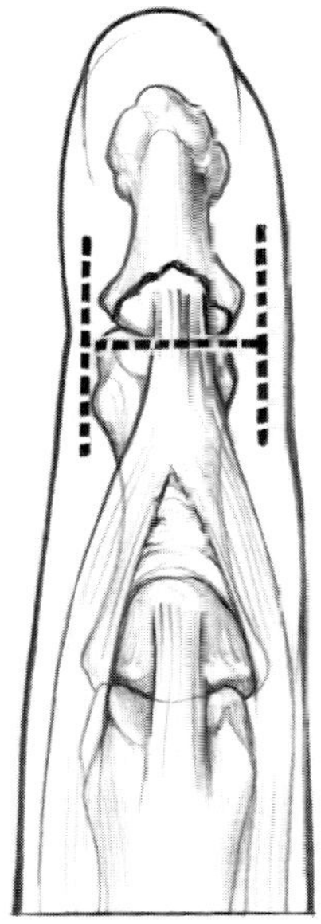

FIG. 64. Exposure of an avulsion fracture in a subluxated mallet finger.

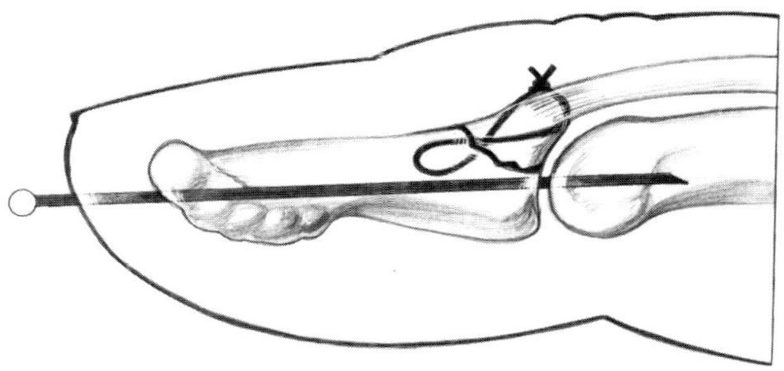

FIG. 65. Repair of an avulsion fracture in a subluxated mallet finger.

to mobilize the PIP joint are begun early with the DIP joint splinted in extension. Splinting is continued for 2 weeks and the Kirschner wire is left in place for 6 weeks. Splinting the finger at night is advisable for an additional month. In patients with ligamentous laxity, the mallet-finger deformity allows volar subluxation of the lateral bands, producing a swan-neck deformity. In addition to a DIP joint splint, a dorsal-block splint is applied to prevent the last 30° of extension in the PIP joint for 3 weeks. This deformity usually corrects itself once the DIP joint returns to a neutral position.

COMPLICATIONS

Complications can arise from incorrect splinting of a mallet-finger deformity. Inadequate splinting that does not correct the flexion attitude produces a permanent mallet deformity. Excessive splinting that restrains motion in the PIP joint can cause loss of motion in this joint.

SKELETALLY IMMATURE PATIENTS

Open Salter-II fractures of the DIP joint are usually associated with mallet-finger deformities. Inadequate visualization and debridement at the time of reduction can result in deep infections. Salter-III and -IV fracture–dislocations of the DIP joint can occur and usually require open reduction.

REFERENCE

1. Stark E, Gainor BJ, Ashworth CR. Operative treatment of intra-articular fractures of the dorsal aspect of the distal phalanx of digits. *J Bone Joint Surg* 1987; 69A: 892–96.

Orthopaedic Trauma Protocols, edited by
Sigvard T. Hansen, Jr., and Marc F. Swiontkowski,
Raven Press, Ltd., New York, © 1993.

CHAPTER 17

Soft-Tissue Injuries in the Upper Extremity

Marc F. Swiontkowski

BRACHIAL PLEXUS INJURIES

Brachial plexus injuries usually result from application of force distal to the shoulder, with resultant deviation of the neck in the direction opposite the force. Motorcyclists or unrestrained passengers in motor vehicles are most commonly injured by this mechanism. Associated injuries include scapular, clavicular, and proximal humeral fractures, chest injuries, and scapulothoracic dissociations. The most common mechanisms injure the plexus at the level of C-5 or C-6 rather than distally, and frequently compromise shoulder girdle function.

The brachial plexus is a network of cervical nerve roots from C-5 to T-1, which forms the major cords of the plexus proximal to the clavicle. Brachial plexus palsies are classified according to the involved nerve roots and cords. Because the exits of the nerve roots are fixed in the spinal cord and the insertions of the peripheral nerves are relatively fixed in the muscle bellies, excursion of the plexus from stretching is limited.

Careful assessment of the motor and sensory function during the initial evaluation of an upper extremity injury reveals any abnormalities consistent with a brachial plexus injury. Crepitus over the clavicle, multiple rib fractures (with or without a pneumothorax), or swelling around the scapula suggestive of a scapulothoracic dissociation are all consistent with injury to the brachial plexus caused by one of the mechanisms described earlier. The radial pulse must be carefully assessed and the upper extremities must be evaluated by a Doppler examination.

Radiographs and other diagnostic studies are obtained to define the brachial plexus injury and to diagnose associated injuries. The admitting AP chest radiograph must be scrutinized for rib fractures and clavicular fractures. Similarly, the radiograph of the lateral cervical spine should be carefully screened for a possible associated fracture of the cervical spine. If a patient complains of tenderness to palpation around the neck, a spinal radiographic series should be done. Anteroposterior and lateral radiographs of the scapula or the upper humerus should be obtained as dictated by the clinical examination. Arteriography is indicated when abnormal blood flow is identified on a Doppler examination. When a scapulothoracic dissociation has been identified, injury to an axillary artery should be suspected. Cervical myelography is indicated in brachial plexus injuries to determine the location of the injury.The decision to explore the plexus is made in part from the results of a myelogram.. Root injuries which are identified on the myelogram, have no potential for recovery. A histamine test is useful to determine whether the plexus disruption is pre- or postganglionic. The triple response of Lewis (blanch, wheal, flare) within the dermatome in the early phase of treatment signifies a preganglionic injury and a poor prognosis. Early management of axillary arterial injuries and associated open fractures is essential for a good prognosis.

The definitive management of a brachial plexus injury depends on the type of injury and its location. Root avulsions at the level of the cord are associated with a poor prognosis and are managed by early reconstruction. If an injury does not significantly involve the nerve roots between C-7 and T-1, shoulder arthrodesis may be considered along with a procedure to restore elbow flexion, such as a Steindler flexoplasty or a latissimus dorsi or pectoralis major transfer. If the lesion is located at the level of the plexus cord, the plexus should be explored and the injured segment should be repaired by microsurgical techniques using cable grafting or intercostal nerve transfer. Neuropraxia that is managed by observation is followed by serial EMGs. Physical and occupational therapy are instrumental in keeping joints supple. When the entire plexus is involved, the optimal procedure becomes an above-elbow amputation and fitting of a prosthesis.

Loss of useful upper extremity function is a major complication of brachial plexus injuries. If neuropraxial involvement is limited to the upper trunk, reconstruction by a staged shoulder arthrodesis and elbow flexoplasty will reliably

Department of Orthopaedics. Harborview Medical Center, University of Washington, Seattle, Washington 98104

restore useful function. Because neural injuries in children heal much more quickly than in adults, operative exploration and reconstructive procedures in children may be delayed significantly longer.

COMPARTMENTAL SYNDROMES

Compartmental syndromes in the upper extremity can occur with or without fracture after crushing injuries. Compartmental syndromes are most commonly associated with forearm fractures, but they can also occur in association with revascularization of an ischemic arm. The forearm contains three compartments: a superficial compartment, a deep volar compartment, and a dorsal compartment (Fig. 1). Compartmental syndromes are named after the affected compartment.

Diagnosis is made from the physical examination of a patient who is awake and alert; the primary symptoms are pain that does not respond to standard management, pain on passive stretch of the musculotendinous units within the compartment, hypesthesia in the distribution of nerves running through the compartment, and tenseness of the compartment. Pain and hypesthesia are the earliest symptoms. Compartmental syndromes in the upper arm are much less common than compartmental syndromes in the forearm but are diagnosed in the same manner. If the diagnois is suspected, the limb is placed at the level of the heart and the cast, dressings, or splint is split to the skin. The physical examination is repeated after 15 to 20 min. A suspected diagnosis, especially in an unresponsive patient, is confirmed by pressure monitoring

Treatment of compartmental syndromes consists of fasciotomy under general anesthesia so that the results of postoperative serial examinations are not masked by regional anesthesia. Any fractures in the limb should be stabilized at the time of the fasciotomy. Diaphyseal fractures in the forearm or the humerus are treated by open reduction and plate fixation. Two arm compartments can be released by the standard anterolateral approach used to visualize the humeral shaft. The forearm compartment can be released by a single ulnar incision (Fig. 2). Release of the deep volar compartment may be more difficult through this approach because the flexor carpi ulnaris muscle must be protected. A surgeon who is unfamiliar with this interval might prefer the more direct volar approach of Henry. When the volar approach is used, a second incision is required to release the dorsal compartment as a prophylactic measure after high-energy upper extremity trauma. Because emergent carpal tunnel release is frequently required after a distal radial fracture, the volar approach is favored after this injury. The wounds are dressed open and delayed primary closure or split-thickness skin grafting is performed 5 days after the fasciotomy. If a carpal

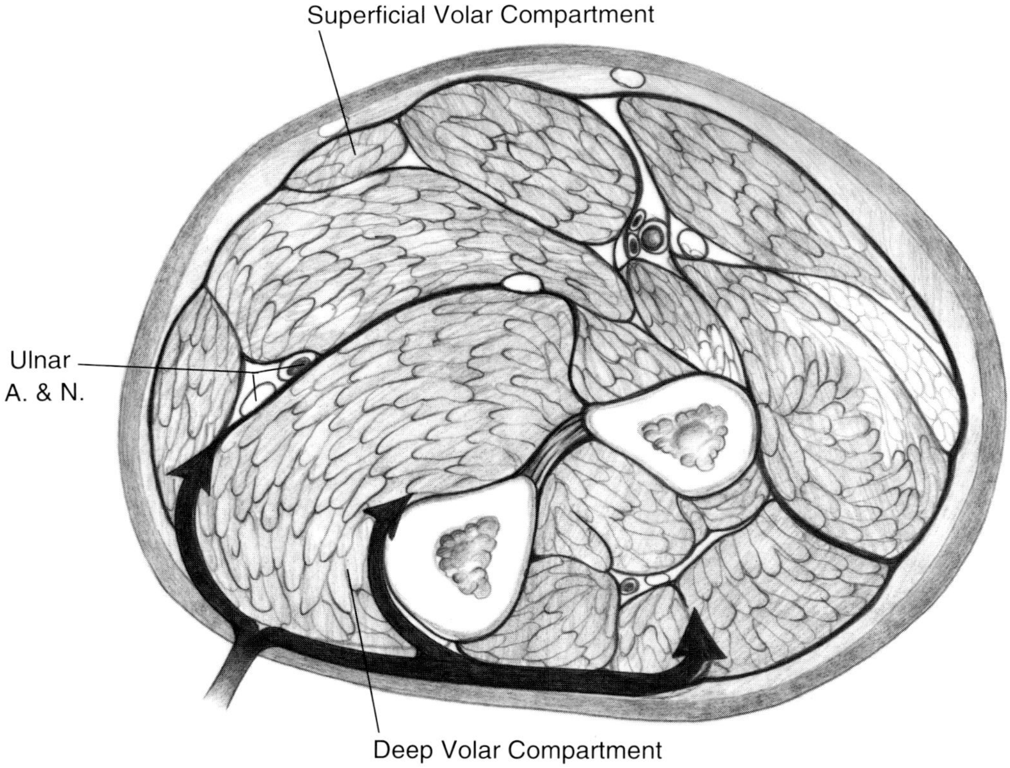

FIG. 1. Cross-section of the forearm, revealing the three compartments of the forearm and the pathways for surgical decompression.

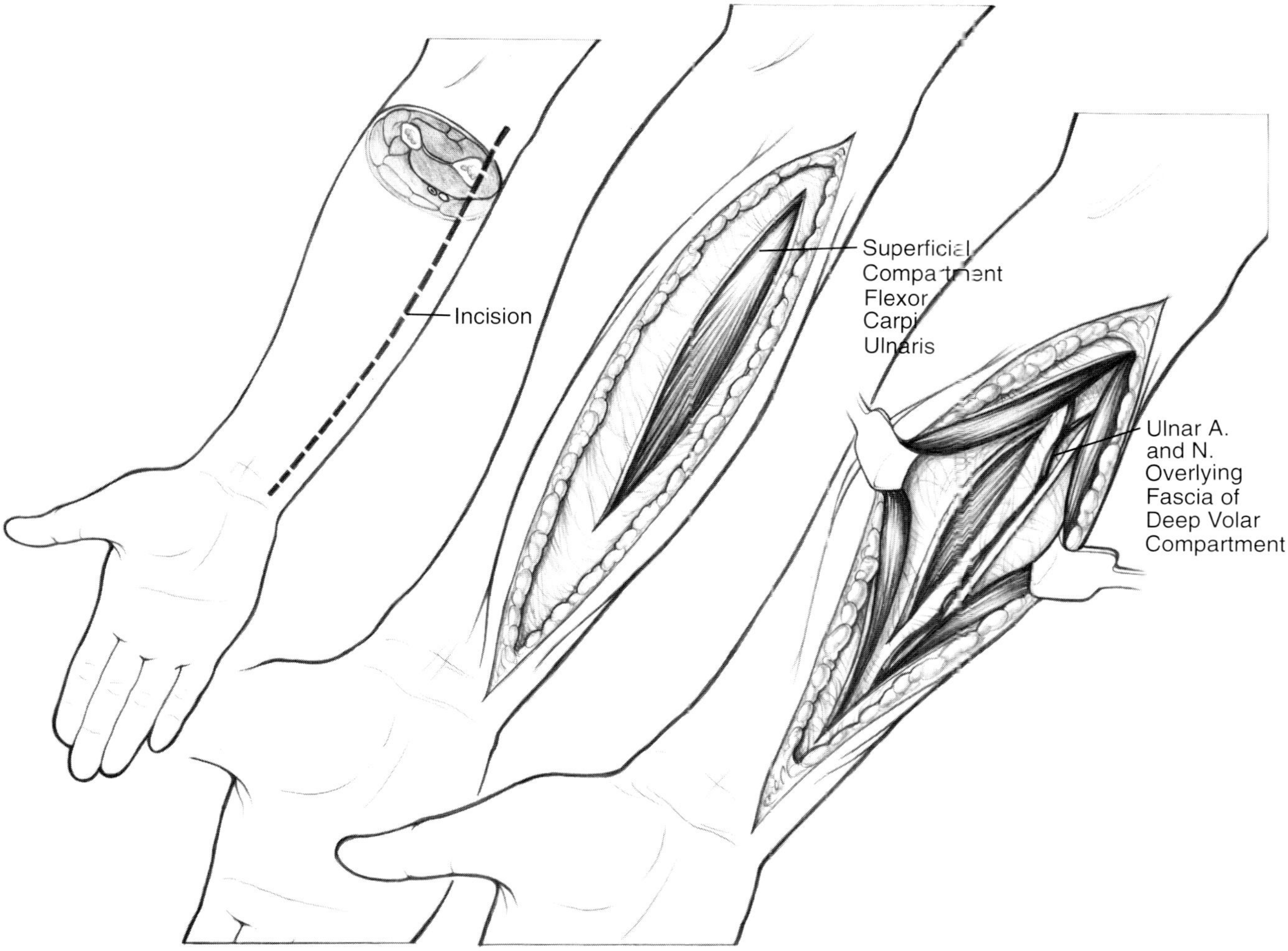

A

B,C

FIG. 2. The ulnar approach for three-compartment fasciotomy. **A:** Skin incision. **B:** Incising the superficial volar compartment directly in line with the skin incision. **C:** Incising the extensor fascia on the dorsal side of the ulna and the deep volar compartment on the volar side of the ulna.

tunnel release has been performed, tissue must be brought forward over the median nerve or this section of wound must be loosely closed. Aggressive rehabilitation is initiated after the wound has epithelialized.

Deep infection and fibrosis of the muscle bellies are consequences of delayed diagnosis and are best managed by prevention. Compartmental syndromes in children and adolescents are treated in the same manner. Upper extremity fractures in children are usually managed by Kirschner-wire fixation or external fixation; fractures in adolescents are managed the same as fractures in adults.

OPEN FRACTURES

Open fractures in the upper extremity are caused indirectly by high-energy trauma or by crushing; they are not commonly associated with penetrating trauma. The most important anatomic factors related to prognosis in the upper extremity are the muscle origins and insertions. Most morbidity associated with fractures in the upper extremity is due to loss of blood supply to the bone.

The classification of open fractures by Gustilo and Anderson (1) is the most useful grading system for soft-tissue injuries (Table 1).

The closed fracture classification of Tscherne (see Chapter 1) is also useful for grading upper extremity injuries. The AO system of grading soft-tissue injuries associated with fractures may prove useful in the future (2). It consists of separate grades for the integument injuries, musculotendinous injuries, and neurovascular injuries. This comprehensive approach may prove the most useful for clinical research.

Table 1. *Classification of open fractures*

Grade I	Small wounds (1 cm or less) caused by low-energy trauma, e.g., the protrusion of a bony fragment through the skin or the entrance wound of a low-velocity bullet lodged in the soft tissues, resulting in minimal soft-tissue damage
Grade II	Extensive wounds with little or no avascular or devitalized soft tissue and relatively little contamination by foreign material
Grade III	Moderate or massive wounds with considerable area of devitalized soft tissue and/or contamination by foreign material, or a traumatic amputation
Grade IIIA	Wounds with extensive soft-tissue lacerations or flaps, or high-energy wounds with adequate remaining soft tissues to cover the fractured bone
Grade IIIB	Wounds with extensive soft-tissue injury or loss, periosteal stripping, and bone exposure
Grade IIIC	Open fractures associated with arterial injuries requiring repair

Emergent management consists of grading the injury and controlling hemorrhage. Extremities that were splinted at the site of the accident are uncovered and the wounds are inspected. Wound inspection should be done only once because the possibility of deep infection increases with repeated manipulations in the emergency department. Wound cultures are not necessary at the time of admission. The wound is probed gently with sterile cotton swabs or with a gloved finger to determine the extent of injury, and profuse arterial bleeding is managed by application of direct pressure to the wound over sterile dressings. Alternatively, a tourniquet can be applied above the injury if the injury is not located extremely proximal for the short period of time it takes to move the patient to the operating room. Instruments such as hemostats should not be placed into wounds for risk of injuring nerves or muscles. After the wound is inspected, it is dressed with a sponge soaked in Betadine solution, wrapped in a sterile manner, and splinted. Wound coverage with antibiotics is continued for 3 to 5 days, depending on the degree of contamination. Treatment of the open fracture is planned after the skeletal injury is graded. Intravenous first-generation cephalosporin is administered on admission and then every 4 to 6 h. In grade III wounds, an aminoglycoside should be added; when contamination with anaerobic bacteria is a possibility (e.g., farm injuries), penicillin should also be included (Fig. 3).

The most important factor in preventing deep infection is immediate aggressive debridement. Patients are taken to the operating room as soon as they are cleared for general anesthesia. As a rule, debridement should take as long as the time required to stabilize the injury. All bone fragments without adequate soft-tissue attachments must be removed, regardless of their size. All contaminated tissue and muscle with a dusky appearance must be sharply debrided. Depending on its size and the amount of contamination, the wound is cleansed with 3 to 12 L of pulsating lavage, usually without antibiotics.

After debridement, fractures are stabilized immediately by internal or external fixation. The only exceptions to mandatory acute fixation are isolated upper extremity fractures. Extremely severe soft-tissue injuries can be bridged by placing remote 2.5-mm or 4.0-mm Schanz pins and an external fixator frame to allow wound management. Grade III injuries are returned to the operating room after 48 h for repeat debridement and pulsating lavage. Delayed closure or split-thickness skin grafting to close the wound should be done five to seven days after injury. Muscle flap coverage can be performed after 3 to 5 days. In general, bone grafting for fractures with contaminated wounds should be delayed until 4 to 6 weeks postoperatively.

The primary complications associated with open upper extremity injuries are compartmental syndrome, necrosis, and infection. The possibility of a compartmental syndrome must be kept in mind during evaluation, and a suspected diagnosis must be confirmed by compartmental monitoring. Any necrotic muscle associated with a compartmental syndrome must be serially debrided to control sepsis. Deep

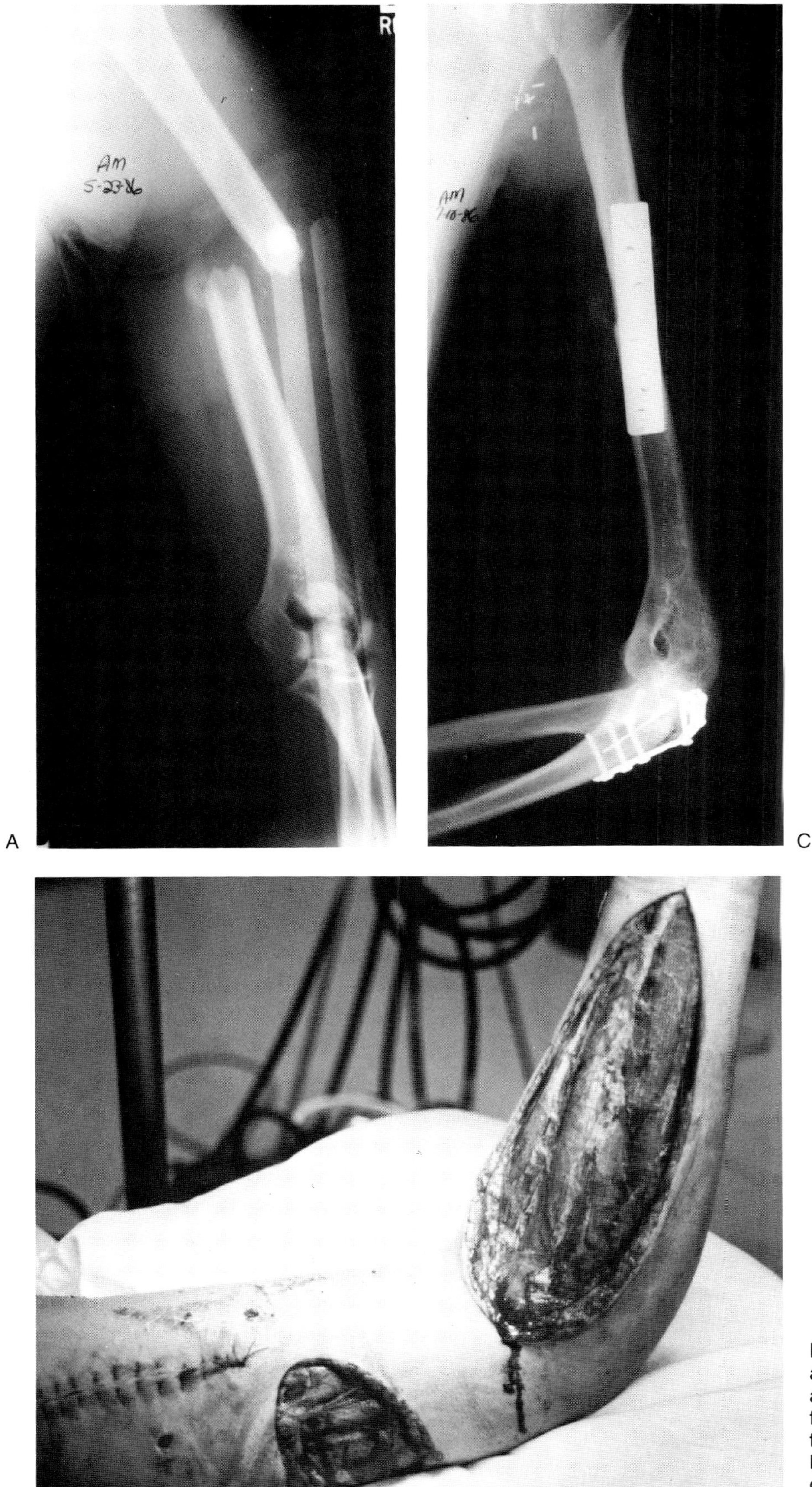

FIG. 3. A: This 22-year-old male sustained a type IIIC open humeral shaft fracture with an ipsilateral comminuted proximal ulnar fracture. After the vascular repair, faciotomies of the forearm were required. **B:** The limb is shown at the time of skin grafting and delayed closure. **C:** Postoperative radiograph.

infections are treated by debridement and the wounds are closed by delayed primary closure or split-thickness skin grafting. Occasionally, free bone or muscle transfers are required to salvage a limb, but these procedures are performed only when the deep infection remains under control after two or more debridements. Internal fixation devices are left in place in the presence of infection if they continue to provide stability. In general, external fixation is used as temporary stabilization to provide stability during soft-tissue debridement and is replaced with internal fixation after wound closure.

The same principles of emergent and acute treatment apply to injuries in children and adolescents, although external fixation is usually preferred for definitive treatment of humeral fractures in children. Cast immobilization can be safely used for low-grade soft-tissue injuries associated with fractures of the humerus and the forearm. External fixation and casting are widely used to stabilize fractures in children because fractures in this age group heal faster and are not subject to the deleterious effects of long-term immobilization.

REFERENCES

1. Gustilo RB, Mendoza RM, Williams DM. Problems in management of type III open fractures. A new classification of type III open fractures. *J Trauma 1984;24:742–746.*
2. Müller ME, Allgöwer M, Schneider R, Willenegger H. *Manual of Internal Fixation,* 3rd ed., Berlin: Springer-Verlag; 1991:151–158.

Orthopaedic Trauma Protocols, edited by
Sigvard T. Hansen, Jr., and Marc F. Swiontkowski.
Raven Press, Ltd., New York, © 1993.

CHAPTER 18

Spine

Paul A. Anderson

Spinal Cord Injuries

MECHANISMS OF INJURY

Spinal cord injuries result from mechanical deformations of the spinal column secondary to impaction by bone or disc fragments or to stretching from kyphosis or distraction. These injuries can cause irreparable neural tissue damage and are called primary insults. Injuries from recurrent trauma or from rapid biomechanical, cellular, and vascular changes that occur after the initial injury are called secondary insults. Damage caused by secondary insults can sometimes be minimized by appropriate treatment. The objectives of treatment of spinal cord injuries are to limit secondary insults and to provide an optimal environment for neurologic recovery.

ANATOMIC CONSIDERATIONS

The spinal cord consists of neural cell bodies in the central gray matter and ascending and descending axons in the peripheral white matter. The spinal cord enlarges for outflow to the extremities in the cervical spine and at the lumbosacral junction, and is narrowest and most easily injured at the midthoracic level. In adults, the spinal cord ends at approximately L-1 in the conus medullaris, an important structure containing cells that control sphincter and perineal innervation.

Surgeons who treat patients with spinal cord injuries must understand the function of each major axonal tract. The corticospinal tracts are located laterally and transmit ipsilateral motor function. The anterior spinothalamic tracts, which conduct sensations of pain and temperature, are crossed, and therefore these sensations are experienced contralaterally. The dorsal columns convey proprioception, vibration, and deep pain sensations. The fibers within each tract are laminated so that the cervical tracts are located near the center of the cord, whereas the lumbar and sacral tracts are located peripherally.

Department of Orthopaedics, Harborview Medical Center, University of Washington, Seattle, Washington 98104

CLASSIFICATION

Spinal cord injuries are classified as complete or incomplete neurologic injuries. Patients with complete injuries have no motor or sensory functions below the level of the cord injury; those with incomplete injuries retain some distal motor or sensory functions (Fig. 1).

Central Cord Syndrome

This injury usually results from cervical hyperextension that causes pinching of the spinal cord between the ligamentum flavum and the intervertebral disc. The central aspect of the cord is injured, causing greater neurologic loss in the arms and hands than in the legs.

Anterior Cord Syndrome

Neural function in the anterior two thirds of the spinal cord is absent in this injury. Patients with anterior cord syndrome experience complete loss of motor function and of pain and temperature sensation, but retain sensations of vibration, proprioception, and light touch

Brown–Séquard's Syndrome

Penetrating trauma or unilateral facet dislocations can result in hemitransection of the cord. Patients experience loss of ipsilateral motor and dorsal column functions and loss of contralateral pain and temperature sensations.

The level of neurologic injury is determined by identifying the level of the most caudad nerve root, which retains at least

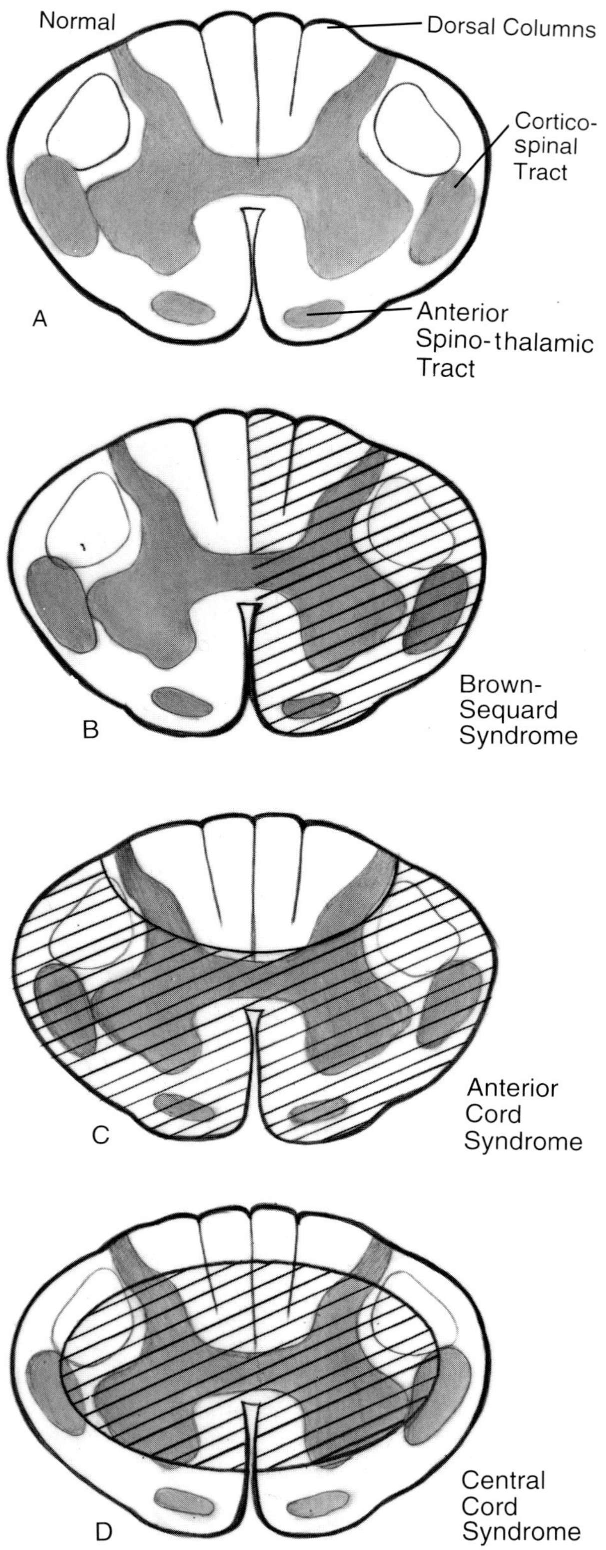

FIG. 1. **A:** Cross-sectional anatomy of normal cervical spinal cord at C-5. **B:** Brown–Séquard's syndrome. **C:** Anterior cord syndrome. **D:** Central cord syndrome.

antigravity strength. Frankel (1) classified the extent of spinal cord injuries according to the following functional criteria:

Frankel A: complete loss of motor and sensory functions below the level of injury
Frankel B: partial distal sensation but absent motor function
Frankel C: retained limited but useless motor functions
Frankel D: retained useful motor and sensory functions
Frankel E: neurologically normal motor and sensory functions.

ASSESSMENT

Physical Examination

Every traumatized patient is presumed to have sustained an injury to the spinal column. After resuscitation in the emergency department, the patient is log-rolled to one side for a physical examination of the spine. The thoracolumbar spine is palpated for kyphotic or gibbous deformity, tenderness, or a gap between the spinous processes. A discernible gap is indicative of a highly unstable fracture that requires surgical stabilization. A careful neurologic examination, including manual muscle testing of the upper and lower extremities, is conducted and the results are documented in the patient's medical record. The sensory evaluation determines sensitivity to pinprick, light touch, and proprioception. Perianal pinprick sensation, rectal tone, voluntary rectal contraction, and the bulbocavernosus reflex also must be noted.

An accurate physical examination of the neck cannot be performed on unconscious patients. In this case, acute spinal injury must be ruled out on the basis of normal AP and lateral radiographs. Patients who are alert but whose radiographs are suggestive of injury to the spine are kept immobilized in a rigid cervical orthosis until the physical examination is repeated after 24 to 48 h. If the second examination reveals no abnormal physical symptoms or neurologic deficits and radiographs are negative, the spine may be cleared of injury and the cervical collar can be removed. Cervical immobilization is continued if symptoms persist.

Radiographic Evaluation

Clearing the cervical spine of potential injury is the responsibility of the general trauma surgeon and the radiologist. Orthopaedists and neurologic surgeons serve as consultants for patients with questionable symptoms or uncertain lesions. Normal radiographic findings from the occiput to T-1 are required to clear the cervical spine. If the cervicothoracic region cannot be visualized on a lateral view, radiographs are obtained with the patient's arms pulled down to the sides or in a swimmer's position. The open-mouth odontoid view is scrutinized for a fracture of the dens (2).

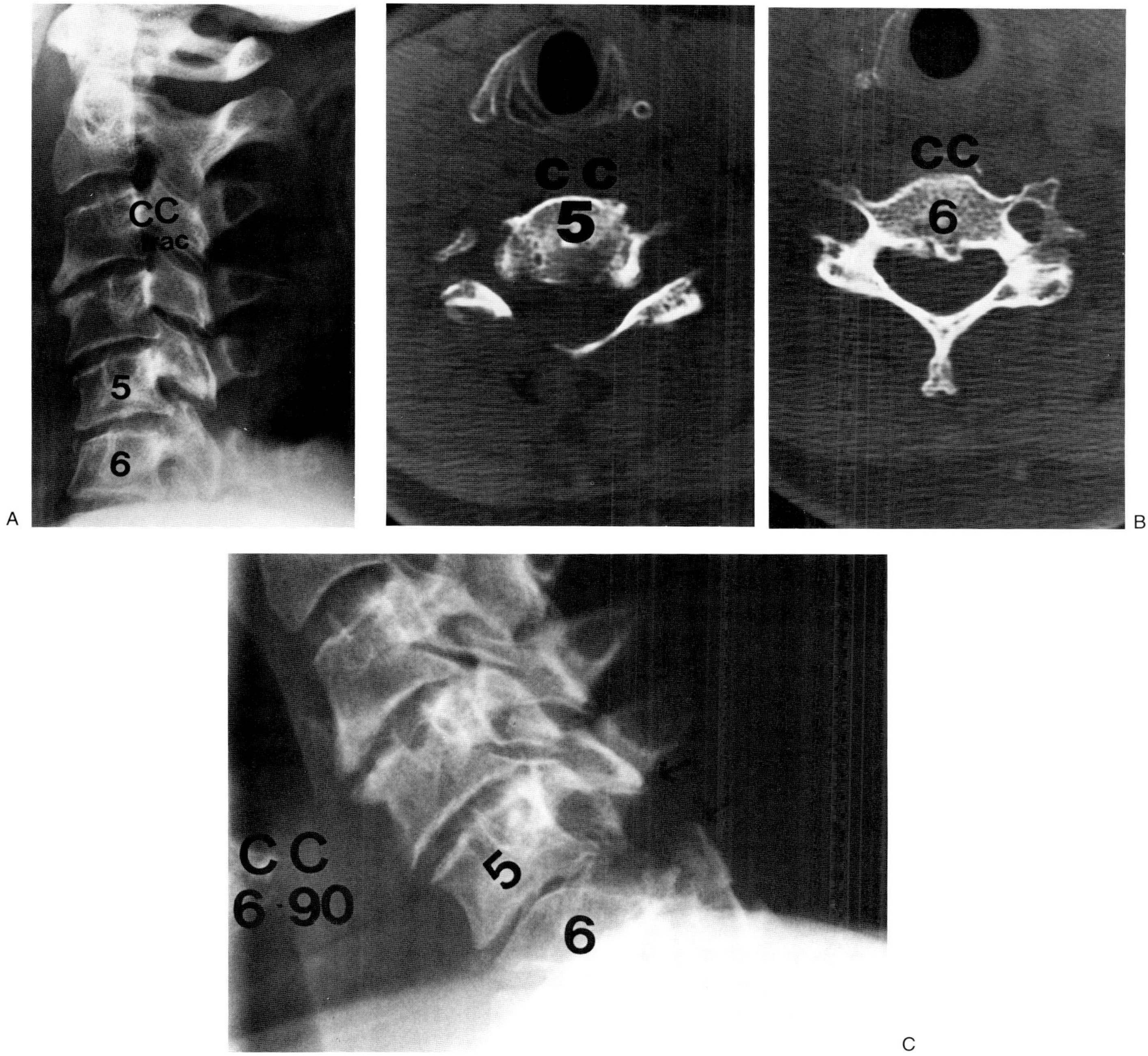

FIG. 2. **A:** Lateral radiograph of 73-year-old woman with neck pain after a motor vehicle accident. Wide separation of spinous processes is present between C5-6 but was overlooked. **B:** CT scan performed to evaluate neck pain and tenderness. No bony injury is noted. **C:** Flexion radiograph demonstrating bilateral facet dislocation at C5-6. The patient developed a central cord syndrome after flexion–extension radiographs.

Radiographs of the thoracolumbar spine are obtained in alert traumatized patients only if they are indicated by clinical symptoms or physical findings. Radiographic evaluation of the thoracolumbar spine is done routinely only on unconscious, intubated, or pharmacologically paralyzed patients. The maxim "a patient cannot injure himself" is not true. Cervical flexion–extension radiographs should not be obtained in an emergent situation because subtle abnormalities, especially ligament instability, can easily be overlooked and movement of the cervical area may result in facet dislocation with spinal cord injury (Fig. 2). Flexion–extension radiographs should be taken only in the outpatient department in patients who complain of persistent neck pain despite normal radiographic findings and no sign of neurologic deficits.

Because a second, noncontiguous spinal fracture is found in 10% to 15% of patients with a single obvious spinal injury, diagnosis of a single spinal fracture warrants obtaining a full spinal radiographic series.

Special Studies

The degree of spinal injury can be underestimated from plain radiographs and may lead to inadequate treatment. Therefore, CT scans are recommended for all patients with obvious spinal fractures on plain radiographs or questionable radiographic findings. Myelography or MRI is performed before surgical treatment of cervical injuries but not necessarily before initial treatment of thoracolumbar fractures.

EMERGENT MANAGEMENT

Traumatized patients are immobilized in a cervical collar immediately after injury and remain immobilized until acute spinal injury is ruled out and the spine is asymptomatic. The collar is applied in the field and the patient is transported to the hospital supine on a backboard. The patient's forehead is taped to the backboard and sandbags are placed adjacent to the head to prevent motion during transport. Patients with spinal cord or cauda equina injuries are given intravenous methylprednisolone within 8 h of injury. A loading dose of 30 mg/kg is given the first hour, followed by a continuous dose of 5.4 mg/kg/h for the next 23 h (3).

Cervical Spinal Cord Injuries

The initial treatment of cervical spinal cord injuries consists of reduction with cranial tong traction. Stabilization procedures are delayed for 5 days to prevent deterioration that has been reported in patients treated by early surgery (4). However, failure to achieve adequate fracture reduction is an indication for immediate open reduction or decompression.

Flaccid or elderly patients and those with ligament injuries can easily be overdistracted by traction, and traction weight should therefore be applied judiciously. In many cases reduction can be facilitated by adjusting the relative position of the head to the thorax instead of adding more traction weight. Special care must be taken in positioning children, whose heads are relatively larger than their chests, and elderly patients with preexisting thoracic kyphosis. Initial traction weight of 2.5 kg is used for injuries in the upper cervical spine and 5.0 kg is used for injuries in the lower cervical spine. Traction weight is increased in increments of 2.5 kg to 5.0 kg at 15-minute intervals, allowing for soft-tissue relaxation. A neurologic examination is performed and a lateral radiograph is obtained after the addition of each increment of weight. Weight is increased until the fracture or dislocation is reduced.

During reduction, radiographs are scrutinized for signs of overdistraction, such as widening of the intervertebral disc or the facet joints. To facilitate unlocking a facet dislocation, the head can be gently flexed by placing towels under the occiput. Burst fractures may require substantial traction weight—we have used up to 70% of the body's weight without incurring complications. However, manual manipulation is not recommended to achieve reduction.

DEFINITIVE MANAGEMENT

The goals of treating any spinal cord injury are to protect the spinal cord from further damage and to provide an optimal environment for neurologic recovery. Although experimental treatments have shown that neurologic recovery can be improved by decompressive surgery in animal models, only the use of corticosteroids and correction of adverse mechanical factors have been demonstrated to be effective in minimizing neurologic deficits in humans.

The benefits of early spinal stabilization include decreased morbidity and a shorter hospital stay, but few reports have demonstrated any neurologic benefits gained by immediate anterior decompression. Jacobs (5), Gertzbein (6), and Anderson (7) have reported improved recovery in patients treated by early fracture reduction, stabilization, and decompression. Bohlman (8) reported improved neurologic function after late anterior decompression in patients with incomplete fractures. Complete quadriplegics may experience some upper-extremity nerve root recovery after late anterior decompression (9).

The timing of surgery for a cervical injury is also controversial. Opponents of early surgical intervention insist that the stress of an operation added to the rapidly changing biochemical, vascular, and cellular events that follow spinal cord injury is harmful to the patient. Conversely, others insist that early operative stabilization enhances neurologic recovery and decreases morbidity associated with long periods of immobilization. The protocols for spinal cord injuries at this institution call for early fracture reduction, stabilization, and decompression of neural tissues.

Gardner–Wells Tong Placement

Gardner–Wells tongs are applied in the emergency department to patients with unstable cervical injuries (Fig. 3). The skin is prepped with a Betadine solution and infiltrated to the level of the periosteum with a local anesthetic. Shaving the scalp is not necessary. The pins are inserted into the skull 1 cm above the tips of the ears and in line with the external auditory meatus. The pins are tightened symmetrically until the spring-loaded plunger protrudes 1 mm from the pin surface. The locking nuts are then tightened and weight is applied via a rope and pulley. The pins are retightened after 24 h and are not disturbed again. When an MRI study is anticipated, for example, in patients with closed head injuries, MRI-compatible tongs are used.

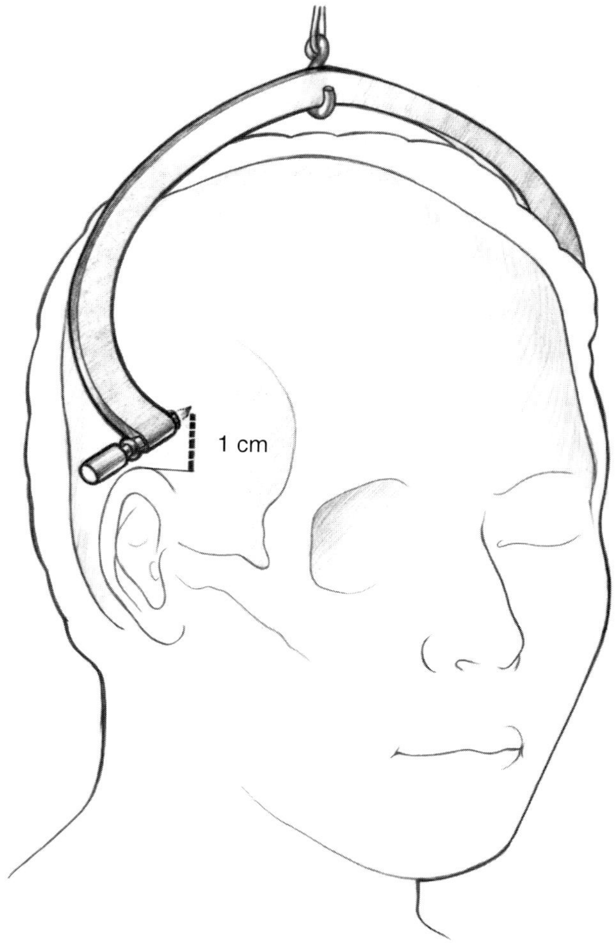

FIG. 3. Placement of Gardner–Wells tongs.

Thoracolumbar Spinal Cord Injuries

Methylprednisolone is administered to patients with neurologic deficits secondary to thoracolumbar fractures according to the previously described protocol. Thoracolumbar fractures cannot be reduced or stabilized nonoperatively and patients with these injuries are candidates for emergent operative stabilization. In patients with incomplete paraplegia, urgent spinal stabilization or decompression is performed depending on the fracture type. In patients with complete paraplegia, the prognosis for neurologic recovery is poor and is not influenced by treatment. Therefore, complete paraplegics with unstable fractures are stabilized electively within 24 to 48 h of injury. This protocol allows early mobilization and decreases morbidity, hospitalization time, and cost (10).

COMPLICATIONS

Complications associated with spinal cord injuries frequently result in significant morbidity and mortality. Hemodynamic complications, including bradycardia and hypotension, can be treated with vasopressors, atropine or, rarely, a temporary pacemaker. Stress ulceration is common after quadriplegia and may be aggravated by the use of corticosteroids. All patients with spinal cord injuries are placed on a regimen of antacid medication, to maintain pH levels over 7, and on H^2 blocking agents. An indwelling Foley catheter is inserted into the urinary tract until fluids are stabilized, at which time the patient is placed on an intermittent self-catheterization program.

Prolonged traction increases the risk of atelectasis or adult respiratory distress syndrome (ARDS). Early spinal stabilization and mobilization appear to help relieve these pulmonary complications. Skin breakdown in insensate areas can be prevented by log-rolling the patient to a different position every 2 h. Patients with neurologic deficits are at high risk for deep vein thrombosis and pulmonary embolism and require prophylactic measures to prevent these complications. All patients wear sequential pneumatic stockings and receive 5000 units of heparin subcutaneously twice daily. The incidence of these complications can also be decreased by early physical therapy intervention that includes mobilization and range-of-motion (ROM) of all joints.

SKELETALLY IMMATURE PATIENTS

Factors that contribute to the difficulty of evaluating a child's spine are incomplete ossification of the vertebrae, the presence of multiple growth centers, and physiologic hypermobility of the spine. Most pediatric cervical injuries occur in the upper cervical spine between the occiput and C-3, because the ratio of mass between the head and the body is disproportionate and the muscles and ligaments supporting the cervical spine are weak. Ligament injuries, particularly atlanto–occipital dislocations, are common.

Spinal cord injuries may be present in children who exhibit no radiographic abnormalities. This phenomenon occurs in cord-traction injuries and is due to greater elasticity in the spinal column than in the spinal cord. Also, injuries at the junction of cartilaginous and bony end plates are not easily identified on radiographs. Children with spinal tenderness or questionable radiographic findings are treated by immobilization until their symptoms resolve or until experienced physicians can review the radiographs.

REFERENCES

1. Frankel HL, Hancock DO, Hyslop G, et al. The value of postural reduction in the initial management of closed injuries of the spine with paraplegia and tetraplegia. *Paraplegia* 1969;7:179–92.
2. MacDonald RL, Schwartz ML, Mirich D, Sharkey PW, Nelson WR. Diagnosis of cervical spine injury in motor vehicle crash victims: how many x-rays are enough? *J Trauma* 1990;30:392–97.
3. Bracken MB, et al. A randomized controlled trial of methylprednisolone or naloxone in the treatment of acute spinal-cord injury. Results of the second national acute spinal cord injury study. *N Engl J Med* 1990;322:1406–11.

4. Marshall LF, Knowlton S, Garfin SR, Klauber MR, Eisenberg HM, Kopaniky D, Miner ME, Tabbador K, Clifton GL. Deterioration following spinal cord injury: a multicenter study. *J Neurosurg* 1987;66:400–4.
5. Jacobs RR, Asher MA, Snider RK. Thoracolumbar spinal injuries. a comparative study of recumbent and operative treatment in 100 patients. *Spine* 1980;5:463–77.
6. Gertzbein SD, Court-Brown CM, Marks P, Martin C, Fazl M, Schwartz M, Jacobs RR. The neurological outcome following surgery for spinal fractures. *Spine* 1988;13:641–4.
7. Anderson PA, Krengel WF, Henley MB. Neurologic recovery in patients with incomplete paraplegia due to thoracic level spinal cord injury. Am Academy Orthop Surg 57th Annual Meeting, New Orleans, Feb. 8–13, 1990.
8. Bohlman HH, Eismont FJ. Surgical techniques of anterior decompression and fusion for spinal cord injuries. *Clin Orthop* 1981;154:57–67.
9. Anderson PA, Bohlman HH. Anterior decompression and arthrodesis in patients with traumatic, complete motor cervical spine cord injury. Long term neurologic recovery in 51 patients. Part II. *J Bone Joint Surg* 1992; 74A:683–91.
10. Schlegel J, Yuan H, Fredericksen B, Bayley J. Timing of operative management of acute spinal injuries. Presented at the 6th Annual Orthopaedic Trauma Association Meeting, Toronto, Nov. 7–10, 1990.

Occipitocervical Articulation: Occipital Condylar Fractures and Atlanto–Occipital Dislocations

MECHANISMS OF INJURY

Occipital condylar fractures and atlanto–occipital dislocations are rare injuries that usually result from severe head trauma. Patients are often unconscious after these injuries and the diagnosis is often made from subtle findings on plain radiographs or incidentally from head CT scans.

ANATOMIC CONSIDERATIONS

The skull is affixed to the cervical spine at the occipitocervical articulation, which includes the atlanto–occipital and the atlantoaxial joints. The strong ligament and bony structures allow a wide range of motion yet are rarely injured. The convex-shaped occipital condyles project downward from the occiput and articulate with corresponding concavities in the lateral masses of the atlas (C-1) (Fig. 4).

The principal ligament structures that limit motion in the occipitocervical articulation are the alar ligaments and the tectorial membrane (Figs. 5 and 6) (1). The alar ligaments attach on the tip of the dens and extend to the medial aspect of the occipital condyles. The tectorial membrane is the uppermost extension of the posterior longitudinal ligament and attaches to the anterior aspect of the foramen magnum. These ligaments span from the occiput to C-2 without attaching directly to C-1, which acts merely as a bushing.

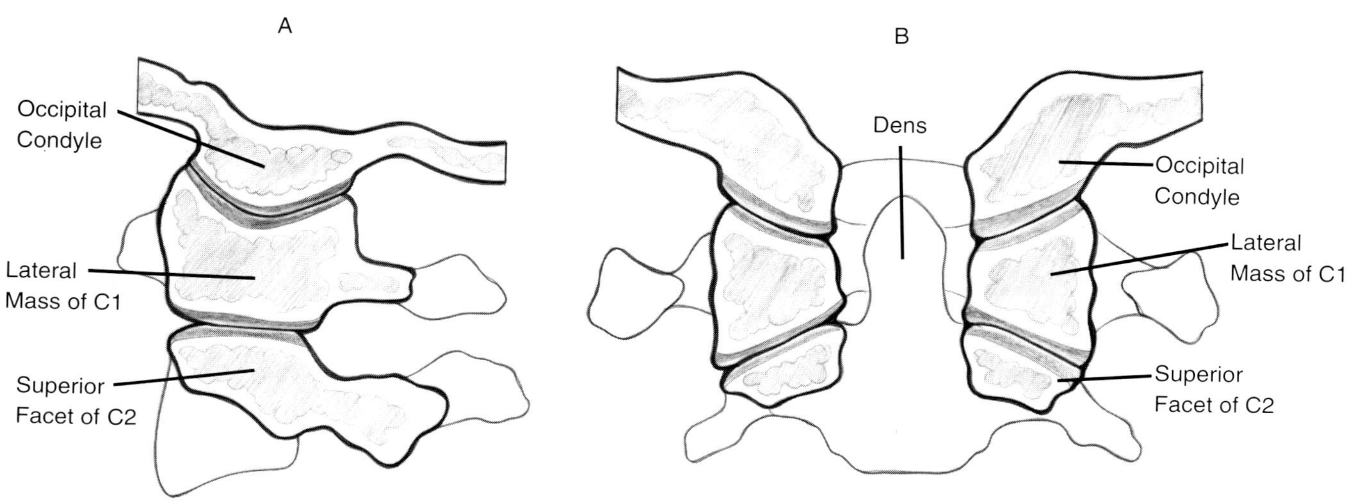

FIG. 4. A: Lateral view of craniocervical articulation. **B:** Anteroposterior view of bony anatomy of craniocervical articulation.

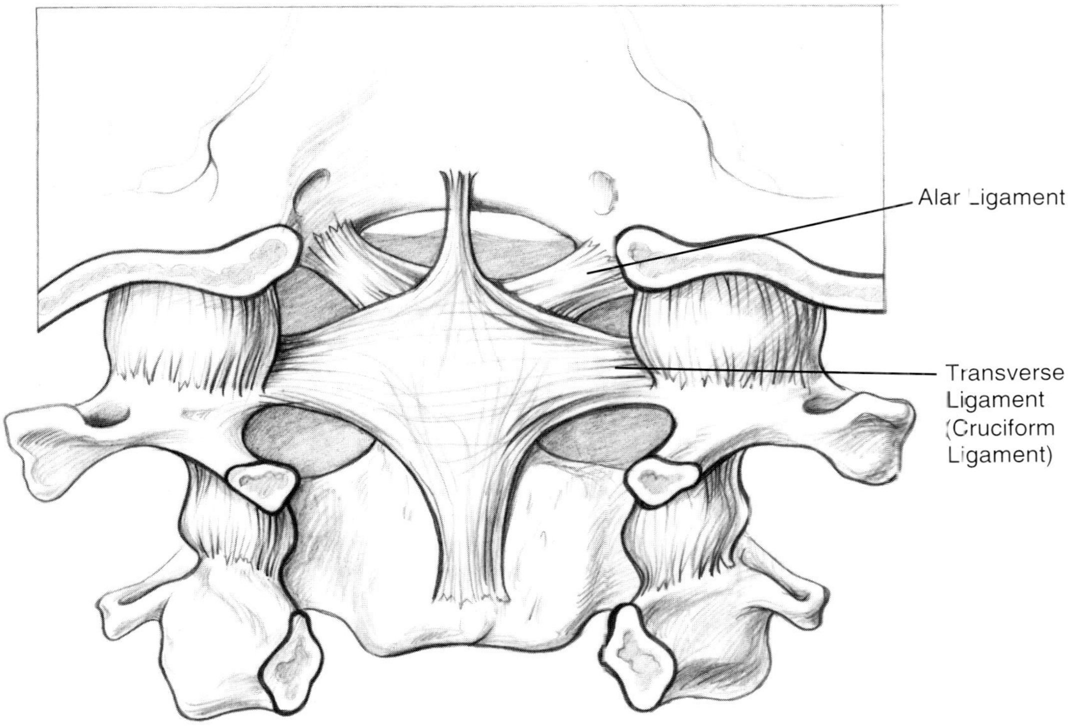

FIG. 5. View of ligamentous anatomy of the craniocervical articulation.

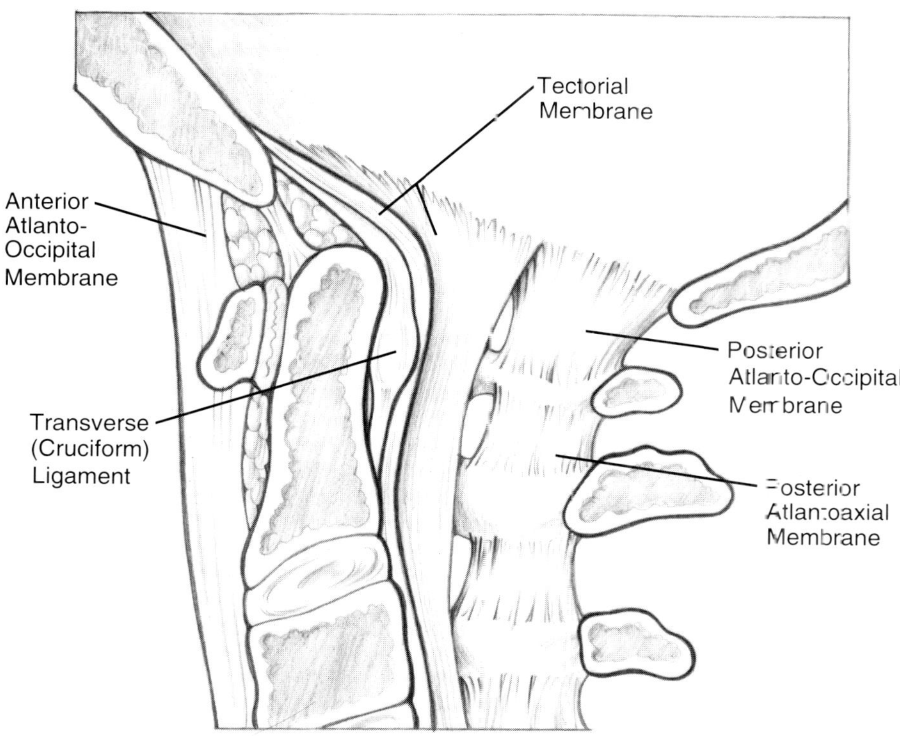

FIG. 6. Lateral view of ligamentous anatomy of craniocervical articulation.

CLASSIFICATION

Occipital Condylar Fractures

Anderson and Montesano (2) have identified three types of occipital condylar fractures based on CT morphology (Fig. 7):

Type I: stable comminuted fractures secondary to axial loading
Type II: stable basilar skull fractures with occipital condyle involvement
Type III: avulsion fractures of the alar ligament (this fracture is potentially unstable and is often associated with an atlanto–occipital dislocation).

Atlanto–Occipital Dislocations

Patients rarely survive atlanto–occipital dislocations because of brainstem and the spinal cord damage. These injuries, which can range from mild instability to complete dislocation with marked vertical distraction, are often initially missed. Atlanto–occipital dislocations are classified by the direction of displacement: anterior, vertical, or posterior (Fig. 8) (3). Pathologically, all the major restraining and alar ligaments and the tectorial membrane are ruptured regardless of the direction of displacement. All injuries are unstable and require posterior occipitocervical fusion.

ASSESSMENT

Physical Examination

Patients who are conscious experience tenderness at the base of the skull and complain of pain in the occipital area. Cranial nerves VI, VII, IX, XI, and XII may be injured and should be examined. Patients with spinal cord or brainstem injury may experience respiratory impairment and require mechanical ventilation.

Radiographic Evaluation

The atlanto–occipital joints are difficult to visualize on routine radiographs because their articulations lie at oblique angles to the x-ray beam. However, indirect evidence of an atlanto–occipital dislocation can be established by confirming the axis of the clivus. The clivus is a bony plate in the base of the skull extending from the sella turcica to the basion at the anterior border of the foramen magnum. Normally the basion lies within 5 mm of the dens tip and the line of the clivus points to the dens (4). This reference line should always be checked to verify the integrity of the atlanto–occipital joint. Disruption of these anatomic relationships may be indicative of an atlanto–occipital dislocation. A later-

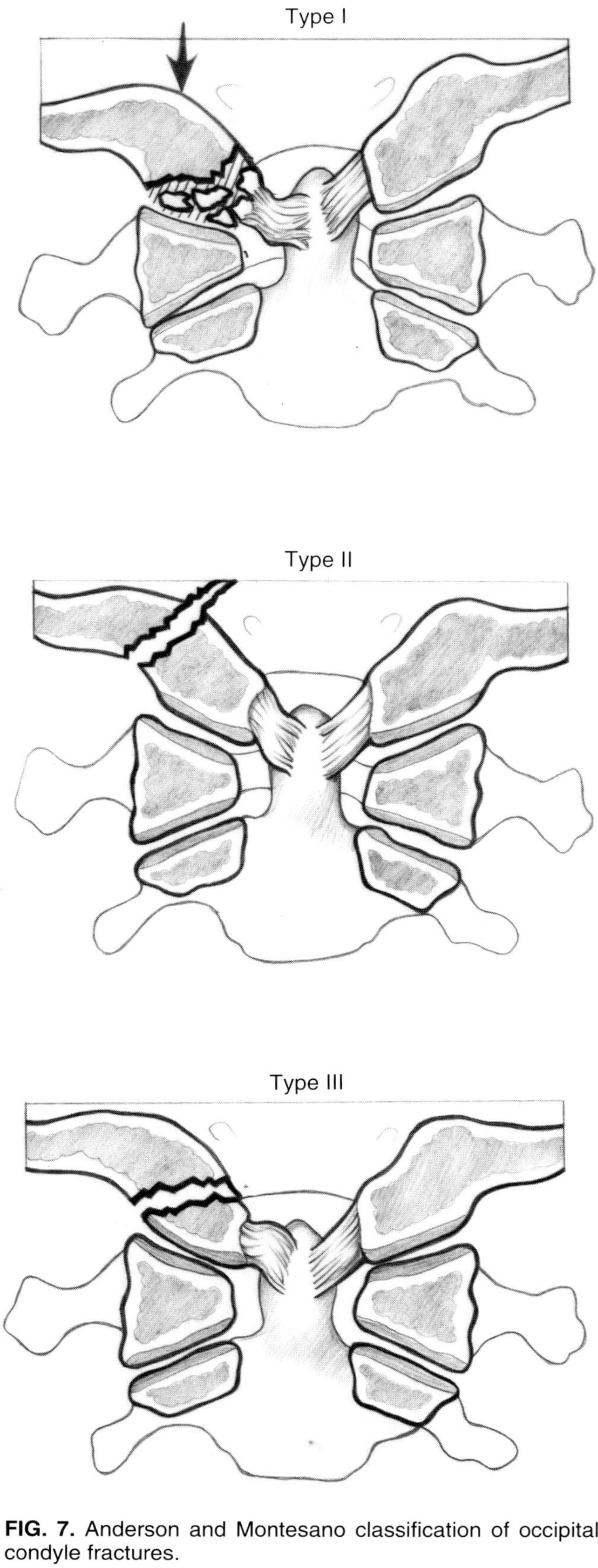

FIG. 7. Anderson and Montesano classification of occipital condyle fractures.

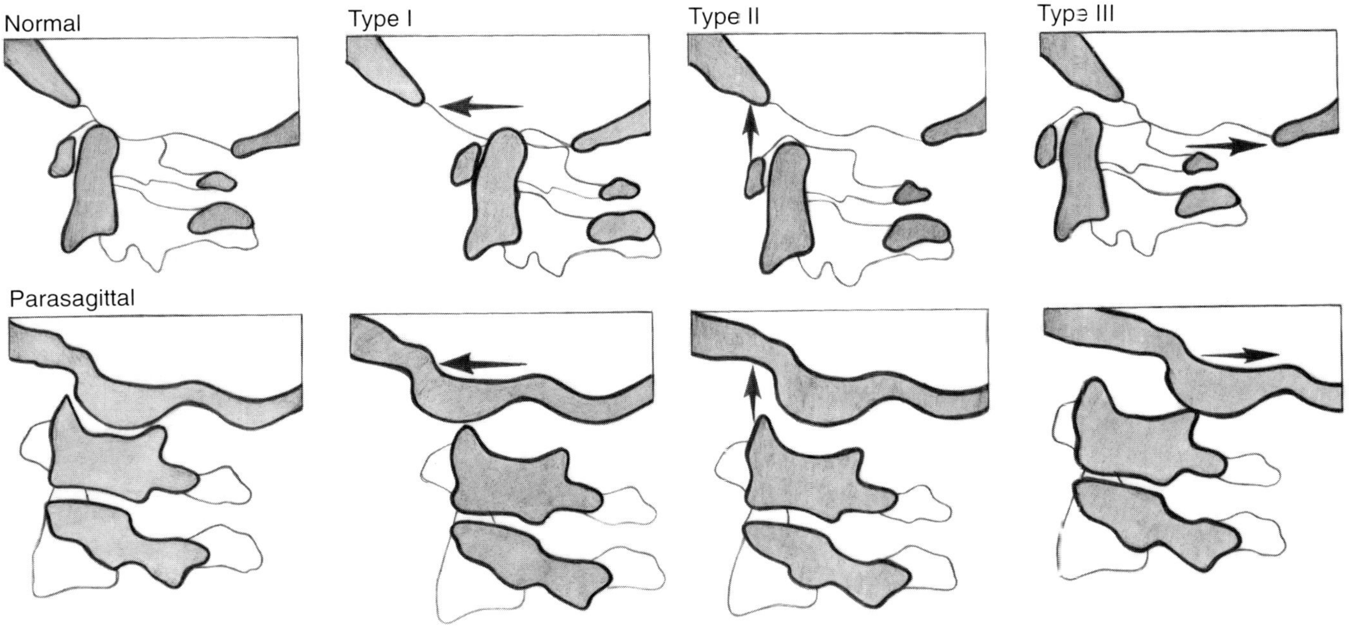

FIG. 8. Classification modified fromTraynelis of atlanto–occipital dislocations.

al radiograph of the skull, rather than of the cervical spine, may be needed for an adequate assessment

Special Studies

Computerized tomography is invaluable for evaluating the integrity of the occipitocervical articulation. Sagittal reconstructions in the plane of the facet articulation document alignment of these joints. Joint diastasis greater than 2 mm is indicative of ligament disruption and a highly unstable spinal column. Occipital condylar fractures frequently occur in patients with atlanto–occipital dislocations.

EMERGENT MANAGEMENT

The initial management of an atlanto–occipital dislocation consists of reduction and stabilization of the head. Because all the restraining ligaments are damaged, applying axial tong traction may be dangerous. Tong traction with 0.5 kg to 1.0 kg of weight can also be applied but is primarily used as a visual reminder of the serious nature of this neck injury. Atlanto–occipital dislocations are best managed by realigning the head with the thorax according to the direction of displacement. Anterior dislocations are realigned by placing blankets under the thorax and allowing the head to fall backwards (Fig. 9). Conversely, posterior dislocations are reduced by placing padding behind the occiput to elevate the head forwards. For realignment of a vertical displacement, the patient is placed in a sitting position and the dislocation is reduced by gravity. A halo vest is applied after reduction.

DEFINITIVE MANAGEMENT

Occipital Condylar Fractures

Type I and type II fractures are stable injuries and are treated in a cervicothoracic orthosis for 6 to 8 weeks. Type III injuries must be carefully assessed for stability of the atlanto–occipital articulation. If the joints are well aligned and diastasis is not evident, treatment consists of a cervicothoracic orthosis. A halo vest is used if the integrity of the joints is questionable.

Atlanto–Occipital Dislocations

All patients with occipitocervical dislocations require posterior fusion of the occiput to C-2. This injury warrants an aggressive surgical approach because the healing potential of ligament injuries is poor and the consequences of loss of reduction are catastrophic. Posterior fusion is accomplished by Bohlman's technique (5), in which autologous iliac bone grafts are wired to the occiput, C-1, and C-2. Postoperatively the patient is immobilized in a halo brace for 12 weeks or until bone union is demonstrated on flexion–extension radiographs (Fig. 9).

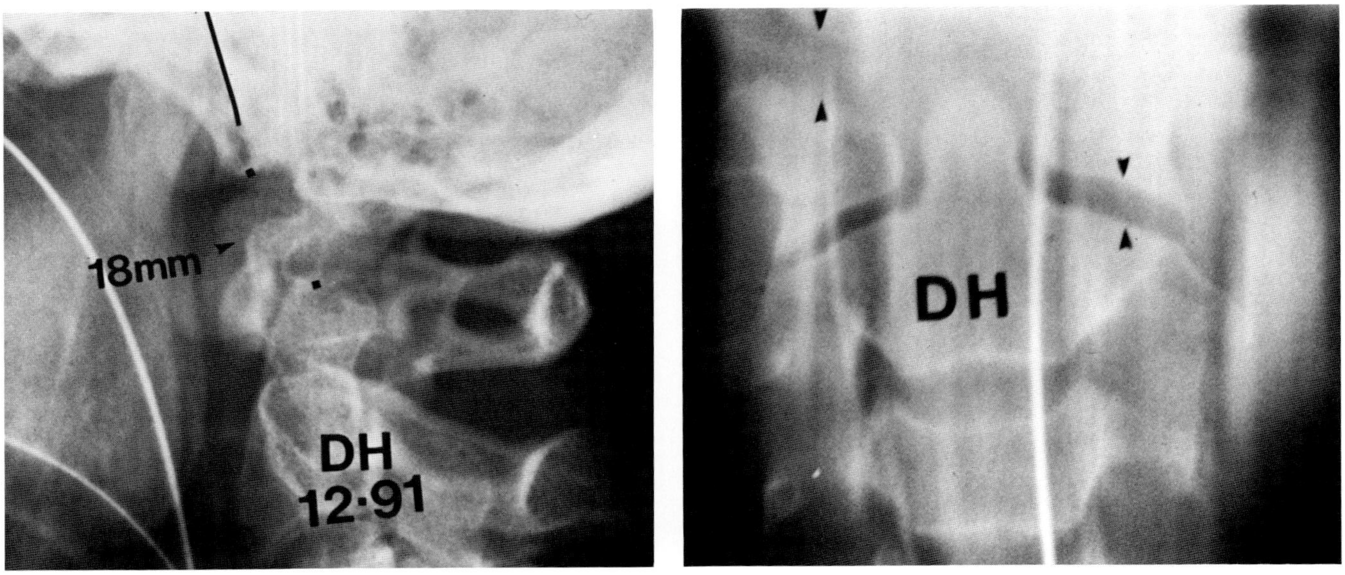

A B

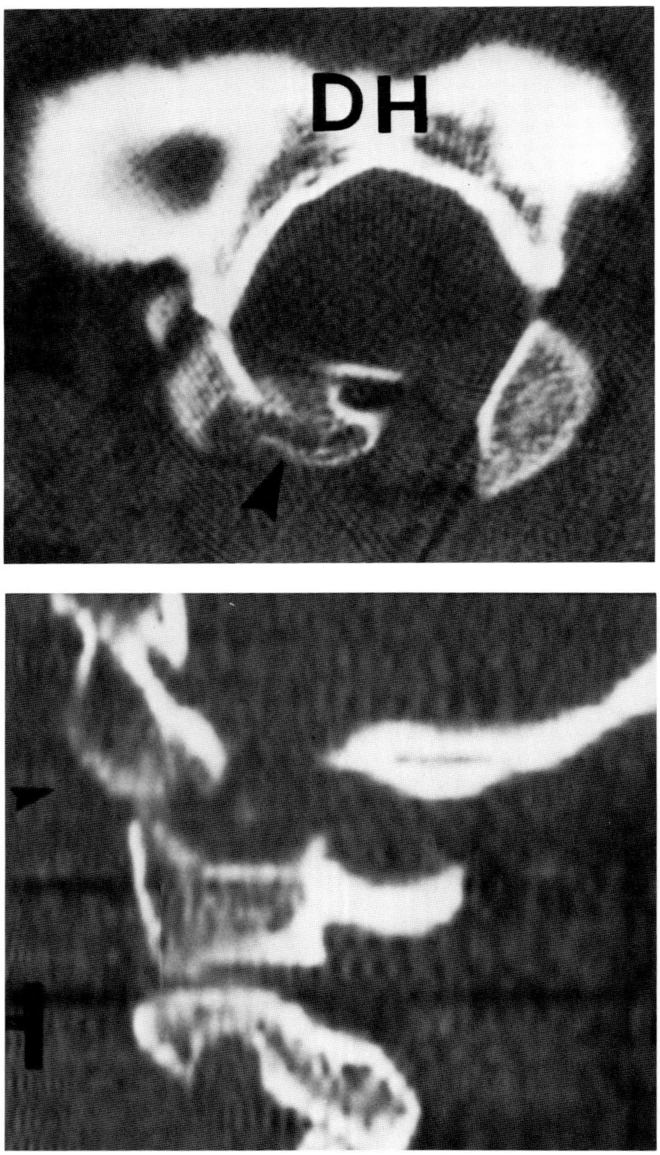

C D

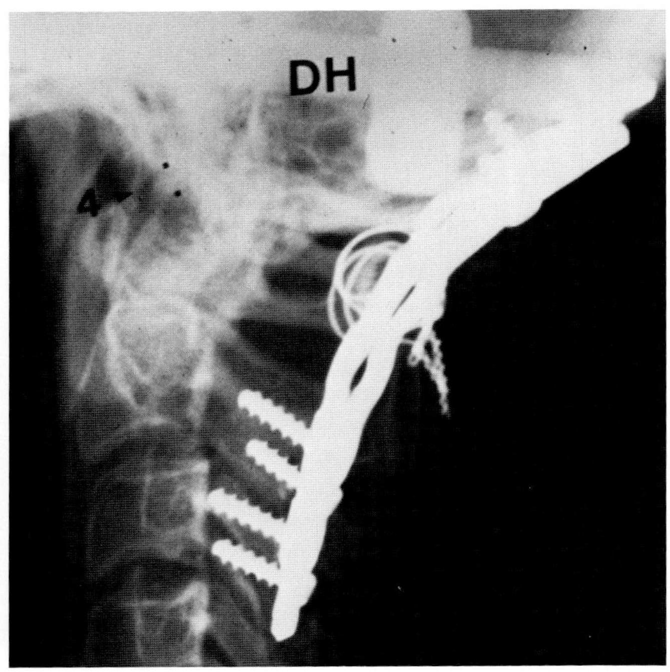

E

FIG. 9. A: Lateral radiograph of 23-year-old woman after a motorcycle accident. The clivus is pointing anterior to the dens and the distance between the basion and dens tip measures 18 mm. **B:** AP tomograms showing distance between the occipital condyles and atlas on the right and between the atlas and axis facet joints on the left. **C:** A displaced right type II occipital condyle fracture is noted on axial CT. **D:** Anterior subluxation of the occipital condyles on C-1 is noted on CT reformations. **E:** Reduction was achieved by gentle head extension. Postoperative radiographs of occipitocervical fusion with AO reconstruction plate.

COMPLICATIONS

These injuries often exhibit subtle radiographic findings and the diagnosis is often delayed. Complete ligament disruption makes atlanto–occipital dislocations highly unstable and, consequently, reduction may be lost during the postoperative period. Radiographs are taken at frequent intervals to ensure maintenance of proper alignment.

SKELETALLY IMMATURE PATIENTS

Atlanto–occipital dislocations are common in children and the occipitocervical articulation must be carefully evaluated in all pediatric trauma patients.

REFERENCES

1. Werne S. Studies in spontaneous atlas dislocation. *Acta Orthop Scand* 1957;23(Suppl):1–140.
2. Anderson PA, Montesano PX. Morphology and treatment of occipital condyle fractures. *Spine* 1988;13:731–6.
3. Traynelis VC, Marano GD, Dunker RO, Kaufman HH. Traumatic atlanto–occipital dislocation: case report. *J Neurosurg* 1988;65:863–70.
4. Wholey MH, Breuwer AJ, Hillier LB. Lateral roentgenogram of the neck with comments on the atlanto-odontoid-basion relationship. *Radiology* 1958;71:350–6.
5. Wertheim SB, Bohlman HH. Occipitocervical fusion. Indications, technique, and long-term results in thirteen patients. *J Bone Joint Surg* 1987;69A:833–6.

C-1 Injuries: Fractures and Transverse Ligament Ruptures

MECHANISMS OF INJURY

Fractures of the atlas usually result from axial loading or hyperextension mechanisms. Associated spinal injuries, especially odontoid fractures, occur in approximately 10% of all cases, but fortunately neurologic injuries are rare. Transverse ligament ruptures with atlantoaxial subluxation occur from hyperflexion or direct blows to the occiput.

ANATOMIC CONSIDERATIONS

The atlas ring is formed by the anterior and posterior arches that connect the lateral masses. The odontoid process of C-2 projects into the atlas ring and is held in place by the transverse ligament. The space between the anterior arch and the dens is called the atlanto–dens interval (ADI). The ADI is normally less than 3 mm in adults and 5 mm in children. Widening greater than 10 mm indicates damage to the secondary ligament restraints, such as the alar ligaments and the tectorial membrane (1). Associated injury of these ligament structures can result in combined atlantoaxial and atlanto–occipital instabilities (2).

Three- or four-part burst fractures of the C-1 ring that occur secondary to axial loading are called Jefferson's fractures (3). Once the ring is fractured, further loading forces the lateral masses into outward displacement, a force that is resisted by the transverse ligament. Rupture of the transverse ligament occurs when the combined displacement of the lateral masses of the atlas is greater than 7 mm (4).

CLASSIFICATION

C-1 Injuries

Fractures of the atlas include posterior ring, anterior ring, lateral mass, and Jefferson's fractures. Posterior ring and lateral mass fractures are stable injuries; anterior ring fractures may be unstable owing to associated posterior atlantoaxial displacement. Jefferson's fractures are stable when the transverse ligament is intact and unstable when it is ruptured (Fig. 10).

ASSESSMENT

Physical Examination

Patients complain of pain in the upper cervical or occipital region and have localized tenderness at C-1 and C-2. Surprisingly, patients with transverse ligament ruptures may have few clinical symptoms at the time of the initial examination.

Radiographic Evaluation

Fracture lines extending into the arches of the atlas are often obscured by overlying bony structures and may not be visible on plain radiographs. An open-mouth odontoid view is essential for assessing outward displacement of the lateral masses of C-1 in relation to C-2. In addition, the symmetry of the dens should be assessed in relation to the adjacent lateral masses.

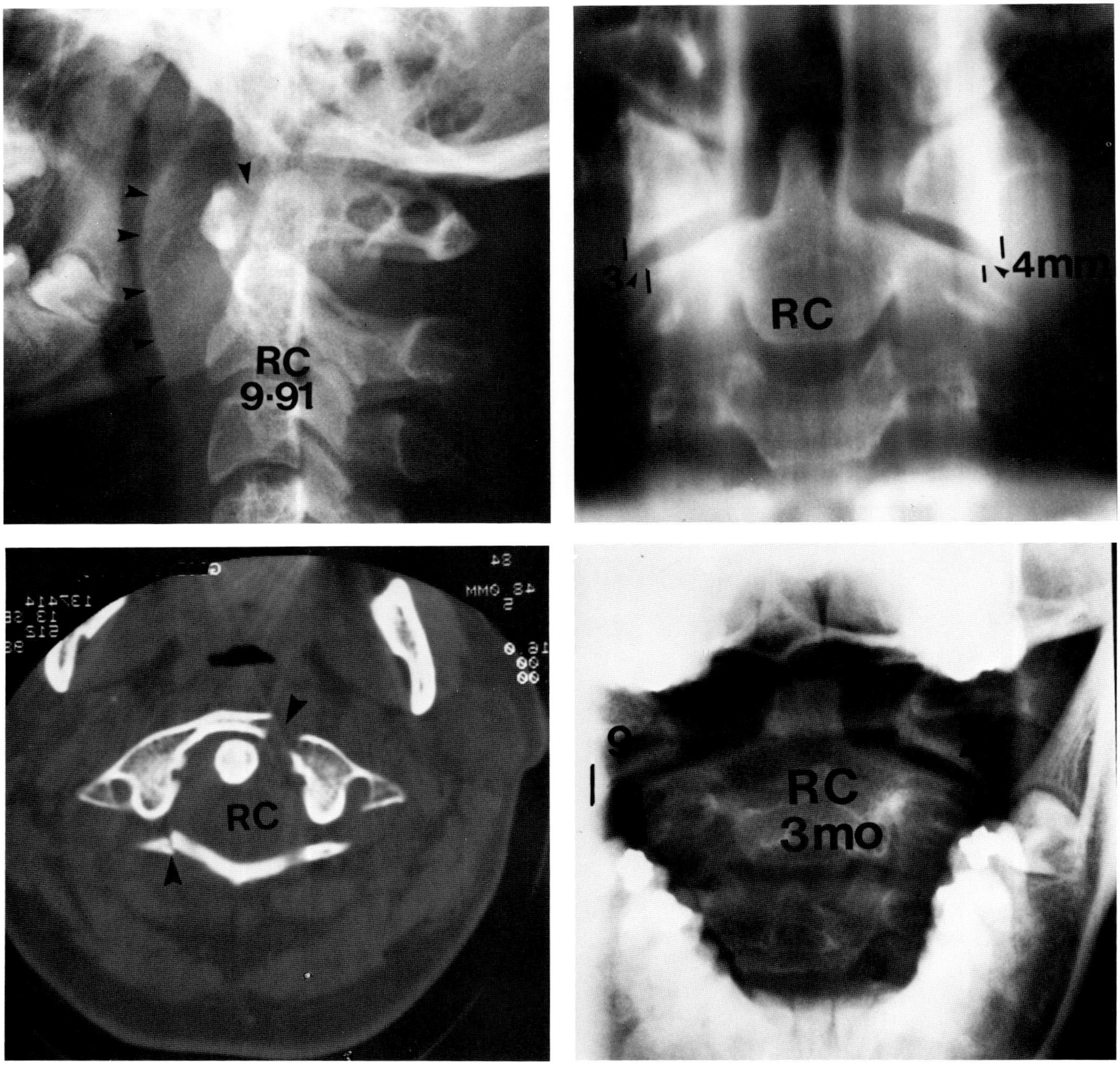

FIG. 10. A: Lateral radiograph of 16-year-old girl. Retropharyngeal soft tissue swelling anterior to C1-2 is noted. Increased ADI is indicative of transverse ligament injury. **B:** AP tomography demonstrates a total of 7 mm spreading of the lateral masses of C-1. **C:** A two-part burst-type fracture of C-2 is noted on CT. **D:** Open-mouth radiograph 3 months after halo treatment. Increased spreading of the C-1 lateral masses to 12 mm is noted.

Special Studies

Axial CT scans with coronal reconstructions are required to properly understand the underlying pathology and to plan appropriate treatment. Occasionally, posterior arch fractures seen on CT scans are, in fact, old injuries or congenital defects. Coronal reconstructions are useful for assessing the amount of outward displacement in Jefferson's fractures and for identifying avulsion fractures at the transverse ligament attachment of C-1.

EMERGENT MANAGEMENT

Patients are managed with tong traction until definitive treatment can be carried out. Reduction of the fracture may be

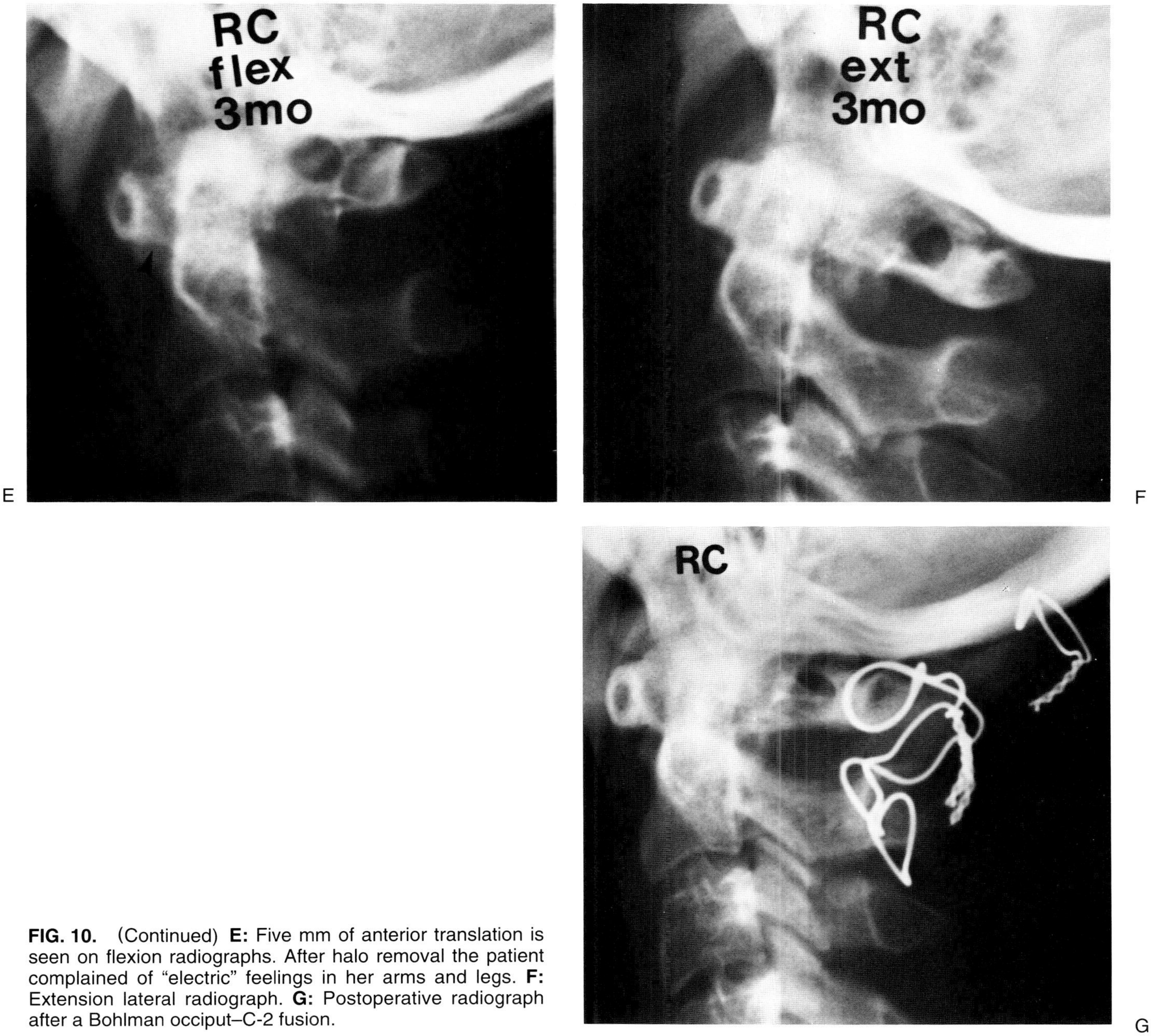

FIG. 10. (Continued) **E:** Five mm of anterior translation is seen on flexion radiographs. After halo removal the patient complained of "electric" feelings in her arms and legs. **F:** Extension lateral radiograph. **G:** Postoperative radiograph after a Bohlman occiput–C-2 fusion.

difficult and often is best accomplished by adjusting the relative position of the head to the thorax. Head extension is required when the transverse ligament is ruptured.

DEFINITIVE MANAGEMENT

C-1 Fractures

Isolated posterior ring fractures are stable injuries that can be treated by immobilization in a cervicothoracic orthosis for 6 to 8 weeks. Anterior ring fractures may be associated with posterior displacement of C-1 on C-2. Treatment of this fracture pattern requires closed reduction and halo-vest immobilization for 8 to 12 weeks.

Stable Jefferson's fractures without transverse ligament involvement are treated by immobilization in a halo vest for 8 to 12 weeks. Unstable Jefferson's fractures are also treated by halo-vest immobilization but require close radiographic surveillance for progressive outward displacement of the lateral masses of C-1. If residual C-1 and C-2 instability remains after the halo vest is removed, late posterior fusion of C-1 and C-2 may be required.

Transverse Ligament Ruptures

Transverse ligament ruptures are highly unstable injuries that require posterior fusion of C-1 and C-2. Posterior arthrodesis of C-1 and C-2 is performed with the fracture reduced and the patient immobilized in a halo vest. The arthrodesis is performed by the Gallie technique (5) and autogenous iliac bone grafting.

COMPLICATIONS

Injuries to the C-1 and C-2 vertebral bodies frequently result in permanent loss of cervical rotation. Patients must be warned of this eventuality early in treatment so that their expectations for future function are realistic.

SKELETALLY IMMATURE PATIENTS

The treatment of upper cervical spinal injuries in children is identical to that in adults.

REFERENCES

1. Fielding JW, Cochran GVB, Lawsing JF III, Hohl M. Tears of the transverse ligament of the atlas. *J Bone Joint Surg* 1974;56A:1683–91.
2. Anderson PA. Occipital cervical instability associated with traumatic tears of the transverse ligament. *Orthop Trans* 12:41. 1988.
3. Schlicke LH, Callahan RA. A rational approach to burst fractures of the atlas. *Clin Orthop* 1981;154:18–21.
4. Spence KF Jr, Decker S, Sell KW. Bursting atlantal fracture associated with rupture of the transverse ligament. *J Bone Joint Surg* 1970;52A:543–9.
5. Fielding WJ, Hawkins RJ, Ratzan SA. Spine fusion for atlantoaxial instability. *J Bone Joint Surg* 1976;58A:400–7.

C-2 Fractures: Odontoid Fractures and Hangman's Fractures

MECHANISMS OF INJURY

Fractures of the odontoid process occur in 7% to 10% of all cervical spinal injuries. The usual mechanism of injury is forced extension of the head and neck secondary to a fall or a collision, e.g., striking the head on the dashboard or windshield of an automobile in a motor vehicle accident. Associated fractures of the atlas occur in 10% to 15% of these cases.

Fractures through the pars interarticularis of the axis are commonly called hangman's fractures because their pathology is similar to fractures caused by judicial hangings. The high frequency of associated facial trauma attests to the mechanism of injury, which is usually hyperextension of the neck. Because the size of the spinal canal is enlarged by this injury, neurologic deficits are rare.

ANATOMIC CONSIDERATIONS

The odontoid process projects from the body of C-2 and is narrowest at the waist, where it is most commonly fractured. The pars interarticularis of C-2 lies between the anteriorly placed superior articular facets and the posteriorly placed inferior facets. This small tubular bone can be easily fractured by forced extension. After fracture, the anterior longitudinal ligament, the C2-3 disc annulus, and the posterior longitudinal ligament are stressed and may progressively fail.

CLASSIFICATION

Odontoid Fractures

Anderson and D'Alonzo (1) based their classification of odontoid fractures on the location of the fracture (Fig. 11).

Type I: rare, stable avulsion fractures of the tip of the dens
Type II: unstable transverse fractures in the cortical bone of the waist of the dens
Type III: unstable fractures in the cancellous bone of the body of C-2.

Hangman's Fractures

Bucholz (2) described hangman's fractures as stable or unstable injuries on the basis of the amount of C2-3 discoligament injury associated with the fracture. Stable hangman's fractures are minimally displaced and the C2-3 disc is intact. In unstable hangman's fractures, the C2-3 disc is disrupted, resulting in C2-3 vertebral body subluxation. A rare third type of hangman's fracture was identified by Levine and Edwards (3). This injury consists of fracture of the pars interarticularis and dislocation of the C2-3 facet joints.

ASSESSMENT

Physical Examination

Patients with C-2 fractures complain of occipital and upper cervical pain and experience tenderness at the C-2 spinous process. Although neurologic injuries are rare, 10% of patients with odontoid fractures have associated spinal cord injuries.

Radiographic Evaluation

An odontoid fracture is the most commonly missed spinal fracture. High-quality lateral and AP open-mouth radi-

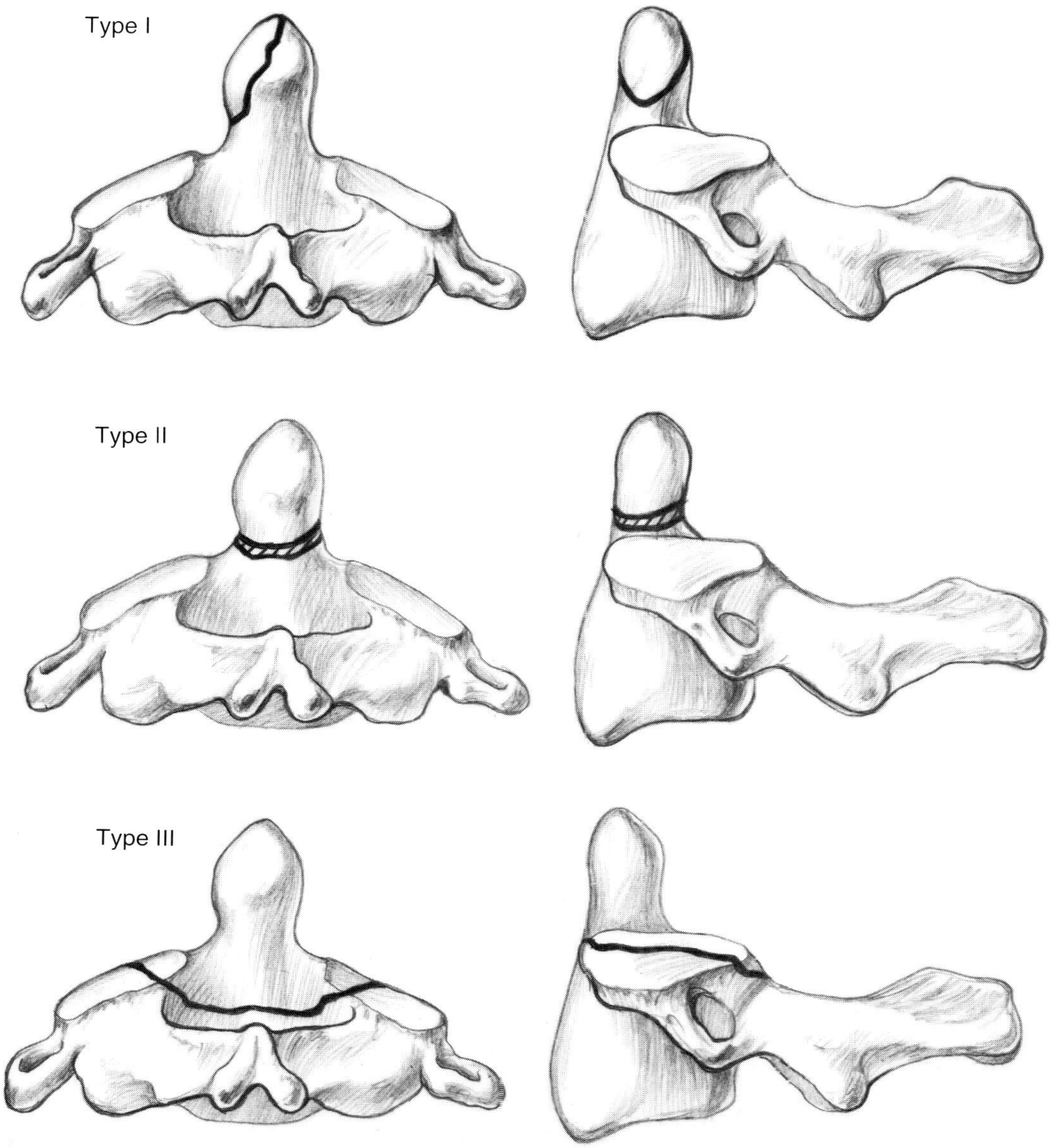

FIG. 11. Anderson and D'Alonzo classification of odontoid fractures.

ographic views are required to evaluate this injury. A subtle but important finding is soft-tissue swelling greater than 5 mm adjacent to the body of C-3.

Special Studies

Nondisplaced odontoid fractures, especially those occurring in the transverse plane, can be difficult to identify on routine radiographs or CT scans. Anteroposterior and lateral polytomography may be warranted in questionable cases.

EMERGENT MANAGEMENT

Patients with nondisplaced hangman's fractures or odontoid fractures are immobilized in a cervical collar until definitive treatment can be provided. Displaced fractures are reduced by cranial-tong traction and careful head positioning.

DEFINITIVE MANAGEMENT

Odontoid Fractures

Type II odontoid fractures are associated with a high incidence of nonunion (15–85%). Risk factors for nonunion include initial fracture displacement of more than 4 mm (4), age greater than 50 years, posterior displacement, incomplete reduction, and inappropriate initial treatment. Treatment of type II injuries is based on the amount of initial fracture displacement and the presence of associated cervical fractures. Patients with nondisplaced or minimally displaced type II fractures are immobilized in a halo\vest for 8 to 12 weeks.

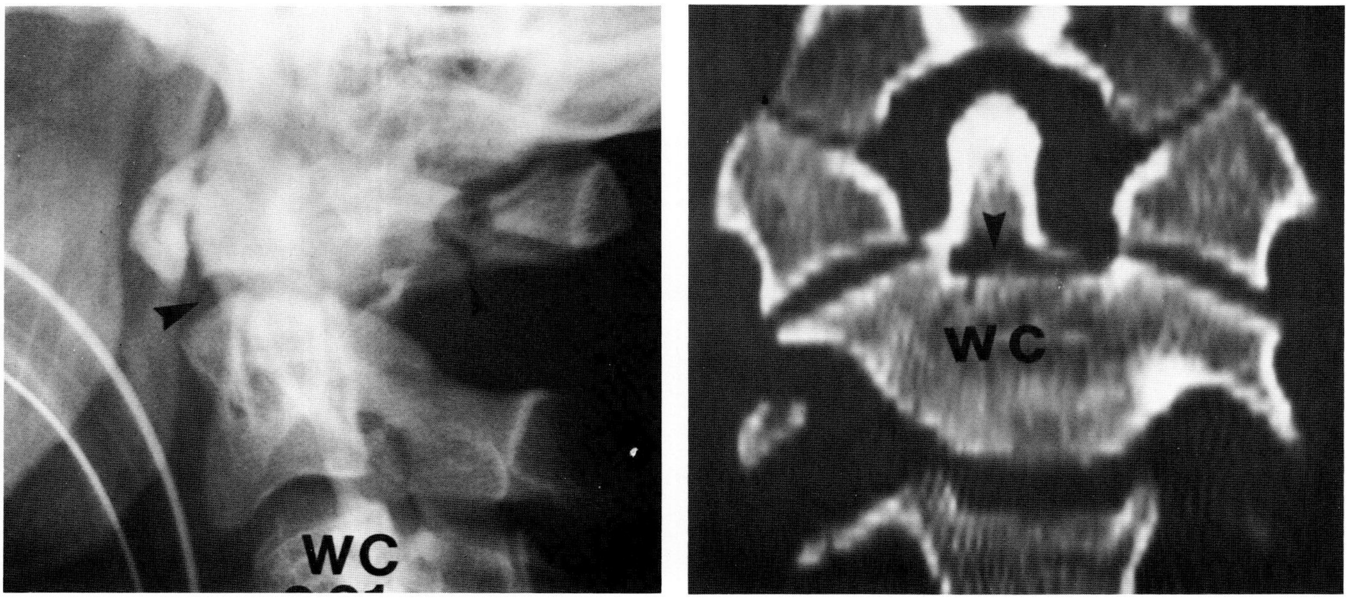

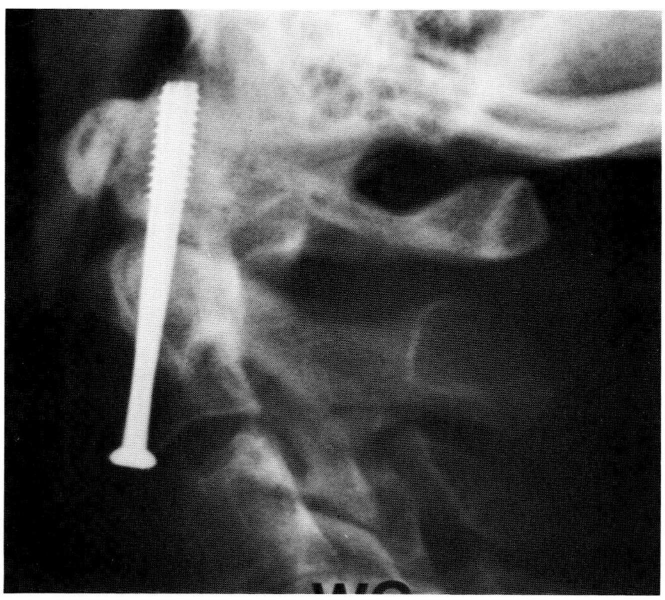

FIG. 12. **A:** Lateral radiograph of 20-year-old respiratory-dependent quadriplegic secondary to type II odontoid fracture and Jefferson's fracture of C-1. **B:** Coronal reconstruction showing fracture of the waist of the odontoid. **C:** Patient was treated with odontoid screw fixation because of skin breakdown in halo vest.

The prognosis for union of displaced type II fractures is poor and they are treated by posterior fusion of C-1 and C-2.

Displaced type II odontoid fractures with associated C-1 ring fractures present a more difficult challenge. These injuries can be treated initially by immobilization in a halo vest, followed by late posterior fusion of C-1 and C-2 in the event of nonunion. An alternative treatment for this complex injury is anterior fixation with two odontoid screws (5). The anterior cervical spine is approached through a Smith–Robinson retropharyngeal incision. Fixation is provided by two cannulated lag screws that are placed from the anterior-inferior corner of the body of C-2 into the tip of the dens (Fig. 12). The patient is immobilized in a halo vest for 6 weeks postoperatively.

Type III odontoid fractures are treated by immobilization in a halo vest for 3 months or until healing occurs.

Hangman's Fractures

The prognosis for union of a hangman's fracture treated with a cervical orthosis is excellent, and this injury should not be overtreated. Stable hangman's fractures are treated in a cervicothoracic orthosis for 8 to 10 weeks. Reduction of an unstable hangman's fracture can be attempted by tong traction and head extension. Absolute anatomic reduction may be difficult to achieve, but fractures healing in 2 mm to 6 mm of displacement are not usually associated with any long-term

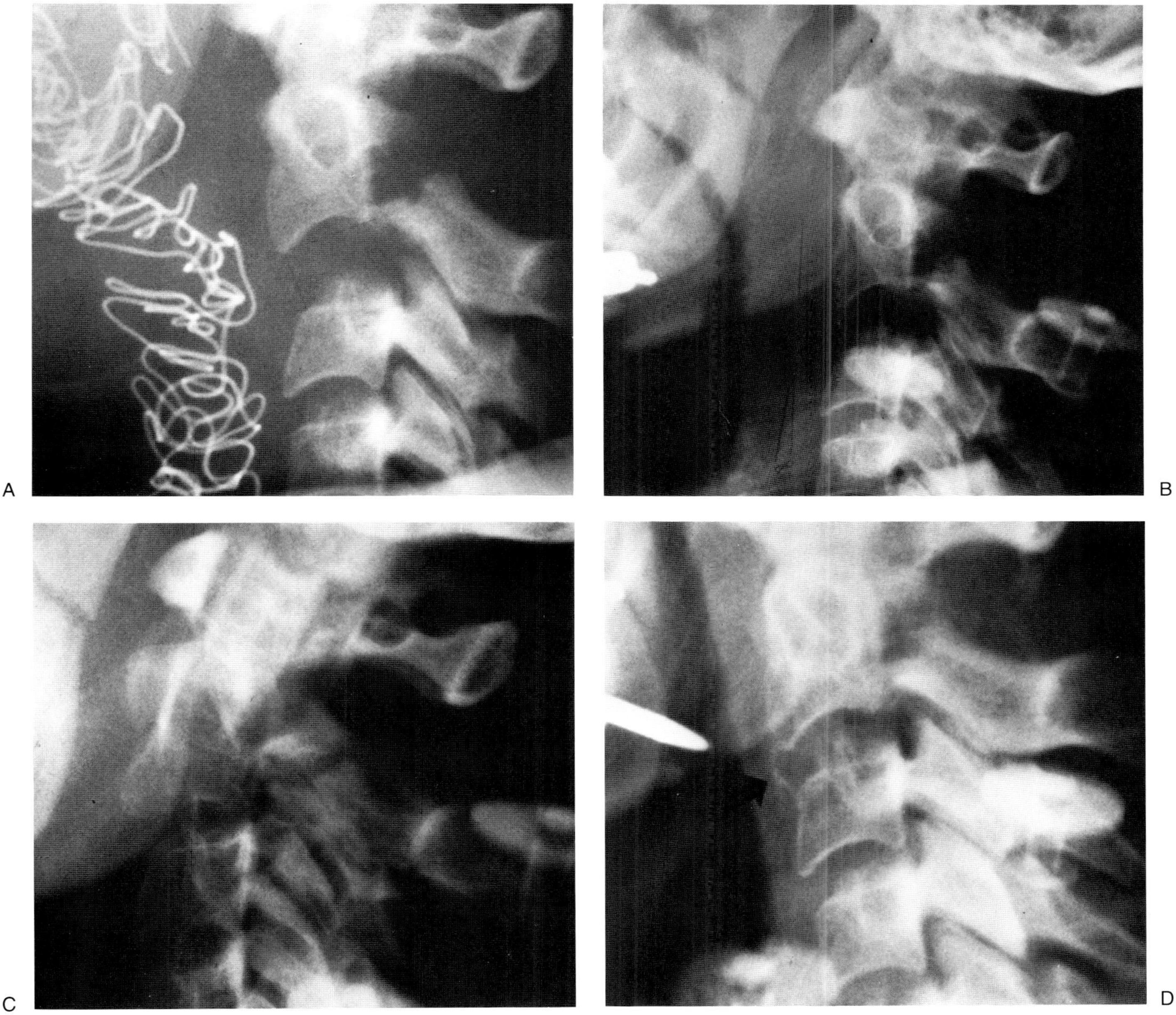

FIG. 13. **A:** Initial lateral radiograph of a distracted unstable hangman's fracture. Gauze packing is noted which controlled life-threatening hemorrhage from oral pharynx. **B:** The fracture remains distracted and anteriorly angulated when patient is supine in a halo vest. **C:** Lateral radiograph taken upright demonstrates excellent reduction. The patient was treated in a halo vest upright for 2 months. **D:** Two months after injury the fracture remains anatomically reduced and a spontaneous fusion of C2-3 is noted.

adverse sequelae. After reduction the spine is immobilized in a halo vest for 12 weeks (Fig. 13).

The halo vest is usually applied 1 or 2 days after injury. This procedure is done in a well-controlled environment. The ring should clear the cranium by 1 cm. The patient's scalp is shaved just behind and above the ears. The skin is infiltrated with local anesthetic to the level of the periosteum and prepared with a Betadine solution. The ring is placed at the level of the skull equator or just below, 1 cm above the eyebrows and just above the tips of the ears. While an assistant holds the patient's head and neck, the ring is positioned with temporary positioning plates. The screws are inserted, tightened by hand, and torqued to 6 inch-pounds (6).

The vest is then applied by log-rolling the patient and attaching the vest to the ring with upright supports. After application, supine and upright lateral radiographs are obtained to rule out excessive motion at the fracture site. The screws are torqued once again 24 h later and the locking nuts are applied. The pins are cleansed with hydrogen peroxide and water twice daily. The patient is mobilized as early as possible and is seen in the outpatient department twice monthly to check the pin care and to tighten the vest hardware. The upright supports are loosened after 3 months and flexion–extension radiographs are obtained at that time. If the radiographs demonstrate healing, the halo vest can be removed and substituted with a soft collar until the neck musculature is rehabilitated.

COMPLICATIONS

Fracture reduction may be lost during treatment and occasionally traction may have to be reapplied. Halo pin-tract infections are initially treated by local wound care and oral antibiotics. Pins that are loose or have persistent drainage can be retightened judiciously once or twice. Persistent loosening requires reinsertion at a different site. Nonunions of odontoid fractures are treated by posterior fusion of C-1 and C-2.

SKELETALLY IMMATURE PATIENTS

In children, the synchondrosis between the dens and body of C-2 may be mistaken for an odontoid fracture. The synchondrosis is present in children up to the age of 7 years and is located in the C-2 body, not at the odontoid waist. The odontoid should not be angulated or distracted at the synchondrosis. No growth center exists posteriorly in the pars interarticularis and a defect at this location is probably a true fracture.

The treatment of odontoid fractures and hangman's fractures in children is approached much more conservatively than treatment in adults because of the greater potential for healing and bone remodeling. Before halo-pin placement in children, a head CT scan should be obtained to ensure adequate bone stock. In young children, just 2 inch-pounds of torque (hand tightened) may be applied, and therefore 6 to 8 pins are required.

REFERENCES

1. Anderson LD, D'Alonzo RT. Fractures of the odontoid process of the axis. *J Bone Joint Surg* 1974;56-A:1663–74.
2. Bucholz RW. Unstable hangman's fractures. *Clin Orthop* 1981;154:119–24.
3. Levine AM, Edwards CC. The management of traumatic spondylolisthesis. *J Bone Joint Surg* 1985;67A:217–26.
4. Dickman CA, Hadley MN, Browner C, Sonntag VK. Neurological management of acute atlas-axis combination fractures. *J Neurosurg* 1989;70:45–9.
5. Böhler J. Anterior stabilization for acute fractures and nonunions of the dens. *J Bone Joint Surg* 1982;64A:18–27.
6. Garfin SR, Botte MJ, Waters RL, Nickel VL. Complications in the use of the halo fixation device. *J Bone Joint Surg* 1986;68A:320–5.

Lower Cervical Spine: Minor Stable Fractures, Facet Dislocations, Burst Fractures, and Extension Injuries

MECHANISM OF INJURY

Injuries to the lower cervical spine or the spinal cord usually occur indirectly as the result of a blow to the cranium or from rapid head deceleration. The mechanisms of injury include flexion, axial loading, rotation, and extension. Fracture patterns depend on the vertebral alignment at the time of injury, the force vector, and the physical characteristics of the patient. It is doubtful that any muscular force can react quickly enough to prevent or lessen such an injury.

ANATOMIC CONSIDERATIONS

All the lower cervical vertebrae (C-3 through C-7) share similar anatomic and biomechanic characteristics. The posterior ligaments, the intervertebral disc and annulus, and the relatively large facet joints are important for stability. These joints project upwards at a 45° angle and prevent anterior translation. White et al. (1) determined that the cervical spine becomes unstable when all the posterior ligaments and one anterior structure are damaged or when all the anterior ligaments and one posterior structure are damaged. Under these conditions, the amount of anterior translation is 3.5 mm or greater and the amount of angulation is 11° or greater in the injured structures than at adjacent levels. Other clinical signs of instability include spinal cord or nerve root injury, vertical distraction, and combined anterior and posterior columnar injuries.

CLASSIFICATION

Minor Stable Fractures

Minor injuries include laminar fractures, spinous process fractures, lateral mass fractures without vertebral body displacement, and avulsion fractures of the anterior longitudinal ligament. These are usually stable injuries that occur with hyperextension and are not associated with neurologic deficits. Flexion injuries include vertebral compression fractures without posterior wall involvement and grade I or II ligament injuries.

Facet Dislocations

Anterior vertebral translation is normally prevented by facet orientation, posterior ligament structure, and the disc annulus. Translation of 25% occurs under three conditions: unilateral facet dislocations, bilateral perched facet fractures, and facet fracture–dislocations. In unilateral dislocations the spinous process is rotated to the side of facet dislocations on AP radiographs. Bilateral facet dislocations result in at least 50% body translation. Interspinous process widening is an important sign of posterior ligament injury. Computerized tomography is useful to identify facet fractures and malalignments. Magnetic resonance imaging has been used successfully to identify intervertebral disc herniation in 35% of bilateral dislocations and in 15% of unilateral cases (2).

Burst Fractures

Axial loading can fracture the vertebral body and retropulse bony fragments into the spinal canal. When this mechanism is combined with flexion (e.g., in diving injuries), a teardrop fracture is produced (3). In this injury, the fractured anterior–inferior corner of the vertebral body forms a teardrop shape and the remaining vertebral body is rotated posteriorly into the canal. In addition, rupture of the posterior ligament structures produces kyphosis and a highly unstable fracture (Fig. 14). Under these conditions, spinal cord damage is often severe.

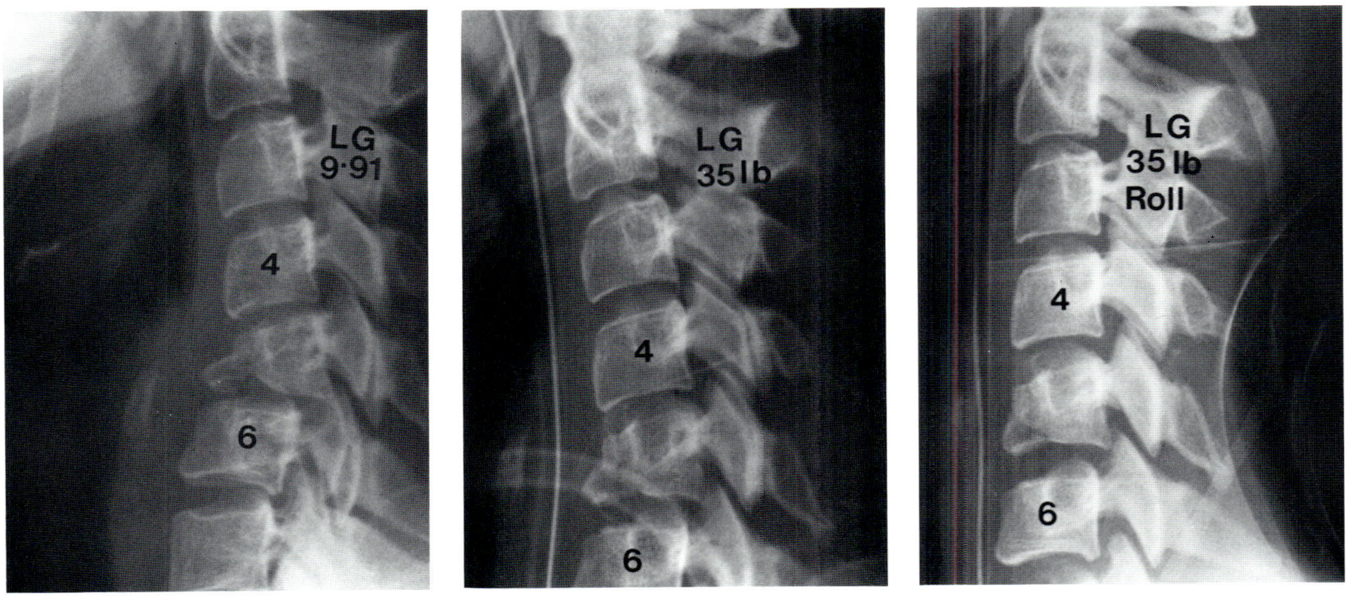

A B,C

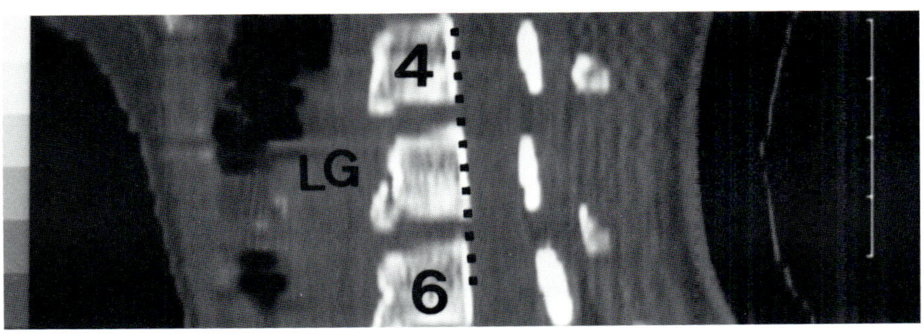

D

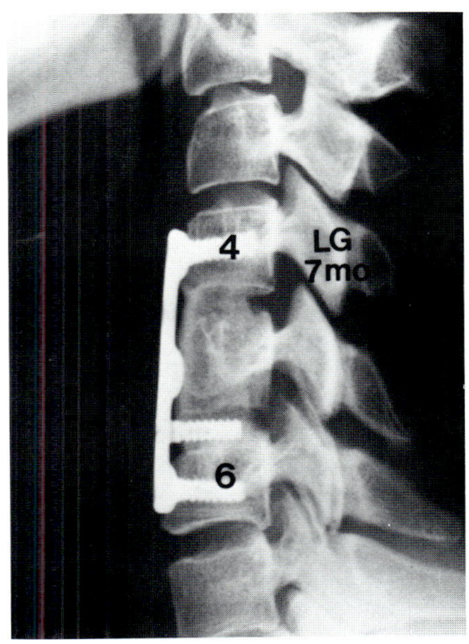

E

FIG. 14. A: Lateral radiograph of a 19-year-old woman with incomplete quadriplegia secondary to burst fracture of C-5. Kyphosis, retropulsion of the C-5 body into the spinal canal, and interspinous widening can be visualized. **B:** Thirty-five pounds of traction reduces the retropulsed bone fragment but not the kyphotic deformity. **C:** A roll placed behind the cervical spinal reduces the kyphotic deformity. **D:** CT reconstruction demonstrating excellent spinal realignment. **E:** She was treated with anterior decompression of C-5 and reconstruction with iliac bone graft and a Morscher cervical locking plate.

Extension Injuries

Schneider and Knighton (4) described a syndrome consisting of damage to the cervical spinal cord in patients without any obvious spinal fractures. Hyperextension occurring in patients with narrow spinal canals results in compression of the spinal cord between the bulging disc and the infolded ligamentum flavum. Neurologically, this injury produces a central cord syndrome in which patients retain better lower extremity function than upper extremity function. The prognosis for recovery in the lower extremities is good, although many patients experience residual loss of hand function.

ASSESSMENT

Physical Examination

The clinical examination of a patient with a lower cervical spinal cord injury is similar to that of a patient with any spinal fracture. Important indications of injury are isolated cervical tenderness, a palpable gap between the spinous process, and neurologic deficits. Special attention must be paid to testing all the muscle groups in the upper extremity to identify subtle radiculopathies.

Radiologic Evaluation

High-quality biplanar radiographs are obtained of the entire cervical spine. Interspinous widening and rotation of the spinous processes are seen on AP radiographic views. Widening of the interspinous process is an ominous sign of posterior ligament instability (see Fig. 2). The alignment of the posterior vertebral body and the spinolaminar line should be scrutinized. The articular facets normally cannot be seen on AP radiographic views and their presence is suggestive of a facet fracture–dislocation.

Special Studies

Computerized tomography is performed on all patients with cervical spinal injuries to identify facet fractures and malalignments. Magnetic resonance imaging or myelography is warranted in patients with progressive or unexplained neural deficits. These diagnostic procedures should be performed before surgical treatment to assess disc pathology, foraminal patency, and possible epidural hematoma formation.

EMERGENT MANAGEMENT

Minor Stable Fractures

Patients with stable injuries are immobilized with a cervical collar. Tong traction is applied only to patients who are to undergo concurrent procedures such as femoral intramedulary nailing or pelvic fixation.

Facet Dislocations

Methylprednisolone is given to patients with spinal cord injuries according to the protocols outlined above. Rapid closed reduction is accomplished by tong traction and weights. Because all the major surrounding ligaments are potentially damaged, overdistraction is possible and must be avoided. If reduction cannot be achieved by closed methods, open reduction and internal fixation are indicated. Closed manual manipulation is not recommended.

Burst Fractures

Spinal realignment and reduction of the retropulsed fragments can be achieved by axial traction. Up to 70% of the body's weight can be used without incurring complications in burst fractures. After reduction, the amount of traction weight can be reduced, but the fracture must be monitored radiographically to ensure maintenance of reduction.

Extension Injuries

Patients who have sustained an extension injury concurrently with a central cord syndrome should be placed in traction even when no evidence of an acute injury is found radiographically. This precaution protects the cord from possible further injury and reduces small malalignments, such as 1 mm to 2 mm of retrolisthesis. Traction can be used to open the canal by applying tension to the ligamentum flavum and pulling it out of the spinal cord.

DEFINITIVE MANAGEMENT

Minor Stable Fractures

Stable cervical injuries are treated in a cervical orthosis for 8 to 12 weeks. After immobilization, flexion–extension radiographs are taken to confirm adequate healing. These minor injuries occasionally displace during treatment and must be monitored by serial radiographs.

Facet Dislocations

Posterior cervical fusion is performed on all patients with bilateral facet dislocations. Surgery is delayed until 5 to 7 days after injury to avoid neurologic deterioration, which occasionally occurs in quadriplegic patients treated within 5 days of trauma (5). Before surgical treatment the status of the intervertebral disc is determined by CT scanning, myelography, or MRI. If the disc is retropulsed into the spinal canal it should be removed before posterior cervical fusion. If the facet cannot be reduced preoperatively, reduction can be easily accomplished during surgery by applying traction to the spinous process or by levering the dislocated facet joint with an elevator. Rarely, a small portion of the facet must be removed to aid reduction.

The treatment of unilateral facet dislocations is controversial. Closed treatment in a halo vest is frequently unsuccessful because reduction can be lost (6). Better results are achieved when anatomic alignment has been maintained; therefore, posterior cervical fusion is recommended for patients with unilateral facet dislocations and those with facet fracture–dislocations (7).

Burst Fractures

Patients with stable burst fractures without associated neurologic injuries are treated in a halo vest for 12 weeks. Anterior decompression and strut fusion are performed in patients who have sustained stable burst fractures with associated neurologic injuries. Late anterior decompression is indicated in patients who fail to improve neurologically and for those with persistent cord compression.

The technique for posterior cervical fusion for burst fractures or facet fracture–dislocations requires coordination between the anesthesiologist and the surgeon. Nasotrachial intubation is performed with a fiberoptic light system on an alert patient. The patient is transferred to a Stryker frame and placed in a prone position. After a neurologic examination is repeated and a lateral radiograph is obtained to confirm adequate alignment, general anesthesia is administered. Spinal cord monitoring is performed when intraoperative reduction is anticipated. A modified Rogers wiring technique provides adequate fixation for ligament injuries with intact bony structures (8). Posterior cervical plate fixation is indicated in fractures with associated posterior ligament instability and in burst fracture patterns (9). With this technique, the fracture is reduced by traction weight and fixed internally with 2.7-mm or 3.5-mm reconstruction plates affixed to the lateral masses with screws (Fig. 15). Autogenous iliac cancellous bone graft is placed in the decorticated facet joint and along the lamina and spinous processes.

Extension Injuries

Patients with extension injuries without fracture can be mobilized in a cervical collar after 5 to 7 days in traction.

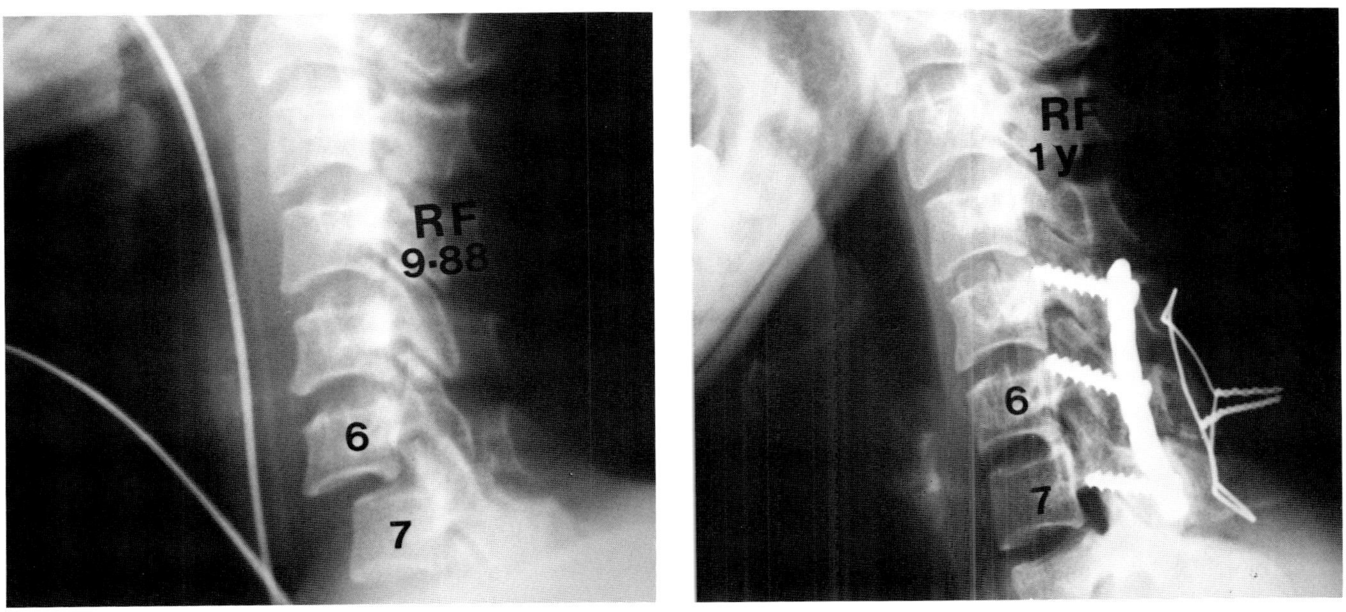

FIG. 15. **A:** Lateral radiograph of a 25-year-old construction worker who sustained a C6-7 bilateral facet dislocation. The patient has a C-6 complete quadriplegia. Reduction was achieved with tong traction within 90 minutes of injury. Immediately after reduction he regained motor function in his legs. Three days later he was neurologically intact. **B:** Posterior cervical plate fixation with AO reconstruction plates.

Because the prognosis for nonoperative management of these injuries is generally good, no initial surgical treatment is required. If a patient fails to make a satisfactory recovery and cord compression is documented by myelography or MRI, late anterior decompression should be considered.

COMPLICATIONS

Complications in lower cervical spine injuries are usually related to the sequelae of quadriplegia. Patients selected for nonoperative treatment must be followed by serial radiography to document maintenance of spinal alignment. Patients with seemingly benign injuries sometimes sustain occult ligament instability and displacement during treatment. Patients with anterior vertebral body compression with concurrent posterior ligament damage are especially prone to failure of closed-treatment methods.

SKELETALLY IMMATURE PATIENTS

Injuries in the lower cervical spine are rare in children. When they occur, they are treated according to the same principles as fractures in adults.

REFERENCES

1. White AA, Southwick WO, Panjabi MM. Clinical instability of the spine. *Spine* 1976;1:15.
2. Pratt ES, Green DA, Spengler DM. Herniated intervertebral discs associated with unstable cervical spinal injuries. *Spine* 1990;15:662–5.
3. Schneider RC, Kahn EA. Chronic neurologic sequelae of acute trauma to the spine and spinal cord. Part I. The significance of the acute flexion or "teardrop" fracture-dislocation of the cervical spine. *J Bone Joint Surg* 1956;38A:985–91.
4. Schneider RC, Knighton R. Chronic neurological sequelae of acute trauma to the spine and spinal cord. The syndrome of chronic injury to the cervical spinal cord in the region of the central canal. *J Bone Joint Surg* 1959;41A:905–19.
5. Marshall LF, Knowlton S, Garfin SR, et al. Deterioration following spinal cord injury: a multicenter study. *J Neurosurg* 1987;66:400–4.
6. Böhler L: Fracture and dislocation of the spine. In: *The treatment of fractures,* 5th ed. New York: Grune and Stratton; 1956;300–467.
7. Beyer CA, Canbanela ME, Berquist TH. Unilateral facet dislocations and fracture-dislocations of the cervical spine. *Orthop Trans* 1990;14:681.
8. Coe JD, Warden KE, Sutterline CE, McAfee PC. Biomechanical evaluation of cervical spinal stabilization methods in human cadaveric model. *Spine* 1989;14:1122–31.
9. Anderson PA, Henley MB, Grady MS, Montesano PX, Winn HR. Posterior cervical arthrodesis using AO reconstruction plates and bone graft. *Spine* 1991;16:572–9.

Thoracolumbar Spine

MECHANISMS OF INJURY

Burst fractures of the thoracolumbar spine most commonly result from falls from heights or from rapid deceleration in vehicular accidents. Fracture–dislocations, especially in the thoracic spine, usually result from direct blows to the back or crushing from industrial accidents or from landing on the back after falling from a motorcycle. Seat-belt–related trauma, associated with Chance-type fractures and flexion–dislocation injuries, has increased since legislation has made the use of seat belts mandatory.

ANATOMIC CONSIDERATIONS

The thoracic (T-2 through T-10), thoracolumbar (T-11 through L-2), and lumbar (L-3 through L-5) segments of the spine are treated as separate entities because their skeletal anatomy, neurologic structure, and biomechanic functions are distinctly different. Although the fracture patterns that occur in all these segments are similar, the optimal treatment and prognosis of each fracture varies according to the level of the injury.

Motion in the thoracic spine is limited except for rotation. This spinal segment is more stable after fracture than other segments because it is supported by the rib attachments to the vertebrae and the rib cage. The thoracolumbar junction, a transitional area between the stiff thoracic spine and the mobile lumbar spine, is the most commonly injured segment. Fractures at the thoracolumbar junction are subject to large bending moments and are the most likely to angulate. The lumbar spine allows a wide range of flexion and extension but only limited rotation. The lordotic angulation in the lumbar spine makes kyphosis appear less important. However, the relative loss of lordosis must be considered when these injuries are treated.

Chest-wall and lung injuries are associated with translational injuries in the thoracic spine, and their presence may contraindicate early stabilization. Mediastinal widening secondary to paraspinal hemorrhage at the site of the spinal fracture is frequently observed and requires aortography to rule out injury to the aorta. Injuries to retroperitoneal structures, such as the pancreas, are associated with injuries to the lumbar spine.

CLASSIFICATION

Holdsworth (1), and later Whitesides (2), divided the spine into anterior and posterior columns. Injuries limited to one column are classified as stable fractures and those with injuries to both columns are unstable fractures. Denis (3) improved this classification with a three-column theory (Fig. 16). In this classification the anterior column consists of the anterior longitudinal ligament, the anterior two thirds of the vertebral body, and the disc annulus; the middle column consists of the posterior longitudinal ligament and the posterior third of the disc and the body; and the posterior column consists of all the posterior elements. Denis defined instability as mechanical and neurologic failure of any two of these three columns. McAfee et al. (4) used Denis' concepts and expanded the classification of thoracolumbar fractures into six patterns based on CT scans. This classification is the most useful for predicting fracture stability and directing treatment.

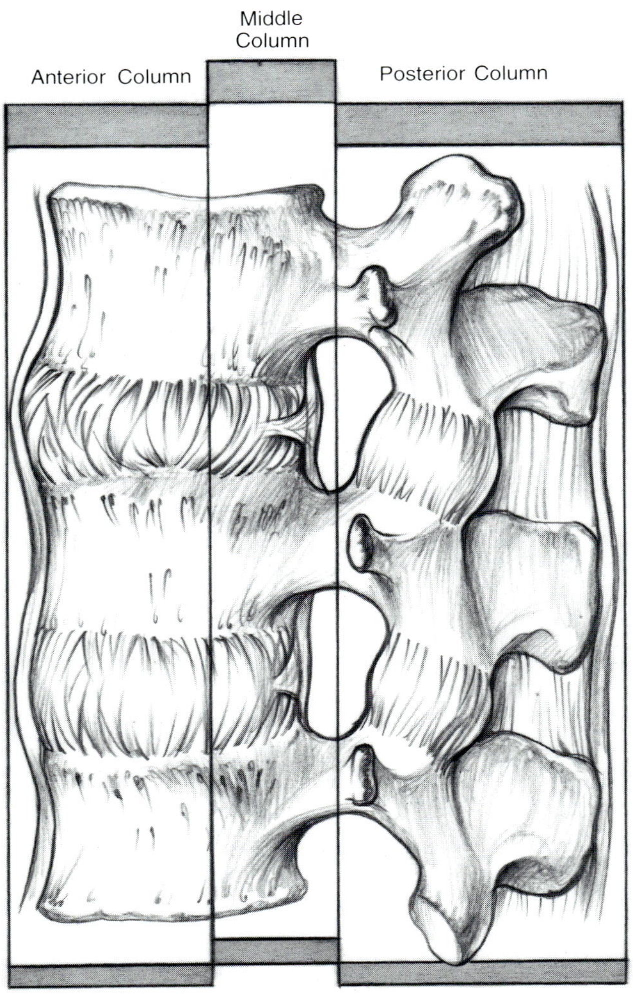

FIG. 16. Denis three-column spine.

Compression Fractures

Compression fractures result from axial loading or flexion forces and are limited to the anterior column (Fig. 17). Kyphotic angulation in these fractures is usually less than 10° and loss of anterior vertebral height is no greater than 40%. The goals of treatment are to prevent the progression of kyphosis and to minimize pain and disability.

Stable Burst Fractures

Burst fractures at the thoracolumbar junction are usually stable injuries. Fractures of both the anterior and middle columns can be seen on radiographs (Fig. 18). Bone is retropulsed into the spinal canal but the resulting stenosis is less than 50%. Kyphosis is limited to less than 15° and loss of anterior vertebral height to less than 50%. Despite the possible presence of a nondisplaced vertical fracture in the lamina, the facet joints and the posterior ligaments remain intact. Clinically, patients with stable burst fractures are neurologically intact.

Unstable Burst Fractures

Unstable burst fractures are three-column injuries consisting of compression of the anterior body, retropulsion of the posterior vertebral wall into the spinal canal, and disruption of the posterior elements (Fig. 19). Radiographs reveal significant kyphosis, often with widening of the posterior elements. Vertebral height is lost in the anterior and middle columns. The hallmark of an unstable burst fracture is pedicular separation on the AP radiographic view. The amount of neurologic involvement varies and depends more on the level of the injury than on the amount of canal compromise. Stenosis up to 80% is tolerated below the level of L-2, whereas stenosis of 30% in the thoracic spine can result in complete paraplegia.

Flexion–Distraction Injuries

Flexion–distraction injuries result in tension failure of the posterior elements and compression of the anterior and, occasionally, the middle columns (Fig. 20) (5). A common mechanism of injury is restraint by a seat belt in a motor vehicle accident. Radiographically, distraction of the posterior elements is seen as separation of the spinous processes and

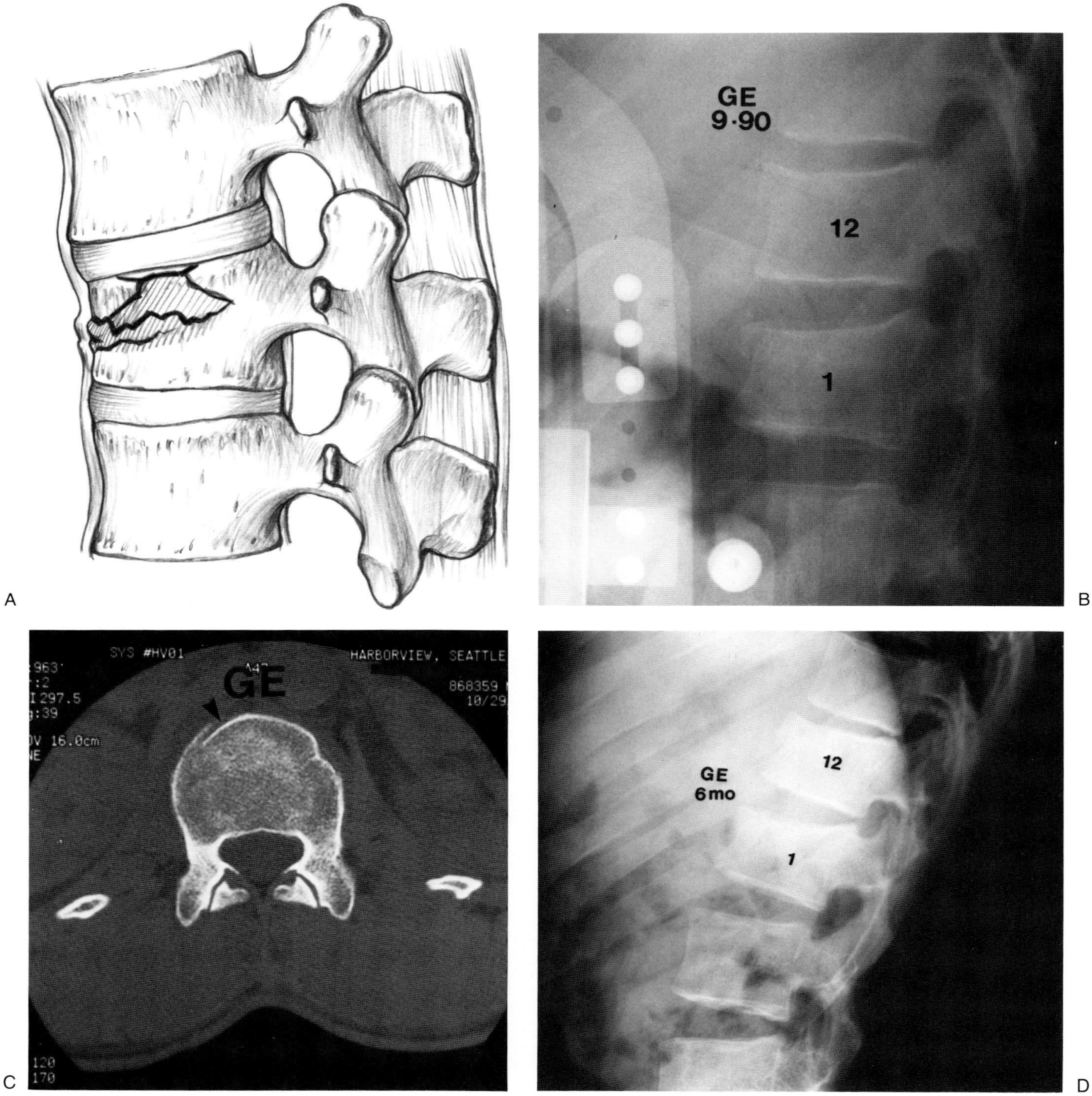

FIG. 17. **A:** Compression fracture of the thoracolumbar spine. **B:** Lateral view of T-12 and L-1 compression fractures in a 25-year-old construction worker who fell 4 meters. **C:** Axial CT at L-1 showing fracture of anterior vertebral body. **D:** Six months after brace treatment the patient has excellent sagittal alignment and has returned to work.

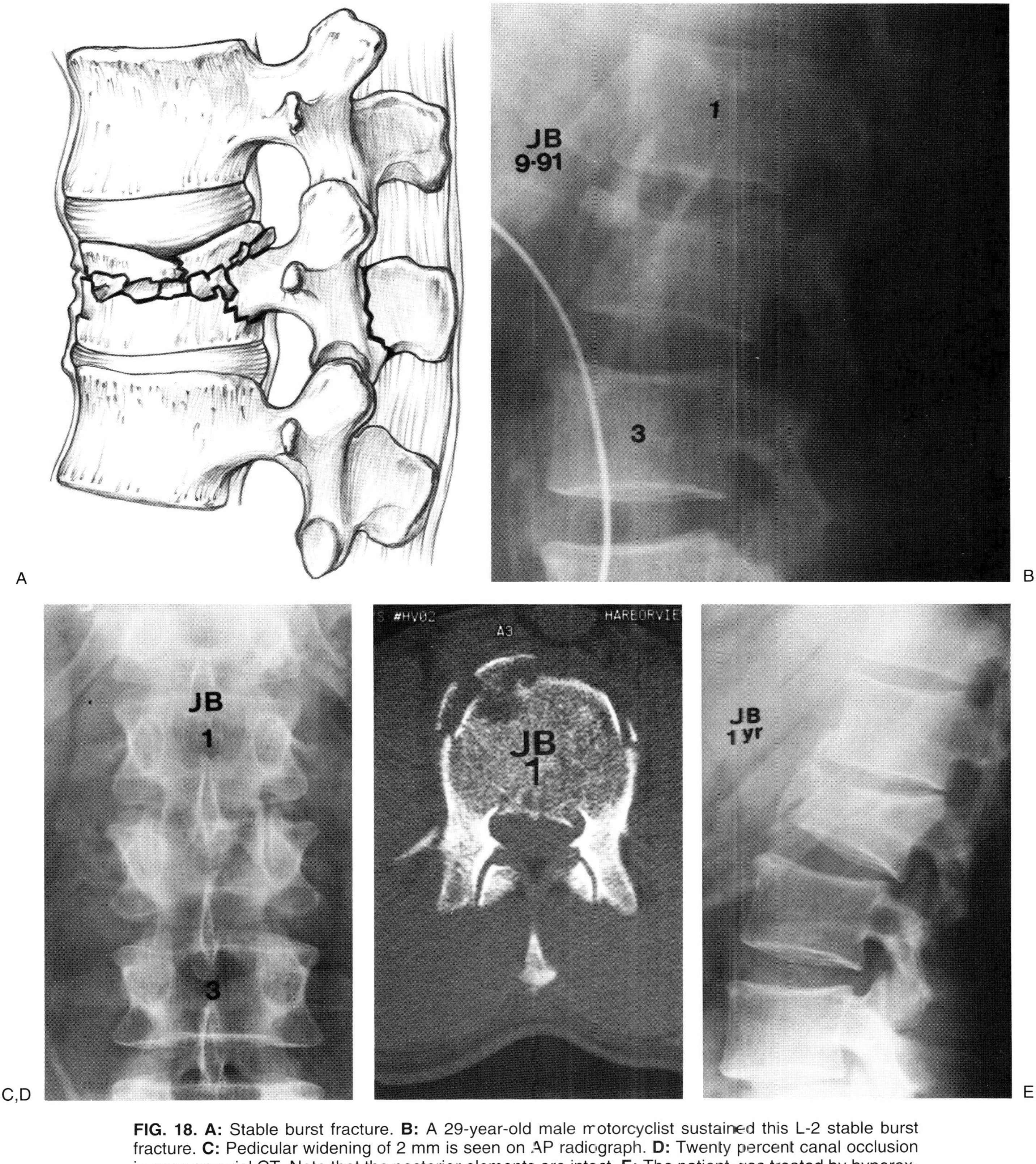

FIG. 18. A: Stable burst fracture. **B:** A 29-year-old male motorcyclist sustained this L-2 stable burst fracture. **C:** Pedicular widening of 2 mm is seen on AP radiograph. **D:** Twenty percent canal occlusion is seen on axial CT. Note that the posterior elements are intact. **E:** The patient was treated by hyperextension casting for 3 months. Lateral radiographs one year after injury demonstrate 3° kyphosis. The patient is pain-free and has returned to work.

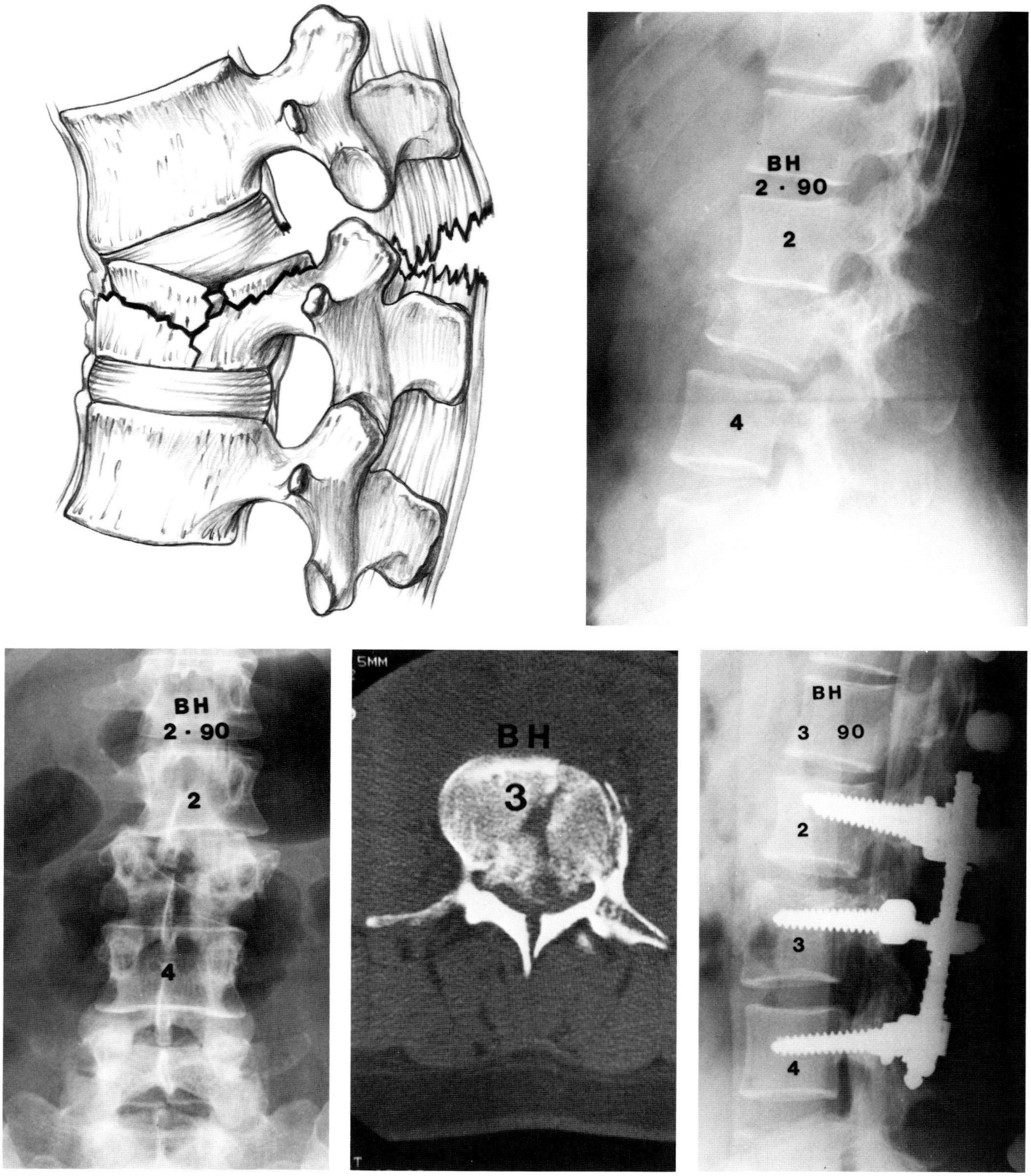

A B C,D E

FIG. 19. **A:** Unstable burst fracture. **B:** Lateral radiograph of 25-year-old woman with an unstable L-3 burst fracture and incomplete paraplegia. **C:** Pedicular widening and lateral translation of vertebral body are seen on AP view. **D:** CT showing 80% canal occlusion and fracture of posterior element. **E:** Excellent restoration of bony anatomy after pedicle-screw fixation.

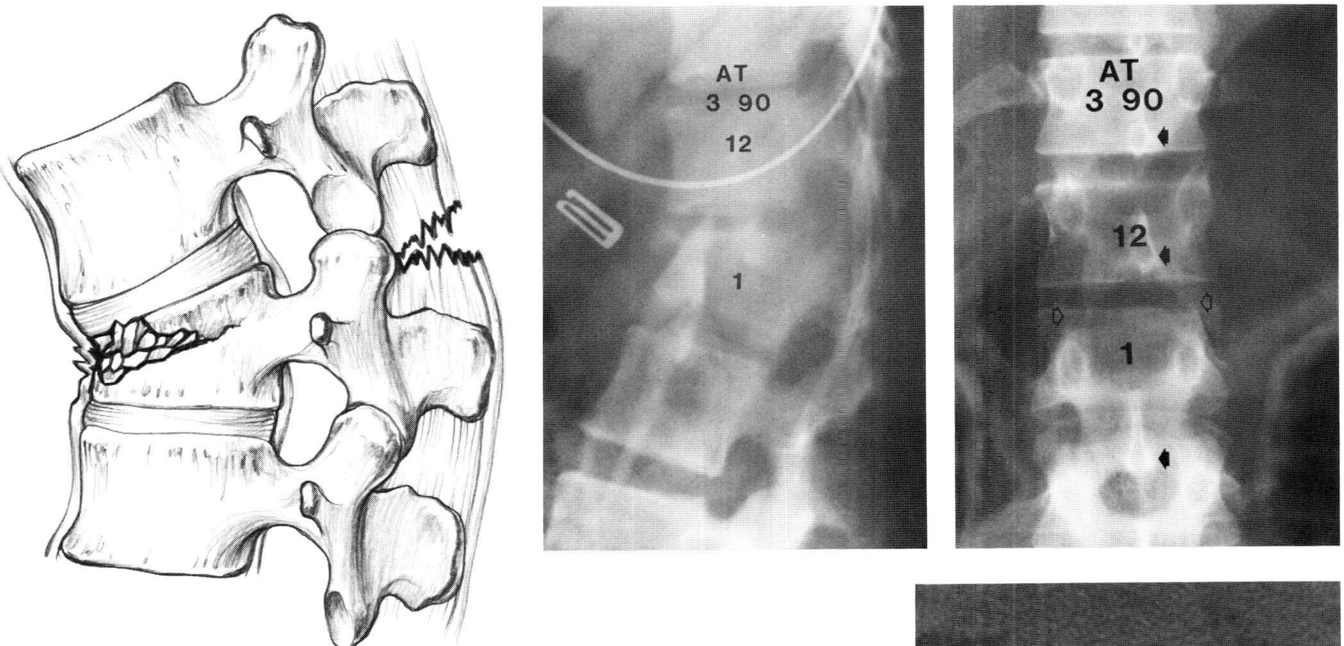

A

B,C

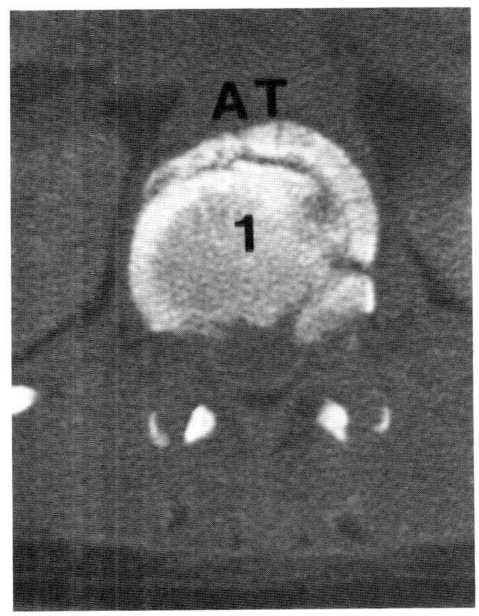

D

FIG. 20. **A:** Flexion–distraction injury. **B:** Flexion–distraction injury at T12-L1 of 22-year-old lap-belt–restrained passenger involved in a motor vehicle crash. **C:** AP radiograph demonstrates interspinous widening and facet subluxation. **D:** Anterior vertebral body compression and disruption of posterior ligamentous complex, hallmarks of flexion–distraction injuries, are seen on CT. **E:** CT of lateral reconstruction. **F:** The fracture was reduced intraoperatively by positioning the patient prone and placing of an interspinous wire. Additional fixation is by Edwards rod–sleeve technique. **G:** Postoperative AP radiograph.

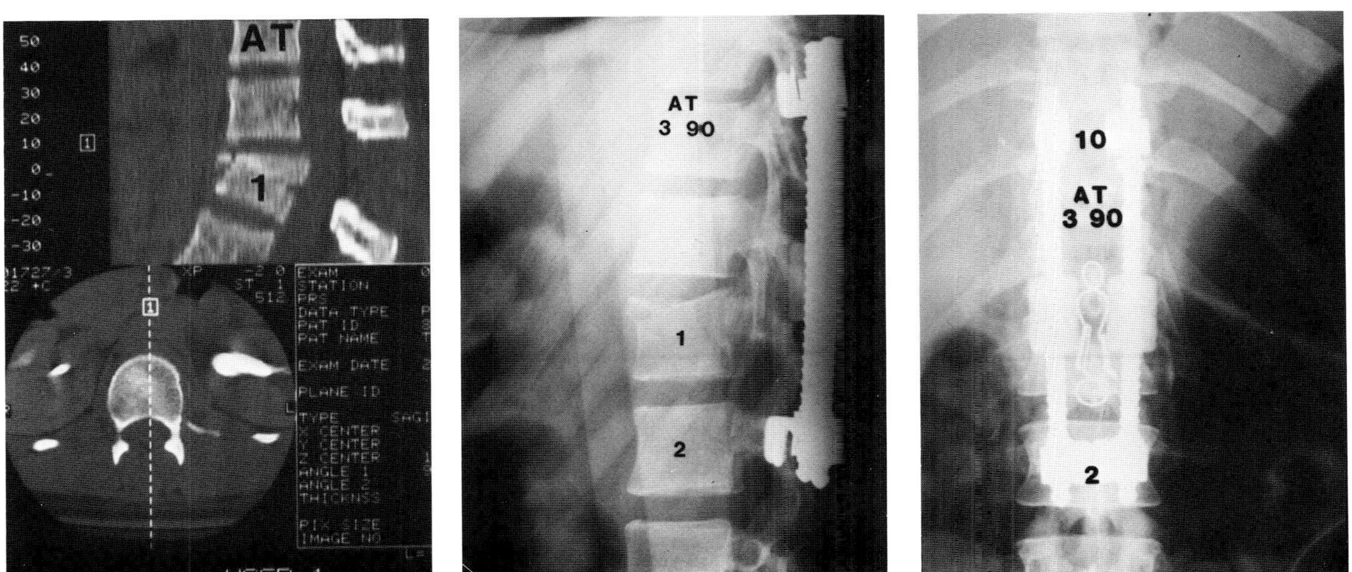

E,F

G

perching or dislocation of the facet joints. A displaced transverse fracture of the pedicles is a common associated injury. The vertebral body is wedged anteriorly, and occasionally a small fragment of bone is retropulsed into the spinal canal. These injuries occur most frequently at the thoracolumbar junction and demonstrate various patterns of neurologic involvement.

Chance Fractures

Chance fractures result from tension failure of all the spinal elements and are usually due to hyperflexion over a lap belt (Fig. 21) (6,7). Bowel injuries occur in 65% of patients with Chance fractures as the result of compression of the abdominal contents between the lap belt and the spine during injury. Consequently, all patients with Chance fractures should be carefully evaluated by a general surgeon. The anterior and middle columns are not compressed in Chance fractures, as they are in flexion–distraction injuries, but are fractured transversely. The injury can be ligamentous, bony, or a combination of both. Soft-tissue damage is usually severe, even in bony Chance fractures, and an aggressive surgical approach is warranted (8).

Translational Injuries

Translational injuries are the most dramatic and unstable of all spinal injuries. They are caused by shear forces that fracture or dislocate the facets, and usually result in complete paraplegia (Fig. 22). In the thoracic spine, injury to the chest wall or the lungs may preclude stabilization; in the lumbar spine, retroperitoneal structures such as the pancreas may be injured. Radiographic evaluation reveals anteroposterior translation of the vertebral bodies and fracture–dislocations of the facet joints.

ASSESSMENT

Physical Examination

Patients with suspected thoracolumbar fractures should be log-rolled for visualization and palpation of the dorsal spine. Acute gibbous deformity, tenderness, and a palpable gap in the spinous process are usually signs of significant injury. The neurologic examination includes manual muscle testing and a sensory evaluation of the lower extremities. A careful examination of perineal function, including perianal sensation, rectal tone, and the bulbocavernosus reflex, is required.

Radiographic Evaluation

High-quality AP and lateral radiographs are taken, centered at the fracture. The upper thoracic spine may be difficult to assess on routine cross-table views and the patient may have to be turned to a lateral position for adequate visualization of the spine.

Special Studies

A spinal CT scan is obtained when plain radiographs are suggestive of a thoracolumbar fracture. Assessments of fracture stability, classification, and canal encroachment cannot be made accurately from plain radiographs and might misdirect treatment. Myelography or MRI is rarely required initially unless the patient experiences neurologic deterioration.

EMERGENT MANAGEMENT

Patients with thoracolumbar fractures who also exhibit evidence of spinal cord or cauda equina syndrome are given methylprednisolone within 8 h of injury. An intravenous loading dose of 30 mg/kg is followed by a dose of 5.4 mg/kg/h for the next 23 h. Because thoracolumbar fractures cannot be reduced by traction, urgent stabilization or decompression is performed in patients with incomplete neurologic injuries. Patients with complete paraplegia secondary to unstable fractures are surgically stabilized within 48 h of injury. Patients with other thoracolumbar fractures are maintained on a regular hospital bed and nursed with log-rolling techniques until definitive treatment can be carried out.

DEFINITIVE MANAGEMENT

The availability of many effective instrumentation systems has led to an increased interest in the surgical treatment of thoracolumbar spine fractures. Current classification systems accurately predict fracture stability and help direct treatment, but indications for surgical treatment and the timing of surgery remain controversial. The long-term results of spinal function after injury are unknown. Treatment of thoracolumbar fractures is directed towards preventing the progression of kyphosis and minimizing pain and disability. The treatment of each injury is planned individually and is based on fracture pattern, patient age, bone quality, biomechanics, neurologic injury, and associated injuries.

Compression Fractures

Single-level compression fractures in the thoracic spine are treated nonoperatively and are observed at monthly intervals. No bracing is required unless the amount of deformity increases. Multiple-level compression fractures in the thoracic spine, compression fractures at the thoracolumbar junction, and fractures in the lumbar spine are treated by immobilization for 3 months in a Jewett brace or a thoracolumbar sacral orthosis (TLSO). A rigorous exercise program under

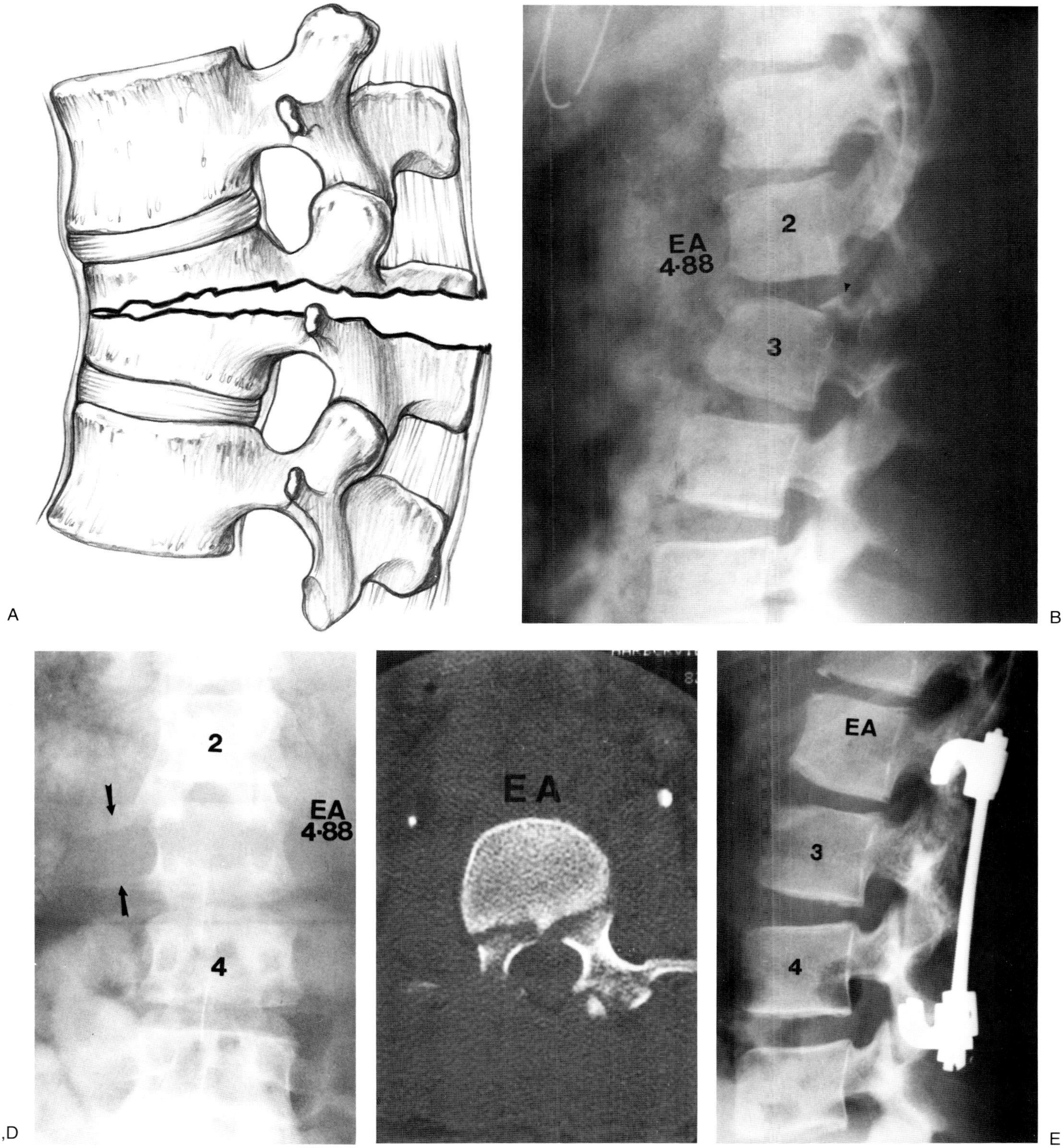

FIG. 21. **A:** Chance fracture. **B:** A 14-year-old female lap-belt-restrained passenger sustained a rupture of the transverse colon and a Chance-type fracture of L2-3. She had incomplete paraplegia. **C:** Fractures of the transverse processes and pedicles are seen on AP radiograph. **D:** Axial CT. Fractures at base of pedicles and comminution of posterior elements are present. **E:** Excellent fracture reduction after insertion of Harrington compression rods.

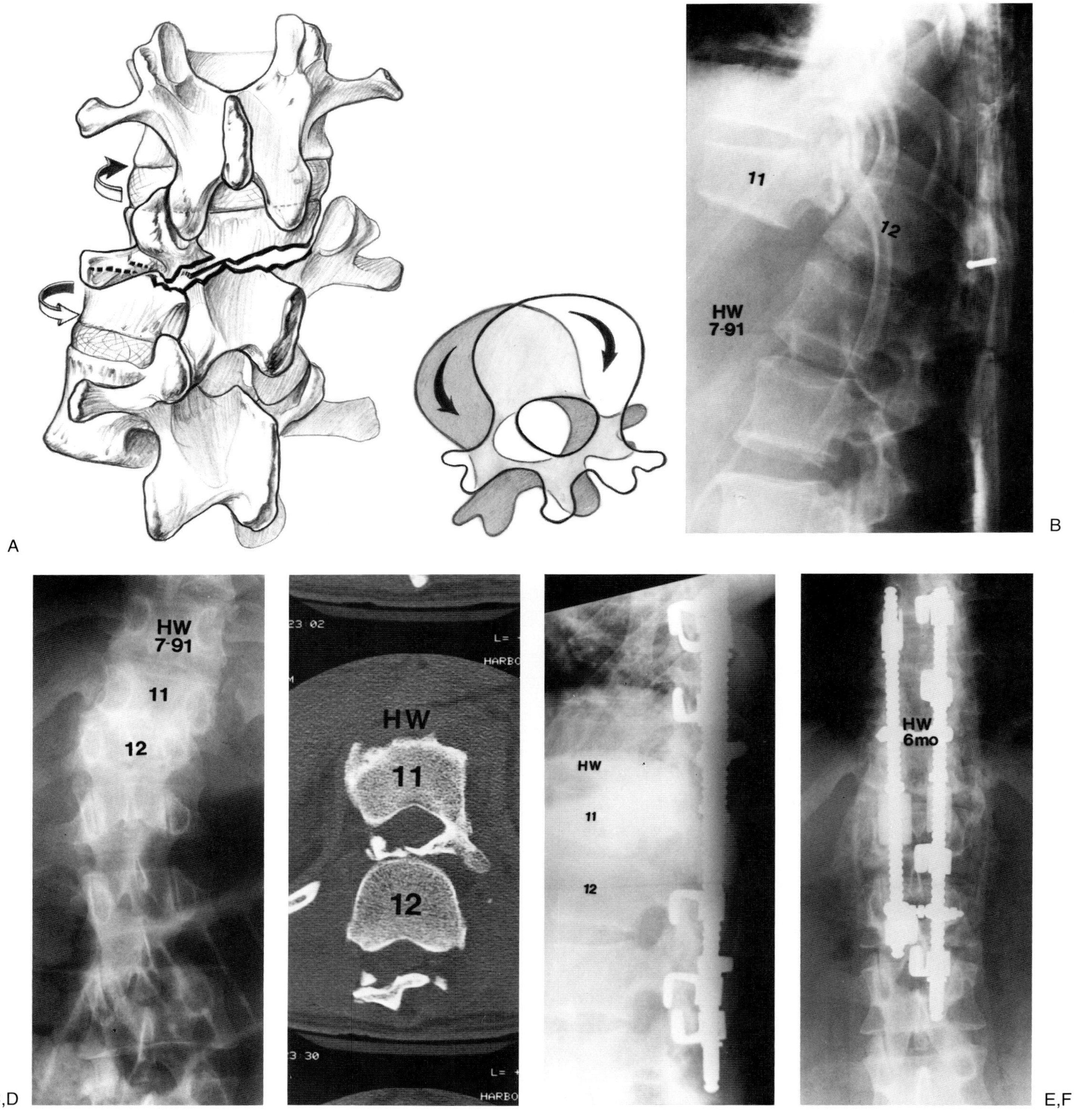

FIG. 22. A: Translational injuries. **B:** Complete dislocation of T11-12 is present. **C:** AP radiograph. **D:** Axial CT demonstrating the double vertebra sign. **E:** Excellent reduction was achieved by intraoperative distraction and manipulation. A multiple hooks–rod system was utilized for stabilization. **F:** Abundant fusion mass is present 6 months postoperatively on AP radiograph.

supervision by a physical therapist is essential during immobilization (see Chapter 9). The exercise program should include aerobic conditioning and isometric strengthening of spinal extensor and abdominal musculature. Posterior instrumentation is indicated for patients with fractures at multiple levels, kyphosis greater than 60°, and deformities that continue to progress despite bracing.

Stable Burst Fractures

Stable burst fractures are treated by the nonoperative technique of Böhler (9), who reported excellent results using closed reduction, body-cast immobilization, and a rigorous exercise program as early as 1935.

The patient is sedated and placed on a Roger Anderson fracture table for closed reduction and body-cast application. Goldthwaith irons, malleable thin bars, are placed between the two table sections and support the patient's spine. The fracture is reduced by adjusting the bend in the bars by opening and closing the table sections. The reduction is monitored by lateral radiographs to confirm adequate alignment. A well-modeled underarm body cast is then applied from the sternum to the pubis. The initial layers of the cast are carefully molded of plaster. Fiberglass is used for the outer layers to reduce weight. The cast is trimmed to allow full range of motion (ROM) at the shoulders and 90° of flexion in the hips. The patient is allowed to ambulate and to begin an aggressive exercise program of daily aerobic and trunk-strengthening exercises immediately after cast application. The cast is worn for 3 months, followed by a Jewett brace for an additional 2 to 3 months.

Unstable Burst Fractures

Unstable burst fractures result in both mechanical and neurologic instability. Treatment of patients with neurologic deficits is designed to correct the deformity, decompress the spinal canal directly or indirectly, and provide long-term stability. Decompression of the spinal canal is rarely warranted in patients without deficits because late neurologic complications are rare and the retropulsed bone is often resorbed.

The treatment of unstable burst fractures is controversial. Posterior instrumentation is the most commonly recommended treatment but is associated with a small incidence of neurologic worsening. In many cases, the spinal canal is not completely decompressed by this method and a second-stage anterior decompression is required. Because two or three levels above and below the injury are stabilized by the instrumentation, low back disorders may appear later in life. Long-term studies have shown that fracture-site kyphosis increases by 10° after posterior instrumentation (10). Pedicle screw systems have been developed to shorten the necessary instrumentation and to improve correction in the sagittal plane. Although the risks associated with screw insertion are acceptable, recurrent kyphosis and a high incidence of hardware failure have been reported when this fixation was used in patients with vertebral body fractures (11). Routine anterior bone grafting has been advocated to decrease bending moments on the pedicle screws.

Fixation of dorsal spinal fractures must achieve lordotic correction and prevent flat-back syndrome. Rod–hook devices usually require stabilization of at least three vertebral levels above and two levels below the fracture. The Edwards rod–sleeve technique is an exception; because the rod sleeves provide lordotic correction and rotational stability, the length of the instrumentation can be shortened to two levels above the fracture and one level below (10).

Anterior decompression treats the offending pathology by removing the retropulsed bone. In experienced hands this procedure has proved to be safe and effective (5). Complications with strut grafts and postoperative kyphosis may occur in patients with unstable burst fractures. Anterior internal fixation devices have been developed to prevent these graft complications, but their safety and efficacy are unknown (3,11).

Posterior instrumentation and fusion are recommended for unstable burst fractures at this institution. Harrington rods are used in conjunction with Drummond spinous-process wires in thoracic fractures. At the thoracolumbar junction, Edwards rod–sleeves limit the length of the fusion and have proved to be a reliable method of fixation (10). Fractures at the level of L-3 or below are treated by pedicle-screw fixation. Spinal cord monitoring is used for patients with some distal motor or sensory functions. Postoperatively, patients wear a custom-molded total-contact orthosis for 4 months. Casting for the orthosis is done intraoperatively, reducing the hospital stay by 2 or 3 days. A chin extension is added for fractures above the level of T-6 and leg extensions are added for fractures at or below the level of L-4. Ambulation or wheelchair transfer is started 2 or 3 days following brace applcation.

When posterior instrumentation is used, a posterolateral fusion is added for the length of the instrumentation. In long instrumentations, the rod-long fuse-short technique is used and the hardware is removed after 1 year. When the pedicle-screw system is used, a second-stage anterior fusion is performed routinely or the patient is confined to bed for 2 to 3 months. Patients who have undergone posterior instrumentation are allowed to sit up in bed to 90° immediately after surgery. Anterior decompression is indicated in patients with unimproved neurologic deficits who have residual spinal cord or cauda equina compression (5). Decompression is performed 1 or 2 days after posterior instrumentation on patients with severe neurologic deficits and high-grade lesions. Patients with mild deficits are closely monitored and anterior decompression is performed only if the deficits fail to resolve completely.

Flexion–Distraction Injuries

These highly unstable injuries require open reduction, posterior stabilization, and fusion. After reduction an interspinous wire is inserted to correct distraction and Edwards rod–sleeves are centered over the injury. However, rod–sleeve placement is contraindicated when unstable laminar fractures are present. The instrumentation is distracted to apply only sufficient tension to the rods to prevent the hooks from disengaging, but not enough to distract the vertebrae. Bone graft is added posterolaterally and in the decorticated facet joints. A TLSO brace is worn for 4 months postoperatively.

Chance Fractures

Patients who sustain bony injuries with minimal kyphosis are treated by extension casting, the same procedure that is used for stable burst fractures. Posterior-compression instrumentation and fusion are performed in patients who have sustained ligament injuries, bony injuries with more than 10° of kyphosis, neurologic deficits, or multiple injuries.

Translational Injuries

Translational injuries require operative reduction and stabilization. Because the amount of ligament damage associated with these injuries is extensive, overdistraction can easily occur with distraction-rod fixation. To prevent distraction, segmental fixation is applied 2 or 3 levels above and below the injury. When possible, interspinous wires are placed across the fracture site before instrumentation. Multiple rod–hook systems or Luque wires are used to provide stable fixation in thoracic fractures; pedicle-screw fixation is used in the lumbar spine.

COMPLICATIONS

Neurologic deterioration is rare in thoracolumbar fractures but must be investigated and diagnosed immediately by MRI or myelography. Patients with neurologic deterioration require immediate operative reduction and neural decompression. Deformity that progresses despite bracing is diagnosed by serial upright radiographs and treated by posterior instrumentation. The size of a patient's body may change during the time spent in a brace and careful attention to the fit of the brace minimizes the possibility of decubitus ulcerations. Hardware failure or increased fracture kyphosis occurs in 5% to 10% of cases and may require further reconstructive surgery.

SKELETALLY IMMATURE PATIENTS

Ligament Chance-type fractures are the most common thoracolumbar injuries seen in children at this institution. Standard instrumentation may be too large for immature spinal canals and alternative methods of fixation, such as interspinous wiring or special pediatric spinal implants, can be used. The management of other thoracolumbar fractures in children is similar to that for fractures in adults.

REFERENCES

1. Holdsworth G. Fractures, dislocations, and fracture-dislocations of the spine. *J Bone Joint Surg* 1970;52A:1534–51.
2. Whitesides TE. Traumatic kyphosis of the thoracolumbar spine. *Clin Orthop* 1977:128:78–92.
3. Denis F. The three column spine and its significance in the classification of acute thoracolumbar spine injuries. *Spine* 1983;8:817–31.
4. McAfee PC, Yuan HA, Frederickson BE, Lubicky JP. The value of computed tomography in thoracolumbar burst fractures. *J Bone Joint Surg* 1983;65A:461–73.
5. McAfee PC, Bohlman HH, Yuan HA. Anterior decompression of traumatic thoracolumbar fractures with incomplete neurological deficit using a retroperitoneal approach. *J Bone Joint Surg* 1985;67A:89–104.
6. Dunn HK. Anterior stabilization of thoracolumbar injuries. *Clin Orthop* 1984;189:116–24.
7. Chance GQ. Note on a type of flexion fracture of the spine. *Br J Radiol* 1948;452–3.
8. Anderson PA, Henley MB, Rivara FP, Maier RV. Flexion distraction and Chance injuries to the thoracolumbar spine. *J Orthop Trauma* 1991;5:153–60.
9. Böhler L. Fractures and dislocations of the spine. In: *The treatment of fractures*. New York: Grune & Stratton; 1956;1:366–71.
10. Edwards CC, Levine AM. Early rod-sleeve stabilization of the injured thoracic and lumbar spine. *Orthop Clin North Am* 1986;17:122–45.
11. Kaneda K, Abumi K, Fujya M. Burst fractures and neurologic deficits of the thoracolumbar spine: results of anterior decompression and stabilization with anterior instrumentation. *Spine* 1984;9:788–95.

Orthopaedic Trauma Protocols, edited by
Sigvard T. Hansen, Jr., and Marc F. Swiontkowski.
Raven Press, Ltd., New York, ©1993.

CHAPTER 19

Pelvic Fractures

M. L. Chip Routt, Jr.

MECHANISM OF INJURY

The etiology of pelvic fractures can vary widely. A pelvic fracture can be caused by a low-impact fall or by a high-speed automobile accident. The direction and energy of the applied load and the quality of the patient's bone determine the fracture pattern, and consequently its clinical management. Although associated hemorrhage can be life-threatening even in a seemingly minor pelvic fracture, it is usually a manageable complication.

ANATOMIC CONSIDERATIONS

The surgical identification of the irregular surfaces of the bony pelvis can be a difficult task. Adding to the intricacy are the many major nerves and blood vessels that traverse the pelvic ring. The greater sciatic notch contains the gluteal neurovascular trunks, the pudendal nerve, and the sciatic nerve. The fifth lumbar nerve root is located very close to the anterior sacral alar region. On the anterior aspect, the femoral nerve crosses the pelvic brim along with the iliopsoas muscle and is separated from the more medial femoral artery, femoral vein, and the lymphatic vessels by the thick iliopectineal fascia. The bladder, which has an abundant vascular supply, is located posterior to the symphysis pubis and is protected anteriorly by the fat within the space of Retzius.

The integrity of certain ligament structures is vital to pelvic stability. The pelvis is supported by the anterior and posterior sacroiliac ligaments and the symphyseal, iliolumbar, sacrospinous, and sacrotuberous ligaments. Each of these structures contributes to the three-dimensional stability of the pelvic ring (Figs. 1 and 2). The muscles that envelop the pelvis produce bony deformity when the pelvic ring is disrupted.

Department of Orthopaedics, Harborview Medical Center, University of Washington, Seattle, Washington 98104

CLASSIFICATION

Pelvic injuries are difficult to classify because of the many fracture patterns that occur. Many authors, including Pennal et al. (1), Letournel (2), Tile (3), and Dalal et al. (4) devised classifications based on fracture patterns, mechanisms of injury, and anatomy. In his classification system, Tile uses the AO schema of types A through C and broadly includes the majority of fracture patterns (Table 1). This system serves as a guide for three-dimensional thought to better understand the dynamics of a pelvic fracture.

ASSESSMENT

Physical Examination

Maintenance of hemodynamic stability is the primary objective during the initial evaluation of a pelvic fracture. After this life-saving goal is achieved, further evaluation and treatment may proceed.

Associated fractures and dislocations are revealed by palpation of the entire length of the spine and the extremities. The status of neurologic function in the lower extremities and the perineal area is documented. Occult or frank bleeding from the rectum or the vagina is investigated by digital rectal and vaginal examinations. Bladder and urethral injuries are suggested by the presence of meatal blood, inability to urinate, or a high-riding or nonpalpable prostate gland on rectal examination. Any of these findings mandate further evaluation before urethral catheterization.

Abraded skin and degloving injuries on the lumbodorsal and flank regions are associated with surgical complications and must be noted. Pelvic instabilities are revealed by direct manipulation of the pelvis; manipulation must be done gently to avoid further injury to soft tissues and the possibility of disrupting an intrapelvic hematoma. The neurologic examination is repeated after the pelvic manipulation.

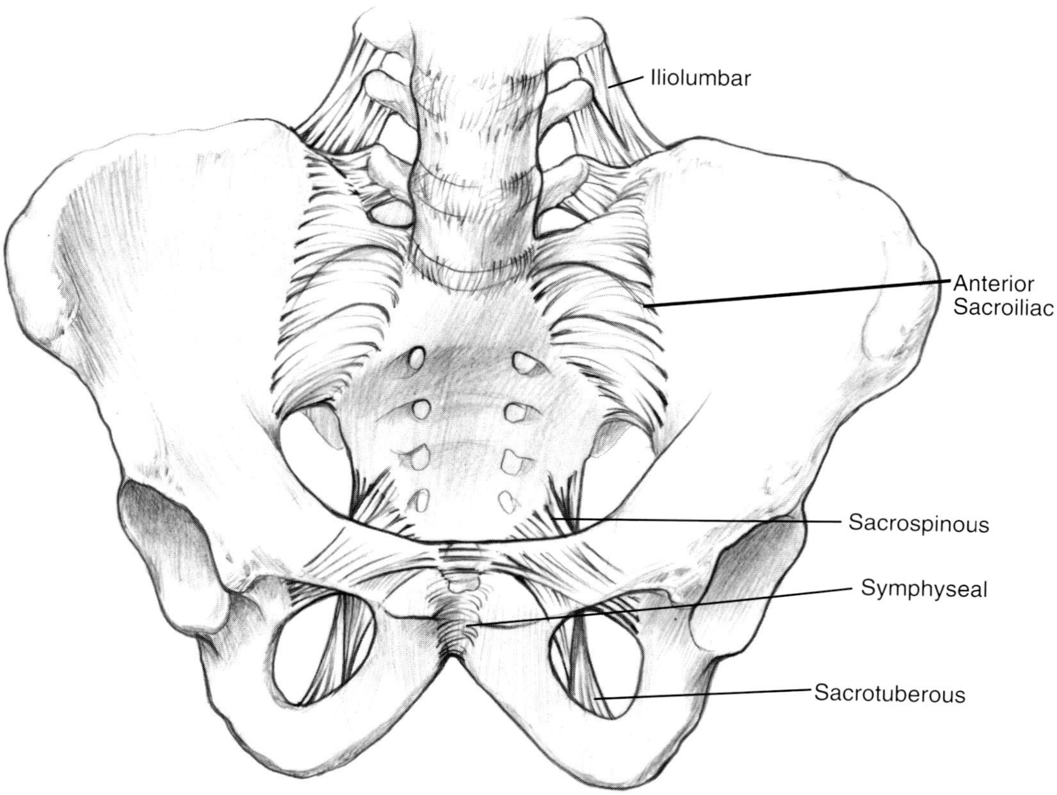

FIG. 1. Anterior view of pelvic ligaments.

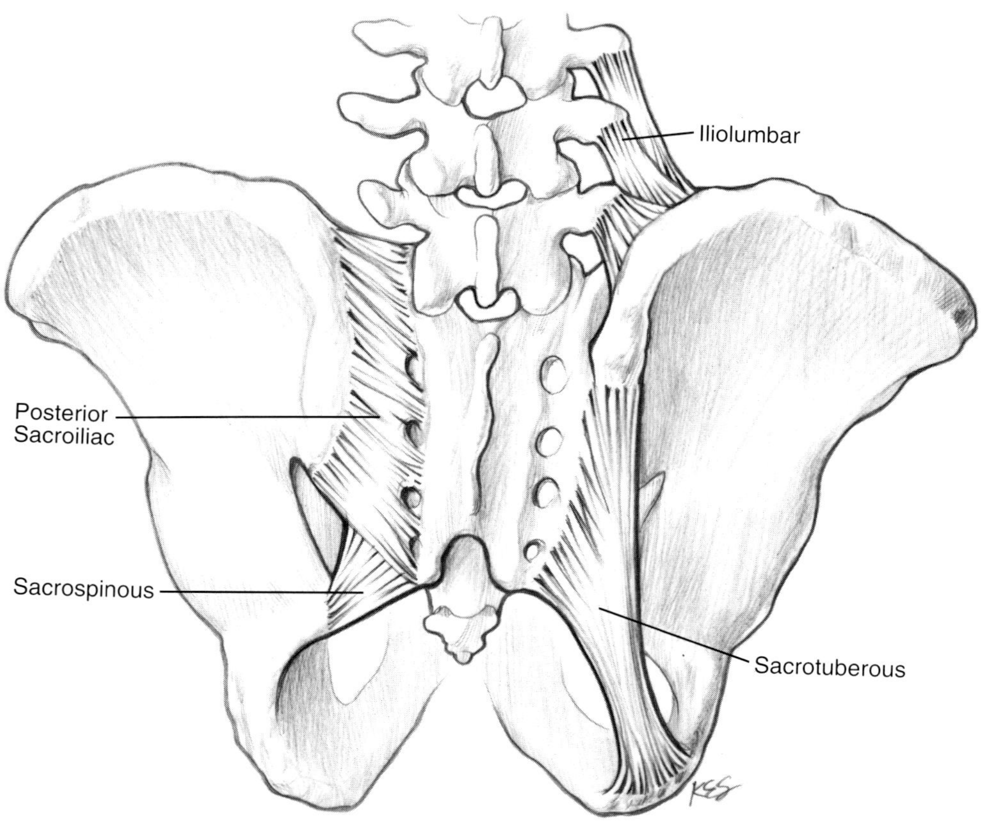

FIG. 2. Posterior view of pelvic ligaments.

Table 1. *Tile's classification of pelvic ring injuries*

Type A:	Includes stable pelvic fractures
Type A1:	Typically an avulsion fracture with no pelvic ring involvement (Fig. 3A);
Type A2:	Nondisplaced pelvic ring fracture (Fig. 3B);
Type A3:	Transverse fractures of the sacrum and coccyx with no involvement of the pelvic ring (Fig. 3C).
Type B:	Rotationally unstable but vertically stable fractures
Type B1:	Anteroposterior compression injury, divided into the following stages:
Stage 1:	Symphysis pubis disruption of less than 2.5 cm with no posterior pelvic ring involvement (Fig. 4A);
Stage 2:	Symphysis pubis disruption of greater than 2.5 cm with a unilateral posterior pelvic ring injury (Fig. 4B);
Stage 3:	Symphysis pubis disruption of greater than 2.5 cm with bilateral posterior pelvic ring injuries (Fig. 4C);
Type B2:	Lateral compression injury (ipsilateral). Unstable in internal rotation anterior and posterior ring involvement of the ipsilateral hemipelvis (Fig. 5A);
Type B3:	Lateral compression injury (contralateral). It is unstable in internal rotation and there is major anterior ring involvement contralateral to the posterior injury (Fig. 5B). The flexion deformity of the affected hemipelvis is associated with unequal limb lengths.
Type C:	Includes rotationally unstable and vertically unstable fractures.* It is subdivided as follows:
Type C1:	Ipsilateral anterior and posterior pelvic injury with vertical and rotatory instabilities in the affected hemipelvis (Fig. 6A);
Type C2:	Bilateral hemipelvic disruptions with significant vertical and rotatory instabilities (Fig. 6B);
Type C3:	Any pelvic fracture with an associated acetabular fracture (Fig. 6C). Each component of the injury must be evaluated individually but treated concurrently.

*This injury usually reflects high-energy trauma with complete bone or ligament instability.

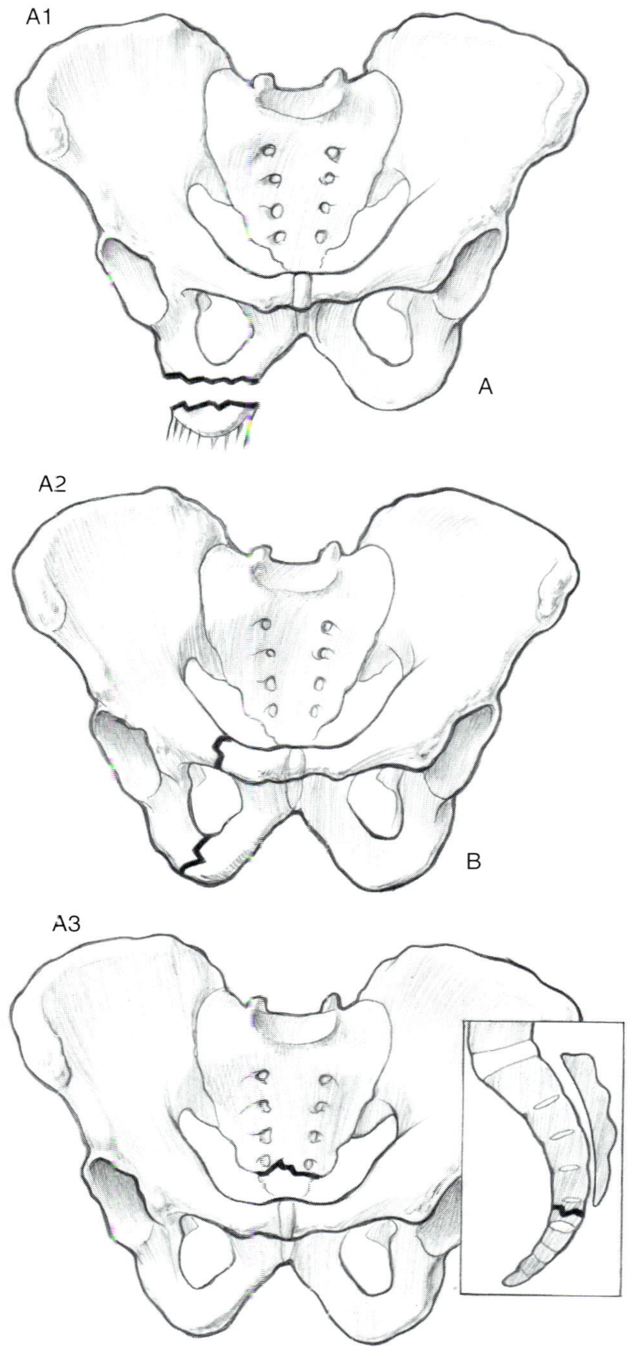

FIG. 3. A:. Type A1 avulsion fracture. **B:** Type A2 nondisplaced pelvic ring fracture. **C:** Type A3 transverse fracture.

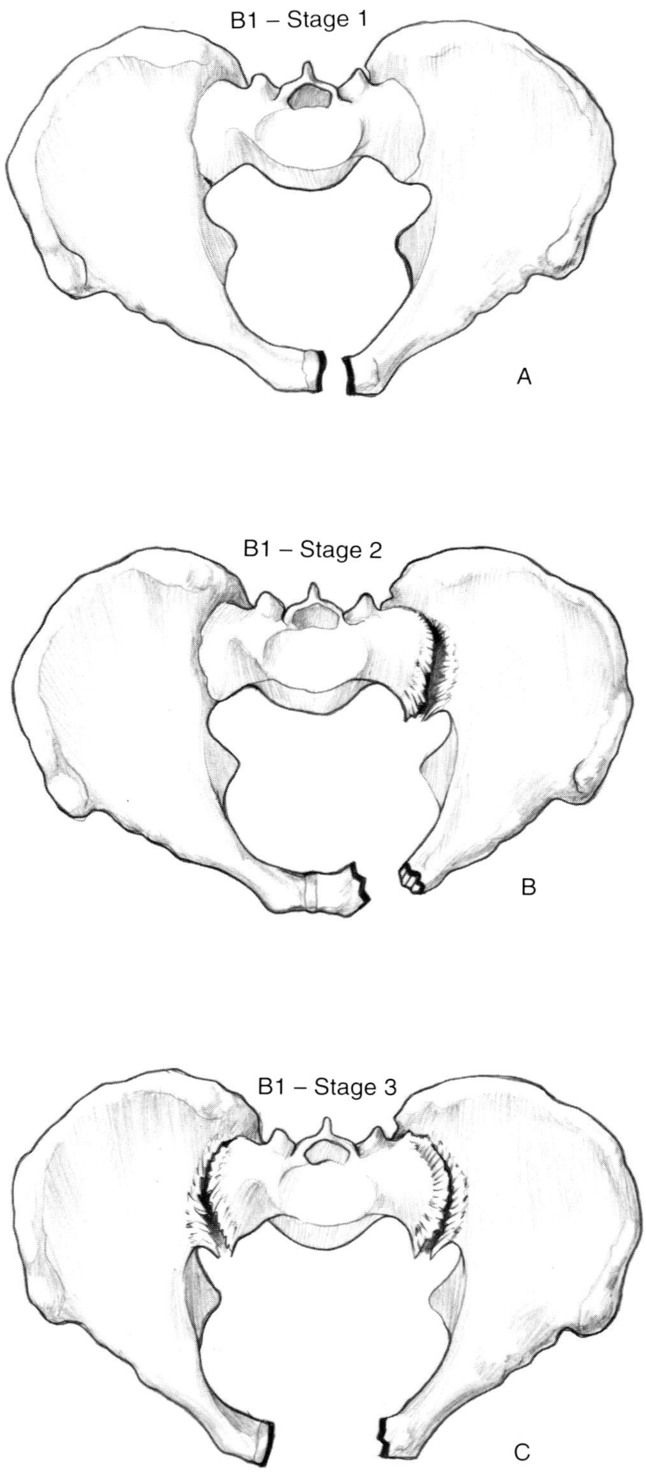

FIG. 4. A: Type B1, stage 1 symphysis pubis disruption. **B:** Type B1, stage 2 symphysis pubis disruption. **C:** Type B1, stage 3 symphysis pubis disruption.

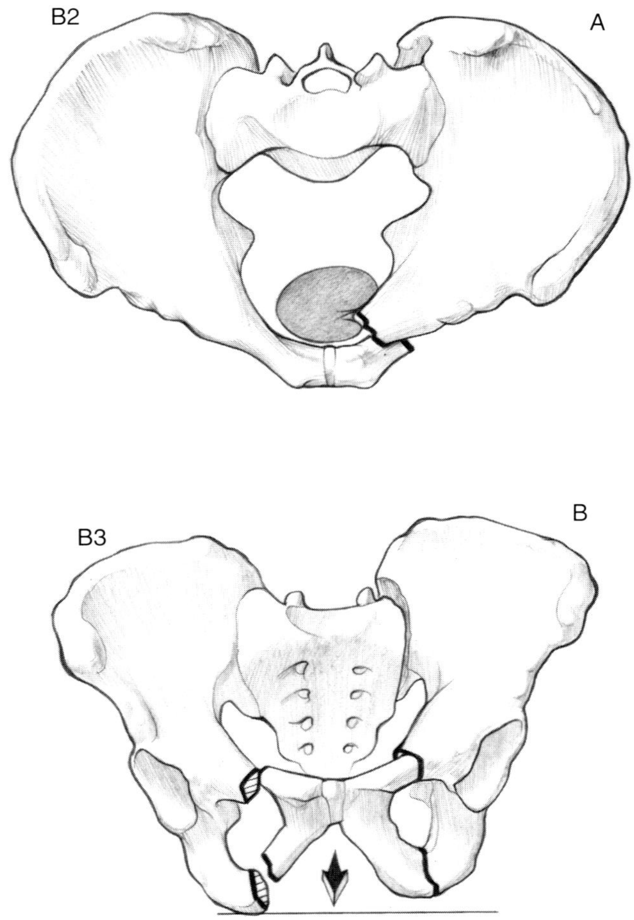

FIG. 5. A: Type B2 lateral compression injury (ipsilateral). **B:** Type B3 lateral compression injury (contralateral).

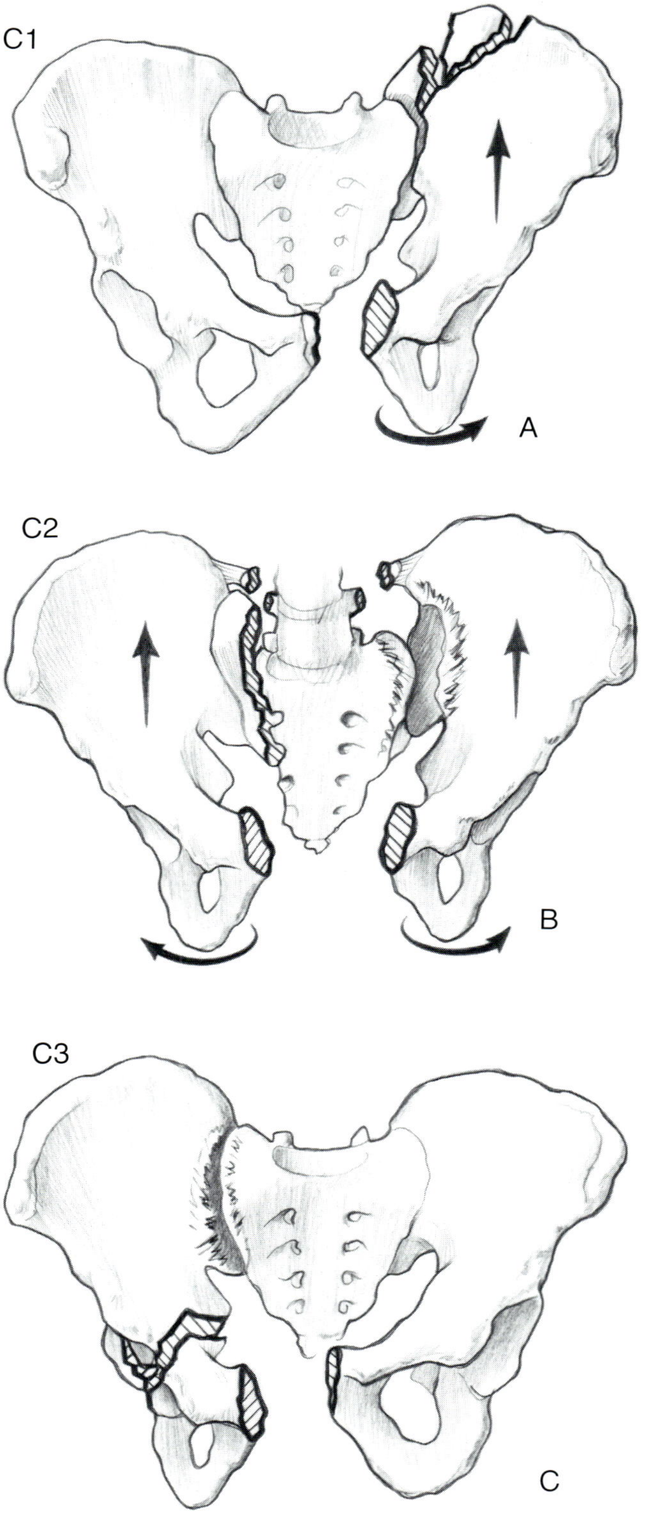

FIG. 6. A: Type C1 pelvic injury. **B:** Type C2 pelvic injury. **C:** Type C3 pelvic injury.

Radiographic Evaluation

A pelvic fracture is usually easily identified on the admitting AP pelvic radiograph and is further delineated with pelvic inlet (45° cephalad tilt) and outlet (45° caudad tilt) radiographic views. A spot lateral radiograph of the sacrum should be obtained. Push–pull radiographs of the pelvis (5) are rarely needed to assess occult vertical instability. Judet–Letournel oblique radiographs are useful for classifying associated acetabular fractures (2). Good quality plain radiographs reveal associated fractures and dislocations in the spine and the lower extremities.

Special Studies

Dynamic retrograde urethrograms, cystograms, and intravenous pyelograms reveal genitourinary abnormalities. Computerized tomography of the pelvis with two- or three-dimensional reconstructions is helpful for delineating the fracture patterns. Pelvic CT scans are done at the same time as the abdominal CT scan if the patient's general condition allows (Fig. 7). Definitive treatment may be complicated when abdominal CT scanning is done first because diagnostic intraabdominal contrast material obstructs the intraoperative fluoroscopic imaging of the pelvic ring.

Angiography is useful when continued hemodynamic instability after bony stabilization is caused by an accessible arterial lesion (Fig. 8). Preoperative duplex scanning is performed at bedside to diagnose deep venous thrombosis.

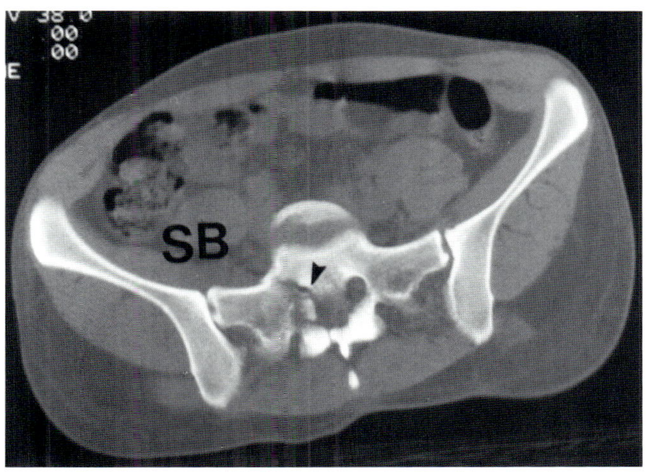

FIG. 7. CT scan demonstrates the right-sided sacral fracture and contralateral minimal sacroiliac joint disruption. Bone fragments obscure the neural foramen on the patient's right side.

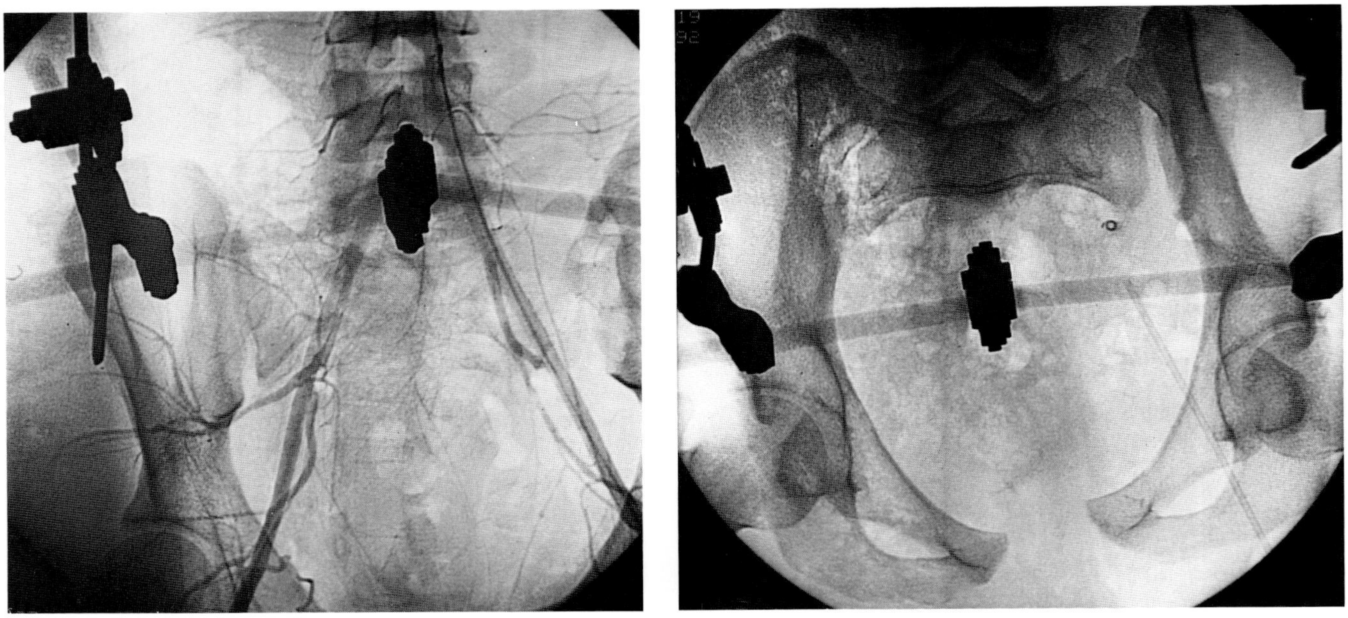
A B

FIG. 8. A,B: This patient was hemodynamically unstable after a high-speed car wreck. A pelvic external fixator was applied at the time of exploratory laparotomy. Angiography demonstrated an avulsion of the left superior gluteal artery, with ongoing bleeding. Embolization arrested the arterial flow.

EMERGENT MANAGEMENT

Despite our best efforts, the mortality rate of patients with major pelvic fractures is approximately 5% to 10%. The cause of death is usually attributed to complications from associated injuries, especially head trauma and hemorrhage, and is directly related to the Injury Severity Score and the age of the patient.

Evaluation and treatment are conducted simultaneously. Early resuscitation efforts include infusions of warmed intravenous fluids, blood, and blood-product replacements (platelets and coagulation factors). Early provisional or definitive pelvic immobilization reduces bleeding from exposed bone surfaces, diminishes pelvic volume, and relieves pain. The fracture pattern suggests the optimal fixation. In general, spica casting, external fixation, or large pelvic clamps are used for emergent stabilization (Fig. 9). Open perineal wounds are irrigated, debrided, and dressed aseptically. A diverting colostomy should be performed emergently to prevent contamination of wounds by the fecal stream. Placement of the colostomy should be done in consultation with the orthopaedic surgeon so that the approaches to delayed reconstructive procedures for acetabular or pelvic ring fractures are not compromised. Angiography is indicated after pelvic stabilization in a hemodynamically unstable patient.

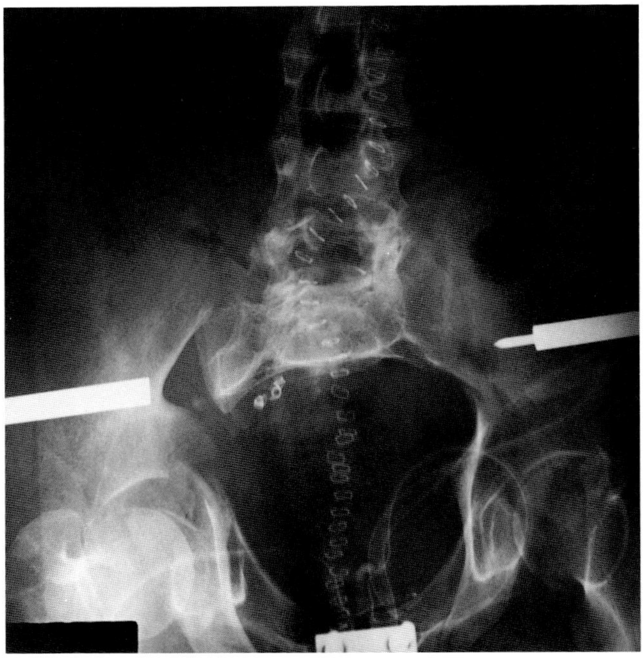

FIG. 9. The emergent application of a pelvic antishock clamp helped to acutely stabilize this patient with a type C3 pelvic fracture. The patient was crushed by a load of logs.

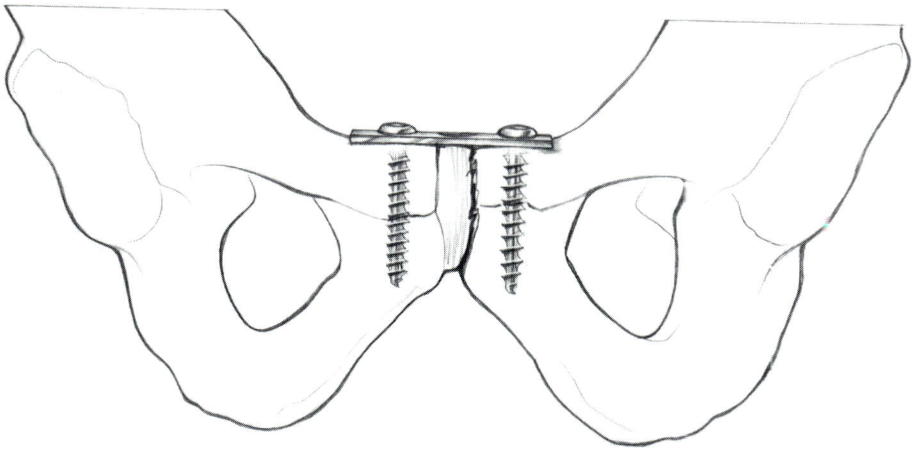

FIG. 10. Location of symphyseal plate.

DEFINITIVE MANAGEMENT

Most pelvic fractures are treated by ORIF; closed management is usually reserved for stable, nondisplaced pelvic fractures. Early anatomic reduction and fixation of the pelvic ring lowers mortality rates in polytraumatized patients and improves their long-term prognoses (6). The method of treatment is determined preoperatively according to the classification of the fracture and the experience of the surgeon.

Type A1 Fracture

An avulsion fracture of the pelvis is usually located in the anterosuperior or the anteroinferior iliac spine. The ischial tuberosity can also be avulsed by strong hamstring contractions. These fractures are usually treated nonoperatively.

Type A2 Fracture

A stable, nondisplaced pelvic ring fracture is treated symptomatically. A patient with this fracture is mobilized as soon as pain tolerance allows.

Type B1 Fracture (Stage 1)

An isolated symphyseal disruption with less than 2.5 cm of displacement is treated operatively only when the symphysis pubis is exposed for other purposes (e.g., for bladder or urethral repair or for exploratory laparotomy). A narrow two-holed 4.5-mm DCP held by 6.5-mm fully threaded cancellous screws is the implant of choice for a simple symphysis pubis disruption. The plate is centered over the symphyseal meniscus and placed along the superior border of the symphysis (Fig. 10). The meniscus remains attached to one of the rami. External fixation is used sparingly for this injury (7).

Type B1 Fracture (Stages 2 and 3)

Minimally displaced sacral fractures or anterior sacroiliac joint disruptions with intact posterior ligaments usually do not warrant operative intervention. A disrupted symphysis pubis with displacement greater than 2.5 cm and with associated unilateral or bilateral posterior ring injuries is treated by plating of the symphysis and posterior fixation if necessary. Associated posterior pathology, such as impingement of the sacral nerve, stenosis of the foramina due to fracture, or retained debris in the sacroiliac joint, requires operative intervention. A posterior approach is used to decompress the nerve root. An anteroiliac exposure is used to debride the joint. ORIF in the posterior region of the pelvis is performed at the time of these procedures. Depending on the fracture pattern defined by radiographic views of the pelvic inlet and outlet and by the CT scans, percutaneous iliosacral screws (Figs. 11 and 12), sacral bars, anterior sacroiliac joint plates, posterior tension-band plates, or a combination of these implants are used for fixation (Fig. 13).

Type B2 and B3 Fractures

Hemipelvic flexion and extension displacements often exhibit subtle symptoms. However, these injuries are unstable in internal rotation and can impinge on soft tissues

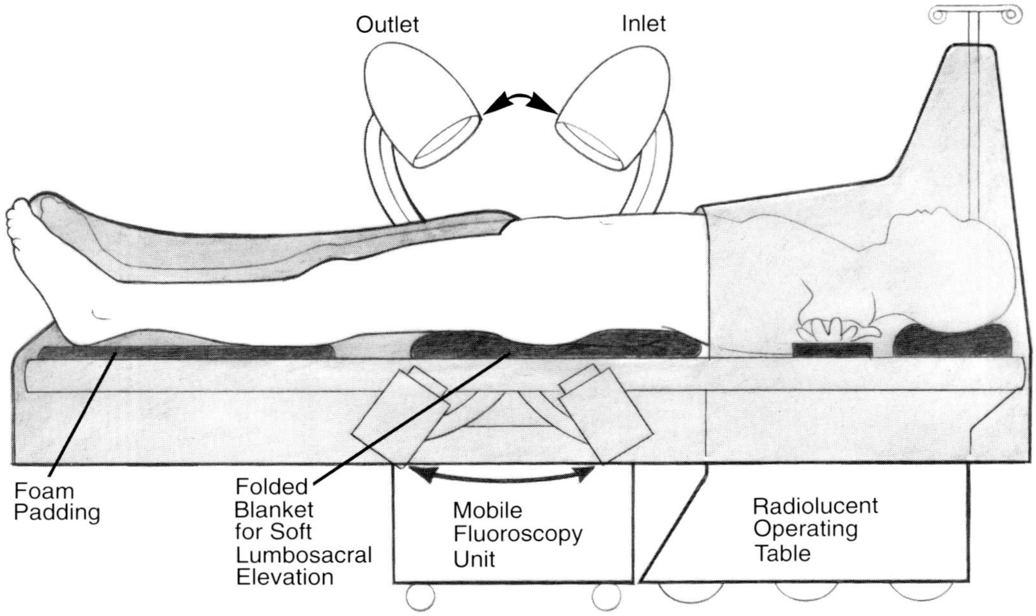

FIG. 11. Patient and fluoroscopic positioning for percutaneous transiliac screw placement into the body of S-1.

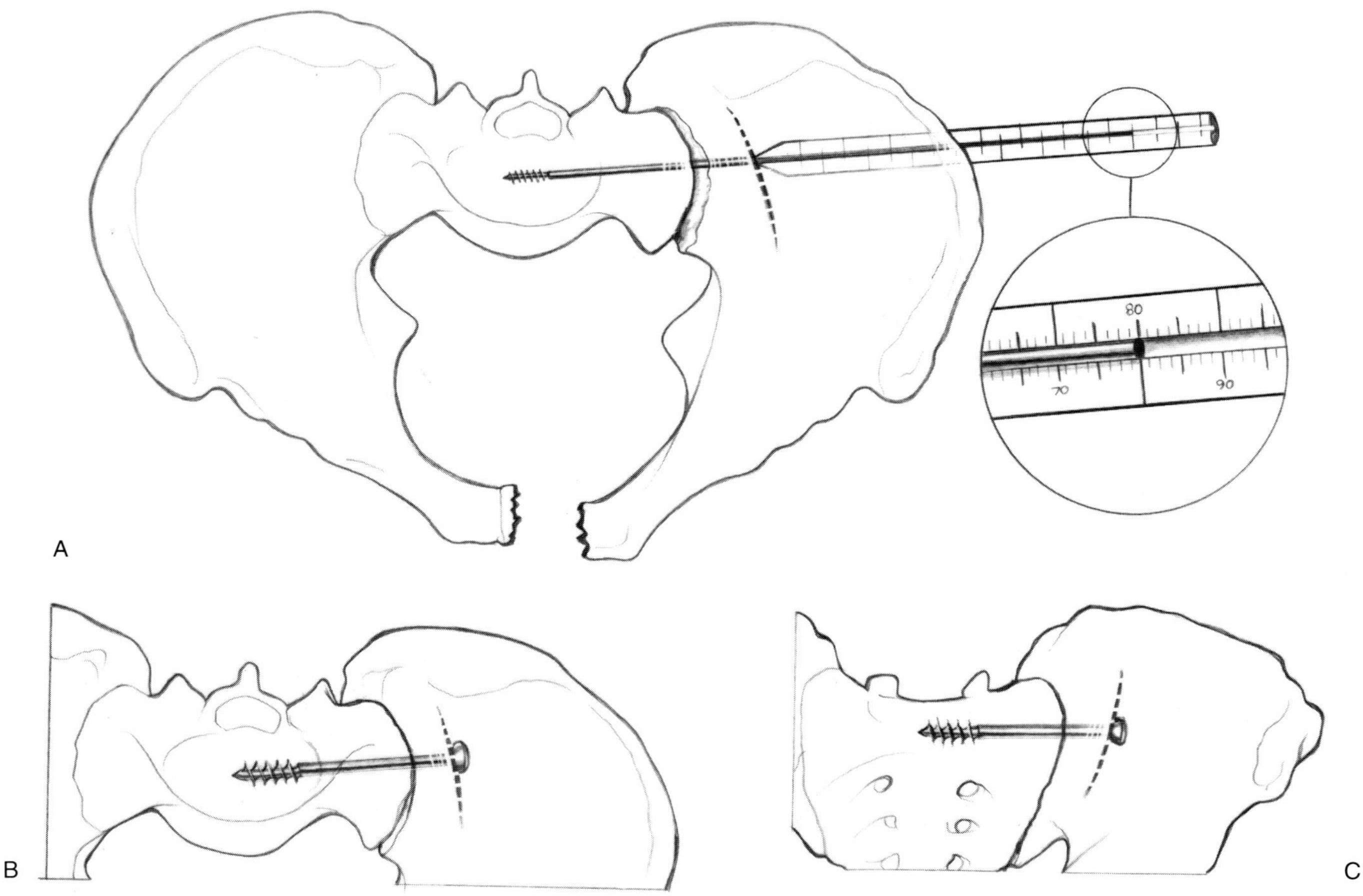

FIG. 12. The guide wire is advanced under biplanar (inlet and outlet views) fluoroscopy into S-1 (**A**). The depth gauge is used to assess screw length; reaming must be 10 mm short of the measured length to avoid removing the guide wire. The final position of the screw must be (**B**) central in the body of S-1 on the inlet view and (**C**) above the S-1 foramen on the outlet (tangential) view.

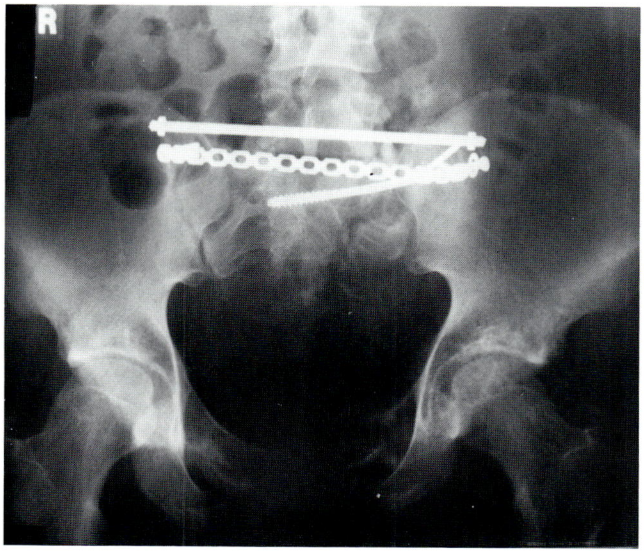

FIG. 13. An atypical array of posterior ring implants were necessary to stabilize this morbidly obese, suicidal jumper.

and vital organs, including the bladder, the vagina, the uterus, and the neurovascular bundle. Occasionally an anterior injury is reduced indirectly during primary reduction of a posterior lesion. Accurate anatomic reduction of a posterior ring deformity may require dislodging an overriding anterior fragment. The anterior ring injury may consist of a symphyseal disruption, a parasymphyseal fracture, or a complex pubic ramus fracture. These injuries are addressed at the same time as the posterior pathology. If necessary, the anterior lesion is fixed by plating, external fixation, or lag screws, depending on the fracture pattern and its location (Fig. 14).

Type C1 and C2 Fractures

Fractures in these categories are caused by high-energy injuries and can result in significant rotatory and shear instabilities and in flexion and extension deformities. Plain radiographs demonstrate the amount of instability and displacement better than CT scans. Unstable anterior and posterior pelvic ring injuries are reduced and stabilized with appropriate implants in the same manner as type B2 and B3 injuries.

Type C3 Fractures

Pelvic ring disruptions with an associated acetabular fractures require special consideration. Perfect acetabular reduction, which is necessary for optimizing hip function outcome takes priority and is dependent on the reduction of the pelvic ring. Concurrent pelvic ring and acetabular injuries are reduced simultaneously (Fig. 15). Combined anterior and posterior approaches are occasionally performed as staged or

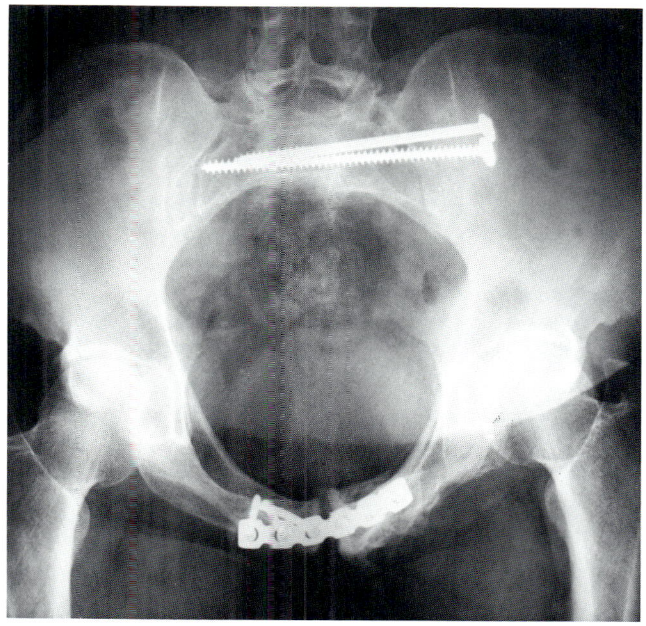

FIG. 14. This patient fell over 100 feet while working on a scaffold. The anterior ring disruption was stabilized with plating, and the posterior sacral fractures were treated using percutaneous iliosacral screws.

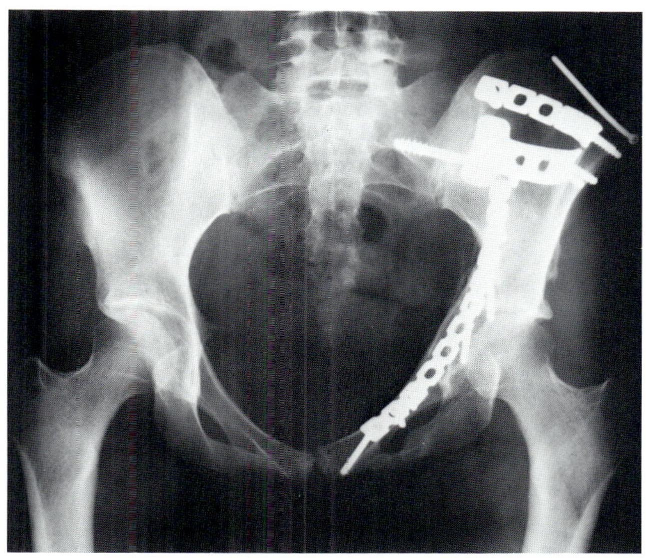

FIG. 15. An occult, complete sacroiliac joint disruption was identified during the ilioinguinal exposure of this acetabular fracture. Significant displacement of an acetabular fracture may mask the sacroiliac joint injury, even on the CT scan. Iliosacral screw fixation was used to stabilize the injury after fixation of the acetabular fracture.

simultaneous procedures. Delayed or late reconstructions are performed when soft-tissue injuries or the patient's clinical condition contraindicate early operation.

Postoperative Care

The stability of a fracture after fixation determines how soon a patient can be mobilized. Transfer from bed to chair is begun as soon as a patient is comfortable sitting in bed. Patients with type A injuries can immediately progress to protected weight-bearing as tolerated, whereas those with unilateral type B or C fractures should remain nonweight-bearing for 6 weeks and gradually proceed to bear weight over the next 6 weeks. Patient with bilateral type B or C fractures are restricted to sitting in a chair for the first 6 weeks and can progress to tandem-crutch or walker ambulation over the next 6 weeks. Active muscle-maintenance exercises are initiated during the rehabilitation period, and progression to exercise with light resistance is allowed within the limits of pain tolerance.

COMPLICATIONS

Complications from pelvic fractures are commonplace, but death secondary to hemorrhage is usually preventable. Associated severe abdominal injuries and head trauma are the most frequent causes of death in patients with major pelvic fractures. High infection rates are associated with open contaminated pelvic fractures and posterior pelvic surgical approaches. The possibility of deep venous thrombosis must be critically evaluated both pre- and postoperatively by duplex scanning. In major pelvic trauma, the use of vena caval filters is preferable to heparin therapy (Fig. 16).

A nonunion or a malunion of the pelvis is frequently painful; malunion can produce pelvic asymmetry with resultant limb length inequality, abnormal pelvic biomechanics, and can cause narrowing of the birth canal and vaginal impingement in female patients.

SKELETALLY IMMATURE PATIENTS

Pelvic fractures in children usually consist of an apophyseal avulsion from a low-energy injury or a pelvic ring disruption from a high-energy injury. A low-energy avulsion rarely warrants operative intervention. A displaced high-energy pelvic ring fracture is treated by reduction and stabilization with spica casting or by internal fixation. The integrity of the triradiate cartilage must be carefully evaluated in a child. Acetabular dysplasia may be a consequence of a physeal bar, which can be located with CT scans, tomograms, and MRI. Resection of the physeal bar is indicated in a young child (Fig. 17).

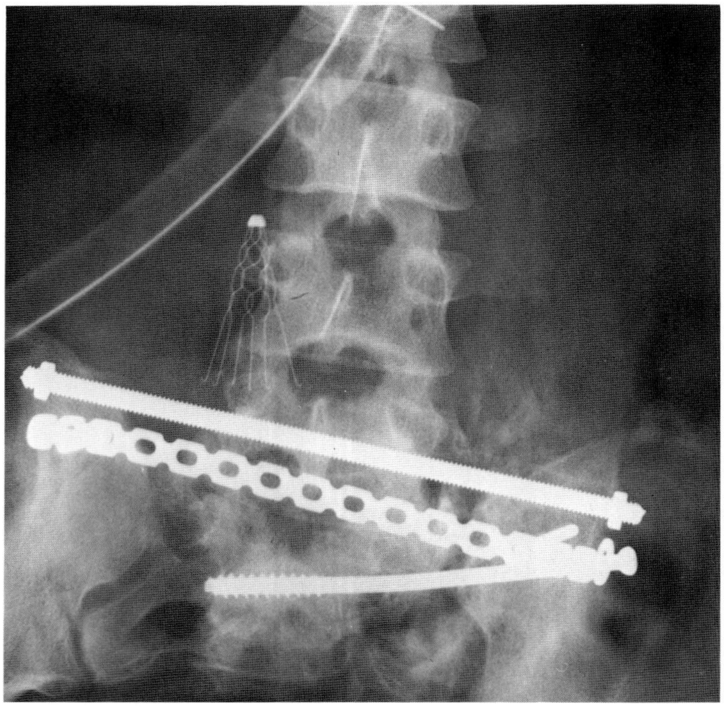

FIG. 16. The vena caval filter is used when pharmacological anticoagulation is impossible. This patient required emergent thoracotomy when the filter migrated to the heart during placement.

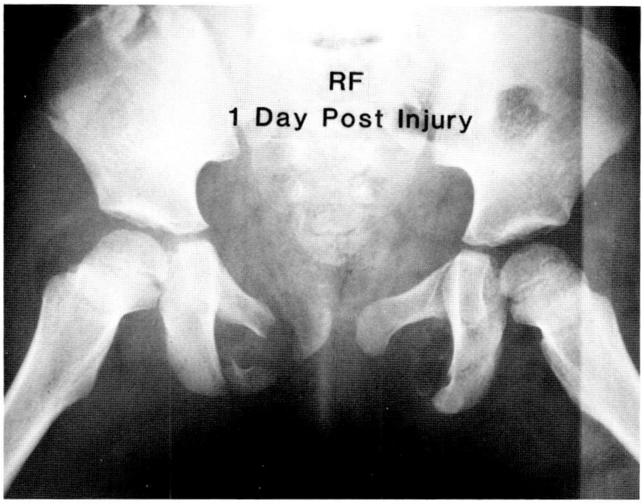

A

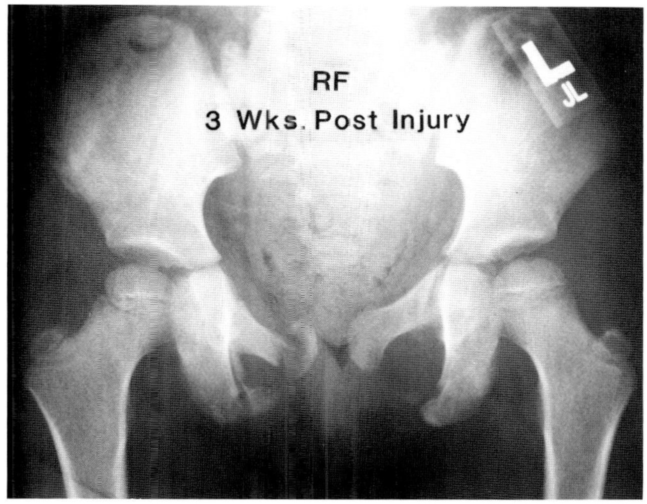

B

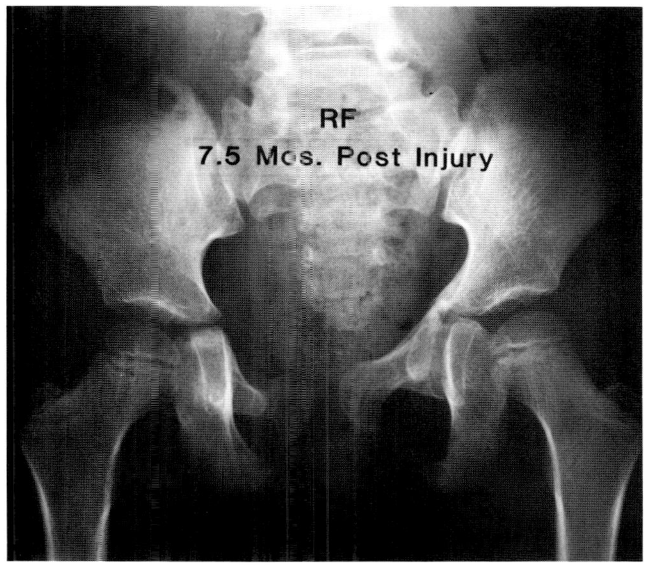

C

FIG. 17. A: This 5-year-old female was crushed by an auto. She sustained an isolated open pelvic injury with vaginal lacerations. The left triradiate growth center was injured. **B:** Three months after injury, periosteal new bone formation was noted at the triradiate cartilage region. **C,D,E:** A physeal bar developed involving the anterior column component of the growth center.

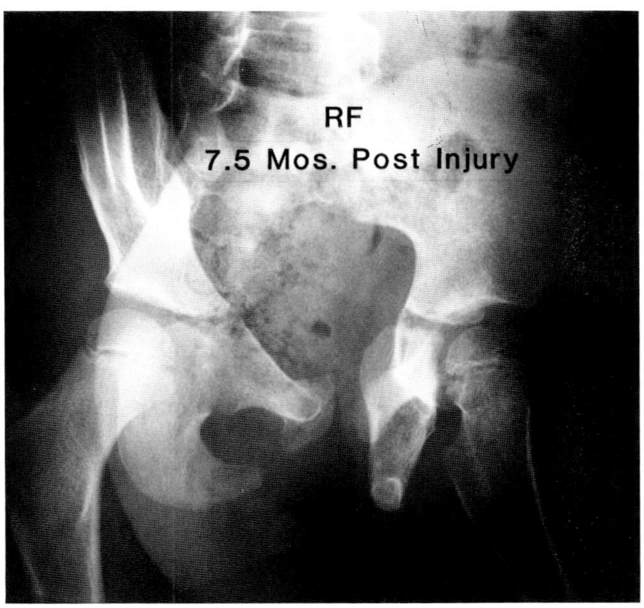

D

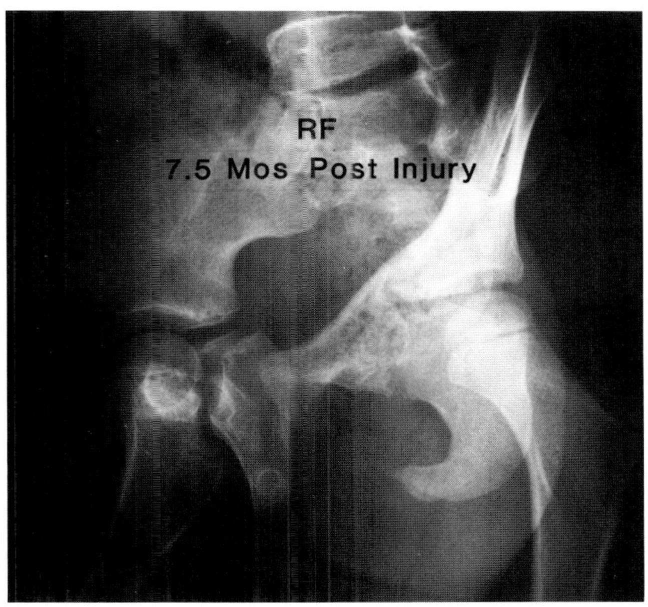

E

REFERENCES

1. Pennal GF, Tile M, Waddell JP, Garside H. Pelvic disruption: assessment and classification. *Clin Orthop* 1980:151:12–21.
2. Letournel E. Acetabulum fractures: classification and management. *Clin Orthop* 1980;151:81–106.
3. Tile M. Pelvic ring fractures: should they be fixed? *J Bone Joint Surg* 1988;70B:1–12.
4. Dalal SA, Burgess AR, Siegel JH, et al. Pelvic fracture in multiple trauma: classification by mechanism is key to pattern of organ injury, resuscitative requirements, and outcome. *J Trauma* 1989;29:981–1000.
5. Peters B, Bucholz RW. Stress testing of pelvic ring fractures. Presented at the Orthopedic Trauma Association Meeting, Oct. 29, 1988, Dallas.
6. Hesp WL, van der Werken C, Keunen RW, Goris RJ. Unstable fractures and dislocations of the pelvic ring: results of treatment in relation to the severity of injury. *Neth J Surg* 1985;37:148–152.
7. Mears DC, Fu FH. Modern concepts of external skeletal fixation of the pelvis. *Clin Orthop* 1980;151:65–72.

Orthopaedic Trauma Protocols, edited by
Sigvard T. Hansen, Jr., and Marc F. Swiontkowski,
Raven Press, Ltd., New York, © 1993.

CHAPTER 20

Hip Dislocations and Femoral Head Fractures

Marc F. Swiontkowski

MECHANISMS OF INJURY

Hip dislocations occur from high-energy trauma. Posterior hip dislocations result from an axial load applied to a flexed hip, whereas anterior dislocations occur from hyperextension or hyperabduction mechanisms.

Femoral head fractures are usually associated with hip dislocations. Ninety percent of all femoral head fractures are associated with posterior hip dislocations (1). Eight percent of all posterior hip dislocations have associated femoral head fractures. Indentation fractures, which have a very poor prognosis, are associated with anterior hip dislocations (2). The usual mechanism of femoral head fractures is axial loading applied to a hip positioned in neutral to slight adduction and in 70° to 90° of flexion, a common position in "dashboard" injuries in motor vehicle accidents.

ANATOMIC CONSIDERATIONS

The most important consideration in the treatment of any hip dislocation is preservation of the vascular supply to the femoral head. The lateral epiphyseal artery, which is the terminal branch of the medial femoral circumflex system, is the principal arterial supply to the femoral head. In adolescents and adults this group of vessels supples blood to two thirds of the femoral head. The artery from the ligamentum teres in the obturator system, which is usually disrupted in hip dislocations, supplies blood to a smaller area of the femoral head, and the lateral femoral circumflex artery vascularizes a small area of the anterior and inferior femoral head in adults.

CLASSIFICATION

Hip dislocations are classified by the position of the dislocated femoral head in relation to the acetabulum.

Department of Orthopaedics. Harborview Medical Center, University of Washington, Seattle, Washington 98104

The classification for femoral head fractures devised by Pipkin is predictive of functional outcome and has been quoted widely since 1957 (Fig. 1) (3). However, this classification describes only those femoral head fractures that are associated with posterior dislocations. Brumback's classification (2) includes femoral head fractures that occur in association with anterior hip dislocations and, therefore, promises to be more widely useful. Brumback classified hip dislocations into five categories (Table 1).

Brumback's classification will be used throughout this section and the corresponding Pipkin classification will appear in parentheses.

ASSESSMENT

Physical Examination

Obvious deformity is seen at the admitting examination if the hip has remained dislocated. In a typical posterior dislocation, the leg is slightly flexed, shortened, adducted, and internally rotated. In an anterior dislocation, the hip is positioned in neutral to slight flexion, abduction, and external rotation. A thorough examination of sciatic nerve function (sensation and motor) must be performed in a patient who is awake and alert. The patient's circulatory status is assessed by palpation and a Doppler examination.

Radiographic Evaluation

An admitting AP radiograph of the pelvis, which is required for all polytrauma patients, is obtained when a hip dislocation is suspected and is used to identify the pathology of the dislocation. In all hip dislocations, the femoral head is examined for indentation or shear fractures and the acetabular fovea is examined for femoral head fragments. Most important, the femoral neck is inspected for nondisplaced fractures. A type IIIB fracture (Pipkin type III) can frequent-

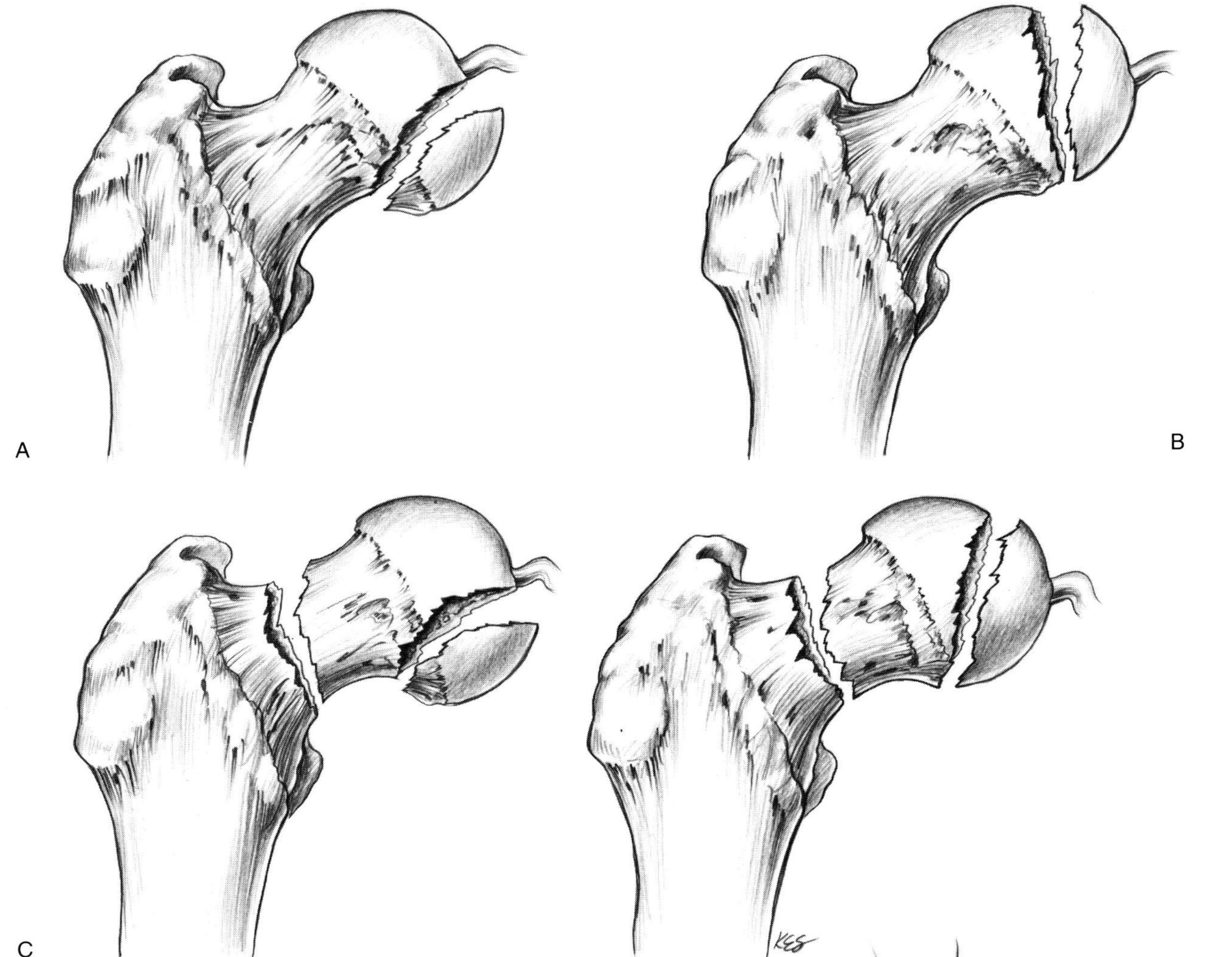

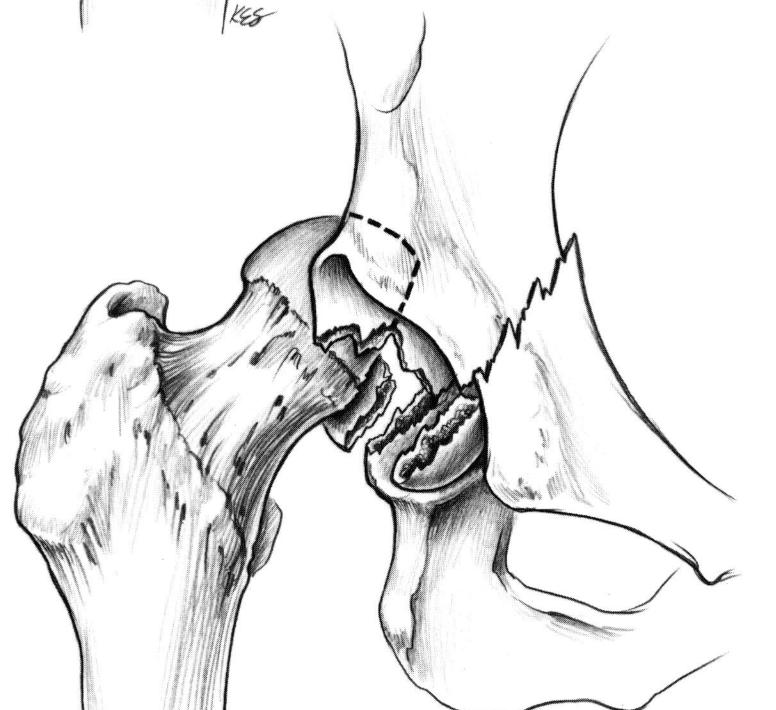

FIG. 1. Classification of femoral head fractures. **A:** Infrafoveal fracture; Pipkin I, Brumback IA. **B:** Suprafoveal fracture; Pipkin II, Brumback IIA. **C:** Either (**A**) or (**B**) associated with a femoral neck fracture; Pipkin III; Brumback IIIB. **D:** Any femoral head configuration associated with an acetabular fracture; Pipkin IV, Brumback IB, IIB.

Table 1. Brumback classification of hip dislocations

Type I	A posterior hip dislocation with a femoral head fracture involving the inferomedial non-weight-bearing portion of the femoral head
Type IA	With minimal or no fracture of the acetabular rim and a stable hip joint after reduction
Type IB	With significant acetabular fracture and hip joint instability
Type II	A posterior hip dislocation with a femoral head fracture involving the superomedial weight-bearing portion of the femoral head
Type IIA	With minimal or no fracture of the acetabular rim and a stable hip joint after reduction
Type IIB	With significant acetabular fracture and hip joint instability
Type III	A dislocation of the hip from an unspecified direction with an associated femoral neck fracture
Type IIIA	Without fracture of the femoral head
Type IIIB	With fracture of the femoral head
Type IV	An anterior dislocation of the hip with fracture of the femoral head
Type IVA	Indentation type, with a depression in the superolateral weight-bearing surface of the femoral head
Type IVB	Transchondral type, with an osteocartilaginous shear fracture on the weight-bearing surface of the femoral head
Type V	A central fracture–dislocation of the hip with fracture of the femoral head

ly be displaced by the reduction maneuver if it is not initially recognized. A postreduction AP radiograph of the pelvis is obtained, and if a femoral head fracture is suspected a pelvic CT scan is performed with 1.5-mm cuts through the femoral head.

Special Studies

A postreduction CT scan, described above, is critical for planning the management of a femoral head fracture.

EMERGENT MANAGEMENT

Closed reduction of a hip dislocation is performed as soon as possible after injury to minimize the risk of posttraumatic avascular necrosis (AVN). The hip can be reduced in the Emergency Department if the patient is cooperative and has not sustained any serious associated injuries. Benzodiazepine and morphine sulfate are administered to provide relaxation. If the initial attempt at closed reduction is unsuccessful, the patient is taken to the operating room, where optimal relaxation can be provided and an open reduction can be performed if necessary. Patients who are taken to the operating room for treatment of other injuries should have the hip reduction performed there after anesthesia is induced.

Reduction of a posterior dislocation requires an assistant to deliver countertraction to the anterior iliac crest. The surgeon flexes the hip to 70° in slight abduction while pulling in line with the femur. This is best accomplished by standing over the patient (it may be convenient to move the patient on a backboard to the floor) and placing the patient's lower leg between the surgeon's legs. The surgeon's quadriceps muscles are able to deliver the force necessary for distal traction. Anterior obturator or inguinal dislocations also require countertraction, and distal traction is delivered in the same manner although more abduction is used. Short-angle rotational movements may help the head back into position through a rent in the capsule. In refractory dislocations or ipsilateral femoral shaft fractures, a 5-mm Schanz pin is inserted percutaneously into the greater trochanter to serve as the point where skeletal traction can be delivered.

DEFINITIVE MANAGEMENT

Plain postreduction radiographs and the CT scan are carefully examined before the treatment plan is finalized. The presence of bone fragments in the joint warrants surgical removal, generally through a Kocher–Langenbeck approach. Operative treatment is indicated for femoral head fractures with displacement of 2 mm or more in type IA or type IIA fractures (Pipkin types I and II), the presence of a type IIIB femoral neck fracture (Pipkin type III), displaced type IVA or type IVB fractures (Pipkin type IV), and in patients with multiple injuries.

When minimally displaced or nondisplaced type IA or type IIA fractures (Pipkin types I or II) occur as isolated injuries, they are treated nonoperatively. Excellent results have been achieved by immobilizing the patient with skeletal traction for 3 to 4 weeks, followed by mobilization with touch-down weight-bearing for 4 to 6 weeks. Hip flexion greater than 60° must be avoided for the first 6 to 8 weeks. Operative treatment of type IA or type IIA femoral head fractures (Pipkin types I and II) that are displaced or occur as components of a multiple-injury complex is done through an anterior incision to visualize the anterior fragment (Fig. 2). Internal fixation is accomplished with countersunk 3.5-mm or 4-mm screws or with Herbert screws.

The Watson–Jones approach is used for type IIIB injuries (Pipkin type III). The femoral neck fracture is reduced anatomically and fixed with three parallel cannulated screws (Fig. 3). Associated femoral head fragments are visualized by rotating the leg externally with the knee flexed (the "figure-of-four" position) and are managed with screw fixation.

Internal fixation of femoral head fragments in type V injuries (Pipkin type IV) that are associated with acetabular fractures must be planned concurrently with internal fixation of the acetabular fracture. The prognosis for Brumback type IV injuries is particularly poor. Elevation and bone grafting

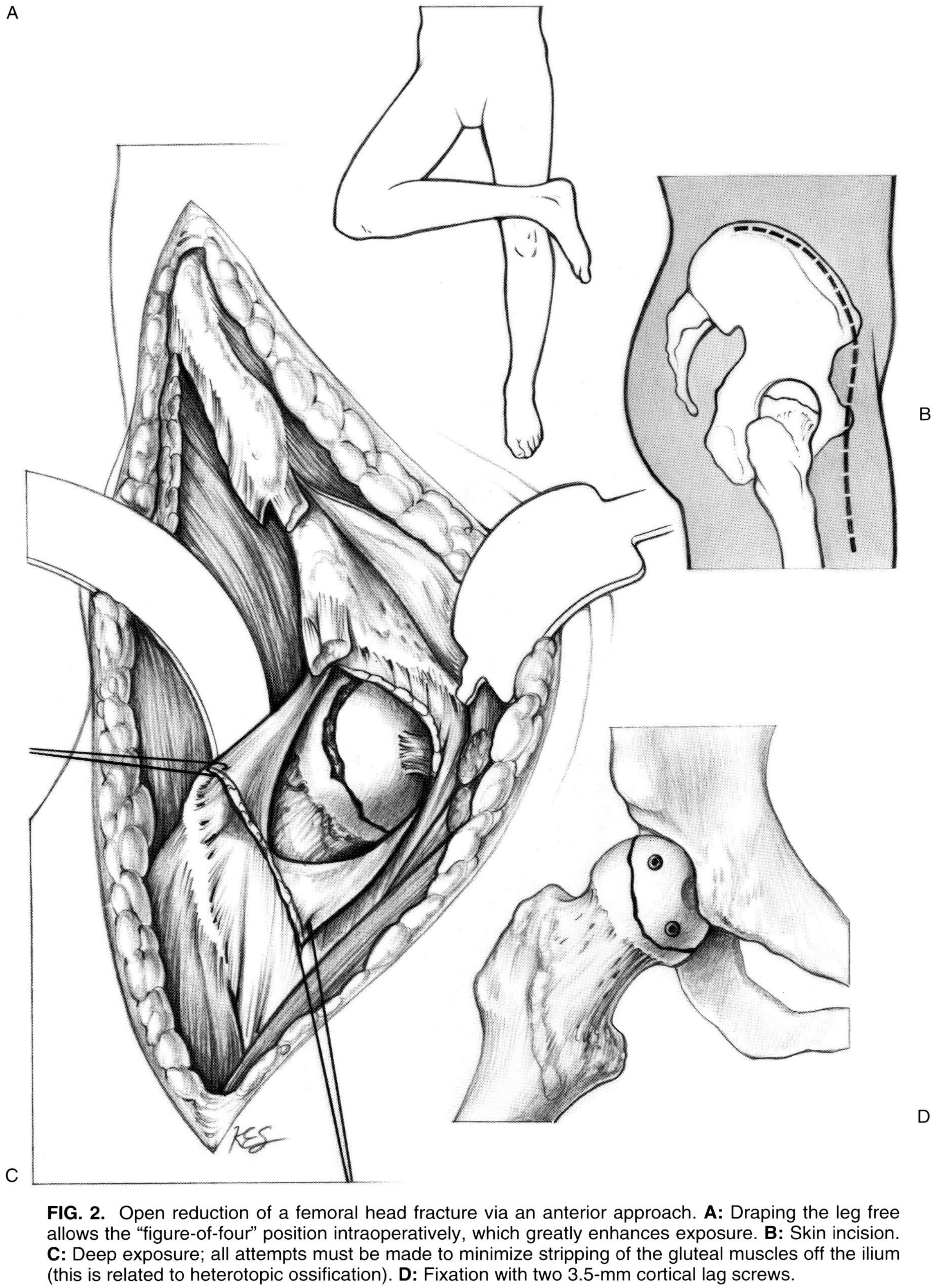

FIG. 2. Open reduction of a femoral head fracture via an anterior approach. **A:** Draping the leg free allows the "figure-of-four" position intraoperatively, which greatly enhances exposure. **B:** Skin incision. **C:** Deep exposure; all attempts must be made to minimize stripping of the gluteal muscles off the ilium (this is related to heterotopic ossification). **D:** Fixation with two 3.5-mm cortical lag screws.

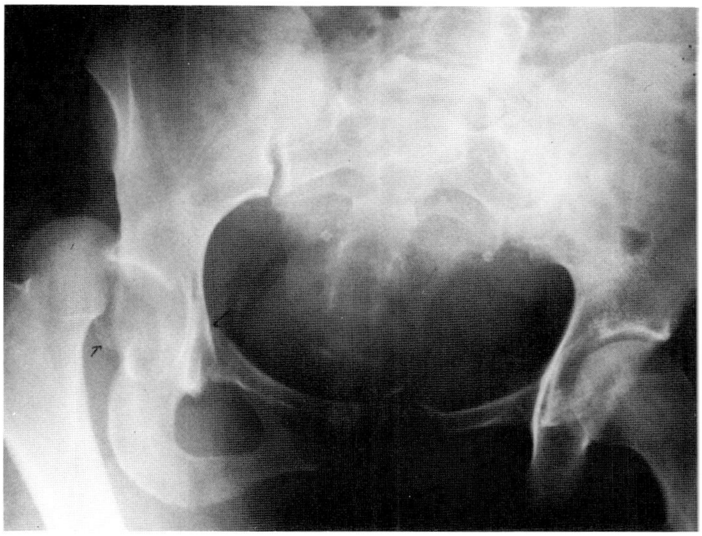
A

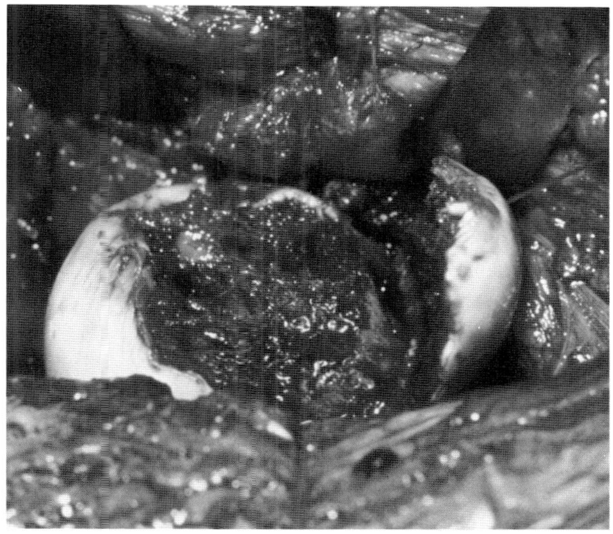
B

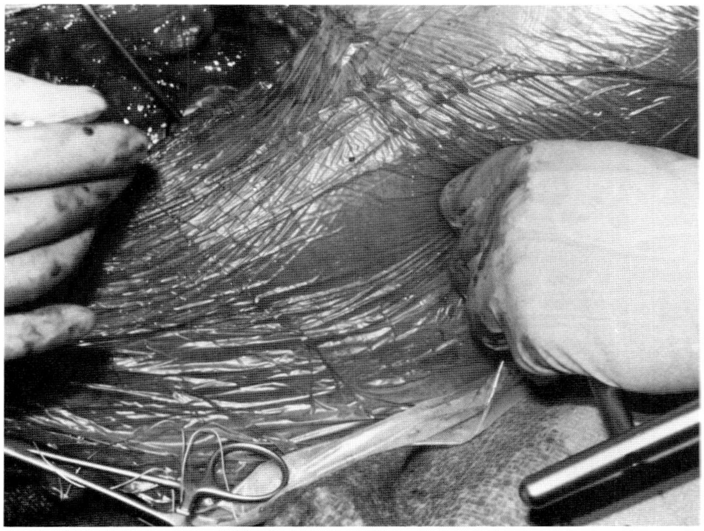
C

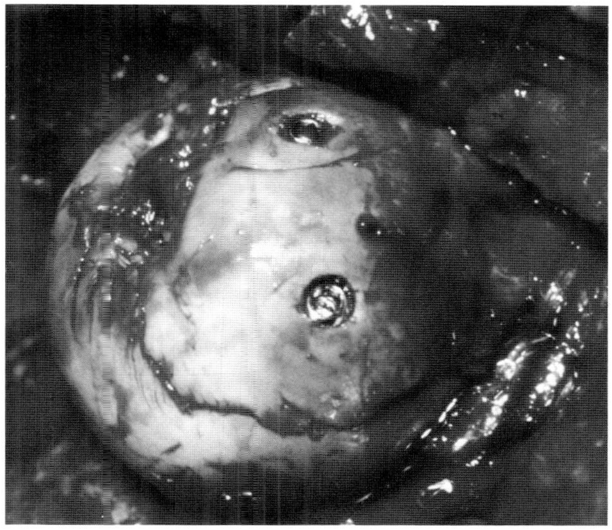
D

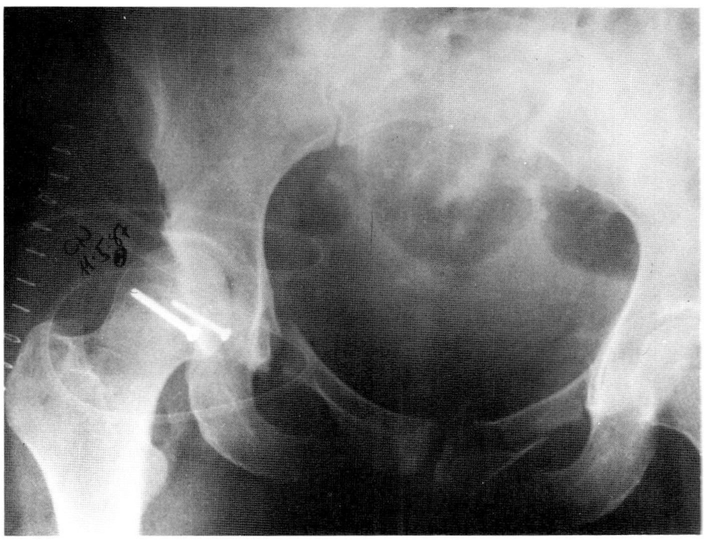
E

FIG. 3. A Brumback IA femoral head fracture in a 22-year-old woman. **A:** Admission pelvic radiograph of the posterior dislocation. **B:** Intraoperative view of displaced fracture. **C:** Exposure and reduction are enhanced by the percutaneously placed 5-mm Schanz screw with a universal chuck attached. **D:** Reduction and fixation with two 3.5-mm cortical lag screws. **E:** Postoperative radiograph.

of the indentation fracture have recently been recommended, but the results are unsatisfactory.

Unless limited weight bearing is contraindicated by other injuries, patients with femoral head fractures of any severity are permitted to ambulate with touch-down weight-bearing for 10 to 12 weeks after internal fixation. No hip flexion precautions are necessary if all the posterior wall fragments have been securely fixed.

COMPLICATIONS

Avascular necrosis is a common complication of hip dislocations and must be treated conservatively whenever possible. Using an anterior approach for open reduction and internal fixation does not increase the risk of AVN (4). Intertrochanteric flexion osteotomy is a possible treatment if a small avascular lesion can be removed from the weight-bearing area by an osteotomy of 40° to 60°.

Heterotopic ossification and subsequent limited function can occur with any hip dislocation or surgical management, but the incidence of these complications increases when an anterior approach is used for fixation of type IA and IIA fractures (Pipkin types I and II). If hip flexion is restricted to less than 90° and rotation is impaired, surgical resection can reliably increase flexion by 20° to 30°. Planning of the resection is based on a preoperative CT scan. The sciatic nerve must be identified and traced into the sciatic notch before any bone is resected. The results of resection are equally good whether they are done early or late, and resection can be considered as early as 6 to 9 months after injury. Low-dose postoperative irradiation to the surgical field (800–1,000 R over 1–5 days) may prevent recurrence.

SKELETALLY IMMATURE PATIENTS

Hip dislocations are fairly common in children may be associated with avascular necrosis and recurrent instability. For this reason, immobilization in a spica cast after closed reduction is recommended in children under the age of 12 years. Great care must be taken to look for joint diastasis in the postreduction CT scan.

Femoral head fractures in children are rare, but when they occur they are treated by the same principles as fractures in adults. Displaced epiphyseal fractures of the proximal femur must not be misdiagnosed as femoral head fractures and require open reduction and fixation with smooth pins.

REFERENCES

1. Epstein HC, Wiss DA, Cozen L. Posterior fracture-dislocation of the hip with fractures of the femoral head. *Clin Orthop* 1985;201:9–17.
2. Brumback RI, Kenzora JE, Levitt LE, Burgess AR, Polk A. Fractures of the femoral head. In: *Proceedings of the 1986 Hip Society*. St. Louis: CV Mosby; 1987:181–206.
3. Pipkin G. Treatment of grade IV fracture-dislocation of the hip. A review. *J Bone Joint Surg* 1957;39A:1027–42.
4. Thorpe M, Swiontkowski M, Seiler J, Hansen ST. Operative management of femoral head fractures. *Orthop Trans* 1989;13:1–51.

Orthopaedic Trauma Protocols, edited by
Sigvard T. Hansen, Jr. and Marc F. Swiontkowski,
Raven Press, Ltd., New York, © 1993.

CHAPTER 21

Hip Joint: Acetabular Fractures

Keith A. Mayo

MECHANISM OF INJURY

Most acetabular fractures are caused by high-energy indirect forces that transmit energy to the acetabulum through the entire lower limb, the femur, or the greater trochanter. Occasionally, anteroposterior pelvic crushing injuries or direct blows to the lateral aspect of the ilium can produce fractures extending into the acetabulum. Many factors influence the fracture pattern, including the position of the hip at the time of impact, the magnitude and direction of the force, and the point of application of force. The injury pattern is influenced by variable conditions such as a patient's bone density and the presence of ipsilateral lower extremity fractures or blunt soft-tissue injuries, particularly in the gluteal area. These last two factors may dissipate the amount of energy delivered to the acetabulum. The most common mechanisms include vehicular trauma, falls from height, industrial injuries, and athletic accidents. In elderly patients with osteoporotic bone, a simple fall with impact occurring directly on the trochanter can produce a serious acetabular injury.

Because high-energy mechanisms are usually involved, a significant number of patients with acetabular fractures sustain trauma to other systems. The most common associated injuries are fractures of the ipsilateral or contralateral lower extremities. Local soft-tissue injuries may reflect primary or secondary sites of impact but are frequently overlooked or underestimated. They are a major problem when peritrochanteric crushing and closed degloving (Morel–Lavale lesion) have occurred. Injuries associated with fracture displacement include disruption of the superior gluteal artery, most commonly seen with medial rotation of a proximal sciatic notch fragment. Associated neurologic trauma may involve injury to various divisions of the sciatic nerve from traction or direct contact with a fracture fragment or a dislocated femoral head. Displaced anterior pelvic ring disruptions may damage the lower urinary tract. In women these injuries are usually restricted to the bladder, whereas in men they may involve both the bladder and the urethra. Rarely, iliac, femoral, or obturator vascular injuries may result from anterior ring displacement or crushing.

Concurrent spinal injuries seldom occur with acetabular fractures. The only exceptions are fracture configurations encompassing complex posterior ring injuries, particularly displaced fractures of the sacrum associated with injuries to the articulation between L-5 and S-1.

Diverse intraabdominal trauma may occur in association with acetabular fractures. Splenic and hepatic injuries are the most common, but bowel injuries can also occur. They can be difficult to diagnose and have direct consequences for acetabular fracture management. Coincident intracranial and thoracic trauma often have a profound influence on acetabular trauma (1). The presence of these injuries is an urgent indication for ORIF of the acetabular fracture to mobilize the patient but, at the same time, constitutes a serious perioperative liability. Balancing these considerations can be a difficult management challenge.

ANATOMIC CONSIDERATIONS

The trabecular architecture of the innominate bone directly influences fracture patterns and implant placement (Fig. 1). The articular surface of the acetabulum can be conceptualized as being enclosed within the arms of an inverted "Y" (Fig. 2). The limbs of the "Y" correspond to the two-column schematic proposed by Letournel and Judet and are the basis of their fracture classification (Fig. 3).

Department of Orthopaedics. Harborview Medical Center, University of Washington, Seattle, Washington 98104

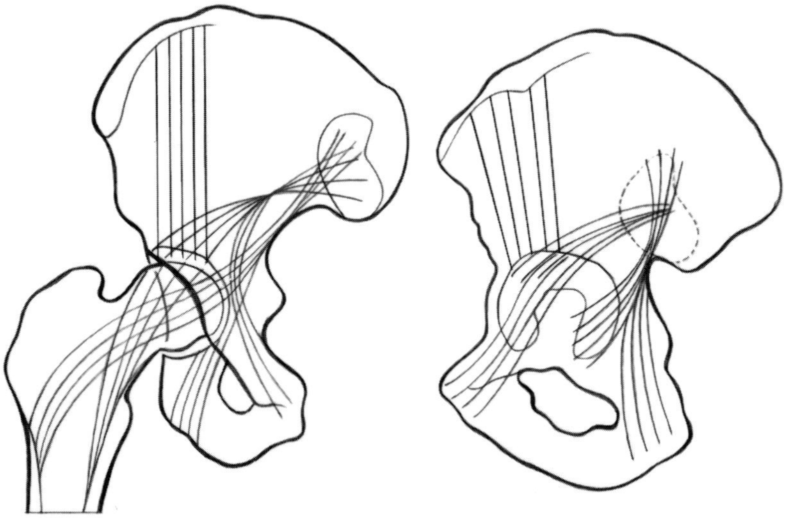

FIG. 1. Trabecular architecture of the proximal femur and innominate bone. Fracture planes frequently follow these trabecular planes.

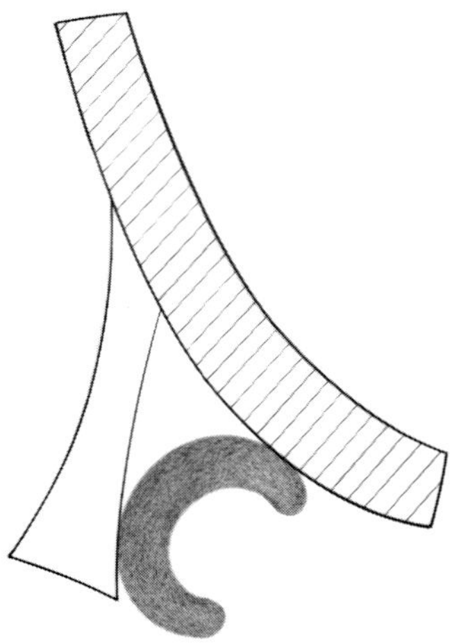

FIG. 2. The inverted "Y" concept of Letournel. The two limbs define the anterior and posterior columns.

The soft tissues surrounding the innominate bone are also very complex. The muscular envelope, the adjacent neurovascular structures, and the pelvic viscera are at risk for both traumatic and iatrogenic injuries. The primary concern with regard to posterior and extended lateral surgical approaches is protection of the sciatic nerve and the superior gluteal neurovascular bundle (Fig. 4). Anterior exposures require precise dissection of the inguinal anatomy and safe mobilization of the external iliac vessels and the femoral and obturator nerves (Fig. 5). The bladder and the urethra must also be protected during an anterior pelvic ring exposure and reduction. These structures are susceptible to injury from fracture displacement or symphyseal disruptions, and sometimes occur in conjunction with blunt abdominal trauma.

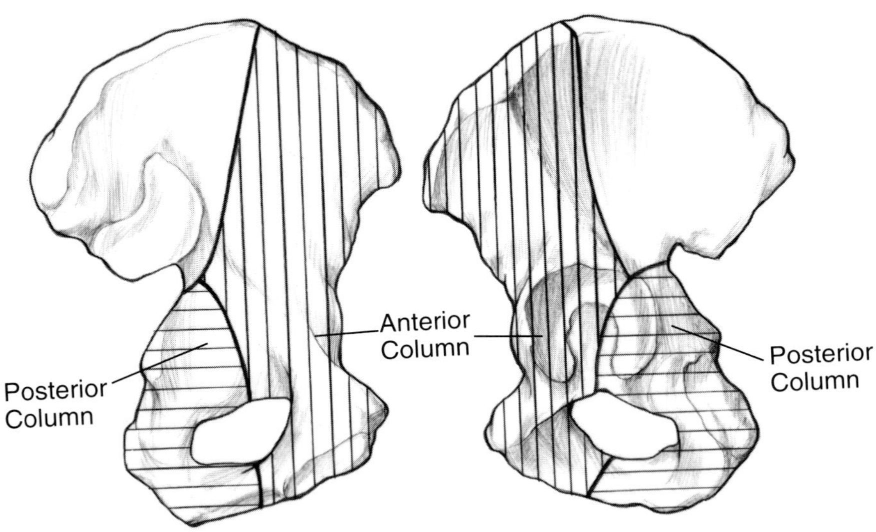

FIG. 3. The two-column schematic.

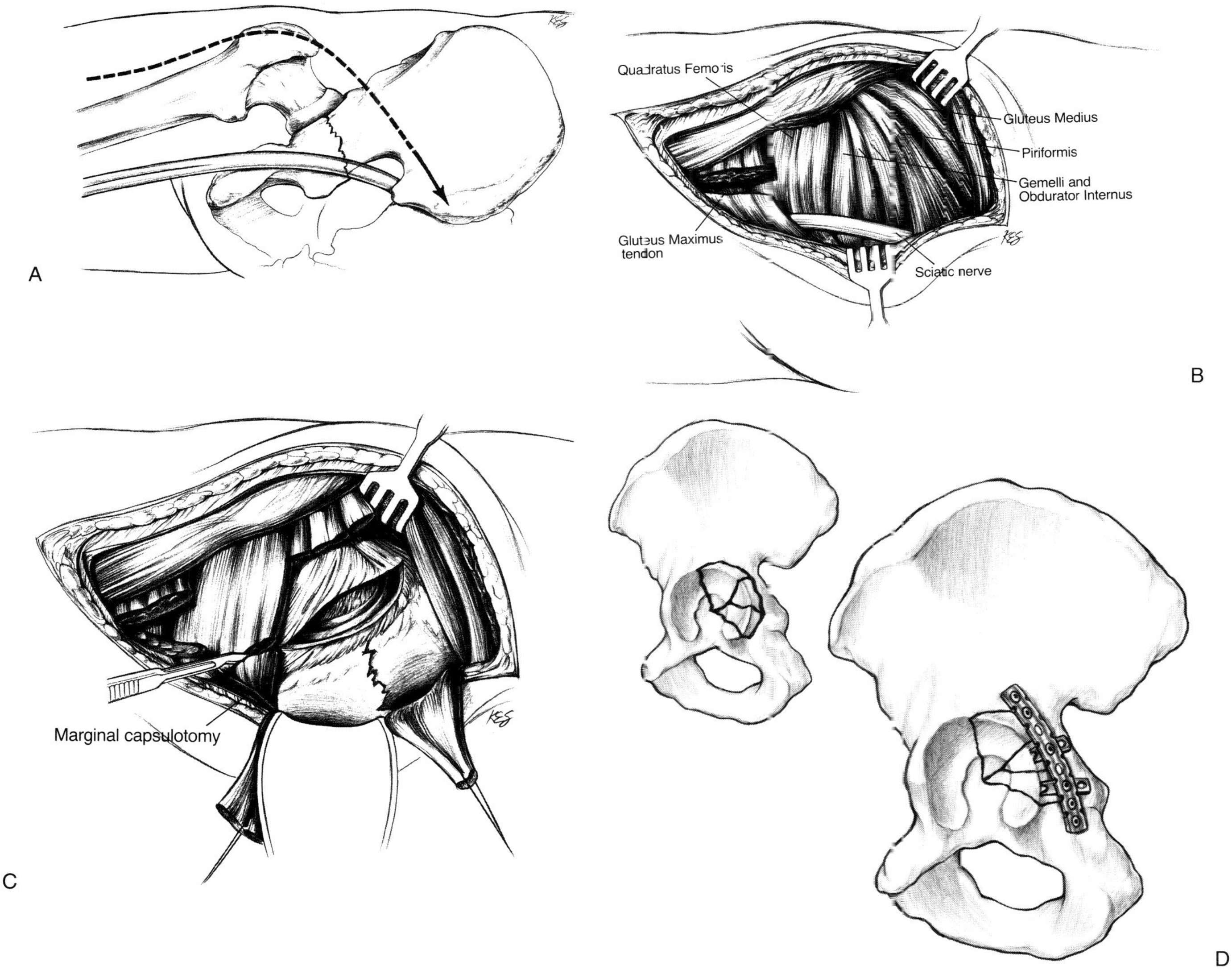

FIG. 4. Kocher–Langenbeck approach. **A:** Skin incision. **B:** Localization of sciatic nerve posterior to short external rotators. **C:** Final exposure following short external rotator tenotomy, partial division of quadratus femoris, and marginal capsulotomy. **D:** Fixation of a comminuted posterior wall fracture with two "spring" plates and a 3.5-mm reconstructed plate in the buttress mode. (**A–C**: Reprinted from Mayo, KA. Surgical approaches to the acetabulum. *Tech Orthop* 1990; 4:28. Used with permission of Aspen Publishers, Inc.)

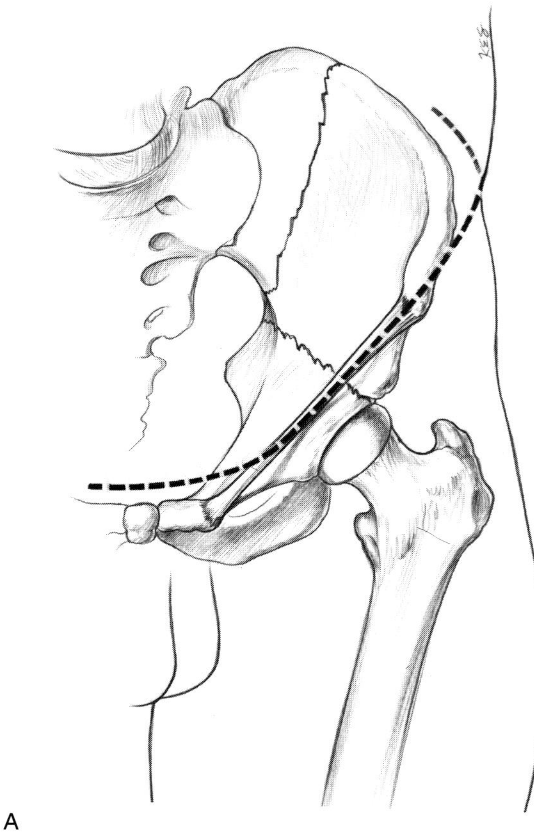

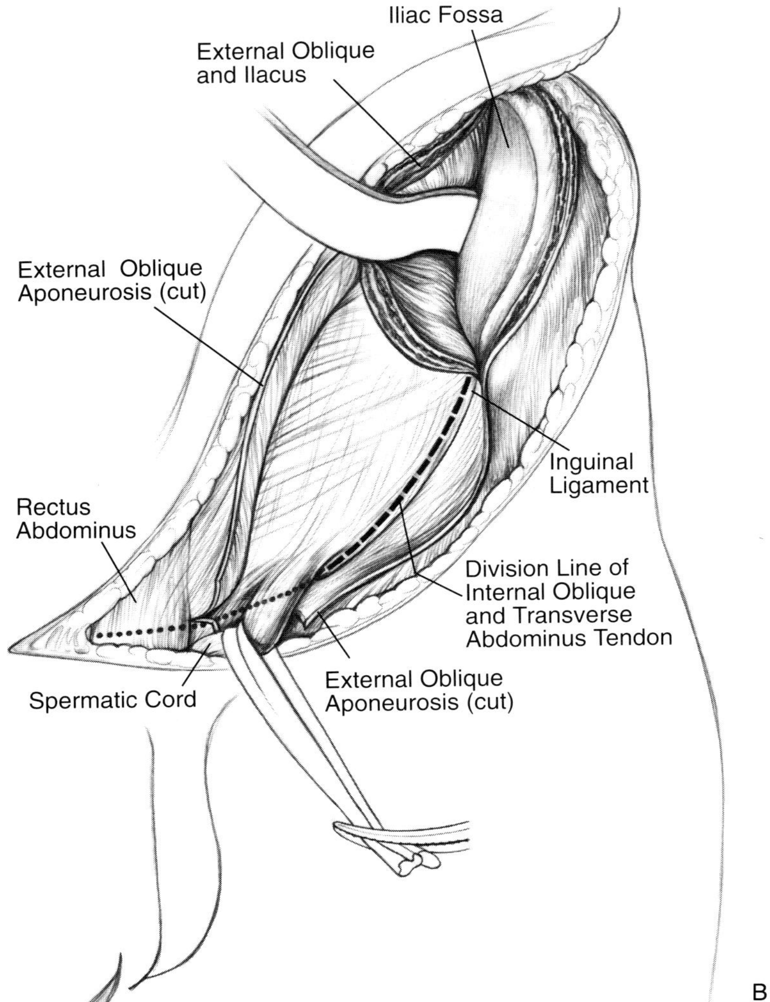

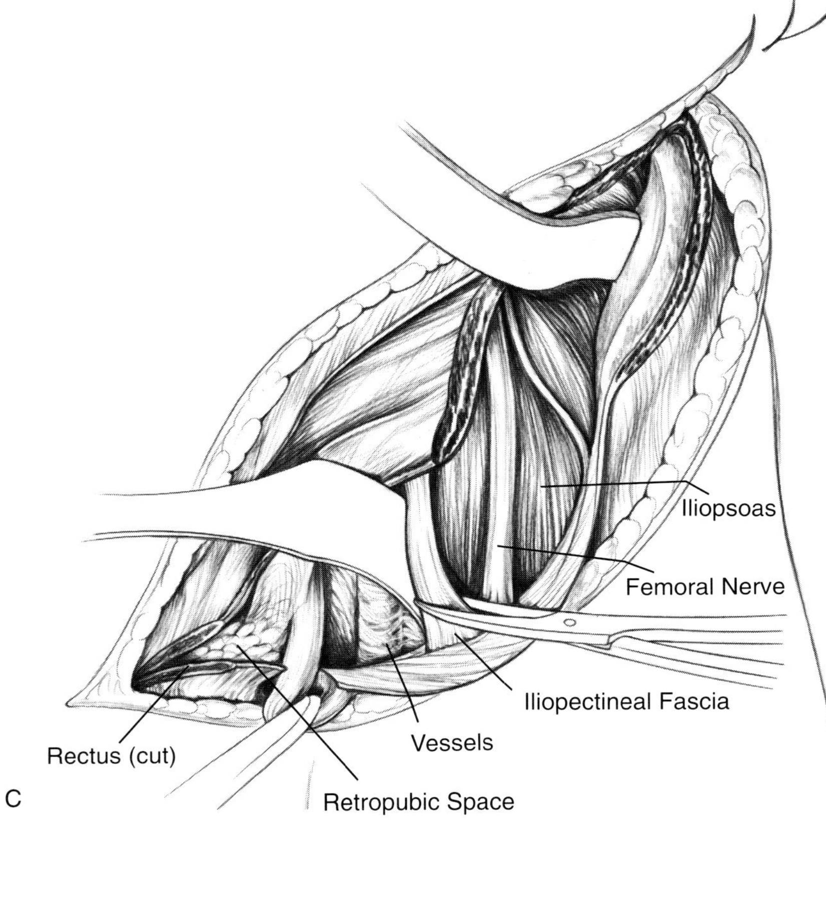

FIG. 5. Ilioinguinal approach. **A:** Skin incision. **B:** Exposure of internal iliac fossa and unroofing of the inguinal canal. **C:** Floor of the inguinal canal has been opened by release of the conjoint tendon and tranversalis fascia. The iliopectineal fascia is released with retraction of the vessels medially. **D:** Lateral wound interval exposing entire internal iliac fossa from sacroiliac (SI) joint to psoas gutter. **E:** Fixation of a both-column fracture with multiple 3.5-mm cortical lag screws and a 3.5-mm pelvic reconstruction plate along the pelvic brain. (**A–D:** Reprinted from Mayo KA. Surgical approaches to the acetabulum. *Tech Orthop* 1990; 4:30–1. Used with permission of Aspen Publishers, Inc.)

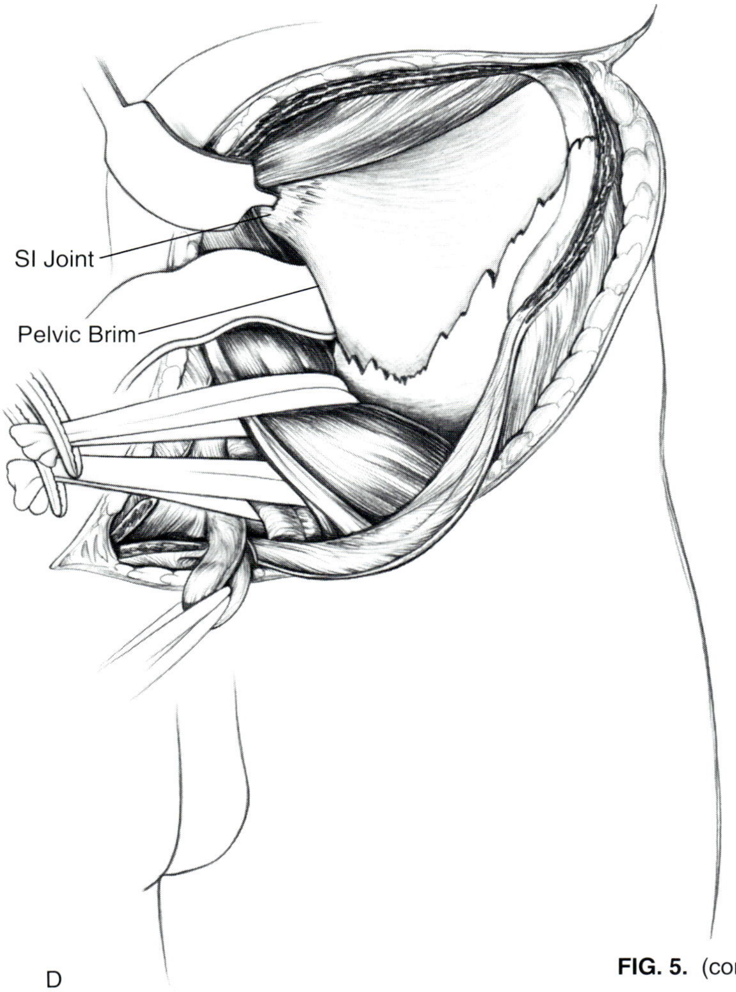

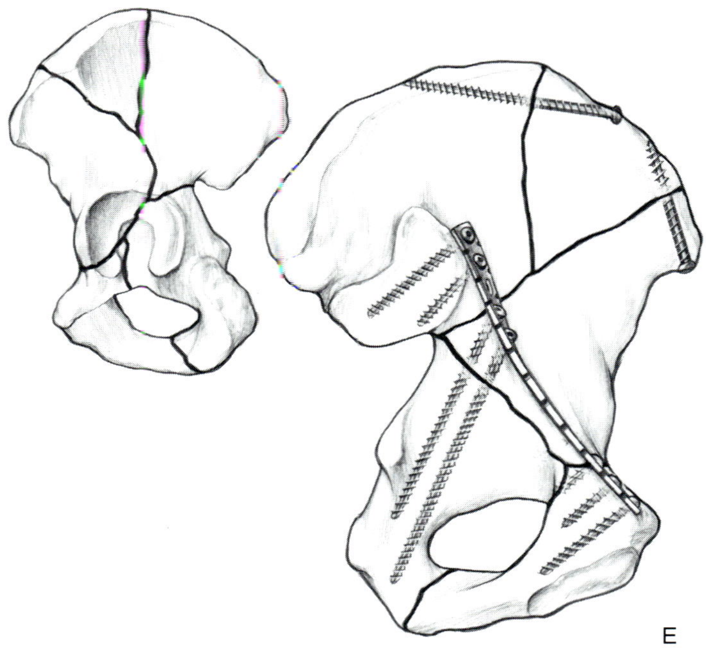

FIG. 5. (continued)

These mechanisms rarely produce bowel injuries, but injuries to the sigmoid colon can occur and have disastrous consequences if they are not detected.

CLASSIFICATION

The classification of Letournel and Judet is based on anatomy and provides guidelines for choosing a surgical approach (Fig. 6). This classification is based on the two-column schematic (inverted "Y") mentioned above (see Fig. 2). By definition, posterior wall fractures become columnar fractures as they extend into the obturator foramen. The transition from an anterior wall pattern to a columnar pattern is somewhat less precise but occurs with involvement of significant portions of the extraarticular pubic ramus or ilium. Confusion can arise when attempts are made to differentiate both-column variants from fracture patterns involving a transverse component. In both-column fractures no articular segment is contiguous with intact ilium, and the acetabulum is free-floating. Both columns are also involved in transverse patterns, but an articular section remains intact in all cases.

ASSESSMENT

Physical Examination

Special consideration should be given to the neurologic examination to detect subtle yet significant deficits, particularly in the peroneal branch of the sciatic nerve. All patients should have a rectal examination, and when marked anterior ring displacement is noted rectosigmoidoscopy may be indicated to rule out an occult open fracture or a retroperitoneal colon injury. In this situation, bimanual and speculum vaginal examination is also indicated. Finally, the soft-tissue envelope is thoroughly assessed for evidence of blunt trauma and closed degloving injuries. The condition of the soft tissues directly influences the choice of surgical approach.

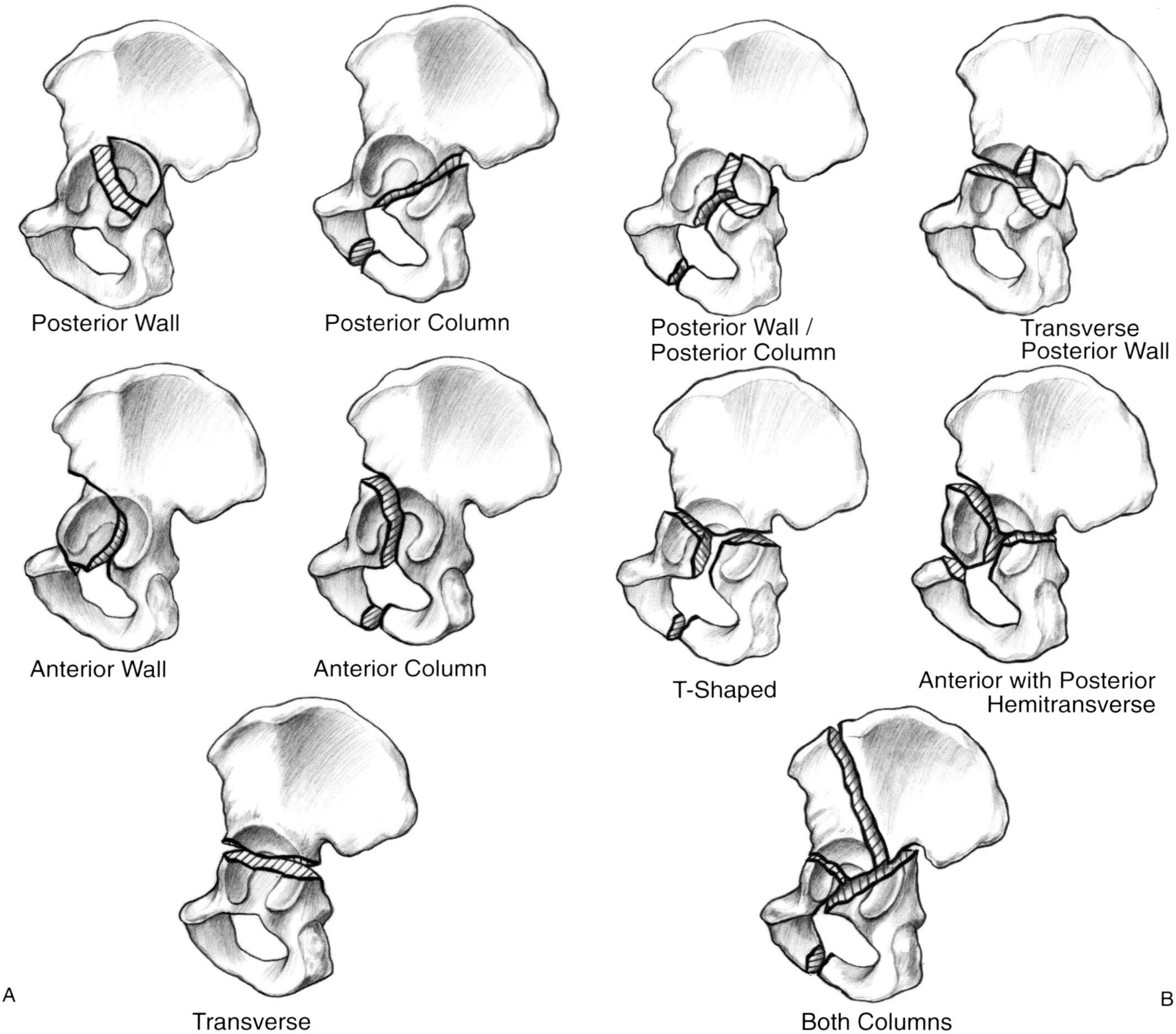

FIG. 6. Classification of Letournel and Judet. Elementary **(A)** and associated patterns **(B)** are based on the two-column schema.

Radiographic Evaluation

Routine plain radiographic projections include an AP of the pelvis, an AP of the involved hemipelvis, and 45° Judet oblique views in which the patient, not the beam, is rotated (Fig. 7). Two-dimensional CT scans are also routinely obtained, usually with 3-mm intervals through the joint and 5-mm intervals both above and below the joint. The CT scan provides additional information about the primary fracture pattern and may also reveal areas of marginal impaction, loose intraarticular fragments, femoral head fractures, and comminution that was unrecognized on standard radiographic views.

Special Studies

Three-dimensional CT reconstructions are useful for delineating complex or transitional injury patterns but should not be substituted for the primary studies. When three-dimensional reconstructions are anticipated, software manufacturers' guidelines regarding scan intervals and overlap must be followed carefully. Angiographic evaluation of acetabular fractures is rarely indicated. An exception is made when an unexpectedly large amount of blood has been lost, a situation usually associated with injury to the superior gluteal artery at the level of the greater sciatic notch. In this case embolization may be warranted, and the vascular injury becomes a

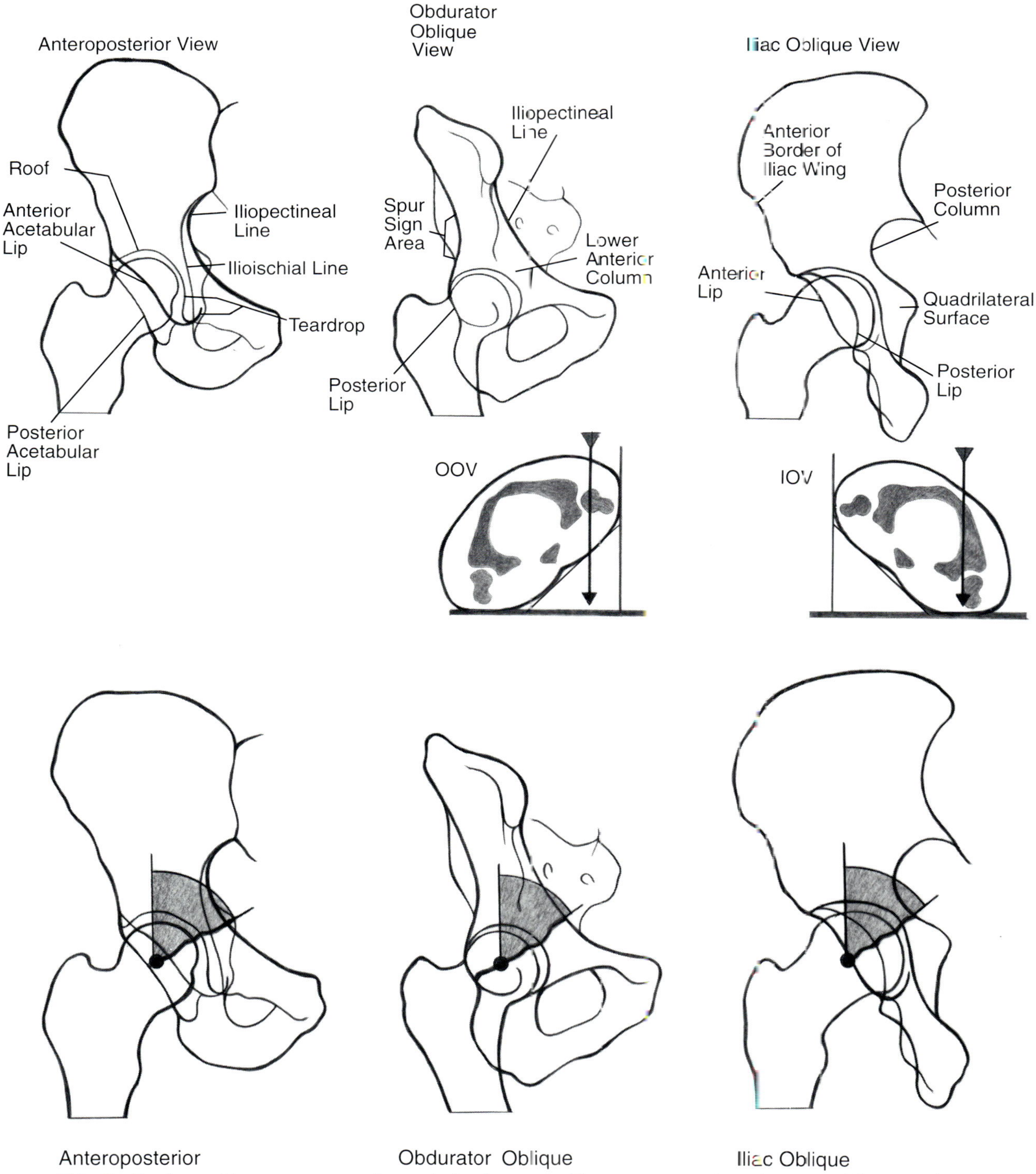

FIG. 7. Radiographic assessment of acetabular fractures. The anteroposterior, obturator oblique, and iliac oblique views are essential for the definition of the fracture.

factor in choosing the approach. Assessment of the lower urinary tract is required for displaced anterior pelvic ring injuries. A retrograde urethrogram should be performed in males and a cystogram should be performed in both sexes. The urethrogram should precede placement of a Foley catheter to avoid conversion of an incomplete lesion into a complete lesion.

EMERGENT MANAGEMENT

Acute intervention is usually focused on reduction of associated hip dislocations. Most hip dislocations are posterior and are associated with various sizes of wall fragments. Every effort should be made to carry out reduction as atraumatically as possible. Optimally, these maneuvers are performed with full muscle relaxation and should not be attempted more than once without relaxation. Occasionally reduction can be difficult even with general anesthesia and skeletal paralysis. Two examples include ipsilateral femoral shaft fractures and soft-tissue impingement secondary to "buttonholing" of the femoral head through a relatively small posterior capsular tear. A percutaneous Schanz screw placed in the proximal femur is a helpful reduction aid in this situation. Using a Schanz screw in this manner allows direct application of force, which is usually successful in reducing the dislocation when it is combined with hip positioning in variable amounts of flexion, adduction, and medial rotation. This maneuver indirectly reduces the ligamentous and capsular attachments between the proximal femur and the acetabular columns, and is useful for reduction of fracture patterns with predominantly medial displacement.

Temporary skeletal traction is indicated in patients with femoral head subluxations who are at risk for injury by pressure from a fracture margin. Traction applied through the distal femur or the proximal tibia reduces the potential for this injury by distracting the joint. Traction is most useful in fracture patterns with displaced transverse components. Temporary, laterally directed traction delivered through a trochanteric screw is rarely indicated.

With important exceptions, emergent ORIF of acetabular fractures is rarely indicated. Secondary nerve (sciatic) palsy after closed reduction warrants emergent neural exploration and primary fracture stabilization. Closed reduction can also result in entrapment of large bony fragments within the joint. These fragments must be removed urgently to prevent further articular trauma. Fractures associated with repairable large-vessel injuries should also be emergently reduced and stabilized to protect the vascular repair. Injuries with large open wounds should be stabilized to enhance wound management. Finally, when suprapubic drainage for a bladder or urethral injury is unavoidable, primary ORIF should be performed if the fracture pattern can be managed through an ilioinguinal approach. These two procedures should be performed in a coordinated or a simultaneous effort to avert potential infectious complications associated with late intervention in the face of established suprapubic drainage.

DEFINITIVE MANAGEMENT

After emergent considerations have been addressed, attention is directed to other preoperative considerations. One of the more important is surveillance and prophylaxis for deep venous thrombosis. Duplex ultrasound has been shown to be an extremely reliable diagnostic modality and has replaced venography in most situations. When thrombi are detected preoperatively, a vena caval filter should be inserted and ORIF should be expedited. Anticoagulation should be postponed until a safe postoperative juncture. Prophylaxis is a more complex issue. Preliminary studies indicate that both pneumatic compression devices and low-dose anticoagulation (heparin) can be valuable. However, either therapy can present problems in the presence of multiple lower-extremity injuries, and their use should be individualized. Operative indications in acetabular fractures vary and are discussed separately according to fracture type (2,3).

Wall Fractures

All wall fractures that allow subluxation of the femoral head should be treated operatively. In addition, fractures with large areas of articular (marginal) impaction and those with incarcerated joint debris are best managed surgically. In other situations, treatment is determined by the location, size, and amount of displacement of the wall fragments, particularly in posterior wall fractures. Patterns extending into the supraacetabular surface involve the lateral weight-bearing surface and are particularly worrisome. They are best treated by ORIF if there is any malrotation or displacement that limits contact between the wall and the femoral head. When involvement is primarily retroacetabular, the size of the fragment and the potential for joint instability become more important considerations. Studies done on cadavers suggest that ORIF is appropriate when more than one third of the wall is involved. However, joint debridement and lavage benefit even fractures with small fragments and no obvious bony debris after reduction of a posterior dislocation. For this reason, an argument can be made for surgical treatment when ORIF is technically feasible.

Columnar and Transverse Fractures

Failure to maintain a concentric reduction between the intact articular segment and the femoral head is the most important indication for surgery in these injuries. Even subtle subluxations completely alter joint congruity and consequently force transmission properties (Fig. 8). When joint congruity is maintained and a significant (2–3 mm) intraarticular step-off exists, roof arc measurements provide a semiquantitative method of assessing the remaining area of intact acetabulum and a preliminary guide for operative intervention.

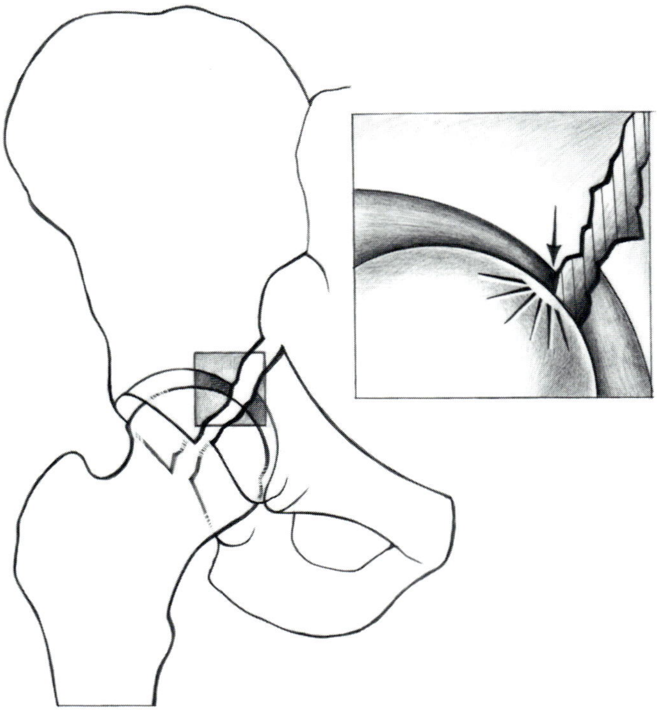

FIG. 8. Articular incongruity. Minimal subluxation of the femor head medially results in high-peak stresses on the acetabular and femoral head articular cartilage.

Both-Column Fractures

Both-column fracture patterns are characterized by complete separation of the acetabular articular segments from the intact ilium. The free-floating joint and the bony fragments can rearrange themselves around the displaced femoral head much like a template. This phenomenon is called secondary congruence (Fig. 9). When the displaced fragments are small, satisfactory functional outcomes are possible from secondary congruence. However, with significant medial and cephalad displacement, the sequelae of pelvic obliquity, leg-length inequality, and disrupted hip mechanics warrant surgical treatment in most cases.

Preoperative planning is critical for acetabular reconstruction and entails a detailed examination of the pertinent radiographic studies. The fracture pattern should be outlined on a pelvic model or diagram, and an alternative plan for reduction and fixation should be chosen and drawn within the constraints of the desired approach (3). A variety of surgical approaches, including the Kocher–Langenbeck (see Fig. 4), the ilioinguinal (see Fig. 5), and the extended iliofemoral (Fig. 10), are widely used. The choice of approach is based predominantly on the injury pattern but a number of other factors should also be taken into consideration. They include the condition of the local soft tissues, the presence of associated injuries (particularly intracranial trauma), the age and functional status of the patient, and the delay until surgical

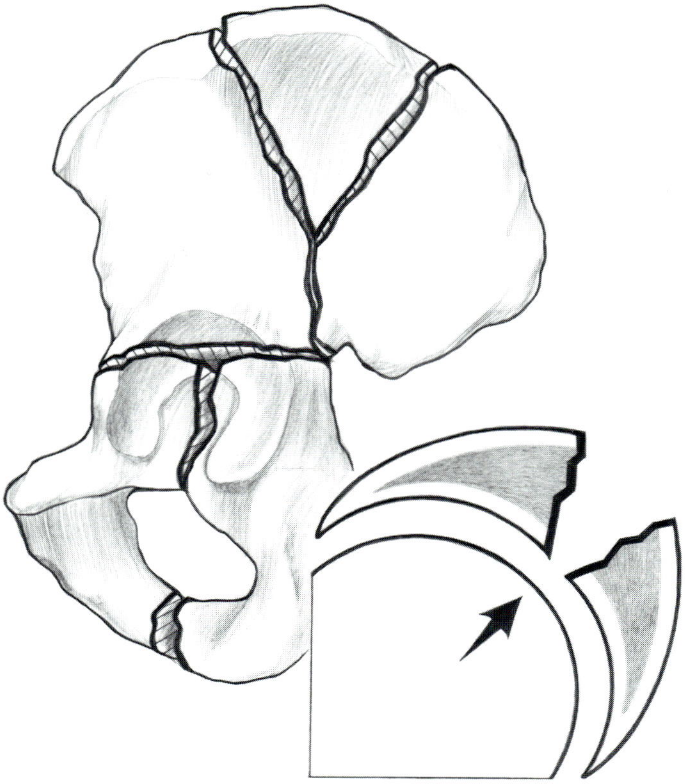

FIG. 9. Secondary acetabular congruence in a displaced both-column fracture.

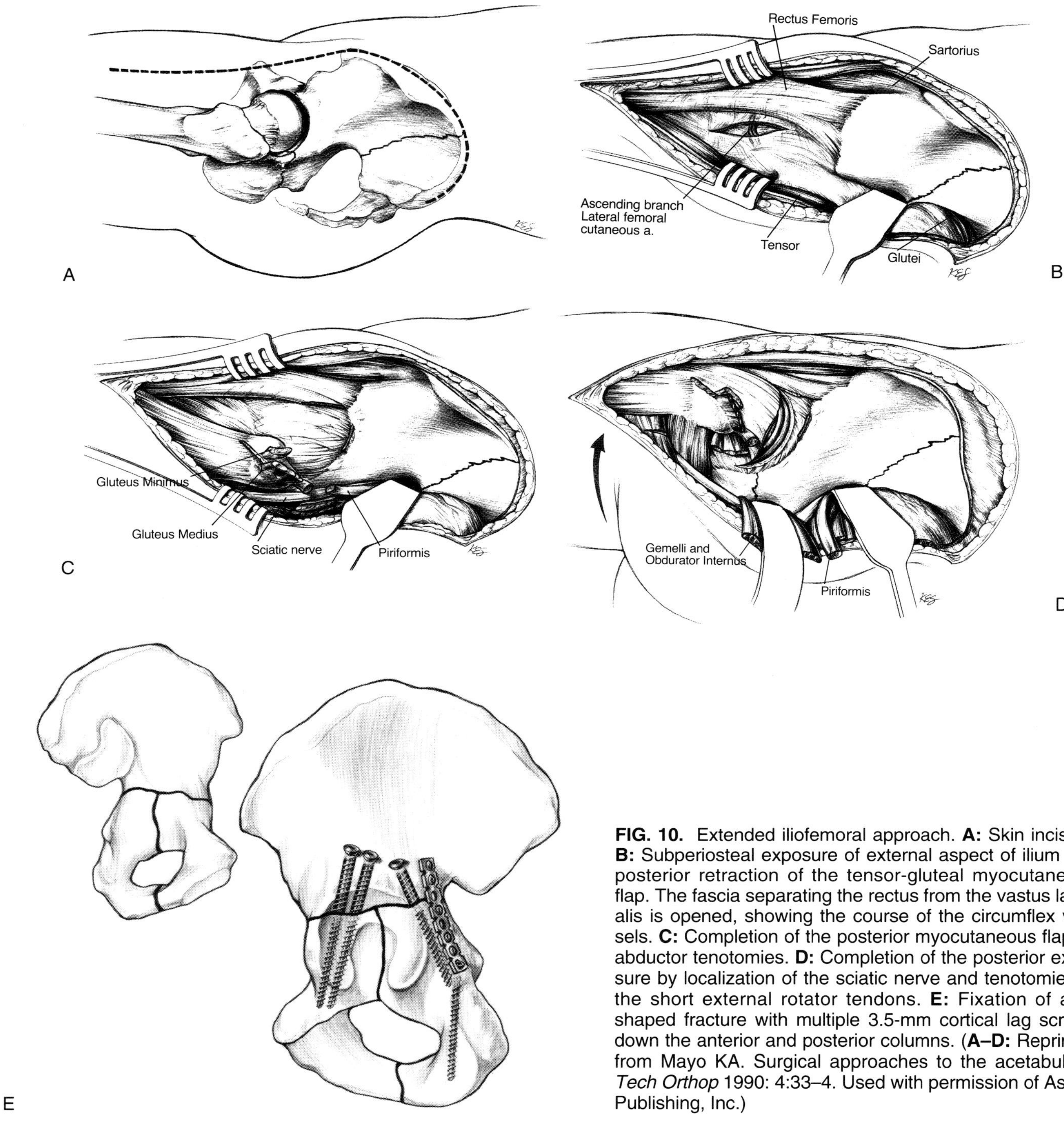

FIG. 10. Extended iliofemoral approach. **A:** Skin incision. **B:** Subperiosteal exposure of external aspect of ilium and posterior retraction of the tensor-gluteal myocutaneous flap. The fascia separating the rectus from the vastus lateralis is opened, showing the course of the circumflex vessels. **C:** Completion of the posterior myocutaneous flap by abductor tenotomies. **D:** Completion of the posterior exposure by localization of the sciatic nerve and tenotomies of the short external rotator tendons. **E:** Fixation of a T-shaped fracture with multiple 3.5-mm cortical lag screws down the anterior and posterior columns. (**A–D:** Reprinted from Mayo KA. Surgical approaches to the acetabulum. *Tech Orthop* 1990: 4:33–4. Used with permission of Aspen Publishing, Inc.)

intervention. The ilioinguinal approach is associated with the lowest overall rate of patient morbidity and is the first choice when the injury pattern is amenable. Primary and alternative approach choices are listed by fracture types according to the Letournel classification in Table 1.

Positioning considerations are guided by the surgical approach. The prone position on a fracture table is optimal for the Kocher–Langenbeck approach (see Fig. 4), especially for treatment of complicated fracture patterns. The Judet table is suitable for this approach and can also be used for ilioinguinal and iliofemoral approaches. Alternatively, the patient can be positioned supine or in the lateral decubitus position on a standard operating table. In this case, the injured hindquarter is prepped and the leg is left free for intraoperative manipulation. Access for plane radiography and fluoroscopy should be guaranteed before prepping. The use of somatosensory-evoked potential monitoring is controversial, but this modality may provide some protection against iatrogenic nerve injury. Routine perioperative antibiotics are administered and a Foley catheter is placed when long operating times are anticipated. An epidural catheter is inserted either before or after induction of a general anesthetic. Combined anesthesia decreases the need for inhalational agents, induces a measure of hypotension, and provides access for postoperative pain management with epidural opiates or bupivacaine. Vascular access and cardiopulmonary monitoring are appropriate for keeping track of a patient's overall condition and anticipated blood loss. Induced hypotension is useful in an appropriate clinical setting and a Haemonetic Cell Saver (Haemonetics, Braintree, MA) is used routinely except for minor wall injuries.

In addition to the standard fracture sets, a variety of instruments should be available. These include specialized clamps, oscillating drills, long drill bits and sleeves, long (up to 130 mm) 3.5-mm and 4.5-mm screws, and both straight and curved pelvic reconstruction plates. A femoral distractor should be available for joint distraction when reconstruction is not done on a fracture table. The techniques for each reduction and fixation are determined by the approach and the specific injuries.

Postoperatively, the leg on the injured side can be placed in a hip CPM machine in the recovery room. Postoperative pain relief is usually provided by epidural anesthesia. Suction drains are left in place until drainage subsides. Sequential compression devices are placed on both legs while the patient is in bed, and additional thromboembolic prophylaxis is administered with low-dose warfarin when there are no contraindications. Mobilization is begun by the second postoperative day and progressed as tolerated. Weight-bearing is limited (between 10–20 kg) for 8 to 12 weeks, depending on the fracture pattern and the fixation. In fracture patterns with significant posterior wall involvement, hip flexion is limited to 70° for the first 6 postoperative weeks. When the extended iliofemoral approach has been used, active hip abduction is deferred for 8 postoperative weeks.

In all patients except women of reproductive age, prophylaxis for heterotopic ossification consists of single low-dose irradiation when an extended iliofemoral approach has been used. In women of reproductive age and in patients who had surgery through the Kocher–Langenbeck approach, indomethacin is used. No intervention is indicated with an ilioinguinal approach.

Table 1. *Surgical Approach Choice*

Posterior wall
Posterior column
Anterior wall
Anterior column
Transverse
Post. column wall
Transverse-PW
T-shaped
Assoc. ant. + post. hemitransverse
Both-column

Primary
K-L
K-L
II
II
K-L
K-L
K-L
EIF
II
II

Alternatives
EIF (extended patterns)
EIF, II
II, EIF (depending on level)
EIF
EIF
II, K-L
EIF

COMPLICATIONS

Complications after acetabular fractures include sciatic retraction neuropraxia, heterotopic ossification, deep venous throbosis, infection, and vascular injuries. Sciatic retraction neuropraxia is the most common complication in an acute injury. The reported incidence of this complication has reached 11% with the Kocher–Langenbeck approach; much lower rates have been reported with the extended iliofemoral approach. Sciatic retraction neuropraxia is not associated with the ilioinguinal approach. The incidence of this complication can be lowered to inconsequential levels by careful leg positioning, meticulous delineation of the nerve path, limited skeletal traction, and prudent retraction. Skilled somatosensory-evoked potential monitoring may also be beneficial, particularly in cases of delayed surgery. Injuries to the lumbosacral plexus and the superior gluteal, obturator, and femoral nerves have been reported but are rare.

Among late complications, heterotopic ossification is very common. Unfortunately, functional grading systems developed for total hip surgery are poorly adapted for acetabular fractures. In most patients the amount of functional impairment caused by development of ectopic bone is not significant enough to warrant resection. The overall occurrence of heterotopic ossification reported with acetabular fractures ranges from 17% to 60%; the incidence of ankylosis or severe limitation of motion ranges from 2% to 12% (1). Differences among the series are largely attributable to use of the extensile approach. Preferred prophylaxis modalities have been described earlier.

Pulmonary embolism can be fatal but is rare (less than 1%) with acetabular surgery. However, the incidence of deep venous throbosis in pelvic ring injuries is very high; rates as high as 30% to 40% have been reported in duplex surveillance studies. Detection and prophylaxis remain the most effective deterrents. As mentioned earlier, preoperative detection of significant thrombi warrants placement of a vena caval filter during the perioperative period, followed by routine postoperative anticoagulation.

Overall infection rates in most series vary from 3% to 5%. Increased risk for infection is associated with local soft-tissue injuries, obesity, adjacent urinary drainage or colostomy, and extended approaches. In many cases joint involvement can usually be averted by early recognition and intervention. Debridement and lavage followed by closure over drains provide adequate treatment in some cases. In other cases, placement of antibiotic beads or delayed closure or flap coverage may be indicated. Optimal intervention is determined by the organisms involved and the condition of the local soft tissues.

Vascular injuries are relatively uncommon; most series report an incidence of less than 1%. The external iliac and superior gluteal systems are most at risk for vascular injuries. Surgery around these vessels requires great care during the initial dissection and the subsequent drilling and implant placement.

SKELETALLY IMMATURE PATIENTS

Acetabular fractures in children are relatively rare, occurring in less than 1% of patients reported in most series. Because the triradiate cartilage persists until early adolescence in most individuals, it is a component of most acetabular injuries. Imaging may be difficult in younger children and requires CT scanning and arthrography. The principles of treatment in children and adolescents are the same as in adults. No significant intraarticular deformity is acceptable. Implants are modified to accommodate the small pelvic size and, in general, implants should be removed early to avoid growth arrest or bone overgrowth. Screws and plates are preferred for pelvic stabilization in children because fixation with pins and wires is less secure and these implants are susceptible to migration. Short-term (3–4 week) spica casting may be indicated if compliance with weight-bearing restrictions is in doubt.

REFERENCES

1. Webb LX, Bossee MJ, Mayo K, Lange RH, Miller ME, Swiontkowski MF. Results in patients with craniocerebral trauma and an operatively managed acetabular fracture. *J Orthop Trauma* 1990;4:376–82.
2. Matta J, Mehne D, Roffi R. Fractures of the acetabulum: early results of a prospective study. *Clin Orthop* 1986;205:241–50.
3. Mayo K. Fractures of the acetabulum. *Orthop Clin North Am* 1987;18:43–57.

Orthopaedic Trauma Protocols, edited by
Sigvard T. Hansen, Jr., and Marc F. Swiontkowski,
Raven Press, Ltd., New York, © 1993.

CHAPTER 22

Femoral Neck Fractures

Marc F. Swiontkowski

MECHANISMS OF INJURY

Low-energy femoral neck fractures usually occur in elderly patients with osteopenic bone who slip and fall from a standing position. The degree of osteopenia can be estimated from the physiological age and the activity level of the patient. Motor vehicle accidents or falls from significant heights are the usual mechanisms of high-energy femoral neck fractures in patients with normal bone density. Although high-energy injuries make up only 5% to 7% of all femoral neck fractures, they are the types most often treated at regional trauma centers.

The force vector that produces a high-energy femoral neck fracture is applied along the axis of the femoral shaft. In a fall or a jump, the force is usually applied to an extended hip; in a motor vehicle accident, it is usually applied to a flexed hip. Injuries to an extended hip are commonly associated with spinal and calcaneal fractures; injuries occurring to a flexed hip are associated with femoral shaft fractures, posterior acetabular wall or femoral head fractures, and ligamentous disruptions or fractures around the knee.

ANATOMIC CONSIDERATIONS

Depending on the nature of the force, the resulting injury can be a vertical fracture. The mean neck-to-shaft angle (valgus) of an adult human femur is 13° (±7°) and the mean anterior angulation of the femoral neck (anteversion) is 10.4° (±4°), with no significant differences between males and females. These data have implications for fracture fixation. Greater valgus (neck–shaft angle) is often associated with fractures beginning at the superior margin of the articular cartilage. These fractures are associated with a higher incidence of disruption of the critical blood supply to the femoral head.

The major blood supply to the weight-bearing portion of the femoral head is provided by the lateral epiphyseal artery complex, which is the terminal branch of the medial femoral circumflex artery (Fig. 1) (1). The lateral femoral circumflex artery, which traverses the base of the anterior femoral neck, vascularizes a large portion of the metaphysis of the anterior neck but only a small area of the femoral head. Limited vascularity in this area has important implications in the management of femoral head fractures. Whereas the posterior lateral epiphyseal arterial system can be disrupted completely in widely displaced fractures, it is more commonly kinked by displacement of the proximal fragment. Complete disruption is associated with high-energy trauma and a high incidence of posttraumatic osteonecrosis in young adults and children.

The location of the capsular origin and its insertions also affect posttraumatic osteonecrosis. The hip capsule originates on the rim of the acetabulum, on the external surface of the labrum. Anteriorly, it inserts onto the intertrochanteric ridge of the femur; posteriorly, it inserts on the ligament of Weitbrecht just distal to the mid-neck. This dense periosteal membrane can accommodate wide angulatory displacement without disruption. Moreover, thick ligament can contain hemorrhage from a fracture within the capsule. When placed under pressure, a hematoma within the capsule can restrict blood flow to the femoral head and further increase the risk of posttraumatic osteonecrosis. The effects of this pathophysiologic phenomenon are probably relevant primarily to minimally displaced or impacted femoral neck fractures (2).

CLASSIFICATION

The Garden classification is widely used for reporting the results of femoral neck fracture management (Fig. 2) (3). Because no significant difference exists in the rates of nonunion and osteonecrosis between type I and type II fractures (impacted and nondisplaced) and between type III and type IV fractures (displaced in varus and totally

Department of Orthopaedics, Harborview Medical Center, University of Washington, Seattle, Washington 98104

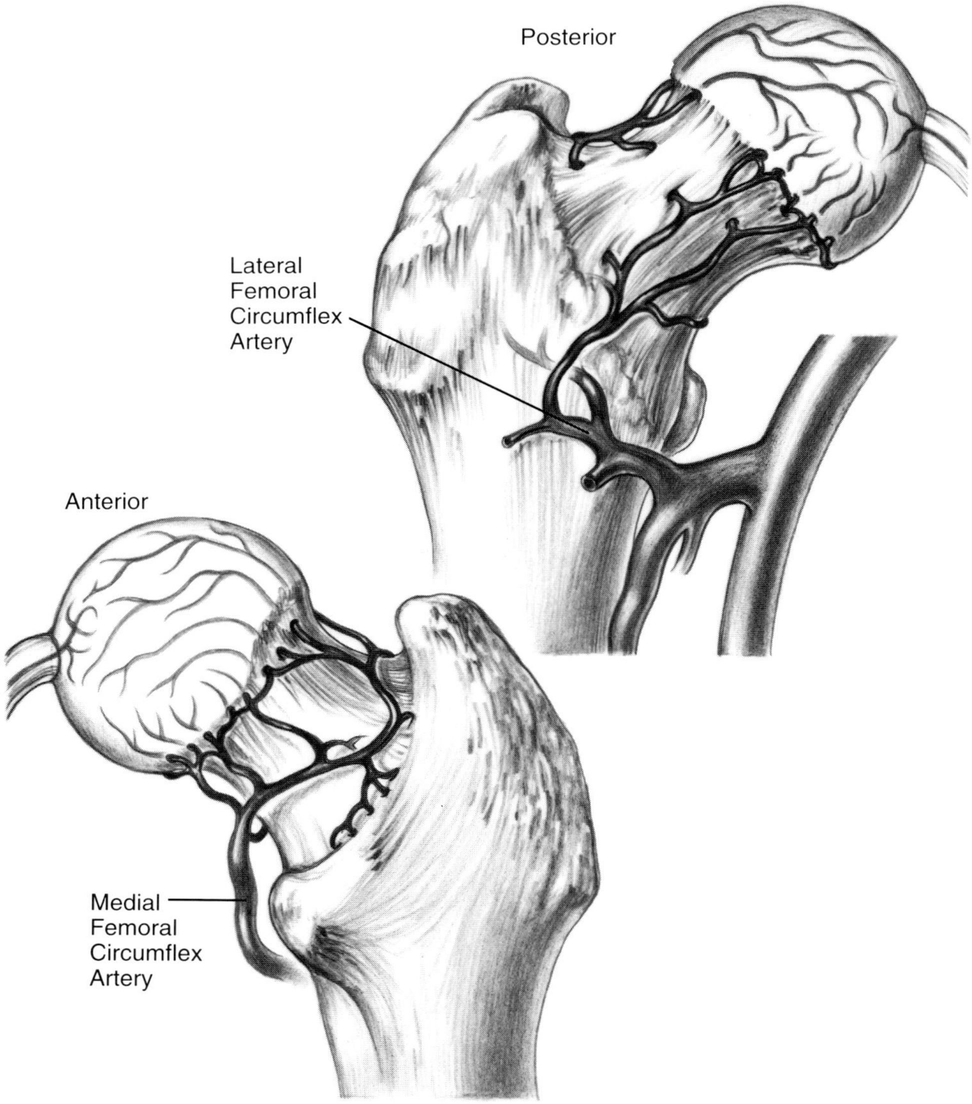

FIG. 1. The vascular anatomy of the proximal femur.

displaced), discussion of definitive management will be limited to two categories of fractures: nondisplaced (impacted) and displaced.

ASSESSMENT

Physical Examination

All patients with femoral neck fractures must be examined for associated injuries. Patients with high-energy femoral neck fractures must be thoroughly evaluated for associated musculoskeletal and internal injuries. Musculoskeletal structures requiring thorough evaluation include the cervical, thoracic, and lumbar spine, the femoral shaft, and the hindfoot. Patients with age-related osteopenia who sustain low-energy femoral neck fractures often have associated injuries, including head injuries, cervical spinal injuries, or distal radial fractures.

Patients with nondisplaced or impacted femoral neck fractures commonly complain of peritrochanteric or buttock pain, even though physical examination may reveal nothing more noteworthy than tenderness in the area of the hip and increased pain on hip rotation or flexion. Because the intracapsular volume might be full, patients with this injury are most comfortable with the hip flexed 20° to 30°. A distal screening examination of the motor, sensory, and circulatory systems is performed. In addition to these findings, patients with displaced femoral neck fractures exhibit shortening and

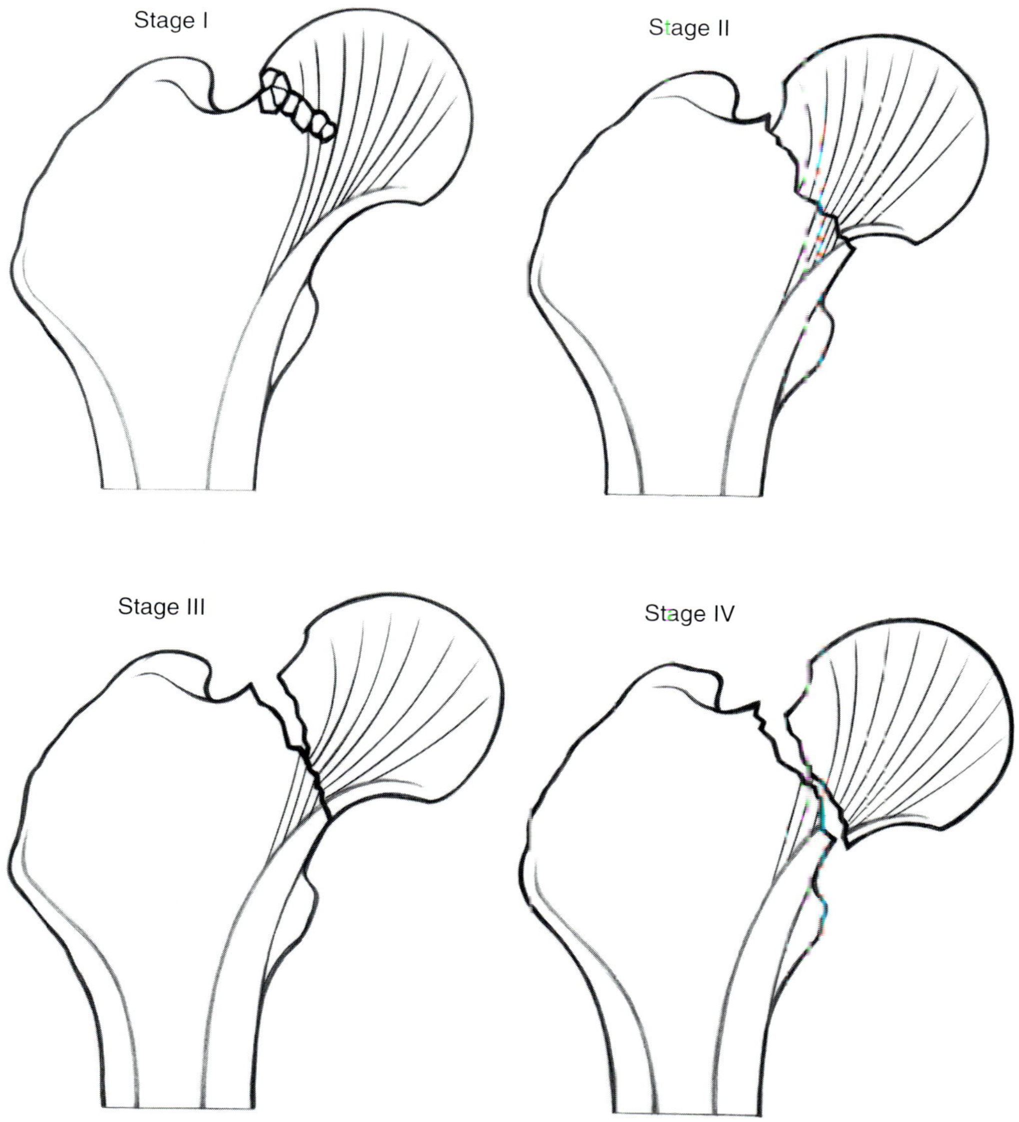

FIG. 2. The Garden classification for femoral neck fractures. Stage I, impacted, valgus position; stage II, nondisplaced fractures; stage III, displaced varus position; stage IV, completely displaced fracture.

external rotation of the limb. Diagnosis of a femoral neck fracture is frequently made from the distorted position of a patient's leg upon arrival at the emergency department.

Radiographic Evaluation

In cases of high-energy trauma, the screening evaluation routinely includes an AP radiograph of the pelvis, a lateral view of the spine, and a chest radiograph. Femoral neck fractures are seen on an AP radiographic view of the pelvis. In low-energy fractures, the patient's history and the physical examination will indicate the need for these radiographic studies.

Diagnosis of a nondisplaced or impacted fracture can be confirmed by a second AP radiograph of the pelvis taken with the hips rotated internally and the feet taped together. Treatment decisions are further guided by a cross-table lateral radiograph of the injured hip, which allows a more accurate assessment of displacement and posterior femoral neck comminution. Abdominal and pelvic CT scans, which are commonly obtained in patients with high-energy injuries, should also be evaluated for displacement and posterior neck comminution. If a prosthetic replacement is planned in an elderly patient, an AP radiograph should be taken of the contralateral hip. This radiograph, taken with a marker to document the percentage of magnification, provides a precise template of the femoral stem and helps determine the size of the femoral head component.

Special Studies

Neither technetium bone scanning nor MRI can predict the risk of AVN preoperatively (4). However, a digitized technetium bone scan can predict the risk of posttraumatic osteonecrosis with 86% accuracy and should be done if this information will be useful (5).

EMERGENT MANAGEMENT

Patients with femoral neck fractures that require internal fixation should be treated urgently. Kinking of the lateral epiphyseal artery and intracapsular tamponade, the two conditions that inhibit blood flow to the femoral head, can be managed by reduction and capsulotomy. The affected limb should be placed in a comfortable position while the work-up is being completed. Traction in extension should be avoided because this position decreases capsular volume and causes discomfort. Medical and surgical evaluations should be completed quickly and the patient taken to the operating room without delay.

DEFINITIVE MANAGEMENT

Elderly patients should be examined by an internist for dehydration and the status of renal, cardiac, and pulmonary functions. The older and more frail a patient is, the more time should be taken to accomplish a thorough preoperative work-up to optimize future function. Patients in this age group typically receive prosthetic hip replacements, and therefore delayed treatment has little effect on the clinical result. Replacement of the femoral head should be reserved for physiologically debilitated patients. A patient's level of physical activity, not age, should be the determining factor for femoral head replacement. Those who have been ambulatory outside the home without severe endurance limitations should be treated by reduction and internal fixation, as should all patients with impacted or nondisplaced fractures. Patients who are home-bound or institution-bound and have a limited life expectancy are candidates for less expensive, fixed-head prostheses instead of bipolar prostheses. A template of the femoral head should be made from radiographs of the normal side to ensure the correct size of the prosthetic head and stem.

Nondisplaced or Impacted Fracture

Patients with nondisplaced or impacted fractures should be positioned supine on the fracture table with the affected limb internally rotated to neutral. A lateral approach is made to the proximal femur, and the fracture is reevaluated for possible displacement during positioning. The vastus lateralis muscle is elevated anteriorly from its origin and off the intertrochanteric ridge. A linear incision is made through the hip capsule to alleviate any hematoma. The fracture is then fixed with three cannulated or cancellous screws inserted in a triangular pattern (6). The implants are placed parallel to each other, using cannulated screw guides. This is an important technologic consideration when bone density is not optimal and the fracture is expected to settle. In general, large-diameter guide wires can be placed more accurately with the screw guide.

Displaced Fractures

Closed reduction of a displaced fracture is attempted after the patient is placed on the fracture table. The affected hip is flexed in abduction and external rotation. Traction is then applied as the hip is extended, adducted to neutral, and internally rotated as far as possible. Traction is maintained by the fracture table and the accuracy of reduction is assessed by fluoroscopy. In the event of an unsatisfactory reduction the reduction maneuver can be repeated once, but if the second attempt is unsuccessful further attempts at closed reduction should be discontinued.

Open reduction of a displaced fracture can be done through a lateral approach as described above. However, a standard Watson–Jones approach is preferred in more muscular or obese patients (Fig. 3). A Hohmann retractor is placed on the anterior acetabular rim to facilitate exposure of the fracture site. The vastus lateralis is detached as described above and the capsule is opened in line with the neck of the femur. The capsule is then released off the intertrochanteric ridge 1.5 cm medially and laterally, and the corners of the capsule are tagged with nonabsorbable sutures to allow retraction. The reduction is assessed visually and by palpation. If residual posterior displacement persists, the fracture can be disengaged by pulling the greater trochanter laterally with a bone hook and lifting the proximal fragment with a curved instrument. An unscrubbed assistant can temporarily decrease the amount of traction and rotate the leg externally to adjust the reduction and then replace the traction and internal rotation. Internal fixation is similar to that for nondisplaced or impacted fractures.

Patients are allowed to get out of bed and sit up in a chair on the first postoperative day. Physical therapy for touch-down weight-bearing is instituted immediately. A walker or crutches are used to assist ambulation for the first 3 postoper-

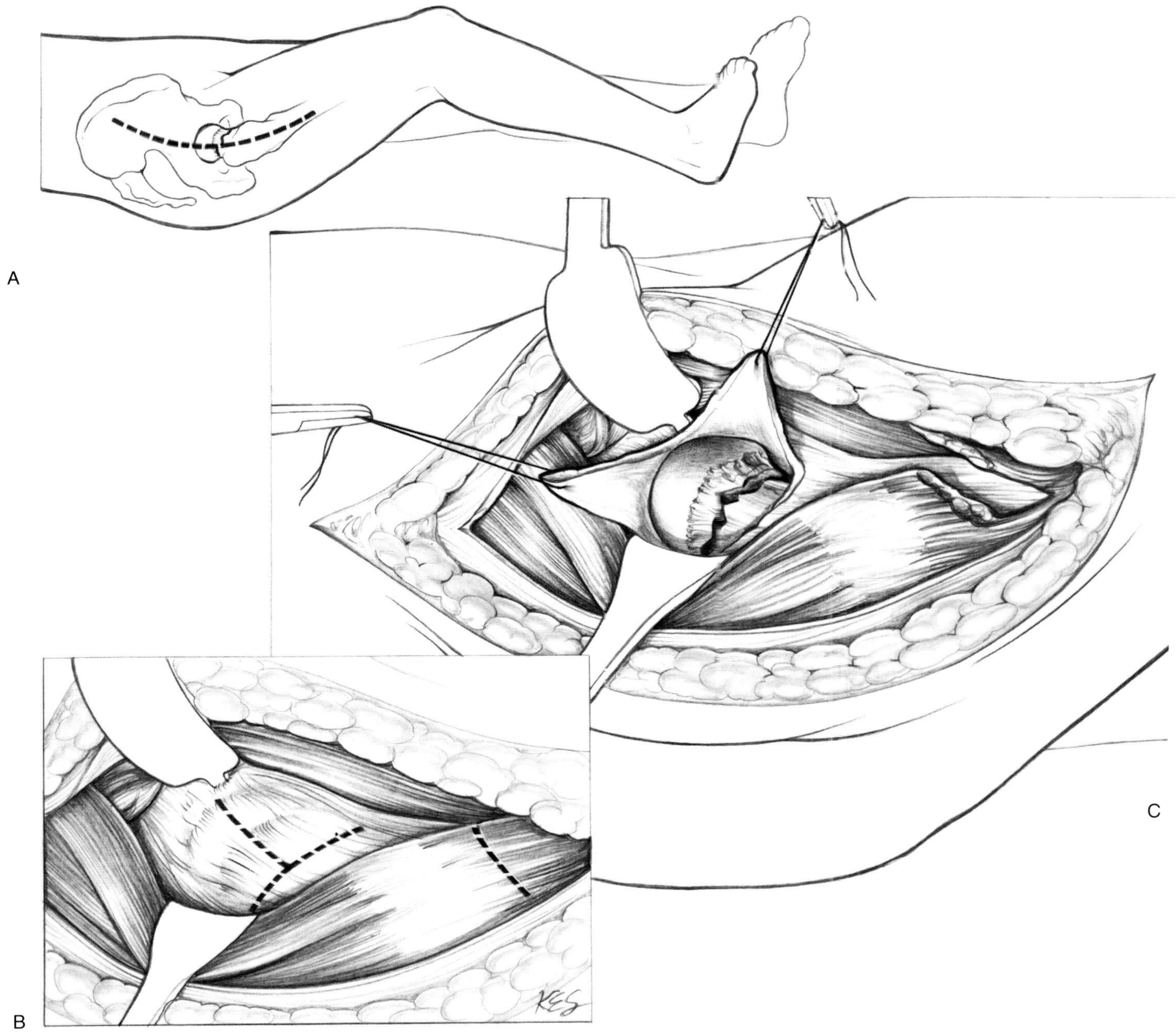

FIG. 3. The Watson–Jones approach for open reduction of femoral neck fractures. **A:** Patient positioned with leg free or on fracture table, skin incision shown by dotted line. **B:** The gluteous mass is retracted posteriorly and the vastus lateralis is detached from the intertrochanteric ridge, exposing the hip capsule. **C:** The capsule is opened in line with the neck and is detached from the intertrochanteric ridge, exposing the fracture.

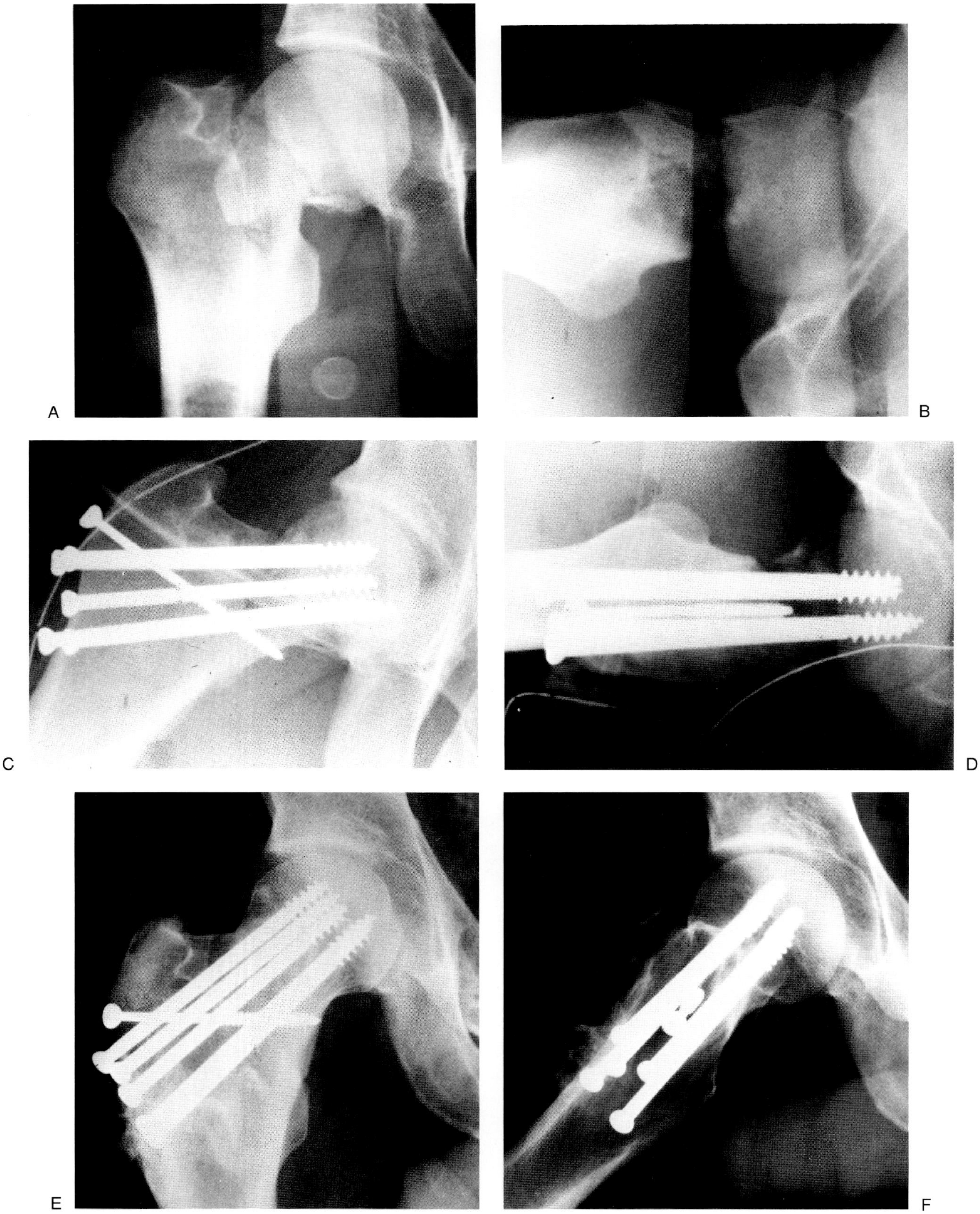

FIG. 4. A, B: Preoperative radiographs of a 23-year-old man with a high-energy femoral neck fracture. **C, D:** Postoperative films after open reduction; the inferior screw was placed with lag technique. **E, F:** Four-year follow-up radiographs.

ative months, by which time fracture union should be confirmed. Sequential compression stockings should be worn until the patient is able to ambulate independently. After a prosthetic hip replacement, a patient is allowed to bear full weight with a walker as soon as possible but must adhere to flexion and internal rotation limitations for the first 6 postoperative weeks. Low-dose Coumadin therapy should be considered for patients with serious medical problems.

COMPLICATIONS

Complications associated with femoral neck fractures (deep venous thrombosis, pulmonary embolism, pneumonia, urinary tract infection, and prolonged ileus) must be managed with medical consultation. Infection after internal fixation of a femoral neck fracture or a prosthetic replacement is rare, but if it occurs it can be managed by a regimen of local wound care and antibiotics. Acute infection is managed by debridement, closure over drains, and antibiotic medications. If the infection becomes recurrent or appears after the patient is discharged from the hospital, the fixation device or prosthesis may have to be removed.

Nonunion

Nonunion of nondisplaced or impacted femoral neck fractures is rare. Nonunion of displaced fractures fixed by the method described above occurs in 3% to 5% of cases. If a patient is physiologically young with fairly good bone density, and if the angle between the neck and shaft remains anatomic, the nonunion is treated by anterior bone grafting or pedicle grafting of the anterior gluteus medius muscle. Any loose or short screws are exchanged at this time. If the neck-to-shaft angle has deflected into varus, a closing wedge subtrochanteric osteotomy is performed and fixed with a 130° angled blade plate or a sliding hip screw. This procedure is successful in 80% to 90% of patients. Elderly patients with significantly deformed nonunions are best treated by bipolar prosthetic replacements. If the acetabulum has been eroded by an intraarticular implant, total hip arthroplasty is recommended.

Avascular Necrosis

Adequate treatment of avascular necrosis after a femoral neck fracture is a dilemma, and prevention remains the best management. As a rule, posttraumatic osteonecrosis that will become functionally limiting becomes clinically evident soon after full weight-bearing is initiated. Patients who complain of persistent pain in the groin or the buttock, despite radiographs that demonstrate a healed fracture and a normal-looking femoral head, almost always experience late collapse of the femoral head. A bone scan is not useful for diagnosis because increased uptake is noted in patients both with and without AVN (4).

Treatment of AVN is based on the extent of a patient's functional limitation, not on the radiographs. Surgical intervention is warranted in virtually all young, active patients, but is desirable in only half the patients aged 65 or over. In this older group, function can be improved by a total hip arthroplasty. A flexion osteotomy can be considered in a younger patient when the area of collapse is small (one third or less of the weight-bearing surface) and when the necrotic process does not progress over time. If a large area of the femoral head is involved but the acetabulum is not damaged, a bipolar prosthesis with an uncemented stem is the most widely accepted treatment. Core decompression, usually a benign procedure when properly performed, does not offer adequate relief to most patients.

SKELETALLY IMMATURE PATIENTS

The prognosis of a femoral neck fracture in a child or an adolescent is poor, and this injury must be treated as a surgical emergency. With operative management, nonunion is less common in children than in adults, but posttraumatic osteonecrosis affects 50% of all cases.

Delbet's classification (7) is used to describe proximal femoral fractures in children and adolescents and to predict the likelihood of AVN. The risk of AVN in type I transepiphyseal fractures approaches 100% when they are displaced. These fractures are treated by immediate ORIF through the lateral surgical approach described above. Fixation is provided by smooth K-wires placed across the fracture. Type II fractures are transcervical and present a 50% risk of AVN. These fractures must be treated emergently, even when they are nondisplaced, because an anterior capsulotomy is needed for decompression. The lateral surgical approach is used and fixation is provided by 3.5-mm or 4.5-mm cortical lag screws that stop short of the physis. Open reduction of a displaced type II fracture is also considered an emergency and should be performed by the same lateral approach and fixation described above. Excellent results with this protocol have been reported in small groups of patients (8). Type III basicervical fractures present a lower risk of AVN (20–30%) and are managed in the same way as type II fractures. In very young or uncooperative children, these fractures are immobilized in a 1-1/2 leg spica cast for 6 weeks. Type IV intertrochanteric fractures are discussed in Chapter 23.

REFERENCES

1. Trueta J, Harrison MHM. The normal vascular anatomy of the femoral head in adult man. *J Bone Joint Surg* 1953;35B:442–461.
2. Stromquist E, Nillson LT, Egund N, Thorngren KG, Wingstrand H. Intracapsular pressures in undisplaced fractures of the femoral neck. *J Bone Joint Surg* 1988;70B:192–194.

3. Barnes JT, Brown JT, Garden RS, Nicoll EA. Subcapital fractures of the femur. A prospective review. *J Bone Joint Surg* 1976;58B:2–24.
4. Speer KP, Spritzer CE, Harrelson JM, Nunley JA. Magnetic resonance imagery of the femoral head after acute intra? fracture of the femoral neck. *J Bone Joint Surg* 1990;72:98–103.
5. Stromquist B. Femoral head vitality after intracapsular hip fracture; 490 cases studied by intravital tetracycline labeling and tc-mdp radionuclide imaging. *Acta Orthop Scand* 1983;54(Suppl 200):5–71.
6. Swiontkowski MF, Harrington RN, Keller TS, Van Patten PK. Torsion and bending analysis of internal fixation techniques for femoral neck fractures: the role of implant design and bone density. *J Orthop Res* 1987;5:433–444.
7. Colonna PC. Fractures of the neck of the femur in children. *Am J Surg* 1929;6:793–797.
8. Swiontkowski MF, Winquist RA. Displaced hip fractures in children and adolescents. *J Trauma* 1986;26:384–88.

Orthopaedic Trauma Protocols, edited by
Sigvard T. Hansen, Jr., and Marc F. Swiontkowski,
Raven Press, Ltd., New York, © 1993.

CHAPTER 23

Intertrochanteric Femoral Fractures

Marc F. Swiontkowski

MECHANISMS OF INJURY

Although intertrochanteric femoral fractures can occur from high-energy trauma, they more commonly result from low-energy injuries. Most intertrochanteric femoral fractures are caused by low-energy falls in elderly patients with visual or neuromuscular problems. Recent findings have implicated the use of benzodiazepine sedatives in the frequency of falls experienced by the elderly (1). Owing to the nature of these injuries and the patient population in which they occur, most intertrochanteric femoral fractures are isolated injuries. Injuries caused by high-energy trauma often have associated ipsilateral femoral shaft fractures. Associated pelvic, knee, and spinal fractures can also occur with high-energy intertrochanteric fractures and must be diligently ruled out, but none of these injuries is common.

ANATOMIC CONSIDERATIONS

The osseous anatomy of the proximal femur is shown in Fig. 1 of Chapter 22. The extracapsular intertrochanteric ridge runs anteriorly and medially between the greater and lesser trochanters. The vastus lateralis tubercle appears as a prominence along this ridge and corresponds to the superior aspect of the femoral neck. The normal angulatory relationships between the femoral neck and shaft should be noted for preoperative planning of internal fixation. The mean neck-shaft angle (varus) is 130° (±7°) and the mean anterior angulation of the femoral neck (anteversion) is 10° (±6°), with no significant differences between males and females. The calcar femorale, a thick plate of bone extending posteriorly from the linea aspera to the posterior aspect of the femoral neck, separates the lesser trochanter from the femoral metaphysis. This structure is instrumental in determining the plane of fracture lines in the intertrochanteric region. The term "calcar" is frequently misapplied to the medial femoral neck by arthroplasty surgeons. The internal trabecular anatomy of the proximal femur with the primary and secondary tension and compression trabeculae are shown in Fig. 1. These structures are critical to mechanical strength and are selectively lost with advancing age. This loss of mechanical strength plays a role in increasing susceptibility to proximal femur fracture with advancing age.

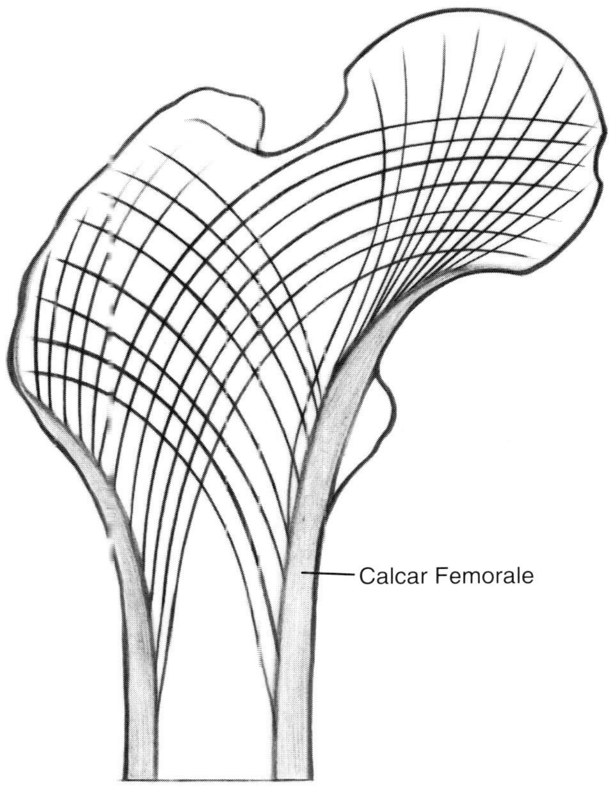

FIG. 1. Trabecular anatomy of the proximal femur.

Department of Orthopaedics, Harborview Medical Center, University of Washington, Seattle, Washington 98104

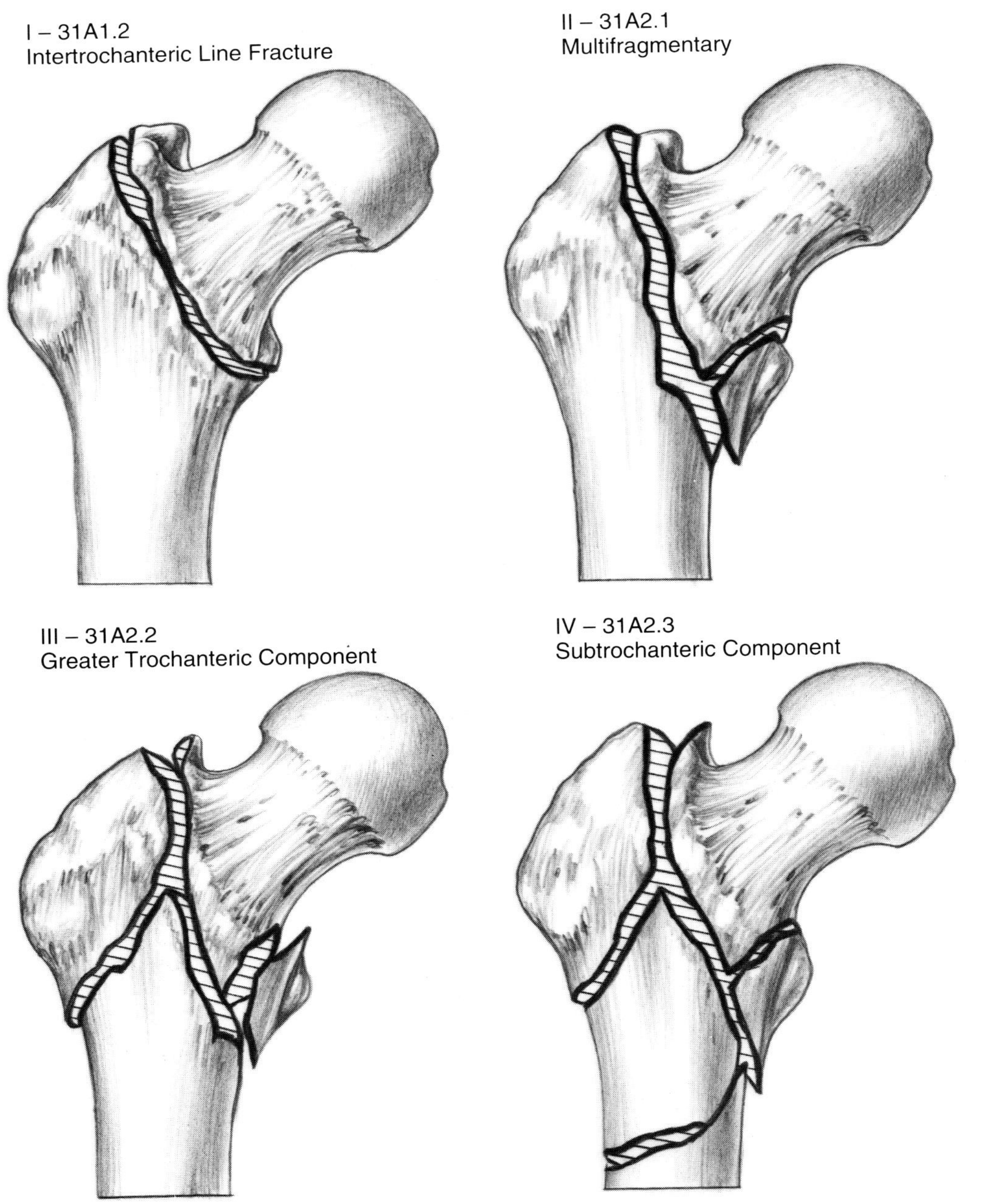

FIG. 2. Kyle's classification of intertrochanteric fracture. Superimposed are the codes for the AO scheme.

CLASSIFICATION

Historically, the classification of Boyd and Griffin (2) was the first to provide a reproducible prognostic framework for these injuries, but Kyle's later classification (3) was more precise (Fig. 2). The system we presently use is a descriptive classification of two-, three-, and four-part fractures that are identified as stable or unstable. Because two-part fractures can be reduced they are almost always considered to be stable; three-part fractures are considered stable if the lesser trochanteric fragment is small and does not compromise the posteromedial support. A fracture that follows the path of the calcar femorale may be unstable if the posteromedial support is compromised. Four-part fractures are almost always unstable because posteromedial support is compromised and the greater trochanter is detached from the distal fragment. This fragment must be stabilized before the abductor muscles can compress the major fracture lines. Other factors that indicate a lack of stability include fracture displacement and diminished bone density. Widely displaced fractures in osteopenic bone are the most unstable and have the worst prognosis of all intertrochanteric fractures.

ASSESSMENT

Physical Examination

The patient should be examined for associated fractures in the ipsilateral femur and knee, the pelvis, and the spine. A distal screening examination must be performed to determine the status of sensory, motor, and circulatory functions. Because an intertrochanteric fracture is usually displaced, the affected limb often lies in an externally rotated position. Since most fractures in the elderly are caused by falls, elderly patients with neuromuscular disease may have lain on the ground or the floor for a long time before receiving medical attention. In such cases, the region of the buttocks and the greater trochanter should be carefully examined for bruises, pressure sores, and chemical burns from urine.

Radiographic Evaluation

High-energy intertrochanteric femoral fractures are evident on the admitting AP radiographs of the pelvis. This radiograph is also indicated in injuries resulting from low-energy falls and when patients complain of pain in the area of the hip, the trochanter, or the buttock. After an intertrochanteric fracture is identified, a cross-table lateral radiograph should be obtained to fully assess the fracture pattern and the degree of instability. Both films should be specifically evaluated for bone density; the AP radiograph can be used to grade osteoporosis according to the Singh Index.

Special Studies

No special studies are recommended. Plain radiographs are used to rule out associated injuries and to assess pulmonary and cardiac function.

EMERGENT MANAGEMENT

Evaluation of low-energy fractures in elderly patients must include a thorough assessment of their pulmonary, cardiac, and renal status. Medical consultations are requested and appropriate diagnostic tests (cardiograms, chest radiographs, coagulation screening) are carried out. Patients with chronic medical problems that have not been managed optimally are admitted to the hospital, possibly to the ICU, for 24 to 36 h of medical treatment to stabilize these problems. Special attention is directed to managing dehydration. Skin traction is applied to provide comfort during this time. High-energy fractures should be treated by immediate operative stabilization after associated injuries have been stabilized or ruled out. Five pounds of skin traction is applied through a foam traction boot to make the patient comfortable during transport and diagnostic evaluations.

DEFINITIVE MANAGEMENT

Radiographs are carefully examined to determine the need for lag-screw fixation of any posteromedial fragments or tension-band wiring of the greater trochanter and for planning the placement of the implant. If poor bone density is noted in a very unstable fracture, an implant with a higher angle placed in valgus over reduction might be necessary. A preoperative plan is made using the radiograph of the normal side as a template to determine the placement of the implant and to plan a surgical tactic. The importance of providing preoperative medical therapy for elderly patients cannot be overemphasized.

The patient is placed on the fracture table in the supine position with both feet in traction boots. The unaffected limb is abducted widely to allow positioning of the fluoroscope. Alternatively, the normal leg can be flexed in the lithotomy position with the table-mounted leg holder. Traction is applied to the affected side with the leg in a neutral position and in slight external rotation. The limb must not be rotated internally, as would be done for a femoral neck fracture. Internal rotation of an unstable intertrochanteric fracture can create a gap in the posterior aspect of the fracture. Consequently, the proximal end of the screw in the femoral head can migrate out of position and reduction would be lost.

After traction is applied, the reduction is assessed with fluoroscopy. If the reduction is unsatisfactory, a closed reduction maneuver is performed by applying pressure over the

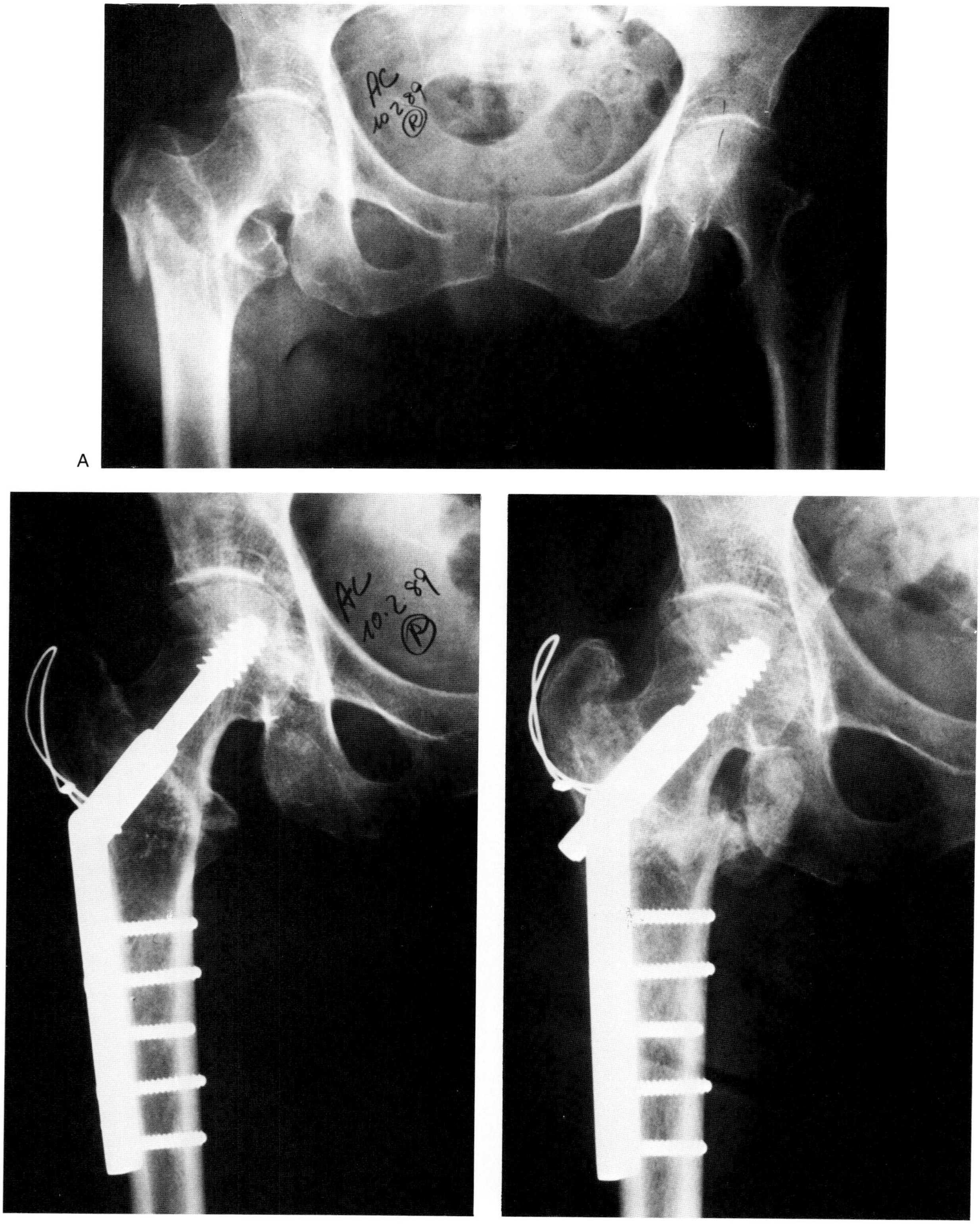

A B C

FIG. 3. A 68-year-old woman sustained this three-part intertrochanteric hip fracture in a fall down some stairs. **A:** Preoperative radiograph. **B:** Postoperative radiograph showing good placement of the sliding hip screw. A tension-band wire loop has been used to stabilize the greater trochanteric component of this fracture noted intraoperatively (making it a four-part fracture). **C:** Follow-up radiograph at 6 months. The patient is ambulatory with a walker and has mild pain in the hip.

greater trochanter posteriorly while an assistant flexes the hip 60° to 70°, extending the limb as traction is applied. In extremely unstable fractures in osteopenic bone, the patient can be repositioned into the lateral decubitus position, similar to that used for femoral intramedullary nailing, to eliminate the posterior sag that occurs in the supine position.

After the fracture is reduced by closed techniques, a straight lateral incision is made over the mid-femur. Unless the greater trochanter is to be reduced with cerclage wires, the incision is not extended proximally beyond the base of the greater trochanter. The posterior sag typical of unstable fractures is corrected by having an assistant lift both fracture fragments with a broad periosteal elevator. The vastus lateralis muscle is detached posteriorly along the linea aspera and minimally elevated.

Under fluoroscopic visualization, the guide wire for the sliding hip screw is placed in the center–center position of the neck and head on both views. The reamer is set to stop 1 cm short of the tip of the guide wire that will be placed in the subchondral bone. A 135° sliding hip screw with a four-hole sideplate is used to stabilize most intertrochanteric femoral fractures. A longer sideplate is needed when the fracture has a subtrochanteric extension or when the posteromedial fragment is exceptionally large. In the latter situation, care must be taken to reduce the fragment and to fix it internally with an anterior-to-posterior lag screw. Tapping the hip screws is done only in bone of normal density. To facilitate reduction, the hip can be flexed 30° to relax the iliopsoas muscle. In rare cases, this tendon may have to be divided.

If a fracture in osteopenic bone is extremely unstable, a sliding hip screw with a 150° sideplate may be applied in 140° to 145° of valgus over reduction. The initial stabilization of a four-part fracture includes passing a cerclage wire around the tip of the greater trochanter and through the iliopsoas tendon in a "figure-8" configuration with a wire-passing guide (Fig. 3). The wire then is passed under the angle of the sideplate before the first shaft screw is placed. The wire is easier to pass while the plate is not close to the bone.

In the presence of a trochanteric pressure sore or a chemical burn, the fracture is stabilized in a valgus position by the retrograde Ender nailing technique. The nails should fan out within the femoral head and the heads of the nails should be buried and locked with inter-eyelet wires. If an intertrochanteric fracture extends far into the subtrochanteric region, fixation with an antegrade second-generation nail or a Zickel nail is recommended. Although a sliding hip screw is the treatment of choice for almost all intertrochanteric femoral fractures, the Gamma nail might be a viable option in this situation. The only exception is a "reverse" intertrochanteric fracture. In this case, a 95° condylar blade plate is recommended because the sole proximal fixation is contained within the proximal fragment. Blade plating enhances stability of the fracture by enabling more screws to be placed into the proximal fragment and lag screws to be placed across the fracture line.

Patients with any type of intertrochanteric femoral fracture should be mobilized as soon as possible after surgery. Sequential compression boots are applied until patients are independently mobile. Physical therapists should see patients on the first postoperative day to assist with early attempts at ambulation. Touch-down weight-bearing is allowed on the affected side with the aid of a walker for the first 8 to 12 postoperative weeks. The level of activity should progress more slowly in unstable fractures. A 1-1/2 leg spica cast is used for noncompliant patients, and the same postoperative regimen is followed for 6 to 8 weeks.

Low-dose Coumadin therapy should be considered in medically impaired patients. When Coumadin therapy is implemented, a screening duplex ultrasound of the venous system should be done soon after admission and every 5 to 6 days thereafter. Special attention is paid to the nutritional status of a patient with a low-energy fracture. The lymphocyte count and serum albumin levels provide an indication of the patient's overall nutritional status. If these diagnostic test results are not within normal levels, consultation with the dietary service for nutritional supplementation may be indicated.

COMPLICATIONS

Many complications, including deep venous thrombosis, pulmonary embolism, pneumonia, and urinary tract infection, are managed with the help of medical consultants. Infection is rare and occurs in less than 1% of all patients with intertrochanteric femoral fractures. If localized superficial infection occurs, it can be treated by local wound care and administration of antibiotics. If the infection is deep, surgical debridement followed by delayed closure over multiple suction drains is indicated. Removal of the implant is not recommended because the resulting instability makes the infection harder to eradicate.

Nonunion of an intertrochanteric femoral fracture is rare. When nonunion does occur, it is most often associated with contralateral fractures and full weight-bearing that was begun too early. Anterior cancellous bone grafting may be sufficient treatment for a nonunion if the femoral neck-shaft angle remains normal and the implant is not loose. However, most nonunions drift into varus as the screw within the femoral head loosens. Under these circumstances, nonunions are treated by removing the sliding hip screw and performing a subtrochanteric (closing wedge) osteotomy to restore the femoral neck-shaft angle and the limb length. A 95° condylar plate may be substituted for the original fixation (Fig. 4).

A proximal femoral replacement is an optional procedure in patients over the age of 65 who have sustained highly unstable comminuted fractures with resultant loss of fixation. Because restoration of normal anatomy can be very difficult, replacement of the femoral head should be performed by a skilled arthroplasty surgeon.

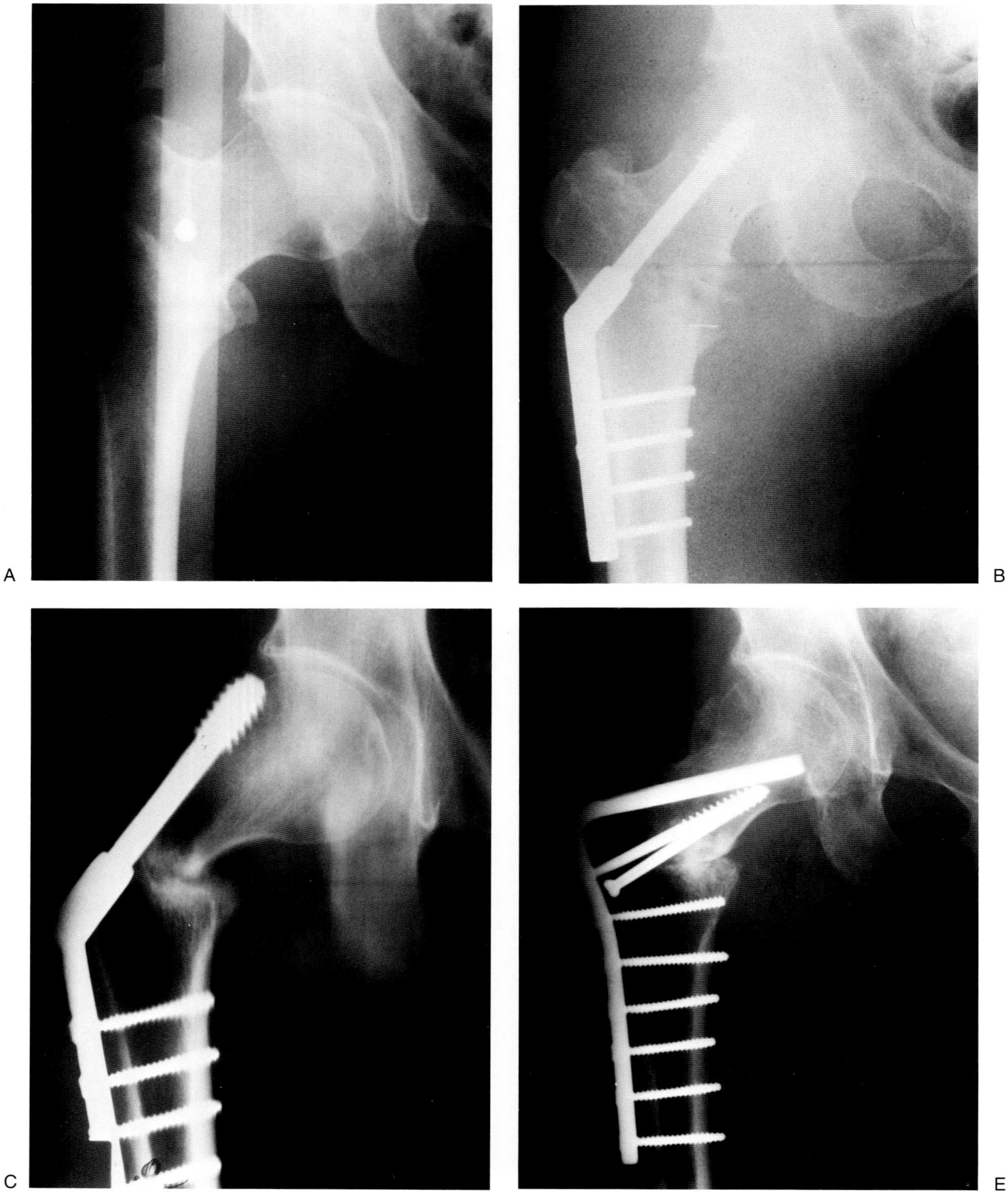

FIG. 4. A: A 49-year-old man was struck by a car and sustained this four-part fracture. **B:** The postoperative radiograph shows a suboptimal placement of the compression screw (high center). **C:** The patient had a contralateral tibial plateau fracture which was treated operatively and was weight-bearing at 8 weeks on the side of the intertrochanteric fracture. The patient experienced hip pain; tomograms revealed the screw "cut out." **D:** (opposite page) Preoperative planning for a subtrochanteric osteotomy. **E:** Postoperative radiograph showing good correction of the varus deformity.

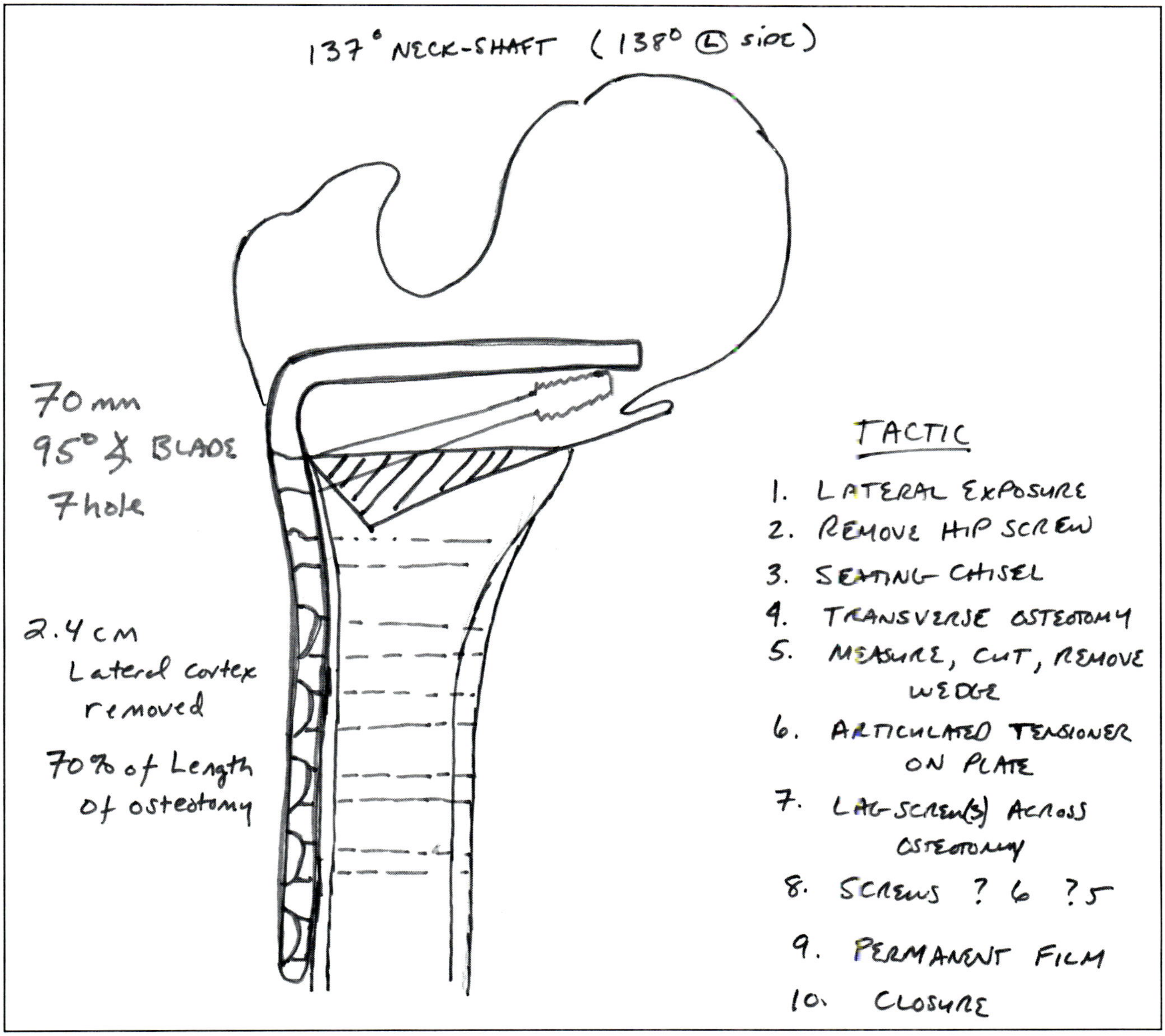

D

FIG. 4. (Continued)

SPECIAL CONSIDERATIONS IN SKELETALLY IMMATURE PATIENTS

In the Delbet classification (4) of proximal femoral fractures in children and adolescents, an intertrochanteric fracture is a type IV injury. Young children (aged 10 years and under) with this fracture can be treated by closed reduction and spica casting. Care must be taken to maintain the femoral neck-shaft angle within 5° of its anatomic position.

The importance of achieving anatomic reduction becomes more critical as the child ages. If an anatomic reduction cannot be obtained and maintained in cast, a Steinmann pin can be used to hold the reduction until the fracture has united. The pin can be placed percutaneously if closed reduction is obtained with fluoroscopic control. Children over 10 years of age and adolescents should be managed with sliding-screw or blade-plate fixation to minimize postfracture deformity and to promote early return to normal function. Blade plating encourages rapid healing in this situation.

REFERENCES

1. Ray WA, Griffin MR, Schaffner W, et al. Psychotropic drug use and the risk of hip fracture. *N Engl J Med* 1982;316:363–369.
2. Boyd HB, Griffin LL. Classification and treatment of trochanteric fractures. *Arch Surg* 1949;58:853-866.
3. Kyle RF, Gustilo RB, Premer RF. Analysis of six hundred and twenty-two intertrochanteric hip fractures. A retrospective and prospective study. *J Bone Joint Surg* 1979;61A:216-221.
4. Colonna PC. Fractures of the neck of the femur in children. *Am J Surg* 1929;6:793-797.

Orthopaedic Trauma Protocols, edited by
Sigvard T. Hansen Jr., and Marc F. Swiontkowski.
Raven Press, Ltd., New York, © 1993.

CHAPTER 24

Subtrochanteric Femoral Fractures

Marc F. Swiontkowski

MECHANISMS OF INJURY

Like other fractures in the proximal femur, fractures in the subtrochanteric region can be caused by high-energy or low-energy trauma. However, unlike intertrochanteric fractures and those occurring in the region of the femoral neck, most subtrochanteric fractures are usually caused by high-energy injuries. Low-energy fractures in this region typically occur as subtrochanteric extensions of intertrochanteric fractures in elderly patients with neuromuscular problems. Age-related osteoporosis in this patient population makes subtrochanteric femoral fractures particularly difficult to stabilize and precludes early functional ambulation.

A high incidence of injuries to the head, chest, and abdomen is associated with all high-energy fractures. Patients with high-energy subtrochanteric fractures must be systematically evaluated to rule out these injuries as well as associated fractures to the cervical and thoracolumbar spine, the pelvis, the patella, the proximal tibia, and the ipsilateral knee. Low-energy falls may be associated with fractures of the upper extremity, particularly of the distal radius.

ANATOMIC CONSIDERATIONS

The subtrochanteric region is subject to very high mechanical stresses. The thick medial and posteromedial cortex of the area distal to the lesser trochanter reflect the high demands placed on this region (Fig. 1). The linea aspera is joined to the posterior femoral neck anterior to the lesser trochanter by a dense plate of bone, the calcar femorale. This plate is often the site of separation of the posteromedial fragment from the posterior femur. When the posteromedial fragment is large, it must be reduced to augment the stability of the proximal fixation or left undisturbed to allow the hematoma to play an important role in rapid early healing of the area.

Before a subtrochanteric fracture can be managed by plating, particularly with a 95° condylar blade plate, the normal relationships of the femoral neck to the greater trochanter and the femoral shaft must be understood. Viewed laterally, the femoral neck lies in the anterior half of the greater trochanter. The mean neck-shaft angle is 130° and the mean anteversion angle is 10°. Restoration of these normal anatomic angles is critical for proper placement of second-generation nails and for obtaining good functional results.

CLASSIFICATION

Because 135° fixed-angle fixation devices were associated with high rates of failure, Fielding et al. (1) developed the first classification of subtrochanteric femoral fractures based on the level of the fracture in relation to the lesser trochanter. In this classification system, a type I fracture is located at or above the lesser trochanter, a type II fracture is 1 cm distal to the trochanter, and a type III fracture is >2 cm distal.

Seinsheimer (2) recognized the correlation between lack of reduction of the posteromedial fragment and fixation failure and developed a more complex classification, defining a type III fracture as one with a large posteromedial fragment (see Fig. 1). The AO classification (3) is the most comprehensive classification that presently exists (Fig. 2). When fracture treatment is planned, two important factors must be noted: whether the lesser trochanter is an isolated fragment or is attached to the proximal or the distal fragment, and whether the fracture lines extend into the piriform fossa.

Department of Orthopaedics, Harborview Medical Center, University of Washington, Seattle, Washington 98104

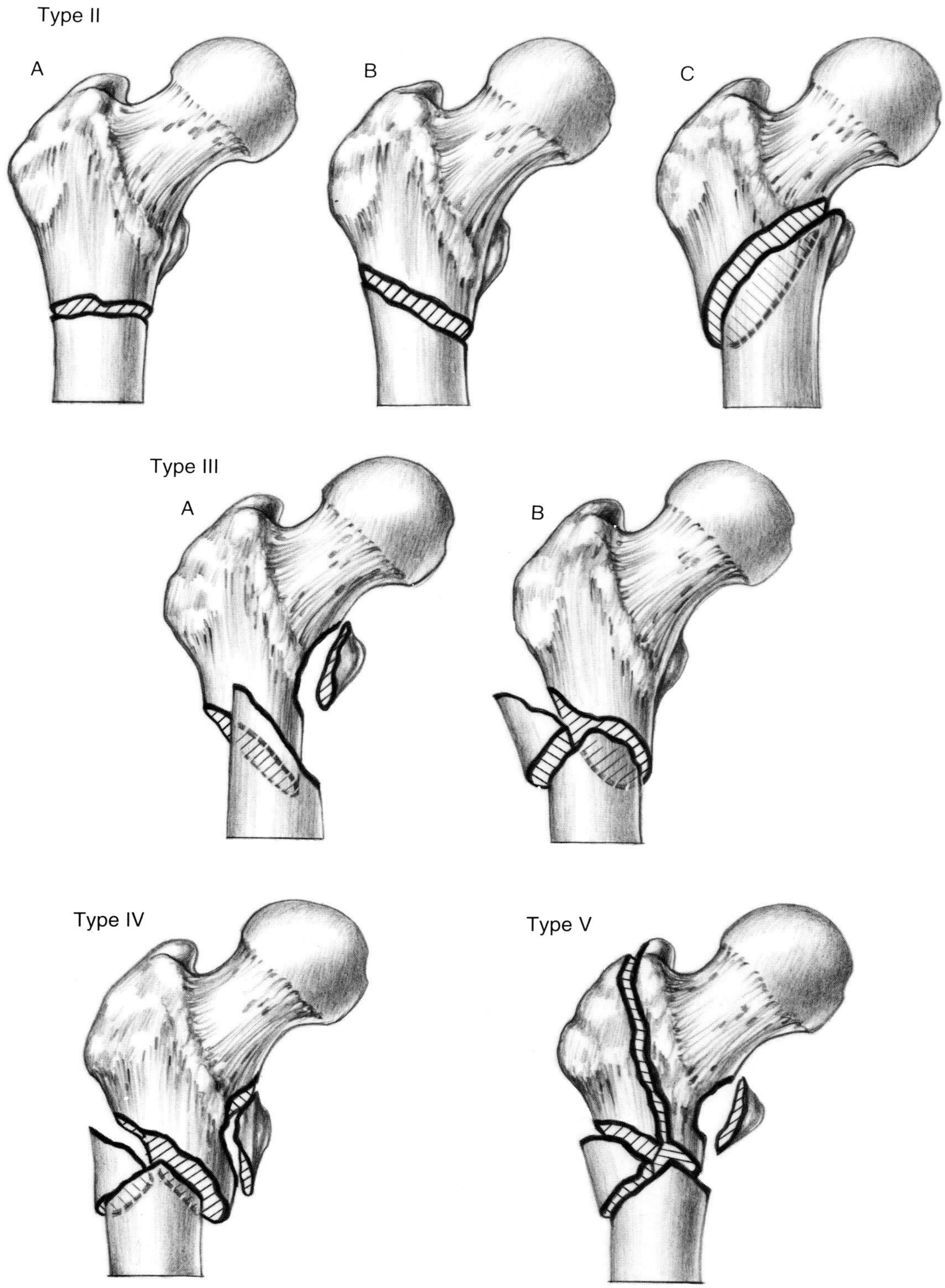

FIG. 1. The Seinsheimer classification of subtrochanteric femoral fractures. The type III fracture has been identified to be at high risk for mechanical failure.

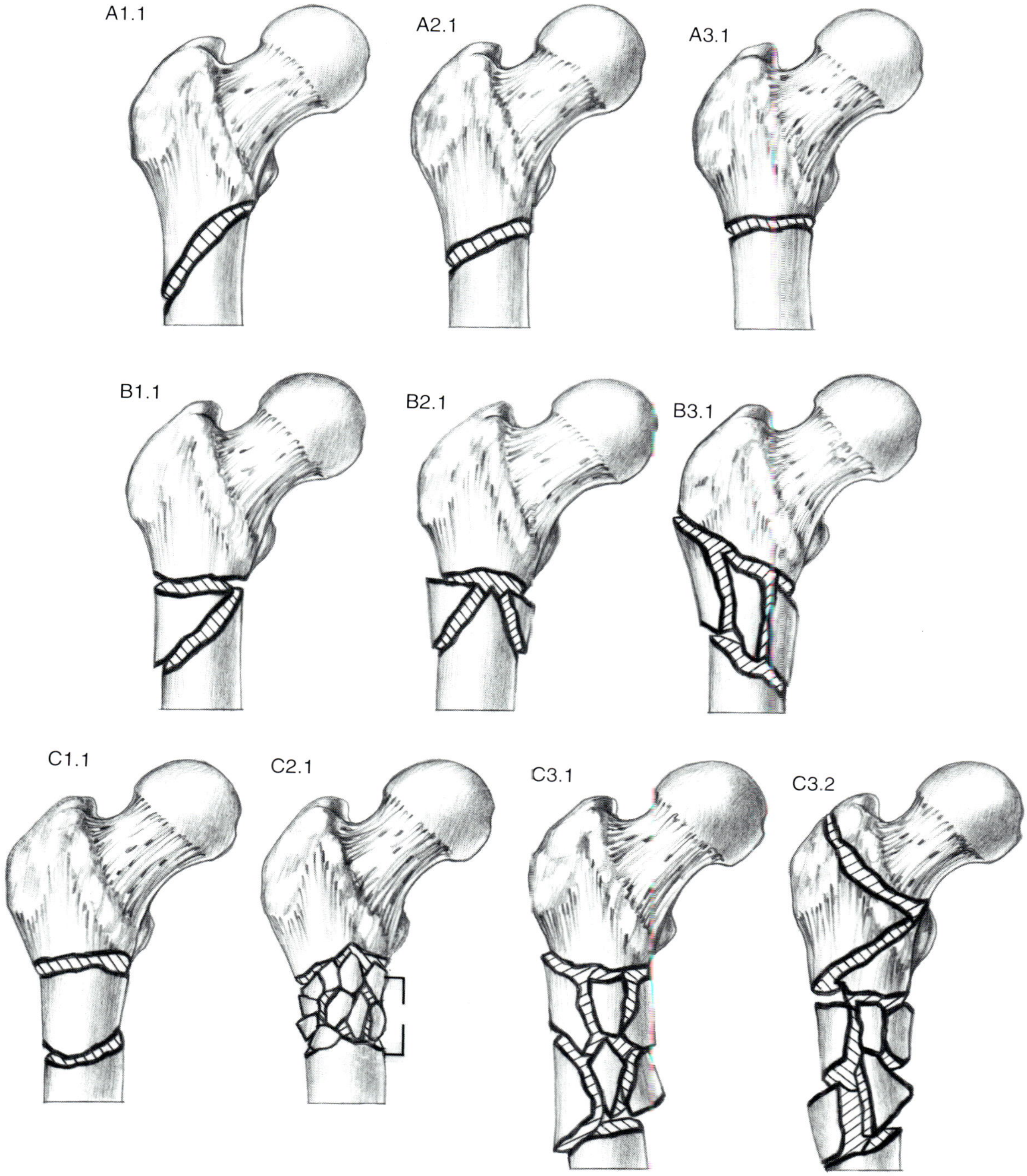

FIG. 2. The AO scheme for classification of subtrochanteric femoral fractures. (Adapted from Müller ME, Algöwer M, Schneider R, Willenegger H. *Manual of Internal Fixation.* Berlin: Springer-Verlag, 1991. Müller ME, Nazarian S, Koch P, Schatzker J. *Comprehensive Classification of Fracture of Long Bones.* Berlin: Springer-Verlag, 1990. Used with permission.)

ASSESSMENT

Physical Examination

In high-energy injuries, the affected limb, the pelvis, and the spine must be carefully assessed clinically. If the patient is alert and cooperative the examination includes an assessment of the circulatory system and the motor and sensory status of the limb. The paramedic team will usually have aligned and splinted the fracture at the scene of the accident. If they have not, a roller splint or a Thomas splint is applied to allow application of traction to the limb during the work-up. In low-energy injuries, the spine, the pelvis, and the upper extremities are carefully assessed. If a patient's existing medical problems preclude early surgery, Buck traction or tibial-pin skeletal traction are applied for comfort.

Radiographic Evaluation

The musculoskeletal pathology of a subtrochanteric femoral fracture is seen on the admitting AP radiograph of the pelvis that includes the upper femoral shaft. Other diagnostic radiographs include full-length femoral and cross-table lateral views of the injured side. A full-length AP radiograph of the uninjured side is obtained for preoperative planning. Both high-energy and low-energy subtrochanteric femoral fractures are evaluated with these radiographs.

Special Studies

Arteriography is indicated when a patient's pulse cannot be palpated or when an abnormal reading is obtained on a Doppler examination. Bone scans, CT scans, and MRI evaluations are not indicated for routine fractures but may be useful when primary or metastatic lesions exist.

EMERGENT MANAGEMENT

The limb is aligned and placed in a portable traction device for the duration of the preoperative workup. Open wounds are evaluated for contamination and are covered with a Betadine dressing. Any suspected arterial injuries are ruled out by duplex scanning or arteriography or else are managed by a vascular surgeon. Fractures in elderly patients who cannot undergo immediate definitive treatment are stabilized temporarily by 5 lb of skin traction applied through a foam boot or skeletal traction via a tibial pin. Whenever possible, elderly patients must be stabilized medically and treated definitively in the operating room within 36 to 48 h of injury.

DEFINITIVE MANAGEMENT

After the injuries have been diagnosed and assessed and a treatment plan has been formulated, an implant must be chosen. Subtrochanteric femoral fractures in adults or adolescents should be managed operatively to prevent pulmonary complications, to limit the hospital stay, and to lessen the degree of deformity in the upper femur, a factor that corresponds directly to improved function. The type of implant to be used is determined by comparing the radiographs of the fractured and normal sides. When the fracture is located distal to the lesser trochanter, a standard interlocked nail is preferred. When the greater trochanter and the piriform fossa are intact in a fracture located above the lesser trochanter, a second-generation interlocked nail is used. This type of nail is also recommended for a "reverse intertrochanteric" fracture. Fixation with an antegrade nail is unreliable in a fracture that involves the piriform fossa. The best choice of fixation for this type of fracture is either a sliding hip screw (in an elderly patient) or a 95° condylar blade plate. A 95° condylar screw is not recommended in elderly patients because a large amount of bone must be reamed to insert this device. In the future, the Gamma nail appears to be a promising alternative to the sliding hip screw, provided that the subtrochanteric extension of the fracture stops within 5 cm of the distal screws. Our experience with this device in this situation is still too limited to recommend its widespread use.

Standard Intramedullary Nailing

A standard interlocked nail is used for fractures in which the lesser trochanter remains attached to the proximal fragment. Nailing systems with oblique proximal-screw orientations are used to manage very high fractures in this region.

The patient is positioned in the lateral position on the fracture table unless an associated pelvic fracture or multiple injuries preclude this position. A distal traction pin is placed anteriorly to reduce the distal fragment to the proximal fragment. This procedure is difficult to perform in the supine position because the proximal fragment is flexed by the iliopsoas muscle. When nailing must be performed with the patient lying supine, precautions must be taken to avoid fracturing the posterior aspect of the proximal fragment at the anterior starting point. The starting point for the nail is developed with a cannulated reamer over a 2.7-mm or 3-mm guide wire. This technique allows the correct location of the wire to be confirmed in both planes by fluoroscopy. Distal locking with only one screw is recommended in stable fracture patterns.

Second-Generation Intramedullary Nailing

Second-generation interlocked nails are used for fixation of fractures located above the lesser trochanter. Radiographs must be carefully examined for any sign of fracture extending into the greater trochanter. If the fracture extends into the greater trochanter, this device might not maintain reduction of the proximal fragment to the distal fragment. The fracture can be nailed with the patient lying in the lateral decubitus position or supine because the iliopsoas muscle does not flex the proximal fragment in this type of fracture. Before the procedure is begun, the femoral head and neck are visualized in AP and lateral radiographic views. A distal femoral pin is placed anteriorly to control traction and rotation. When the procedure is performed with the patient lying supine and the lateral radiographic view is inadequate because the uninjured leg cannot be widely abducted, the leg is placed in the lithotomy position. In the lateral position, oblique positioning of the pelvis (putting the injured hip anterior to the uninjured hip) enhances visualization in the lateral plane.

Second-generation interlocked nails are thicker and stiffer than standard interlocked nails, and the femoral medullary canal must be reamed 1.0 mm to 1.5 mm wider than the diameter of the nail. The guide wires or drill bits used for placing the proximal screws must be adequately visualized in both planes prior to screw insertion. In addition, the locations of the guide wires and the drill bits must be verified in the AP plane to make certain that the nail is driven far enough distally to allow placement of both screws (Fig. 3). Two screws are inserted to decrease the risk of nonunion. Like standard interlocked nailing, second-generation interlocked nailing requires placement of at least one distal screw. The Gamma nail is a type of "condylocephalic nail" but is not recommended because of the risk of creating or extending proximal diaphyseal cracks (Fig. 4). We prefer to splint the entire femur with longer devices

95° Condylar Blade Plating

A 95° condylar blade plate is the best choice of fixation in a young patient with normal bone density, but fixation with this device requires very extensive preoperative planning. The position and length of the blade as well as the length of the side plate must be determined on the preoperative drawing. The surgical tactic should be written out and posted in the operating room for easy reference and for operating efficiency.

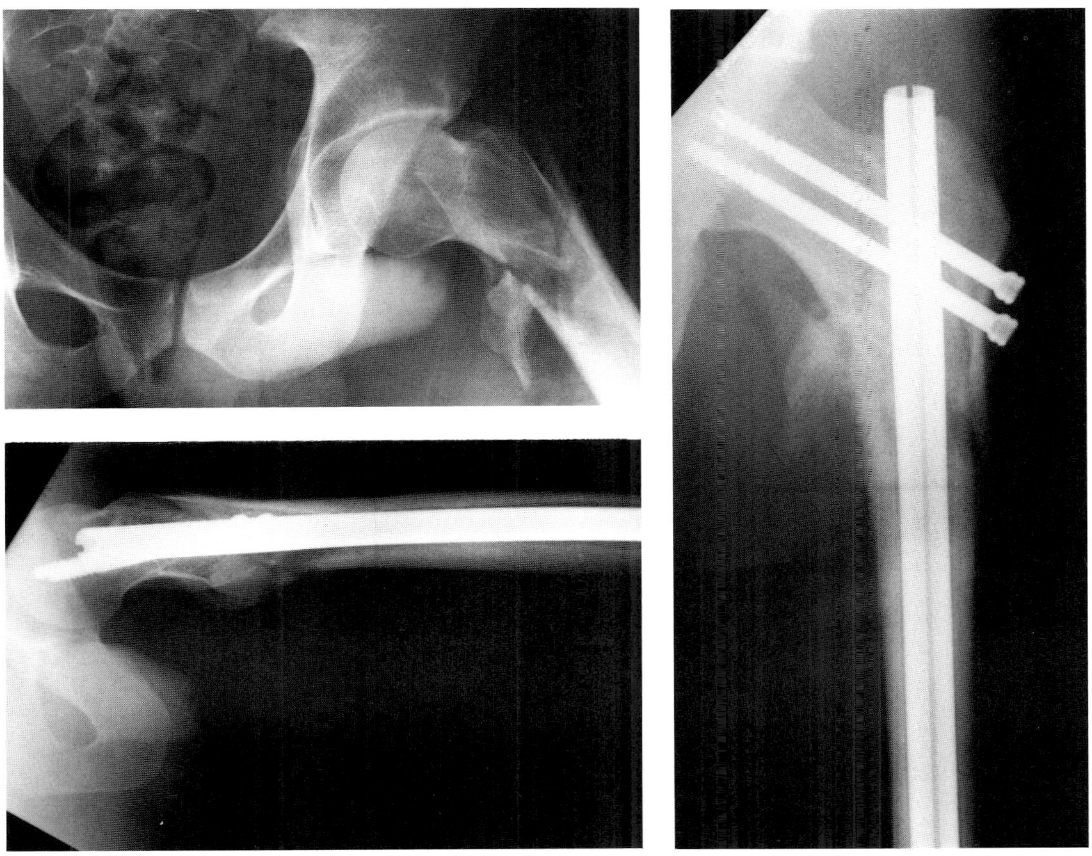

A B C

FIG. 3. Second-generation nailing of a subtrochanteric femur fracture. **A:** Preoperative radiograph. **B, C:** Postoperative lateral views documenting the central position of the two proximal screws.

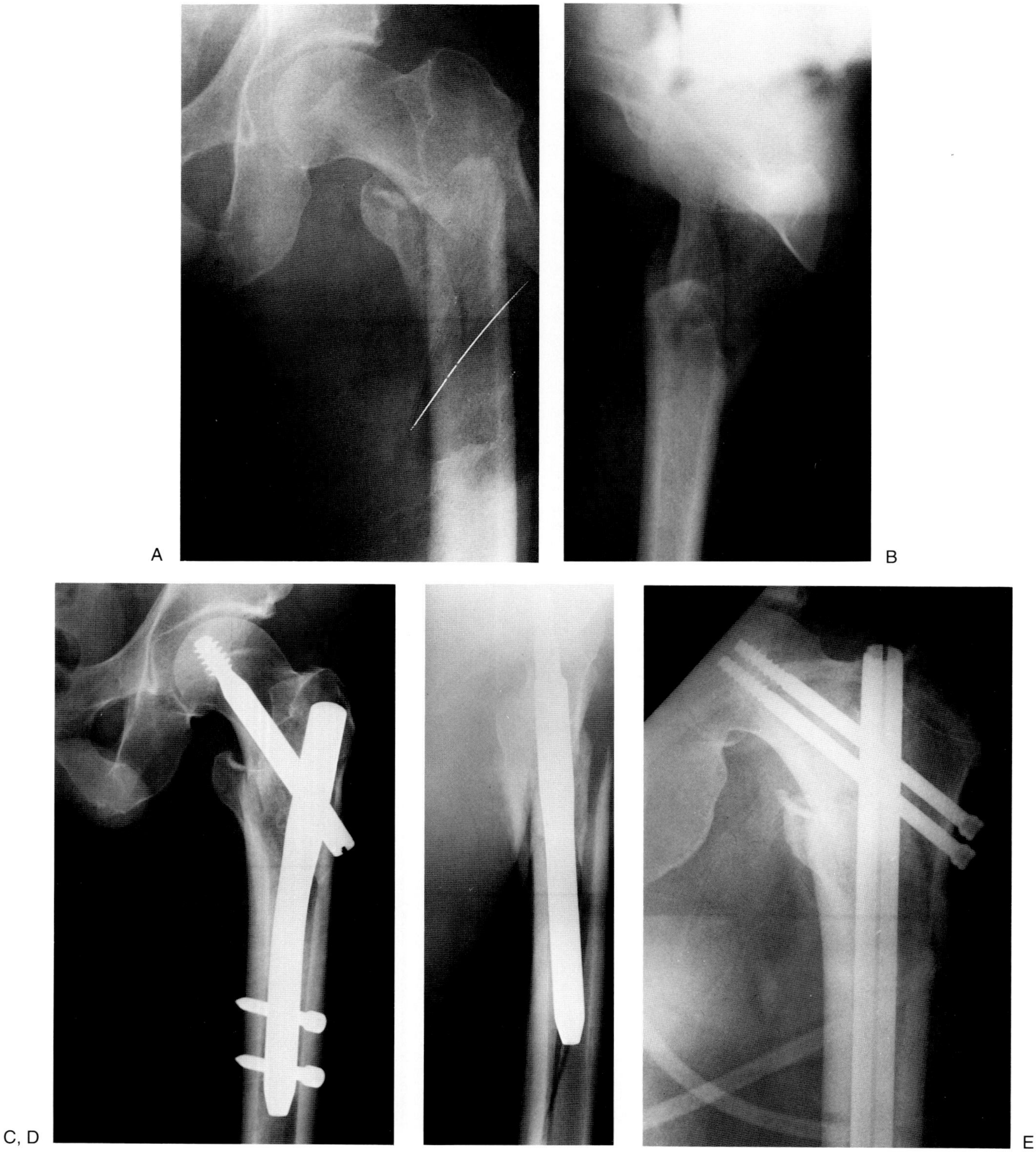

FIG. 4. Failure of a Gamma nail. **A, B:** Preoperative radiographs of a B2.1 fracture. **C:** Postoperative view of the Gamma nail placement. **D:** Failure through cracks created at nail insertion. **E:** Salvage with a second-generation nail.

The patient can be positioned supine on a regular radiolucent operating table or on a fracture table. A fracture table is preferred because the placement of the guide wires and the drill bits for the seating chisel must be confirmed in both planes. The starting point for the seating chisel is marked carefully on the femur. The operating surgeon must be thoroughly familiar with the anatomy of the proximal femur because the neck appears to be located in the anterior half of the greater trochanter when it is viewed from a lateral orientation. The seating chisel must never be inserted without predrilling its path with three 4.5-mm drill bits connected by a router, to avoid splitting the neck of the femur. The position of the seating chisel is confirmed by fluoroscopy in both views and the 95° condylar plate is inserted. The length of the blade on the proximal femur is usually 70 mm to 80 mm; the side plate should be long enough to allow placement of three or four screws distal to the fracture. After the plate is fixed with a single proximal screw, an articulated tensioning device or a femoral distractor is used to regain length and allow indirect reduction of the medial fragments. The number of screws used in the side plate should balance the proximal fixation. Bone grafting may not be necessary if no medial dissection is done, but is usually a good idea if the procedure does not present an unreasonable risk to the patient and if the fixation is stable.

Sliding Hip Screw

When fracture lines extend into the piriformis fossae, the fracture is stabilized with either a sliding hip screw or a 95° condylar blade plate. As mentioned earlier, a 95° condylar screw is not recommended in these highly unstable fractures because its placement requires reaming of a large amount of bone. As a rule, elderly patients with intertrochanteric fractures extending into the subtrochanteric region are managed with sliding hip screws.

The reduction technique is similar to that used for an intertrochanteric fracture. The patient is positioned supine on the fracture table. An assistant lifts up both bone fragments with an elevator to prevent malalignment while the surgeon places a guide wire into the center of the head and neck, confirming the accuracy of placement on both views by fluoroscopy. The only acceptable deviation from completely anatomic placement is below center on the AP view. Accurate hardware placement is critical for a good prognosis and this procedure must not be hurried. A lag screw can be used to reduce and fix a large posteromedial fragment if the screws can be inserted without devitalizing the fragment. In extremely comminuted subtrochanteric fractures, bone grafting (either autogenous or cancellous allograft, depending on the patient's condition and age) is recommended.

The postoperative management for all four types of fixation is similar unless ambulation is contraindicated by injury to an upper extremity or the contralateral lower extremity. Recovery of hip motion can be hastened by CPM. If serous ooze develops, CPM is discontinued until the wound is dry. Touch-down weight-bearing in a walker is indicated for 6 to 8 weeks. Young patients with good balance and upper extremity strength can progress to ambulation with forearm or axillary crutches. Noncompliant patients, especially those with side-plate devices, are managed in a single-leg spica cast with the knee bent at 30° for the initial 6 weeks. When adequate callus is visible on radiographs, the cast can be removed and unrestricted weight-bearing is permitted.

COMPLICATIONS

Systemic complications such as deep venous thrombosis, pulmonary embolus, pneumonia, and urinary tract infection are managed the same as in other proximal femoral fractures. Superficial infections are usually managed successfully with bed rest and administration of intravenous antibiotics. Deep infections are controlled with a regimen of antibiotics, debridement, and delayed wound closure over suction drains. The fixation device should not be removed if the fracture is stable.

Delayed union is rare with an intramedullary device, but if it occurs, it must be managed aggressively to prevent failure of the fixation device. If no signs of healing are seen after 4 postoperative months, bone grafting should be performed. Nonunion occurring in conjunction with implant failure or a varus deformity is usually managed successfully by osteotomy and blade–plate fixation. This procedure has proved successful even when large lucent areas have been created in the femoral head by sliding screws (see Fig. 3). Partial weight-bearing for 12 weeks is recommended after bone grafting.

SKELETALLY IMMATURE PATIENTS

Subtrochanteric femoral fractures in adolescents are managed the same as fractures in adults. Insertion of an intramedullary device is usually advisable, but the diameter of the nail must be small enough for a child's femur. Children under the age of 8 or 9 years are usually managed by 90-90 traction. Rotational deformities and severe flexion-shortening deformities must be avoided. Plate fixation is a good alternative when a child has sustained multiple injuries or a severe head injury. The plates must be removed after 6 to 12 months (depending on the age of the child) to prevent permanent encasement in bone. Very small nonlocked nails can be used initially in children between the ages of 7 and 12 years. Casting is used to supplement this fixation after the patient is clinically stable. Children under the age of 5 years are managed by early spica casting.

REFERENCES

1. Fielding JW, Cochran GB, Zickel RE. Biomechanical characteristics and surgical management of subtrochanteric fractures. Orthop Clin North Am 1974;5:629–50.
2. Seinsheimer F. Subtrochanteric fractures of the femur. J Bone Joint Surg 1978;60A:300–6.
3. Müller ME, Nazarian S, Koch P. The AO classification of fractures. Translated by Schatzker J. Toronto: Springer-Verlag; 1988.

Orthopaedic Trauma Protocols, edited by
Sigvard T. Hansen and Marc F. Swiontkowski,
Raven Press, Ltd., New York, ©1993.

CHAPTER 25

Femoral Shaft Fractures

Sigvard T. Hansen, Jr.

MECHANISMS OF INJURY

In adolescents and young adults, the femoral shaft is usually fractured in high-energy motor vehicle or auto–pedestrian accidents or during rigorous recreational activities such as downhill skiing or competitive contact sports. High-energy injuries caused by direct forces are often associated with significant contusion, degloving, and open wounds. Rarely, femoral shaft fractures may occur as stress fractures from running. Low-energy femoral shaft fractures can be caused by indirect forces in mature adults, whose bones may be weakened by osteoporosis or tumors. Injuries in pathologic bone usually result in rotational or spiral fractures, with very little associated soft-tissue injury.

ANATOMIC CONSIDERATIONS

The femur is very long and is curved in an anterior bow. The radius of the curve is not uniform throughout its length but averages approximately 2.2 meters. Dense peripheral cortex is found in the middle three fifths; the thickest cortex is located on the posterior aspect (the linea aspera) of the upper three fifths, where strong muscle and fascial attachments insert onto the bone. The diameter of the femur increases near the old epiphyseal line in the lower fifth segment near the knee. Here, the metaphyseal cortex is correspondingly thinner and the medullary cancellous bone is increasingly more dense. At the upper end of the femur, the posteromedial lesser trochanter and lateral greater trochanter project from the neck and head anteromedially at an obtuse angle of approximately 140°. Access to the medullary canal is gained easily at the base of the neck, just inside the tip of the trochanter. Access to the femoral medullary canal is also possible through an anatomically "silent" area in the notch in the knee, a site routinely used for inserting the stem of many knee prostheses.

Unlike the tibia, the femur is surrounded by thick muscles that provide excellent potential vascularity and make the femur less dependent on its intramedullary blood supply. The long muscles tend to shorten the femoral shaft significantly after a fracture, and length must be restored by reduction or strong skeletal traction immediately after injury, when pain and muscle spasm are common.

CLASSIFICATION

The purpose of classification systems is to guide treatment and prognosis and to group similar cases for later comparisons of treatment and outcome. To accomplish both of these objectives, we use two classifications, one for fracture patterns (1) and one for the degree of soft-tissue injury (see Chapter 1) (2,3).

The most common fracture patterns are comminuted grade I, II, III, and IV, and longitudinal (spiral) and long oblique fractures (Fig. 1). The fracture patterns most commonly seen in trauma centers are comminuted grade II, III, or IV and segmental fractures. Uncomminuted transverse and short oblique fracture patterns are rare. Soft-tissue injuries are classified into four grades of closed injuries (C-0, C-I, C-II, and C-III) and five grades of open injuries (O-I, O-II, O-IIIA, O-IIIB, and O-IIIC).

ASSESSMENT

Physical Examination

Femoral fractures are easily diagnosed during a physical examination. Femoral shortening, dysfunction, deformity, and tenderness usually correspond to an appropriate history

Department of Orthopaedics, Harborview Medical Center, University of Washington, Seattle, Washington 98104

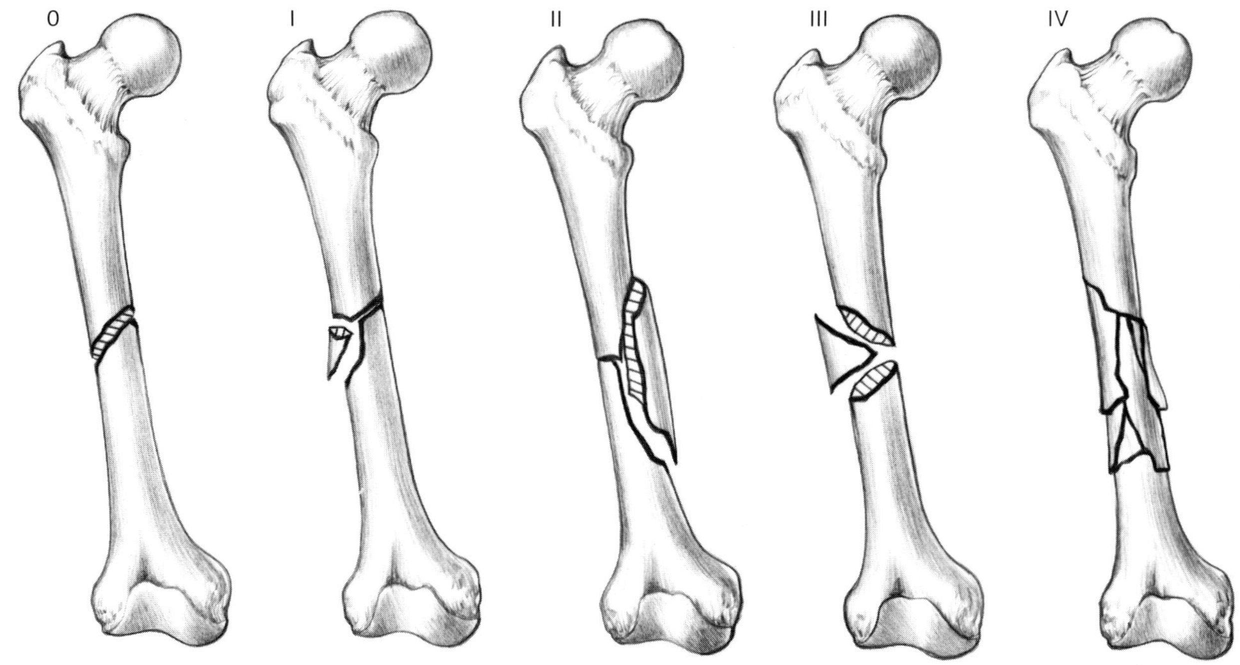

FIG. 1. Fracture stability or comminution must be graded to determine whether a locking nail should be used and, if so, whether it should be locked dynamically or statically. In trauma centers, nails are shtically locked in femoral shaft fractures to ensure control of rohtion. High-energy injuries frequently produce undisplaced cracks in the bone, which can displace and develop into higher grades of comminution when weight is applied postoperatively. Grade 0 and I fractures are stable in length and can be treated without interlocking; grade II fractures are at risk for shortening with rotation, and interlocking is recommended; fractures rated grade m or higher are routinely stabilized with interlocking nails to prevent rotation and malunion.

of injury. Associated injuries, which can be disabling and more difficult to treat than the femoral shaft fracture itself, must be ruled out. Femoral neck fractures occur with approximately 2.5% of high-energy femoral shaft fractures but are often undisplaced and difficult to identify (see Chapter 22). These fractures tend to occur near the base of the neck and are further complicated by a steep Pauwels type III angle. Other common associated injuries include dislocations of the hip, ligamentous injuries of the knee, and avulsions of the tibial attachment of the posterior cruciate ligament.

After associated fractures are ruled out, the femur is evaluated for soft-tissue injuries, fracture location, and fracture pattern, the variables on which treatment is based. Compartmental syndromes are rare, although they may occur in the anterior compartment or in the gluteal area from direct blows. Closed degloving injuries with large areas of hematoma and loose fat in the trauma-induced spaces between the muscle fascia and subcutaneous fat may occur from direct blows and in significantly overweight patients. Muscle may be lacerated by the displaced ends of the fracture, resulting in cavities that fill with hematoma. Multiple injuries, high-grade soft-tissue injuries, compartmental syndromes, and degloving warrant immediate operative stabilization of the femur and management of the soft-tissue injuries.

Radiographic Evaluation

Associated injuries are diagnosed by evaluation of the joints above and below the shaft fracture with good-quality preoperative radiographs. Ligamentous injuries in the knee are diagnosed from radiographs taken preoperatively and by careful physical reexamination after femoral stabilization.

Special Studies

In addition to thorough physical and radiographic evaluations, a useful special diagnostic study is a preoperative arterial blood gas. Marginal PaO_2 levels warrant immediate intramedullary nailing with minimal or no reaming. Alternatively, stabilization by plating or external skeletal fixation may be indicated in this situation.

EMERGENT MANAGEMENT

When immediate surgery is planned, the femur can be temporarily stabilized in the field or the emergency department with a soft skeletal traction loop placed around the ankle and attached to a Thomas splint. In the absence of a knee injury, skeletal traction can be applied to the proximal tibia with a Kirschner wire and bow; if a knee injury is suspected or if surgery might be delayed more than 12 hours, skeletal traction is applied to the distal anterior femur. A balanced traction system, a fixed traction device, or a Böhler–Braun frame can be left in place for several days in patients with isolated femoral fractures who are in excellent health. The femur must be kept at length or slightly distracted to facilitate reduction for closed nailing.

DEFINITIVE TREATMENT

Long-bone fractures have a direct negative influence on patient morbidity. For this reason, an important goal of fracture fixation is to minimize the detrimental systemic effects caused by long-bone fractures. Although closed pre-reamed intramedullary nailing is the ideal method of stabilization for most femoral fractures, reaming is potentially dangerous in patients with compromised pulmonary function. When intramedullary nailing is the treatment of choice, pulmonary damage can be minimized by using small locking nails that require minimal reaming or, in very proximal fractures, by venting the femur distally before reaming. Venting is preferred by drilling a large 6-mm to 8-mm hole in the distal metaphysis to allow egress of the medullary contents (Fig. 2). Plating and external skeletal fixation are not commonly used to stabilize femoral fractures, but each of these techniques is useful under certain circumstances.

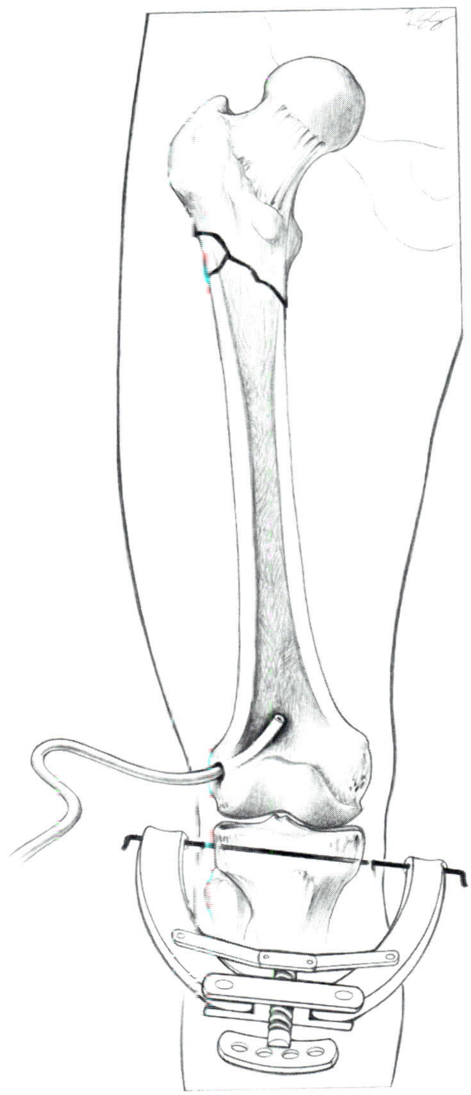

FIG. 2. Venting of the femoral shaft prior to reaming. High intramedullary pressures can develop during reaming when the fracture is closed or located high in the femoral shaft. The pressure is vented through a small incision made over the lateral condyle and a 6-mm or 8-mm hole drilled upward into the distal medullary canal. A large plastic tube is inserted to visualize egress of fluid from the canal, but the tube is less important than the venting hole. Venting is particularly important in the presence of pulmonary dysfunction or when dull reamers are used. Fractures occurring low in the femur are vented intrinsically and do not require a lateral condylar vent.

Intramedullary Nailing

Closed intramedullary nailing with interlocking screws is the core of musculoskeletal traumatology and the ideal fixation for most diaphyseal femoral fractures. When done with indirect reduction techniques, stabilization by this method restores and maintains anatomic alignment, causes few complications, and allows full range of motion (ROM) in adjacent joints and muscles for functional rehabilitation. The femur can tolerate reaming for insertion of a flexible, full-length intramedullary device because it is surrounded by thick circumferential muscles. This muscle cover not only acts as a heat sink to disperse potentially intense heat caused by reaming but also provides osseous blood supply to compensate for damage to the medullary blood supply.

Entry into the long, anteriorly bowed medullary canal is gained through the angled proximal extension of the trochanter. The patient can be placed either in the supine or a lateral position on an operating table (Figs. 3 and 4). We prefer to position patients with chest trauma and spinal or pelvic fractures in the supine position. A Kirschner wire is placed into the distal femur. The wire must lie anterior to the middle of the canal, yet be distal enough to be near the upper fourth of the patella when the knee is partially bent. This traction wire will be left in place as the nail is driven in just behind it. The slightly bowed nail will follow the guide rod into the middle or the posterior portion of the condyle.

When nailing is done in a lateral position for fractures in the distal third of the femoral shaft, the Kirschner wire must be angled slightly so that it lies more proximal on the lateral side than on the medial side. The wire will thus neutralize the femur's gravitational sag into valgus when skeletal traction is

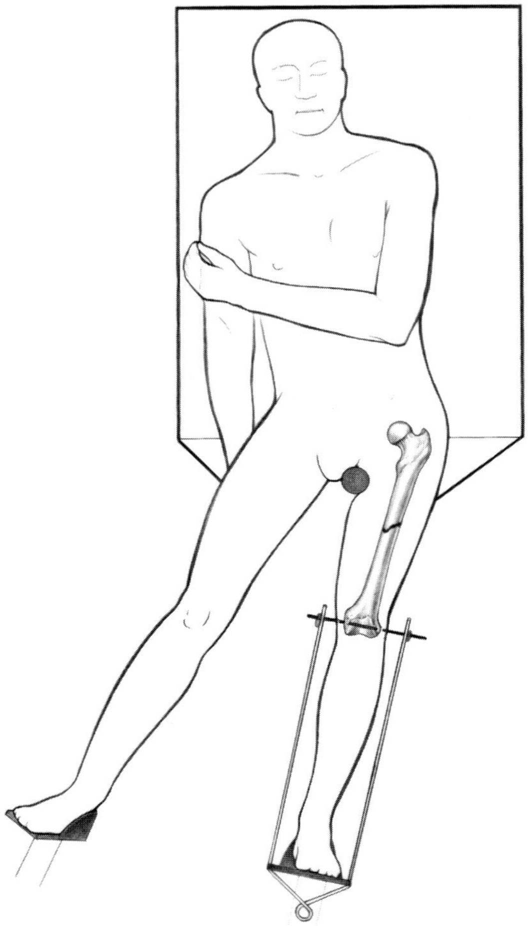

FIG. 3. Supine positioning requires a well-padded perineal post and a table broad enough to accommodate bending the patient away from the entry site of the nail and slightly adducting the leg around the post. In this position, the greater trochanter is accessible even in obese patients. Contrary to the illustration, the table should not protrude laterally but leave room to work proximally. Care must be taken to not contaminate reamers and other instruments when they are withdrawn with the patient in this position. In some cases, the leg is flexed significantly at the knee to avoid hyperextension at the fracture site. A traction pin may be placed either in the distal anterior femur or in the proximal tibia.

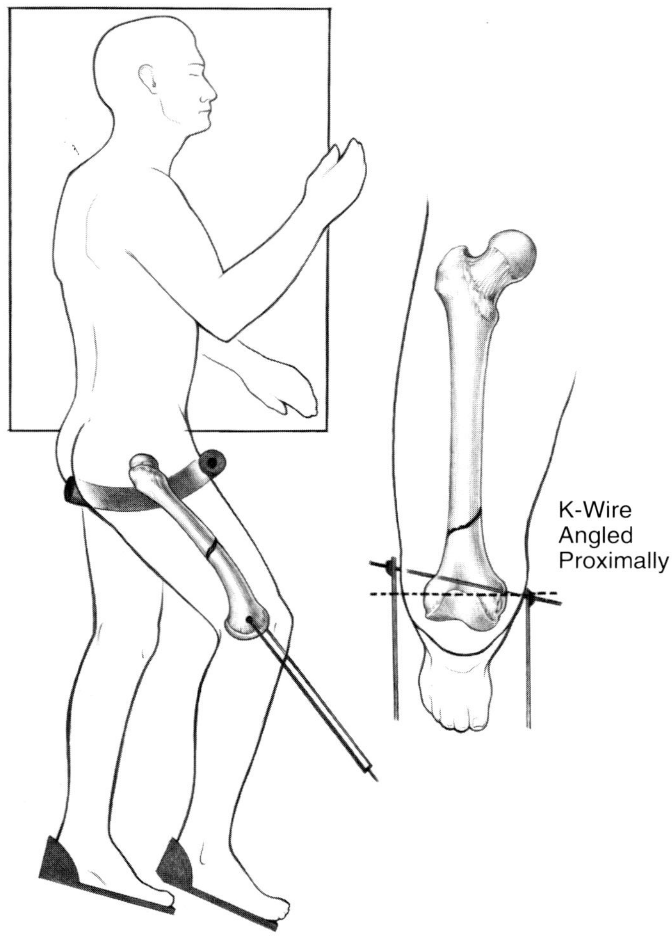

FIG. 4. For lateral nailing the patient is rotated slightly forward and a support is placed under the foot and ankle to position the thigh in slight internal rotation. This position is appropriate for heavy patients with adequate pulmonary function because it allows the soft tissues to be moved aside during access to the femoral canal. The lateral position must not be used if the status of the patient's spine is in question. For distal fractures, the Kirschner wire may be angled slightly to control the tendency of the femur to sag into valgus. Intramedullary nailing is best accomplished immediately after injury, before the onset of swelling, muscle spasm, and pulmonary complications.

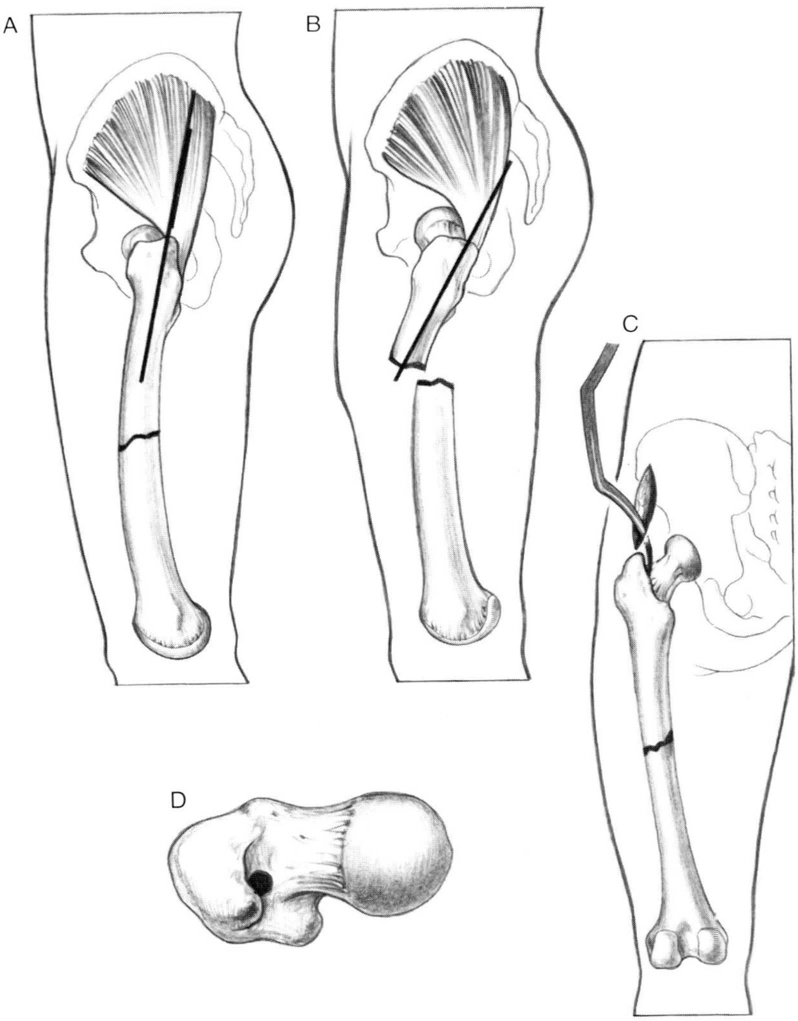

FIG. 5. A: Lateral view of the alignment of the upper femur, usually seen in distal fractures located at the middle third of the diaphysis. This alignment must be kept in mind as the incision is made and the awl or reamer is aligned to enter the bone. **B:** Posterior-to-anterior alignment seen in proximal fractures. These fractures require a more posterior starting point. **C:** The location of the skin incision in relation to the tip of the trochanter is seen on a posterior view. **D:** The top of the upper femur. The ideal location for the starting point is seen in relation to the trochanteric tip and the femoral neck and it is found on a line projected proximally from the center of the upper femoral medullary canal. Minimal hoop stresses are produced in the bone when nails are inserted at this point and directed in perfect alignment with the upper femur. Ideally, the curve of the nail should approximate the normal anterior bow of the femur, producing minimal stress inside the bone at all levels.

applied. The patient must be moved gently and extremes of position must be avoided. Hip flexion should not exceed 30°, the knee should be flexed less than 60°, and hip adduction should range between 15° and 20°. Excessive hip flexion causes the hamstring muscles to tighten, and extreme knee flexion causes the quadriceps muscles to tighten. Both muscle contractions make fracture reduction difficult. Greater adduction may be required in a very heavy patient, but nailing a supine patient who is positioned in more than 15° or 20° of adduction may also be difficult. Patients placed in a lateral position tend to roll forward slightly, and an adjustable Mayo stand with a pillow can be placed under the ankle to hold the femur in approximately 20° of internal rotation. The amount of femoral anteversion on the normal side is measured to appropriately adjust the amount of rotation on the injured side. Rotation is slightly easier to adjust with the patient in the supine position.

A critical factor in this procedure is locating the correct position for the incision (Fig. 5). The osseous starting point should be on a line projected from the center of the upper third of the femoral shaft in both planes. This point usually falls slightly posterior in the fossa just inside the greater trochanter at the extreme lateral end of the base of the neck. The incision is started at the tip of the trochanter in line with the femur and is extended proximally for 2 to 6 inches, depending on the thickness of the soft tissues. The cortex is opened with a sharp awl or with a reamer over a guide wire. A long 8-mm T-handled reamer can be used to enlarge the opening and to align the awl or the drill into the proximal third of the femur. A slightly bent bulb-tipped guide wire is then inserted into the proximal femur and manipulated across the fracture site. This maneuver is easily done immediately after injury if the patient has been positioned appropriately on the fracture table.

Very proximal femoral fractures are the most difficult to reduce. The proximal end of the femur may have to be reamed up to 11 mm before reduction can be attempted. After reaming, a 10-mm-diameter nail containing the bulb-

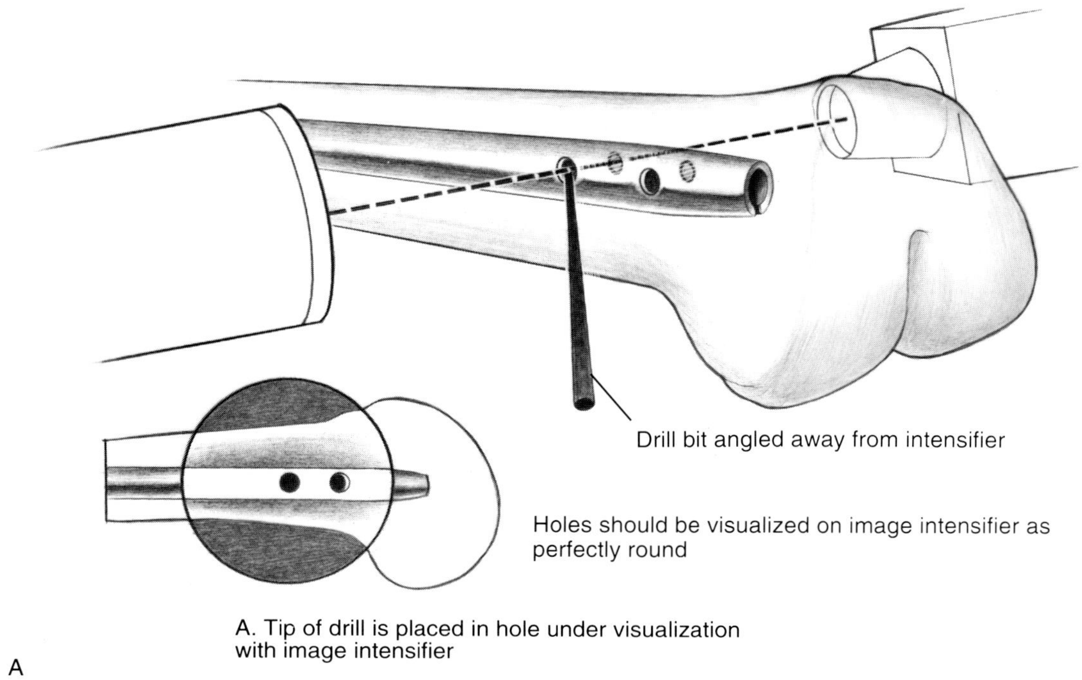

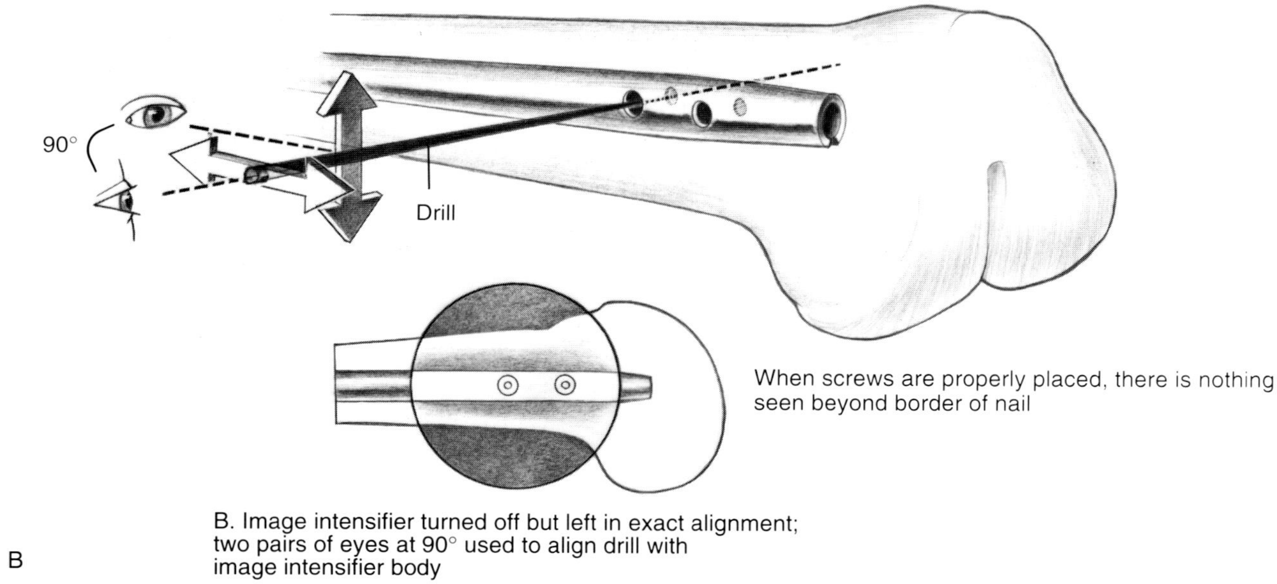

FIG. 6. Free-hand technique for locating distal drill holes. **A:** The most important step for placing screws across the distal drill holes is to accurately locate the first hole as perfectly round on the image intensifier screen. A drill is used in very hard bone and a sharp Steinmann pin in a radiolucent holder is used in soft bone. The point of the drill or the pin is placed directly in the center of the hole located on fluoroscopy or multiple radiographic pictures taken at short intervals. **B:** Once accurately centered, the image intensifier may be turned off and the drill or pin may be lined up by triangulation. The surgeon and the assistant surgeon stand at 90° angles to the image intensifier and ensure that the tip of the drill or pin does not move when drilling is initiated. The second screw can be placed in exactly the same way or with the assistance of a jig.

tipped guide wire is placed into the proximal femur and the proximal fracture fragment is aligned with the distal fragment by manipulation with the nail. Reduction is achieved by advancing the bulb-tipped guide wire into the distal fragment. Finding the correct starting point may be difficult in very proximal fractures, especially if the proximal fragment is abducted and flexed. Because the entire isthmus is contained in the distal fragment of a proximal fracture, venting the femur may be required to avoid excessive pressure in the distal fragment during reaming (see Chapter 1).

Reamers must be well-maintained and used correctly to avoid complications. The reamer bit used to begin reaming must be smaller in diameter than the narrowest portion of the isthmus from measurements taken on preoperative radiographs. As reaming progresses, the size of the reamer bit can be increased by 1-mm increments until contact is made with cortical bone. Reaming then proceeds more slowly, and the size of the reamer bits is increased by 0.5-mm increments until the canal is reamed the desired amount. The optimal amount of reaming and the appropriate diameter of the nail are determined by the size of the patient. A 11-mm to 12-mm nail is used in an average-sized woman and a 12-mm or 13-mm nail is used in an average-sized man. Larger nails can be used in very osteoporotic bone with large medullary canals, and small locking nails, which require little or no reaming, can be used when pulmonary compromise contraindicates reaming or a long surgical procedure. The principles of nailing are basically the same for all types of nails. Some nails (for example, more flexible open-section nails) must be overreamed by 0.5 mm or 1 mm; stiffer closed-section or solid nails may require overreaming by 1.5 mm to 2 mm.

The 3-mm ball-tipped reamer guide is exchanged for the 4-mm straight-tipped nail guide using the medullary tube and its correct positioning is confirmed radiographically in both planes. The nail is advanced over the guide wire until the upper end is flush with or slightly inside the tip of the trochanter and the distal end is within a centimeter or two of the old epiphyseal scar. The proximal locking bolt is applied through the proximally mounted jig according to the manufacturer's recommendations. The distal screw is placed freehand in the distal locking hole after the tip of the drill is aligned on the fluoroscopic image (Fig. 6). Locking nails are used routinely in trauma centers because the majority of fractures treated there are comminuted or contain a split and are potentially unstable in length.

After the nail is inserted, the wound is closed and the patient is placed on a stretcher next to the operating table for evaluation of femoral rotation and the status of the knee ligaments. If the results of the examination are satisfactory, isometric strengthening exercises are begun on the ward the very next day, and ambulation is encouraged as soon as the patient is able to lift the leg from the bed. The amount of weight-bearing that is allowed depends on the amount of stability at the fracture site. With good linear bone contact, a patient can proceed to full weight-bearing within 1 month. Weight-bearing on a markedly comminuted fracture or on a long spiral fracture, where length is maintained solely by the screws, is limited to less than 50 pounds until callus formation is evident on radiographs. Knee ROM and quadriceps-strengthening exercises are encouraged during partial weight-bearing (Figs. 7–10) (4).

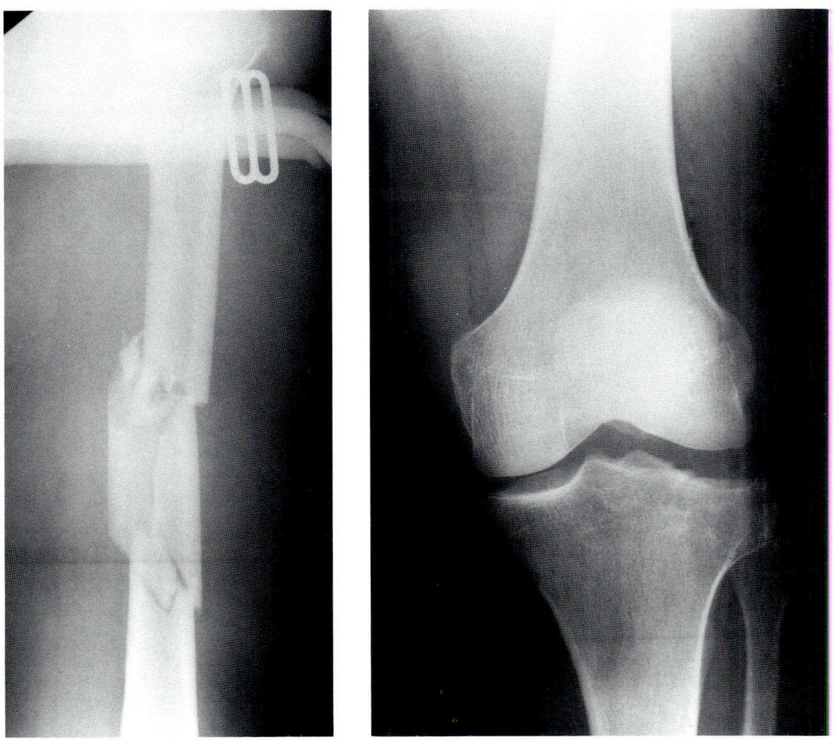
A,B

FIG. 7. This multiply injured trauma patient sustained a comminuted segmental midshaft femoral fracture (**A**) and a slightly depressed and widened lateral plateau fracture of the tibia in the same leg (**B**).

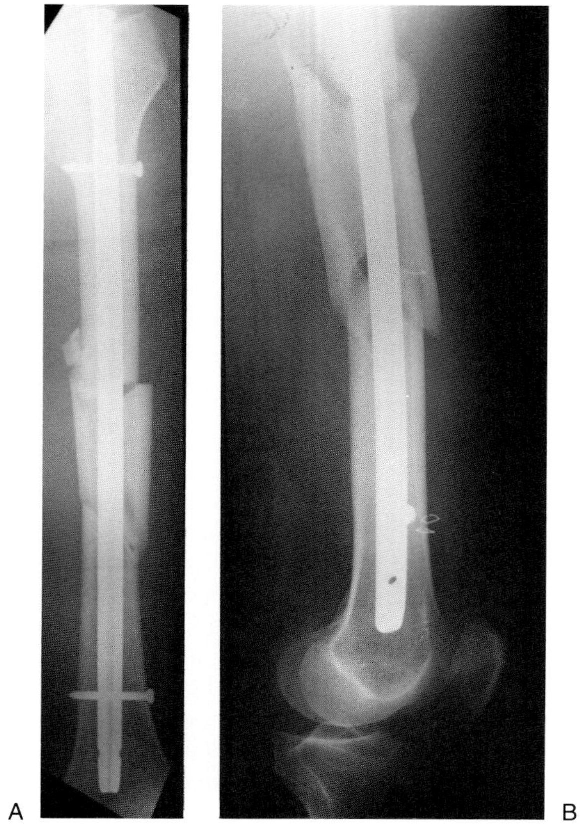

FIG. 8. Anteroposterior (A) and lateral (B) radiographic views of the femoral fracture after a femoral nail was placed by closed technique and statically locked. The starting point is slightly more medial than ideal, but note that the split segmental fragment is not reduced snug against the nail. This is of no particular consequence because overall femoral length and rotation, particularly the anatomic anterior bow, have been well reestablished.

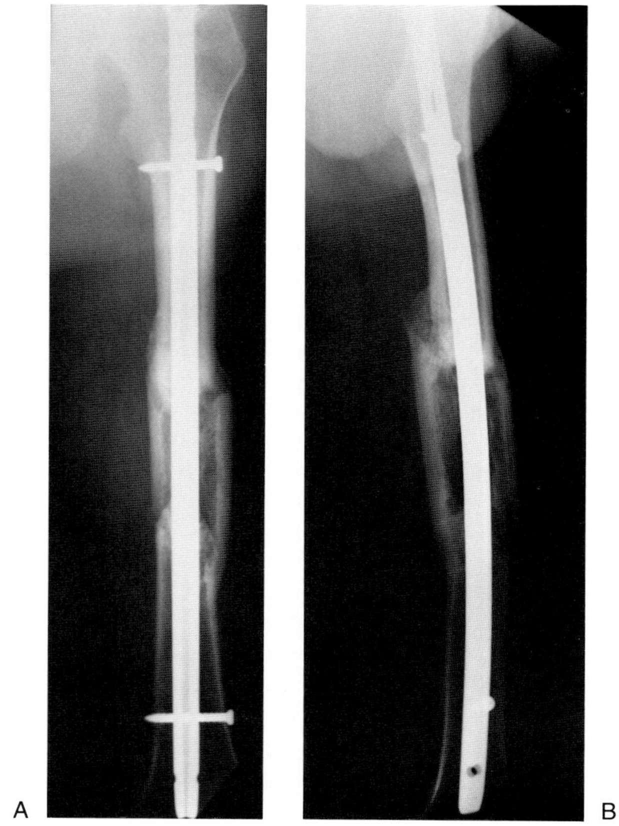

FIG. 9. A: Four months postoperatively, excellent fracture union is seen on radiographs. B: Note the slightly posterior starting point proximally on the lateral view. Using this starting point keeps the nail in the center of the femur and maintains an antomic anterior bow.

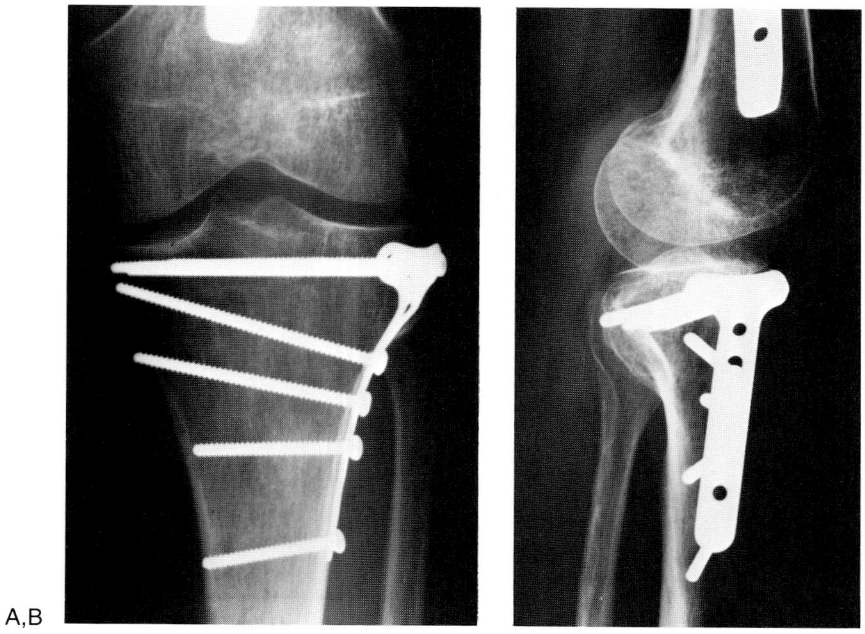

FIG. 10. Anteroposterior (A) and lateral (B) radiographs of the knee joint, in which the articular surface was restored by internal fixation shortly after femoral nailing. Early continuous passive motion in the hospital followed by early physical therapy and gradual resumption of weight bearing allowed the patient to have a relatively short hospital stay and to return to the activities of daily life. Nearly total anatomic and functional reconstruction of the limb after a serious high-energy injury makes internal fixation extremely cost-effective.

Plating of the Diaphyseal Femoral Fractures

Compared to its obvious value in proximal and distal metaphyseal injuries, plating is rarely indicated in femoral diaphyseal fractures. In some circumstances, however, diaphyseal plating may be preferable to nailing. Candidates for plating include multiply injured patients, especially those with pulmonary contusions, who may be unable to tolerate a long surgical procedure or the special positioning required for nailing. When the diaphysis is opened by an open injury, plating is technically and biologically desirable if the soft tissues are already stripped from the bone. Rarely, access to the femoral canal is blocked by an implant or by hardware placed to stabilize a previous fracture. Done correctly, plating can be a quick, safe, and reliable procedure that inflicts no further injury to the medullary blood supply.

Application of the plate to the lateral surface of the bone allows the most direct approach with the least mechanical impact. A straight posterolateral approach is made by following the lateral intermuscular septum to the lateral surface of the bone. The perforating veins are isolated, ligated, and the vastus lateralis is lifted forward. Later, the vastus lateralis will be returned intact to its normal position and secured loosely to the fascial layer with running resorbable monofilament sutures to reduce the risk of necrosis or compartmental syndrome. In open fractures, the muscles are approximated loosely in their anatomic positions and the traumatic wound is left open.

An obvious anatomic problem associated with femoral plating is inability to contour the plate to accommodate the anterior bow in the femur. However, the physiologic anterior bow can be reproduced by applying the plate slightly anterior at the fracture ends and slightly posterior in the center (Fig. 11). When the fracture is transverse, adequate contact with the medial cortex can be provided when the eccentrically placed screws are tightened and the middle of the plate is contoured out from the bone. A 4.5-mm DCP or LC-DCP with four screws grasping eight cortices on either side of the fracture usually provides adequate fixation. A slightly longer plate may be required for a comminuted fracture. Angled interfragmentary compression screws are ideal for short oblique fractures. Indirect reduction techniques should be used extensively to protect the soft tissues from further damage. Retractors and bone- or plate-holding forceps that strip soft tissues from bone should be avoided.

To avoid soft-tissue stripping during plate application, a 3.2-mm hole is drilled through a fragment near the fracture site, tapped, and the plate is applied. The plate is then aligned on the same fragment with a second screw, taking care to accommodate the anterior bowing. Using indirect reduction techniques or a pointed bone-holding forceps or bone hook, the opposite end of the fracture is positioned and fixed with a 4.5-mm screw placed using the AO yellow loading guide for compression when the fracture pattern permits. Only one screw hole can be filled and fixed initially. The external compression device can be attached and stronger compression applied before filling the remaining screw holes. The disadvantage of greater soft-tissue dissection must be weighed against the advantage of external compression. The presence of significant comminution contraindicates compression altogether. Before the remaining holes are filled, flexion angulation and rotation in the femur must be assessed very carefully. Although all the screw holes in cancellous or osteoporotic bone should be filled, this is not necessary in

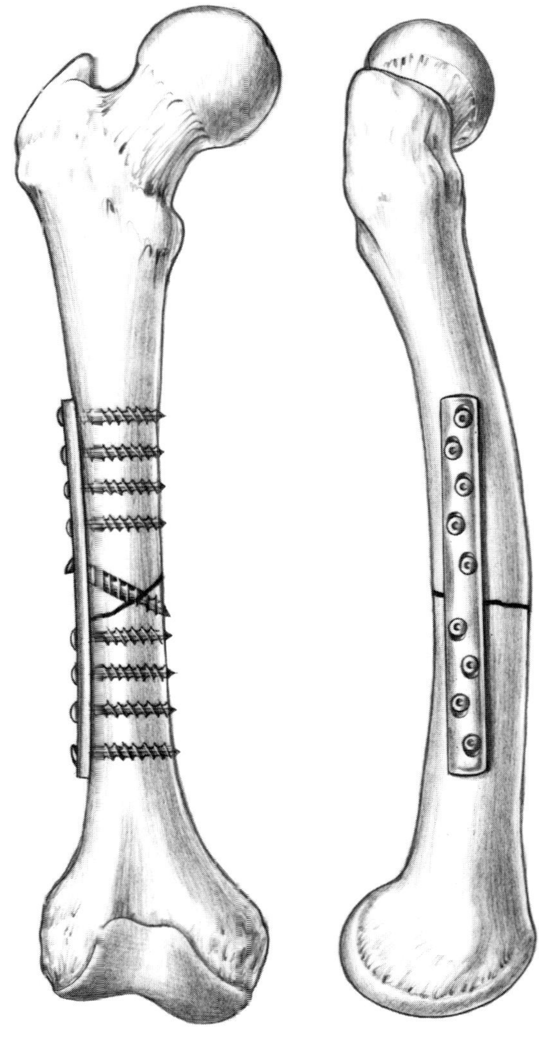

FIG. 11. Femoral plating. Note that positioning of the femoral plate requires maintaining the anterior bow of the femur and the use of an adequate number of screws. Whenever possible, an interfragmental screw is inserted through the plate as well. Cancellous bone graft may be placed on the medial side of the fracture to ensure that healing occurs before the plate loosens or breaks from stress fatigue. Grafting is ideal for open fractures, patients with associated vascular injuries, and where there are lesser degrees of fracture communications.

hard cortical bone. Rarely, the medullary canal in patients with joint replacements, rheumatoid arthritis, or severe disuse atrophy requires supplementation with methylmethacrylate injected in liquid form into the screw holes before placement of the screws. Except in children, cancellous bone graft should be applied to the medial cortex opposite the fracture site in almost all cases. An exception is made for highly comminuted fractures in which indirect reduction techniques are used.

External Fixation of Femoral Fractures

External skeletal fixation of diaphyseal femoral fractures is rarely indicated in traumatology, but this procedure is warranted under certain circumstances. Plating or nailing techniques require longer surgical times and technically demanding procedures. When rapid stabilization and soft-tissue protection are major concerns, external skeletal fixation can be used. Open fractures can be reduced through the open wound as the pins are inserted. Because the femur is subject to high stresses, particularly in large patients, at least two widely spread, 5-mm diameter Schanz pins are usually inserted at each end of the fracture and fixed to a lateral double-bar frame. A narrow-angled Delta frame or the addition of more pins may be required in rare cases.

Like intramedullary nailing, external skeletal fixation requires insertion of a distal femoral traction pin and reduction of the fracture by indirect reduction techniques. The external fixator can be left in place for 5 to 7 days until the patient is stabilized, and the pins can be removed and replaced with an intramedullary nail. A drawback of definitive management by this method is restricted motion at the knee, which may require a quadricepsplasty in the future.

COMPLICATIONS

Intramedullary Nailing

Complications associated with intramedullary nailing are caused by poor patient selection, technique failure, or inadequate postoperative management. Problems attributed to poor patient selection include unrecognized fractures at the base of the femoral neck, pulmonary deficiencies, and grade IIIB or IIIC injuries with severe damage to the extraosseous blood supply. Intramedullary nailing in patients with these problems can aggravate ARDS, infection, and bony necrosis, and can markedly delay union or result in nonunion. Patients with markedly decreased PaO_2 before reaming may be susceptible to fat embolism syndrome. Teenagers, in particular, may exhibit no signs of a low PaO_2 even when the level is marginal. The risk for fat embolism syndrome is highest when nailing is done between the second and fifth postinjury days, when PaO_2 is typically low.

Complications caused by use of an inappropriate surgical technique, such as making a starting point that is too lateral or too anterior, can produce comminution in a short proximal fragment. Starting too far medially can fracture the femoral neck or damage the blood supply to the femoral head and subsequently cause avascular necrosis, but these complications are rare. Reaming can be followed by serious complications; dull reamers can cause either femoral necrosis or mechanical plugging necrosis. Excessive pressure can build up in the long distal femoral fragment from using improper reamers or reaming technique, and the lungs can be damaged when marrow contents are forced into the veins and canaliculi. As noted earlier, the potential for this complication decreases when appropriate reaming techniques and sharp reamers are used and when the distal femoral medullary canal is vented. Improper hardware (e.g., a nail that is too large in diameter, too stiff, or too straight) can cause fracture comminution or loss of anterior curvature with subsequent slight hyperextension of the knee. Nonunion is rare but may be related to soft-tissue stripping from the bone at the time of the initial injury or thermal damage from reaming. The intraoperative decision to treat a fracture with dynamic (nonlocked) nailing can lead to malunion in rotation or shortening. Motion in the knee may be lost because of an inadequate physical therapy regimen to strengthen the quadriceps and extend knee ROM. More commonly, knee motion is limited because of a missed knee injury during the pre- and postoperative evaluations.

Plating

Complications that may occur with plating include infection, osteonecrosis, malunion, nonunion, and hardware failure. Because plating is often done in open fractures with damaged soft-tissues, infection is most likely to occur as the result of inappropriate patient selection. Infection in open fractures can be aggravated by poor soft-tissue techniques. These include excessive stripping, failure to use indirect reduction techniques, and the formation of heat necrosis around the screws from using dull drills. A thin area of necrosis develops underneath the plate when a broad plate is tightened firmly along the shaft. This may be related to refracture after plate removal. The degree of necrosis can be reduced by using low-contact plates. Malunion can occur when the normal anterior bow of the femur has not been restored or when femoral rotation has not been carefully realigned. Nonunion is common with plating when the amount of original damage to the osseous blood supply is extensive. The potential for nonunion can be minimized by adding an onlay bone graft on the medial side. Hardware failure can occur when a patient resumes activity too early, particularly if a cancellous bone graft had not been placed on the side opposite the plate. In spite of potential complications, plating can be a highly successful method of treatment when proper techniques are used.

External Skeletal Fixation

Two major complications are associated with external skeletal fixation of femoral fractures: pin-tract infections and limited knee motion. External skeletal fixation is most successful when the pins penetrate only skin and subcutaneous tissue before reaching bone. Motion in the muscles and soft tissues around the pins damages soft tissues and increases the potential for pin-tract infection. For this reason, external skeletal fixation is not well suited to the femur, which is surrounded by thick soft tissues on all sides, but is an ideal form of fixation for the tibia. When the pins are left in place until the bone heals, approximately 4 months or longer, scarring in these tissues decreases full ROM at the knee. A quadricepsplasty may be required to loosen the adhesions. Malunion can occur because of failure to maintain anatomic alignment while the external fixator is applied. These complications can be avoided by early (within the first 10 days) conversion to an intramedullary nail.

SKELETALLY IMMATURE PATIENTS

Open reduction and internal fixation are rarely used to stabilize femoral fractures in children under the age of 6 years. However, lateral plating with a low-contact 3.5-mm titanium DCP may be effective in certain patients with severe head injury or open wounds. Fractures stabilized with external skeletal fixation heal fairly rapidly in this age group; the advantage of external skeletal fixation over plating is avoidance of a lateral scar and the need for a second operation to remove the plate.

In multiply injured children between the ages of 6 and 8 years, and up to age 10 or 12 years, depending on the maturity and size of the child, femoral fractures can present difficult management problems. Treatment with skeletal traction and spica casting is inappropriate because muscle spasms can shorten the fracture. Although external skeletal fixation is minimally invasive and poses no threat to the trochanteric epiphysis, the device is awkward and maintaining the fixation frame and the pin tracts can be tedious work. Standard intramedullary nailing with minimal reaming is acceptable treatment in mature children in the 9- to 12-year-old group and for those with severe multiple injuries or soft-tissue injuries. Effective methods of intramedullary stabilization in this age group include solid nails, such as Rush nails, or two Ender nails inserted antegrade from the upper lateral femur just below the epiphysis or retrograde from the distal metaphysis (Fig. 12). Minimal reaming must be done in children. Plating through a lateral approach, using the new titanium LC-DCP, is a very safe and effective procedure that facilitates the management of children with multiple injuries, open fractures, or head injuries. Except for a residual scar and the need for plate removal, plating is remarkably free of complications when used with indirect reduction techniques.

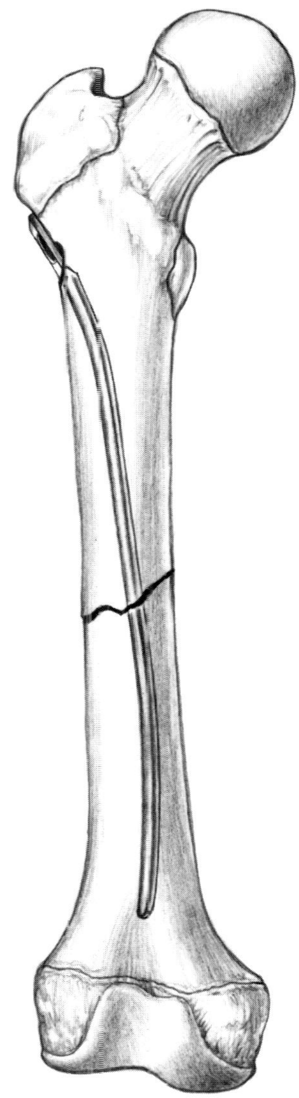

FIG. 12. Placement of Ender or Rush pins in children ages 6 to 10. This technique can be used for patients with multiple injuries or head injuries or when the trochanteric apophysis must be avoided. A small hole is made just below the lateral apophysis. One or two Ender pins or one Rush rod are inserted through this hole until they are within 2 cm or 3 cm of the distal epiphysis. The nail is left short of the distal epiphysis because medullary bone, particularly distal bone, is dense and longer nails may cause distraction. Overall management of patients is facilitated and shortening or major malalignment of the femur is prevented by this technique. Rotation must be prevented by other means.

In adolescents, nonoperative management of isolated fractures can cause financial, behavioral, and social problems. Adolescents are extremely difficult to manage with skeletal traction and spica casting, both in the hospital and at home. The cost for a single working parent to care for an injured child is enormous. In general, management of femoral fractures by intramedullary fixation is by far the most cost-effective and easiest method for the surgeon, the patient, and the family. Closed intramedullary nailing requires a short hospitalization and allows early return to normal function; high priorities in these emotional, highly vulnerable young patients (5). Plating is an acceptable, although limiting, second choice in immature boys. Femoral nailing is recommended as strongly for adolescent patients with high-energy trauma who are within 2 years of completing skeletal growth (girls around age 12 and boys of 13 or 14) as it is for adults.

REFERENCES

1. Winquist RA, Hansen ST. Comminuted fractures of the femoral shaft treated by intramedullary nailing. *Orthop Clin North Am* 1980;11:633–48.
2. Tscherne H, Oestern H-J. Pathophysiology and classification of soft tissue injuries associated with fractures. In: Tscherne H, Gotzen L, eds. *Fractures with Soft Tissue Injuries.* Berlin: Springer-Verlag; 1984:1–9.
3. Gustilo RB, Mendoza RM, Williams DM. Problems in management of type III open fractures. A new classification of type III open fractures. *J Trauma* 1984;24:742–6.
4. Winquist RA, Hansen ST Jr, Clawson DK. Closed intramedullary nailing of femoral fractures: a report of five hundred and twenty cases. *J Bone Joint Surg* 1984;66A:529–39.
5. Kirby R, Winquist R. Femoral shaft fractures in adolescents: a comparison between traction plus cast treatment and closed intramedullary nailing. *J Pediatr Orthop* 1981;1:193–7.

Orthopaedic Trauma Protocols, edited by
Sigvard T. Hansen, Jr., and Marc F. Swiontkowski,
Raven Press, Ltd., New York, © 1993.

CHAPTER 26

Knee

Stephen K. Benirschke and Marc F. Swiontkowski

Tibiofemoral Dislocations

MECHANISMS OF INJURY

Tibiofemoral (knee joint) dislocations usually result from high-energy sports activities or vehicular trauma. Although dislocations may be limited to soft-tissue injuries, they are frequently associated with proximal tibial fractures and minor avulsion fractures of the tibial rim, the fibular head, and the intercondylar eminences. These severe injuries can be associated with neuropraxia or axonotmesis of the common peroneal nerve, and the popliteal artery is sometimes damaged. Left undiagnosed, this injury can deteriorate and eventually require amputation of the limb (1).

ANATOMIC CONSIDERATIONS

Stability in the knee is provided by the cruciate ligaments (primary restraints) and the collateral ligaments and the joint capsule (secondary restraints). The popliteal artery and vein are intimately apposed to the posterior joint capsule and are restrained distally by the soleus fascia. The common peroneal artery is constrained tightly around the fibular neck and therefore is vulnerable to varus forces crossing the knee joint (Fig. 1).

CLASSIFICATION

Knee dislocations are classified by the direction of the tibial dislocation in relation to the femur. Posterior dislocations are the most common and are subdivided into pure posterior, posteromedial, and posterolateral injuries; anterior dislocations are rare.

Department of Orthopaedics, Harborview Medical Center, University of Washington, Seattle, Washington 98104

ASSESSMENT

Physical Examination

A potentially dislocated knee is examined carefully, keeping in mind that it might have reduced spontaneously, either completely or partially. The screening examination includes palpation of the distal pulses, assessment of motor function with the toe and the ankle in plantarflexion and dorsiflexion, and evaluation of the patient's sensation to light touch. Significant tense distal swelling may herald a compartmental syndrome.

A dislocation must be suspected when a patient presents with a swollen, unstable knee after a high-energy injury. In this case, the knee is also examined after an intraarticular injection of 10 ml of 1% lidocaine under sterile conditions. Several tests should be performed under this anesthesia: the Lachman test, tests for anterior and posterior drawer sign in 90° of flexion (if attainable), varus and valgus stress tests in full extension and 30° of flexion, and the "sag" test (genu recurvatum in full extension). Positive diagnosis of a knee dislocation on presentation warrants immediate reduction.

Radiographic Evaluation

In addition to standard AP and lateral views, varus and valgus stress radiographs may be obtained to test the integrity of the collateral ligaments. Stress radiographs are taken routinely whenever patients are anesthetized for operative treatment.

Special Studies

An arterial injury must be suspected if the knee is dislocated or significantly subluxated. Duplex Doppler ultrasound (duplex scanning) is a reliable screening tool when used with Doppler ankle and arm indices comparing the injured limb to the uninjured limb (2). If duplex scanning is unavailable,

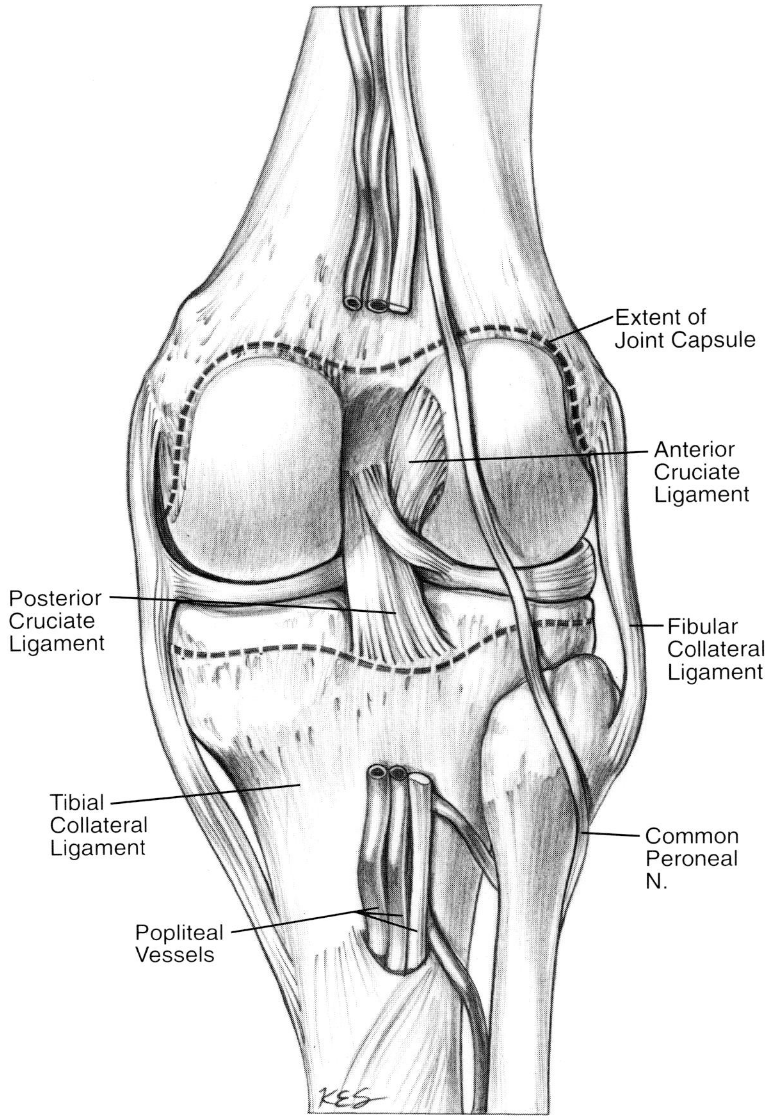

FIG. 1. Ligamentous anatomy of the knee.

arteriography is indicated. Magnetic resonance imaging may be useful for evaluating ligamentous, capsular, and meniscal integrity.

EMERGENT MANAGEMENT

The proximity of the popliteal vessels and the tibial and peroneal nerves to the knee makes reduction of a dislocation an emergent procedure. Minor instabilities with intact secondary restraints can be reduced nonoperatively by applying gentle longitudinal traction after the initial screening examination is performed. After reduction the leg is splinted and the neurocirculatory examinations are repeated. Emergent angiography and operative repair are indicated if an arterial injury is noted; angiography should be omitted if the patient presents with a pulseless limb and no detectable pulse by Doppler examination. The patient should be prepared for emergent operative arterial repair.

DEFINITIVE MANAGEMENT

The treatment is planned after the degree and direction of instability are determined by a thorough examination under anesthesia with stress radiographs. Preoperative duplex arterial scanning or angiography is mandatory if a tourniquet is to be used intraoperatively.

The general principles of operative management include: repair of all repairable meniscal tears; repair of all collateral ligament injuries; and reconstruction of all complete anterior cruciate ligament (ACL) and posterior cruciate ligament (PCL) injuries (3).

Arthroscopy can be performed intraoperatively to identify pathology in the knee joint. In elderly or sedentary patients, partial ACL and PCL tears can be treated nonoperatively or the ACL can be reconstructed arthroscopically. The preferred reconstruction for PCL injuries is the bone–patellar tendon–bone technique using the central third of the patellar tendon. Nonrepairable central-third cruciate tears can be resected during the arthroscopic examination. If an arterial repair must be done by a vascular surgeon, an orthopaedic surgeon should be present to ensure that critical structures required for ligament reconstruction are not sectioned during the surgical approach to the injured artery.

Postoperative management is dependent on the integrity of adjacent ligamentous and meniscal structures. Bracing, weight-bearing restrictions, or ROM limitations may be indicated if the meniscus has been repaired or if the ACL, the PCL, or both structures have been reconstructed.

COMPLICATIONS

Arterial injuries are common with knee dislocations (1). Inflation of a tourniquet days or weeks after a dislocation can result in an acute arterial occlusion from an intimal flap tear. Neural injuries, particularly of the common peroneal nerve, are also associated with knee dislocations. Recovery of complete function may not be possible after a neuropraxic injury, and the patient may require an orthosis. Although some knee instability is expected after a dislocation, the amount of disability is usually greater after nonoperative treatment.

SKELETALLY IMMATURE PATIENTS

Knee dislocations are rare in children. When they occur they are usually treated nonoperatively because the presence of an open physis contraindicates ACL or PCL reconstruction.

REFERENCES

1. Green NE, Allen BL. Vascular injuries associated with dislocation of the knee. *J Bone Joint Surg* 1977:59A:235–9.
2. Johansen K, Lynch K, Paun M, Copass M. Non-invasive vascular tests reliably exclude occult arterial trauma in injured extremities. *J Trauma* 1991:31:515–22.
3. Sisto DI, Warren RF. Complete knee dislocation. A followup study of operative treatment. *Clin Orthop* 1985;198:94–101.

Patellofemoral Dislocations

MECHANISMS OF INJURY

Patellofemoral dislocations usually occur as isolated injuries in women with anatomic malalignments and are seen rarely in trauma centers. Dislocations can also occur from external rotation and acute flexion. A dislocation from high-energy trauma is usually due to a laterally directed blow to the medial side of the patella.

ANATOMIC CONSIDERATIONS

The anatomic variations that predispose a patient to this injury include weakness of the vastus medialis obliquus (VMO), hypoplasia of the lateral femoral condyle, an increased femoral–tibial angle, anteversion, and a history of patellar subluxation or chondromalacia patella.

CLASSIFICATION

Patellofemoral dislocations are classified according to the direction of the patellar dislocation in relation to the femur. The terms *dislocation* and *subluxation* are used to differentiate severe soft-tissue injuries (dislocations) from less severe, often recurrent injuries (subluxations).

ASSESSMENT

Physical Examination

The status of distal sensory and motor functions and the circulatory integrity are evaluated in all knee injuries. When a patellar dislocation is examined soon after injury it is readily evident to palpation. If the patella has reduced spontaneously, as is usually the case, a tense hemarthrosis and tenderness may be present along the VMO insertion on the patella or a palpable deficit may be felt at the site of the medial muscle complex insertion. In high-energy patellofemoral dislocations, the ACL and PCL must be examined in addition to the collateral ligaments.

Radiographic Evaluation

Sunrise and tunnel radiographic views are obtained in addition to AP and lateral views of the knee. A sunrise view is particularly useful to provide additional information about predisposing physical factors and the nature of the injury.

Special Studies

Additional information may be provided by a CT scan. Magnetic resonance imaging and plain radiographs provide similar information, and MRI offers no significant advantages. Arthrography or arteriography is occasionally useful—arthrography when arthroscopic equipment is unavailable and arteriography when the injury is associated with severe ligament disruption or abnormal distal circulatory findings.

EMERGENT MANAGEMENT

After the screening examination is completed, the knee is aspirated and injected with 5.0 ml to 10 ml of lidocaine. Stability testing can be done at that time and the patella may be reduced if it is still dislocated. Reduction is accomplished by applying medial pressure to the patella with both thumbs.

DEFINITIVE MANAGEMENT

Factors that influence treatment are the severity of trauma and the presence of predisposing conditions such as lateral condylar hypoplasia, muscle imbalance, and anteversion. In general, patients with underlying anatomic factors who sustain patellofemoral dislocations from low-energy injuries are treated nonoperatively, and patients with normal anatomy whose injuries are caused by high energy are candidates for operative repair.

The presence of osteocartilaginous loose bodies in the knee is a key factor in this decision. Dislocations without loose bodies in patients with normal anatomy may be treated nonoperatively. Arthroscopy is indicated when loose bodies are present (1). When loose bodies are associated with a history of dislocations or subluxations, open lateral release is indicated with advancement of the VMO from 5 mm to 8 mm over the medial patellar border. Recurrent subluxations and dislocations with excessive anteversion are treated by closed derotational osteotomy. This procedure is associated with a lower incidence of complications than procedures designed to realign the tibial tubercle. If the loose bodies have been removed arthroscopically and the patient has no anatomic abnormalities, the knee is treated in cast extension for 6 weeks. Quadriceps rehabilitation, consisting of short-arc or terminal knee extension exercises and extension quadriceps sets done against progressively greater resistance, is initiated after the cast is removed.

COMPLICATIONS

The most frequent complication is recurrence of the dislocation, especially when the injury resulted from minor trauma. The anatomic factors noted earlier should be carefully assessed and, if intensive quadriceps rehabilitation fails to stop the recurrence, an open lateral release and VMO repair or advancement should be considered.

SKELETALLY IMMATURE PATIENTS

Patellofemoral dislocations in children are usually treated nonoperatively unless physeal closure is imminent.

REFERENCE

1. Morscher E. Cartilage-bone lesions of the knee joint following injury. *Reconstruct Surg Traumatol* 1971;12:2–26.

Supracondylar Femoral Fractures

MECHANISMS OF INJURY

Supracondylar femoral fractures usually result from high-energy trauma, such as direct blows to a flexed knee or motor vehicle accidents. Less commonly, they result from axial loading on an extended knee joint, a common mechanism in tibial plateau and femoral shaft injuries. Vascular injuries are not usually associated with supracondylar femoral fractures because the popliteal artery is tightly constrained more distally at the level of the knee joint and the proximal tibia. Common associated bony injuries include ipsilateral patellar and femoral shaft fractures. The cruciate ligaments, the capsular origins and insertions, and the meniscus and its supports are also commonly injured. Approximately 25% of all supracondylar femoral fractures are associated with open wounds.

ANATOMIC CONSIDERATIONS

The osseous anatomy of the distal femur must be understood for proper insertion of an internal fixation device. Viewed on end, the distal femur is sloped in a rhomboid shape and the lateral condyle is more prominent than the medial condyle (Fig. 2). The anterior half of the distal femur is in line with the femoral shaft; the posterior condyles project posteriorly.

CLASSIFICATION

Despite the existence of several classification systems for fractures of the distal femur, we have used the AO classifica-

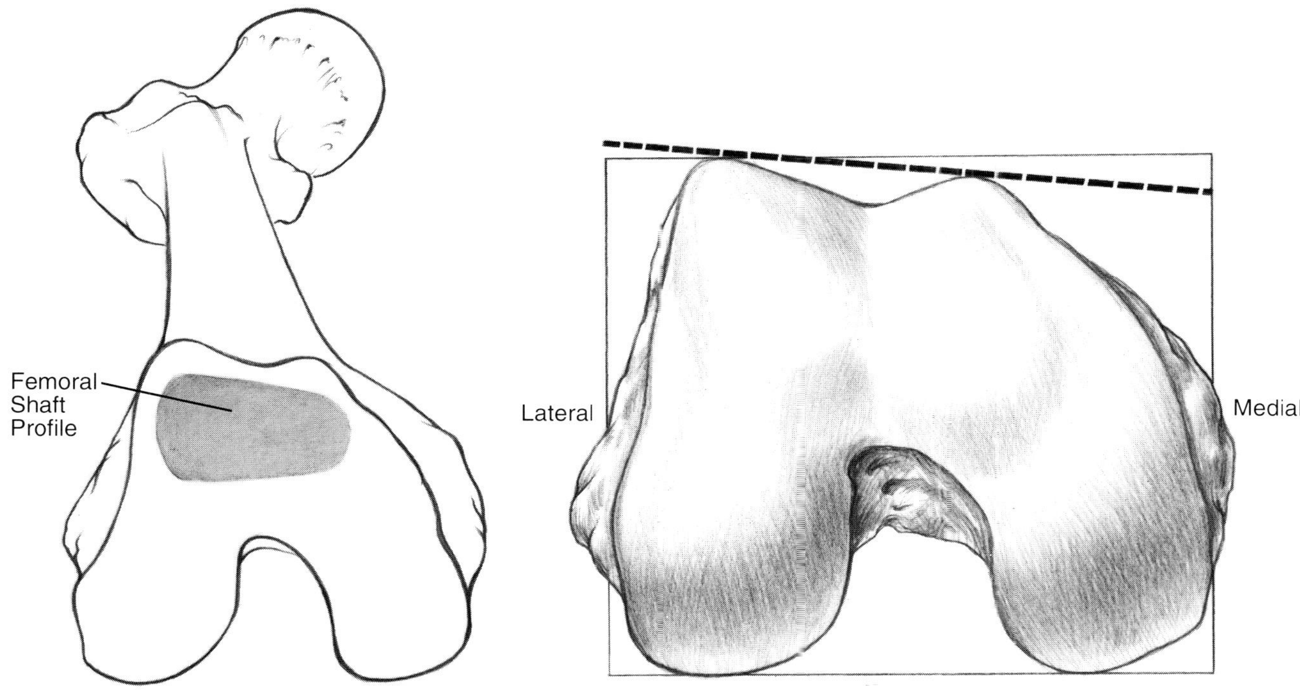

FIG. 2. The osseous anatomy of the distal femur.

tion (1) exclusively for 20 years. This system, which is included in the comprehensive classification of long-bone fractures and which was adopted formally by the Orthopaedic Trauma Association, is valuable for suggesting treatment options and prognoses (Fig. 3). Distal femoral fractures are divided into three types:

Type A: extraarticular supracondylar fractures.

Type B: unicondylar fractures.

Type C: intraarticular or bicondylar fractures.

For grading of open fractures, the system of Gustilo and Anderson (2,3) must also be applied.

ASSESSMENT

Physical Examination

The clinical examination of a knee fracture is the same as the examination of a dislocation. The limb is exposed and examined for deformity, open wounds, and effusion. The circulatory status (pulses and capillary refill), motor function, and sensation to light touch and pinprick are assessed in the distal limb. The knee is palpated for crepitus and tenderness. If the examination is not indicative of a fracture, ligament integrity is tested. The limb is resplinted after the examination. Neurocirculatory status and motor function are reevaluated at 60- to 90-min intervals during the workup.

Radiographic Evaluation

Anteroposterior and lateral radiographic views are centered over the knee joint and fracture lines extending into the knee joint are noted. Radiographs of type A extraarticular fractures are superimposed on AP and lateral radiographs of the opposite side to accurately measure the diameter of the canal and the length of the femur for an interlocked nail. Tomograms may be obtained of isolated closed injuries to aid with preoperative planning. Injuries caused by major blunt trauma require urgent operative stabilization.

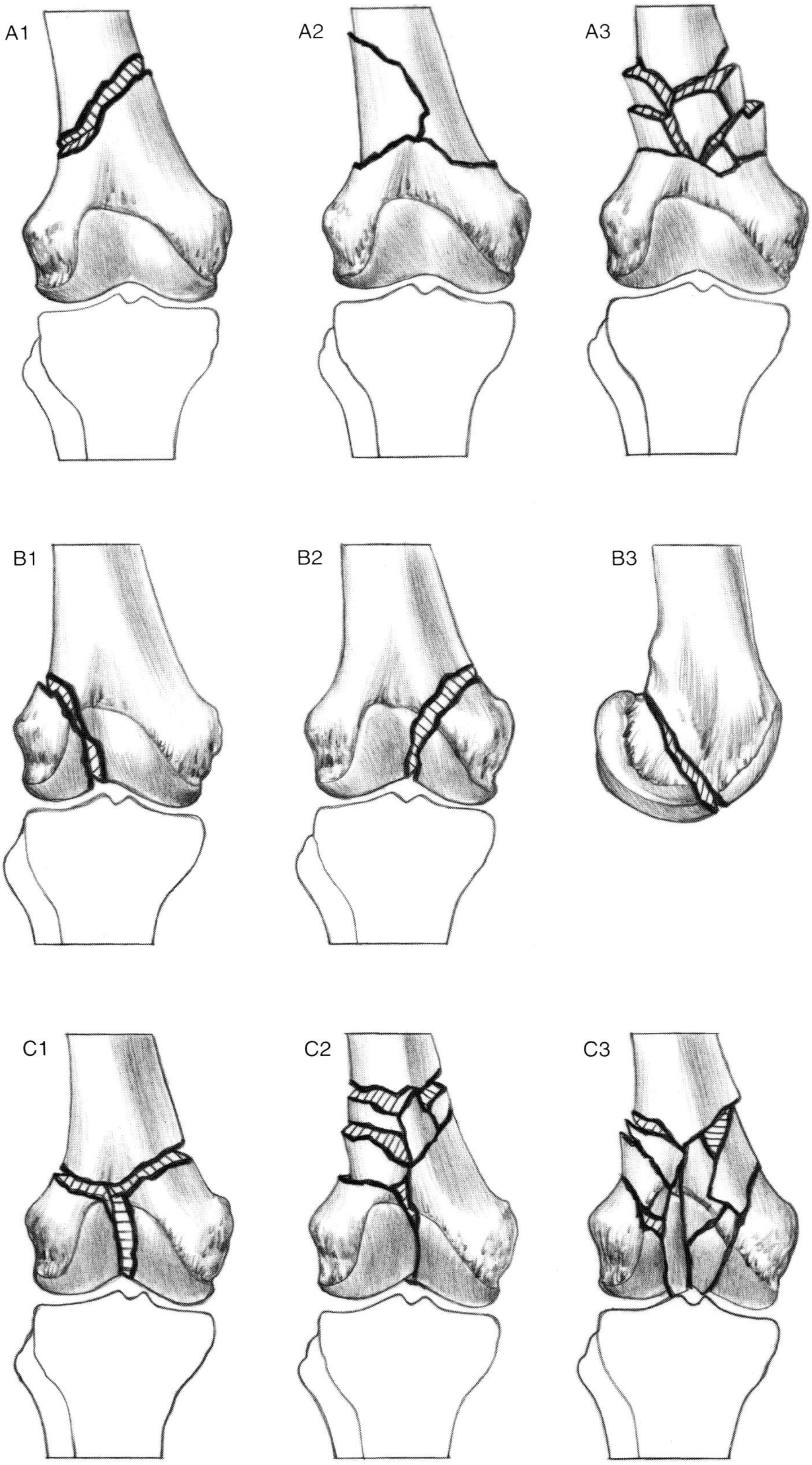

FIG. 3. The AO classification of distal femur fractures. **A1:** Extraarticular fracture, simple. **A2:** Extraarticular fracture, metaphyseal wedge. **A3:** Extra- articular fracture, metaphyseal complex. **B1:** Partial articular fracture, lateral condyle, sagittal. **B2:** Partial articular fracture, medial condyle, sagittal. **B3:** Partial articular fracture, frontal. **C1:** Complete articular fracture articular simple, metaphyseal simple. **C2:** Complete articular fracture articular simple, metaphyseal multifragmentary. **C3:** Complex articular fracture, multifragmentary. (Adapted from Müller ME, Algöwer M, Schneider R, Willenegger H. *Manual of Internal Fixation*, 3rd ed. Berlin: Springer-Verlag, 1991. Müller ME, Nazarian S, Koch P, Schatzker J. *Comprehensive Classification of Fractures of Long Bones*. Berlin: Springer-Verlag, 1990. Used with permission.)

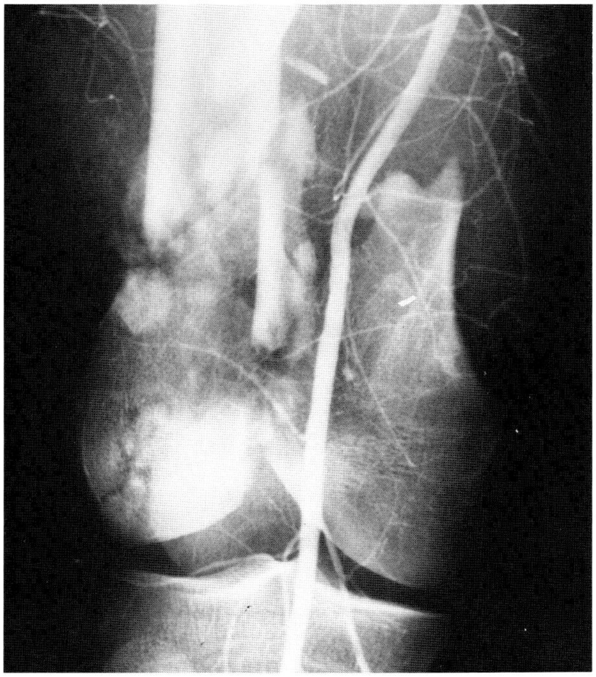

FIG. 4. AP roentgenogram demonstrates intact popliteal artery following markedly displaced supracondylar fracture of the femur.

Special Studies

Arteriography is indicated when an arterial injury is suggested by abnormal findings during clinical examination or abnormal results on the Doppler examination (Fig. 4). Although bone scans, CT scans, and MRI may be useful when a pathologic fracture is suspected, these diagnostic modalities are of limited use in the management of traumatic injuries.

EMERGENT MANAGEMENT

All displaced supracondylar femoral fractures in skeletally mature patients require operative stabilization and early motion to minimize deformity and joint fibrosis. Exceptions to this protocol are made under two circumstances: contaminated isolated grade IIIB and IIIC fractures, and isolated open fractures seen more than 24 h after injury. Contaminated isolated grade IIIB and IIIC fractures are managed by debridement and immediate fixation of the articular component and delayed stabilization of the supracondylar region. Isolated open fractures seen late are initially treated only by debridement, followed by repeat debridement after 2 to 5 days, internal fixation, and delayed closure of the open wound at a third operation 5 days after the internal fixation.

DEFINITIVE MANAGEMENT

Extraarticular Fractures (Type A)

Radiographs of the injured femur are scrutinized for intraarticular fractures. The injured femur is measured to determine the distance between the most distal part of the fracture and the most distal femoral articular surface. Comparing this measurement to the distance between the tip of the femoral nail and the more proximal of the two distal holes determines the feasibility of using an intramedullary device for stabilization. Intramedullary nails can be customized for this application by trimming the tips of the nails (Fig. 5). The nail must not be cut closer than 1 cm to its distal hole. If a distal femoral traction pin had been inserted into the

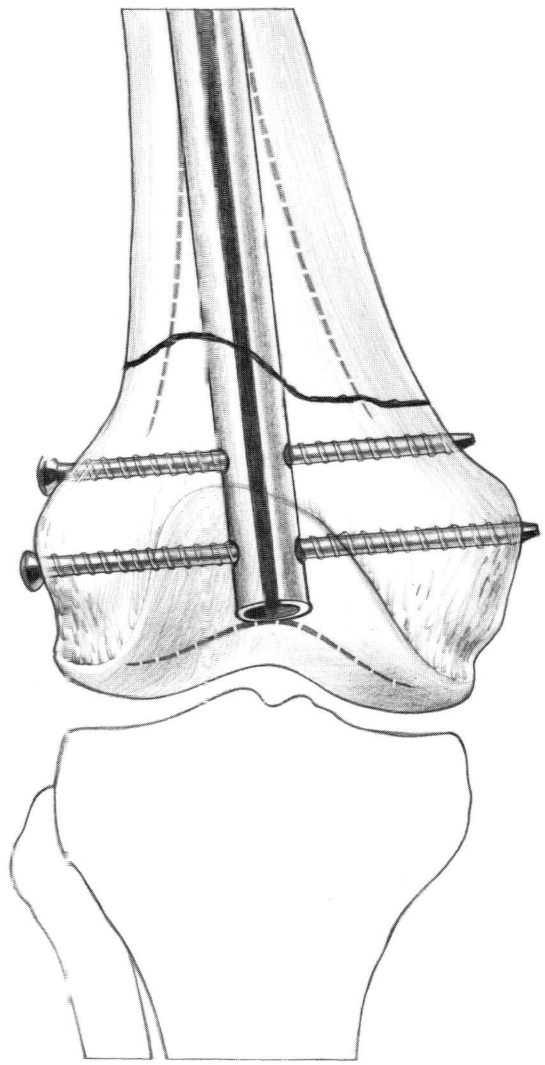

FIG. 5. An intramedullary nail can be customized by shortening the end of the nail and the distance between the screw holes.

distal fragment before the patient arrived in the emergency department, it must be removed during the initial evaluation. A proximal tibial pin can be substituted if immediate fixation will not be performed.

Patients with extremely distal femoral fractures are positioned supine on the fracture table. Traction should be applied with the knee flexed to prevent an extension deformity from the pull of the gastrocnemius muscles. An object such as a crutch can be placed under the distal fragment to support the femur but must not be placed in the popliteal fossa. If an obese patient is placed in the lateral decubitus position for intramedullary nailing, the fracture will sag into a valgus position. This problem is overcome by inserting an oblique 7/64-in Steinmann pin starting more proximal laterally (see Chapter 25). The pin is inserted under fluoroscopic control to ensure placement well anterior in the distal femur. It is then attached to a Kirschner bow and, when traction is applied, the distal fragment is pulled out of valgus. Other positioning suggestions for femoral nailing are discussed in Chapter 25.

Because intramedullary interlocked nails tend to fatigue from stress when they are used for this purpose, nails that are 1 mm or 2 mm larger than those used for mid-shaft fractures are preferred. The femoral canal is reamed 1.0 to 1.5 mm wider than the nail. The closer a fracture is located to an articular surface on the distal femur, the more important it becomes to drive the tip of the nail far enough that it abuts subchondral bone. The static locking technique is performed to securely stabilize the distal fragment. In general, fractures closer than 7 cm to the joint are not stabilized with interlocked nails. Fractures with no joint involvement are treated with 95° condylar blade plates, the same as type C fractures.

Continuous passive motion can be used in fractures with optimal fixation. Ambulation is started in a hinged knee brace that limits flexion to between 30° and 60°, and the patient is allowed to progress to full ROM over 3 to 4 weeks. Bracing is not necessary when fixation is stable enough to tolerate CPM, but patients are limited to touch-down weight-bearing for 6 to 8 weeks until fracture healing is demonstrated radiographically.

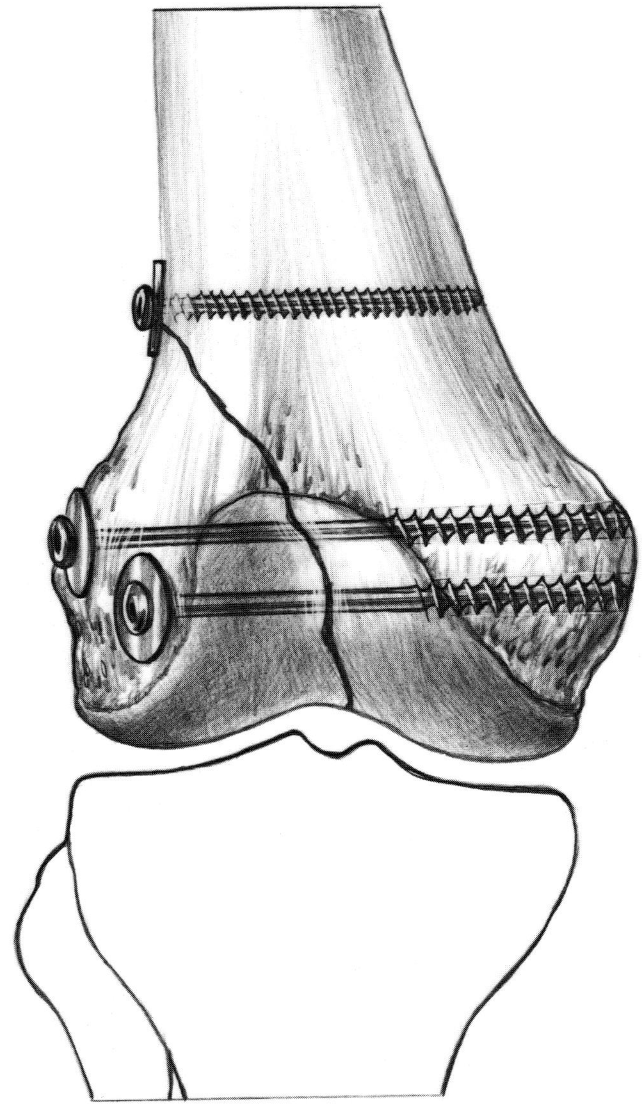

FIG. 6. A lateral condylar fracture is fixed with lag screws.

Unicondylar Fractures (Type B)

Like other distal femoral fractures, type B fractures may be open or closed injuries. In closed injuries, the plane of fracture is defined on tomograms or CT scans. This information is critical for planning the surgical approach and choosing the type of fixation. Preoperative planning of an open injury is done from plain radiographs.

The surgical exposure is suggested by the location of the fracture. A lateral incision is preferred for a lateral condylar fracture. The fascia lata is split and the joint anterior to the vastus tubercle is incised (Fig. 6). A medial condylar fracture requires a medial incision and retraction of the VMO to the anterior side. Exposure and reduction of the posterior condyles are more difficult. A medial incision is used to expose the fractured medial posterior condyle and the VMO is retracted anteriorly. Schanz screws (4 mm) or large smooth Steinmann pins are used as levers to reduce the fracture fragments and the reduction is held with Kirschner wires. Large cancellous screws or cannulated screws are used to stabilize fractures in adults (Figs. 7–9). Fixation with 3.5-mm cortical lag screws is reserved for posterior condylar fractures or for unicondylar fractures in small patients (Fig. 10). Stability must be assessed before the wound is closed over a drain. Continuous passive motion is beneficial for stable fractures. A hinged knee brace is ordinarily used without motion restrictions for the first 6 postoperative weeks to provide external buttressing for a fracture stabilized with screws. Full weight-bearing is delayed for 8 to 12 postoperative weeks.

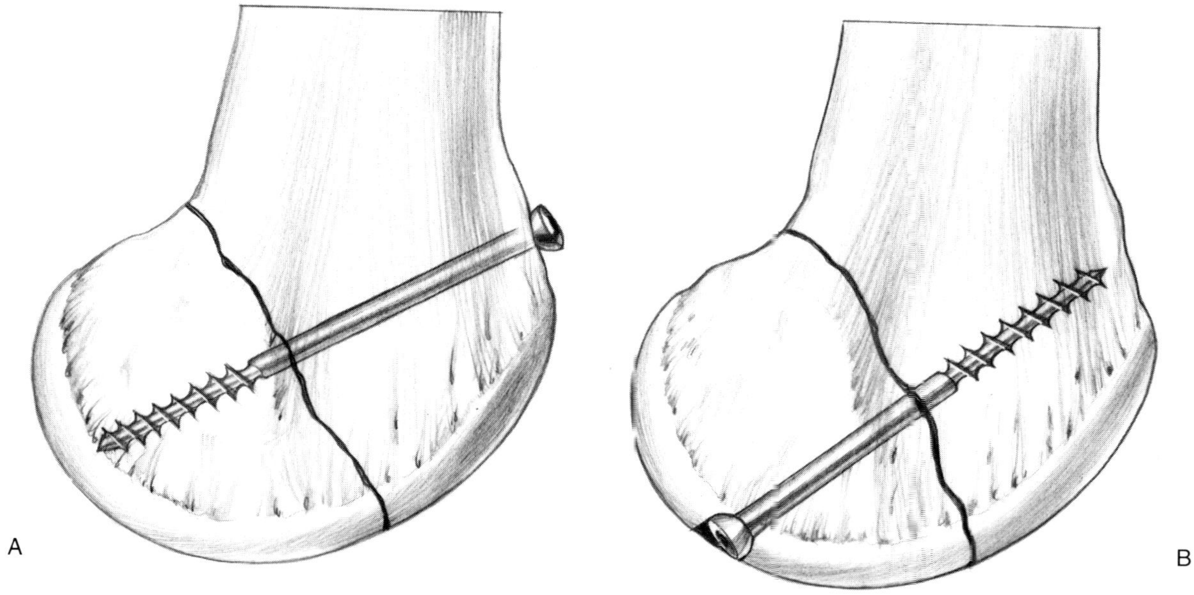

FIG. 7. Internal fixation of a posterior condylar fracture using an extraarticular lag screw (**A**) and a transarticular lag screw with a countersunk head (**B**).

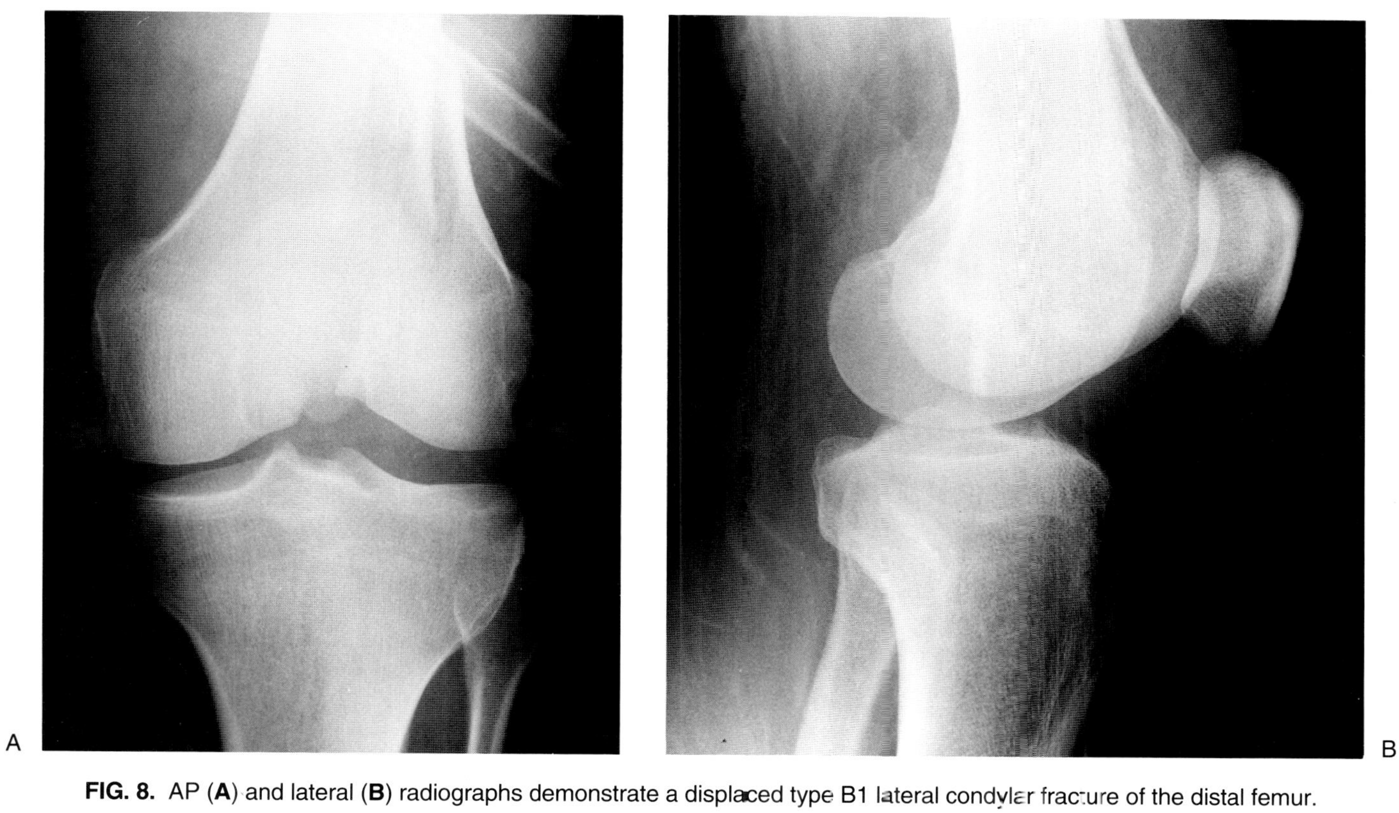

FIG. 8. AP (**A**) and lateral (**B**) radiographs demonstrate a displaced type B1 lateral condylar fracture of the distal femur.

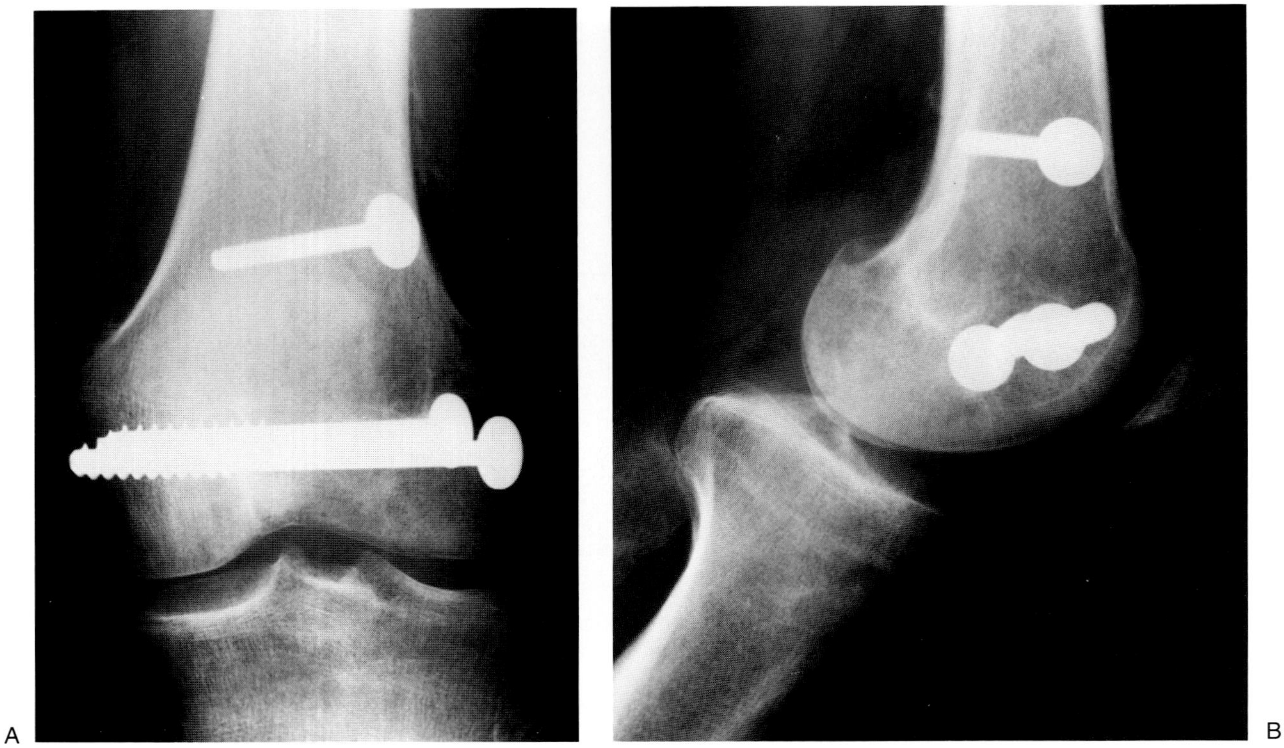

FIG. 9. AP (**A**) and lateral (**B**) radiographs demonstrate cannulated lag screw fixation of articular surface with superiorly placed antiglide screw and washer at the apex of the fracture.

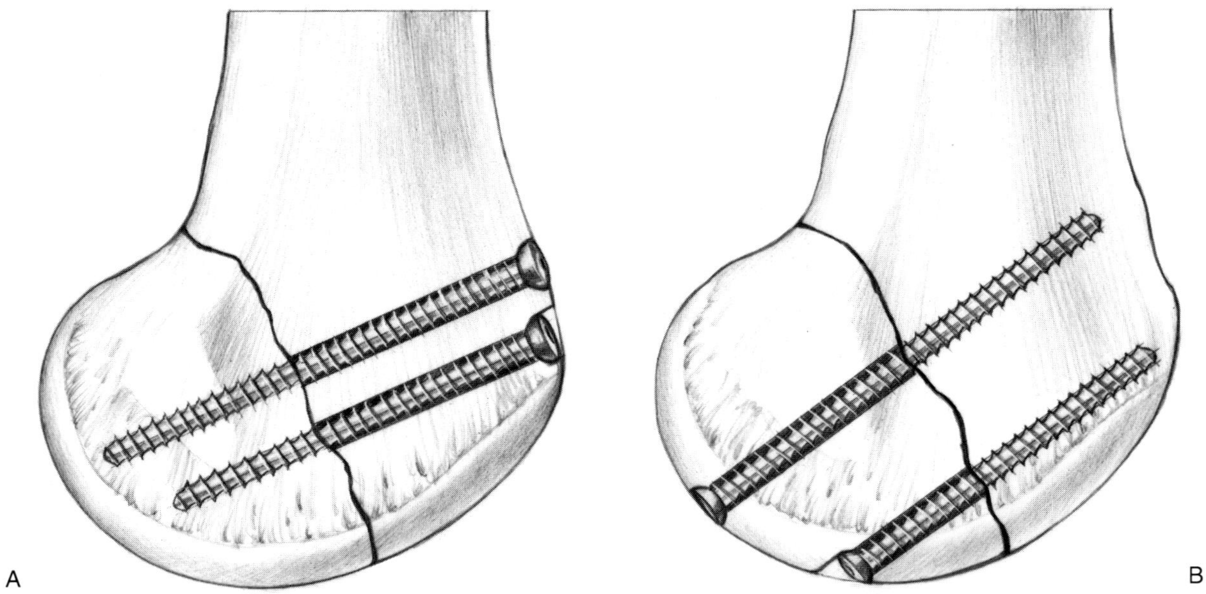

FIG. 10. Internal fixation of a posterior condylar fracture using 3.5-mm extraarticular cortical lag screws (**A**) and transarticular lag screws (**B**). The drill holes have been overdrilled and the heads of the screws are countersunk.

A, B

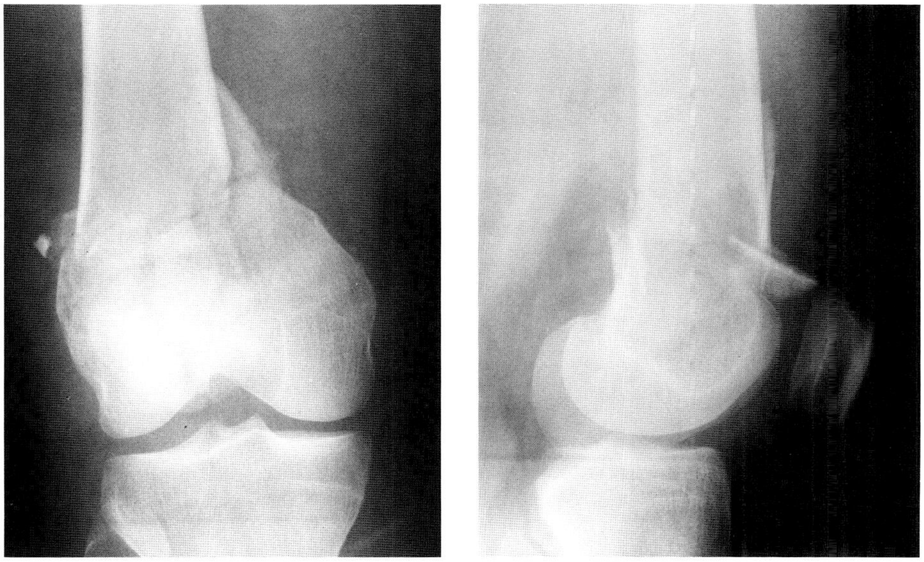

FIG. 11. AP (**A**) and lateral (**B**) radiographs of displaced C2 fracture of the distal femur.

Intercondylar Fractures (Type C)

The level of the supracondylar fracture suggests the type of fixation that should be used. In general, plating is the preferred method of stabilizing type C fractures. Lag screw and intramedullary nail fixation are not appropriate for type C2 intraarticular extension fractures. A 95° blade plate allows early knee motion but requires at least 1.5 cm to 2.0 cm of intact proximal bone (Figs. 11–13) (4). A condylar buttress plate is used when a blade plate or a condylar screw cannot be positioned within 1.5 cm of the articular surface (Figs. 14–16).

A, B

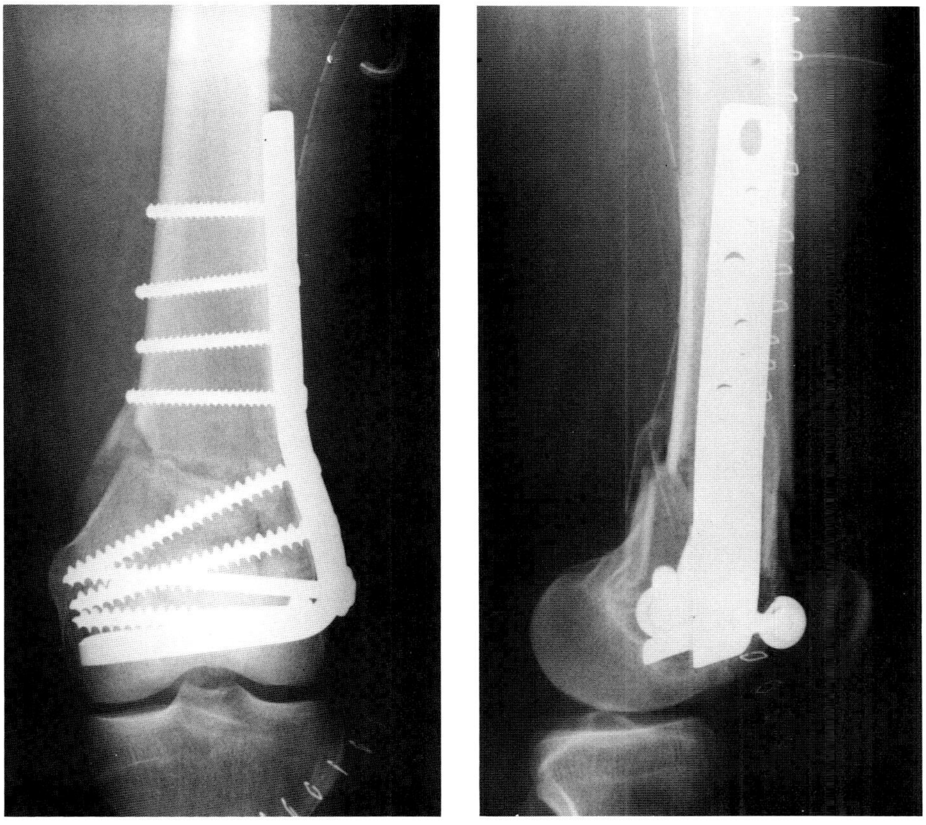

FIG. 12. AP (**A**) and lateral (**B**) roentgenographs show internal fixation with 6.5-mm lag screw fixation for intercondylar split, followed by fixation of the condylar block to the shaft with a 95° condylar blade plate.

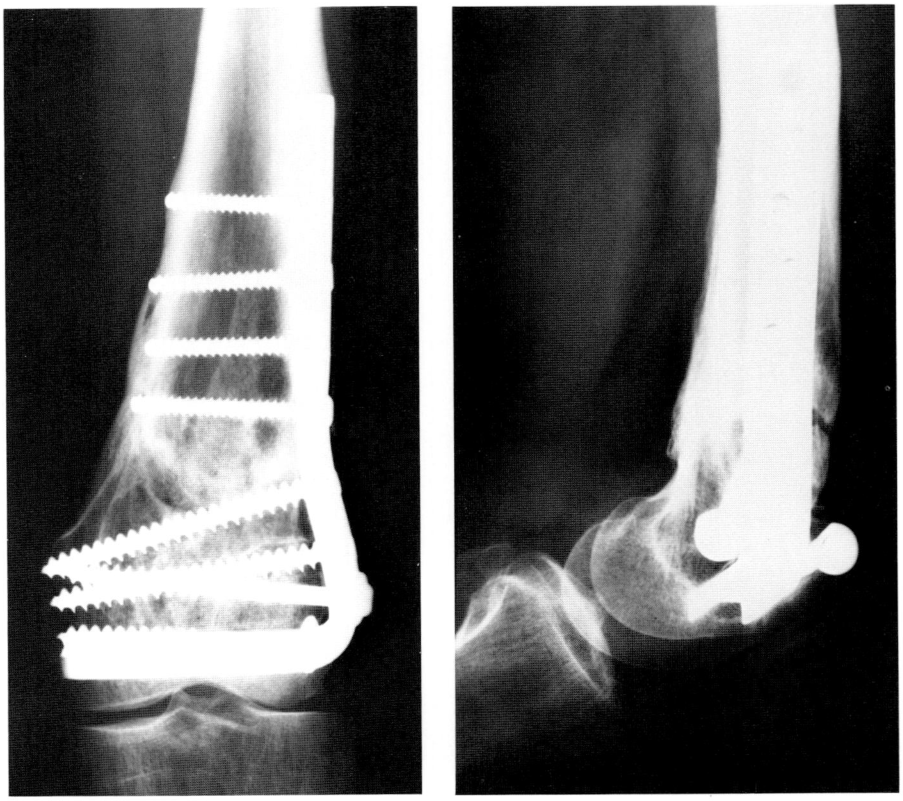

A, B

FIG. 13. AP (**A**) and lateral (**B**) roentgeograms of distal femur demonstrate the healed fracture. The patient had full range of motion of the knee.

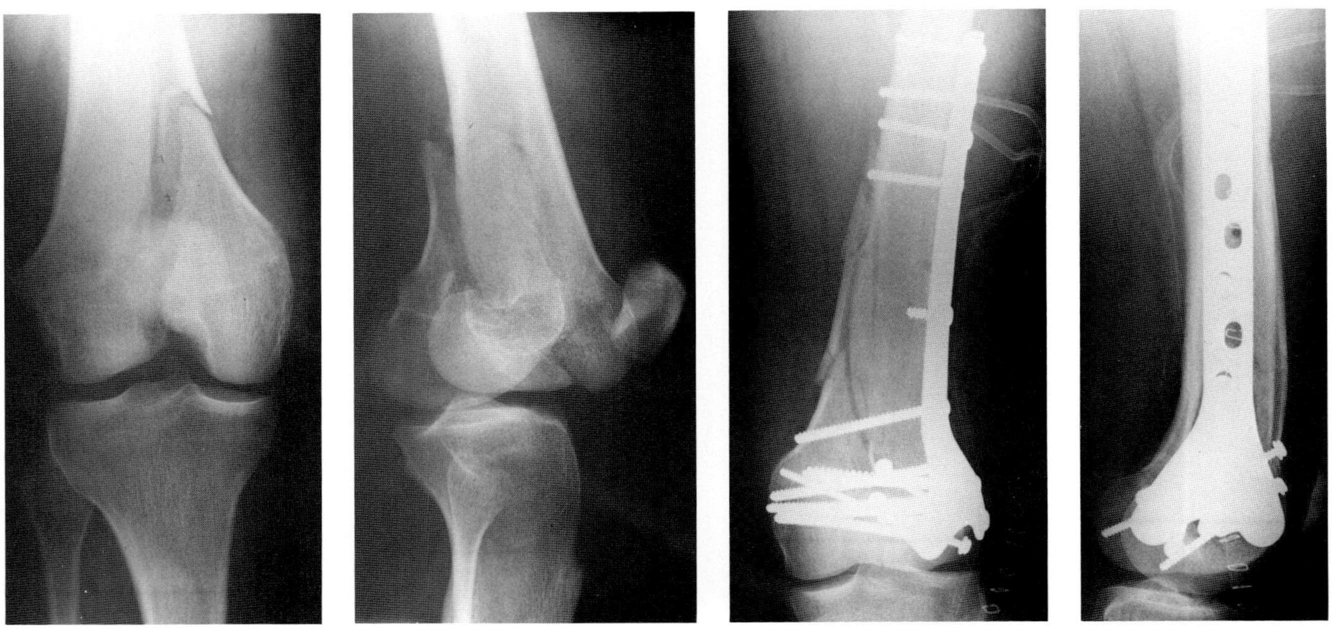

A, B C, D

FIG. 14. AP (**A**) roentgenogram of a C3 fracture of distal femur. Lateral view (**B**) demonstrates the classic Hoffa fracture of the lateral condyle. AP (**C**) and lateral (**D**) roentgenograms show operative fixation of femur fracture using 3.5-mm screws for the Hoffa component of the lateral condyle with stabilization of the distal condylar block to the shaft using a condylar buttress plate.

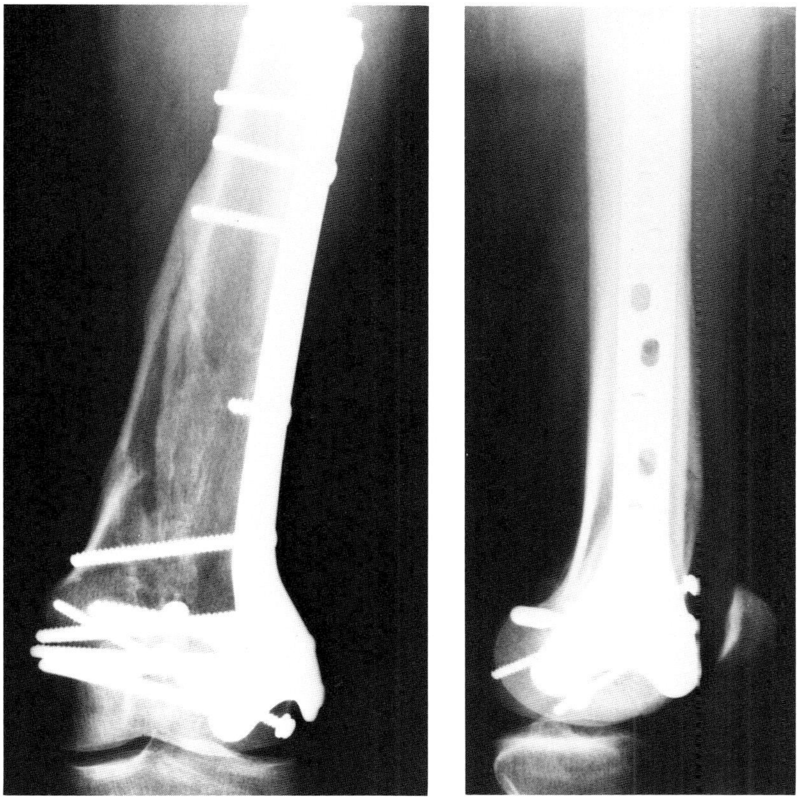

A, B

FIG. 15. A: AP roentgenogram demonstrates healed fracture without the use of bone grafting (no stripping of the medial side). **B:** The lateral radiograph demonstrates healed fracture.

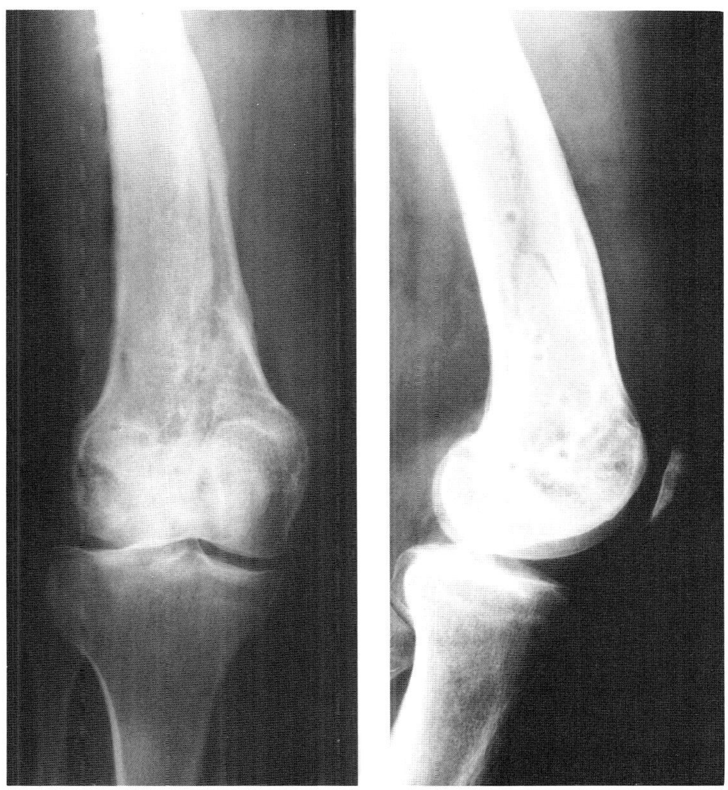

A, B

FIG. 16. AP (**A**) and lateral (**B**) roentgenograms show the osseous anatomy after hardware removal. Hardware removal is often necessary in the case of condylar buttress plate due to prominence at the lateral femoral condyle interfering with iliotibial band function.

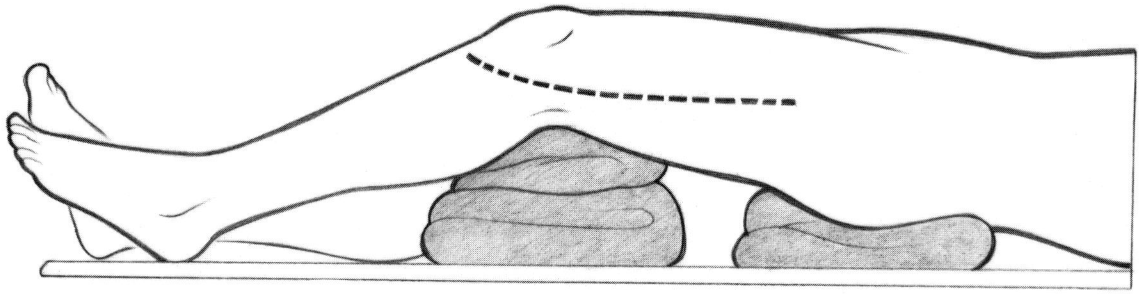

FIG. 17. Positioning a patient with a type C intercondylar fracture.

A patient with a type C intercondylar fracture is positioned supine and a roll is placed under the ipsilateral pelvis (Fig. 17). The injured limb is draped free. A sterile tourniquet can be used during this procedure. A straight lateral incision is made anteriorly, ending between the distal pole of the patella and the tibial tubercle. The iliotibial band is split and the fracture is exposed. Only the anterior half of the distal femur is visible from the lateral side unless the fibular collateral ligaments are taken down for visualization. The condyles are reduced and stabilized with Kirschner wires. An osteotomy of the tibial tubercle is seldom necessary. The articular surface is visualized by shortening the limb through the supracondylar fracture site. After the condyles are provisionally stabilized, the intercondylar fracture is fixed with 6.5-mm lag screws. Fractures in the coronal plane (Hoffa fractures) are reduced and stabilized with 3.5-mm cortical lag screws or 4-mm cancellous screws (Fig. 18). The fixation device for a supracondylar fracture, usually a 95° condylar blade plate, must be inserted correctly in all three planes (Fig. 19) (4). The correct starting point for the seating chisel is the middle third of the anterior half of the lateral femoral condyle. A 95° condylar blade plate can be applied without removing a large amount of bone from the condyles and, in the event of nonunion, the fracture is more easily managed than with 95° condylar screws.

This type of fracture can also be stabilized with a 95° condylar screw (Fig. 20). The screw requires accurate placement in the varus–valgus and the coronal planes but is adjustable in the sagittal plane. Condylar screw fixation can be accomplished more easily by a surgeon with little experi-

A, B

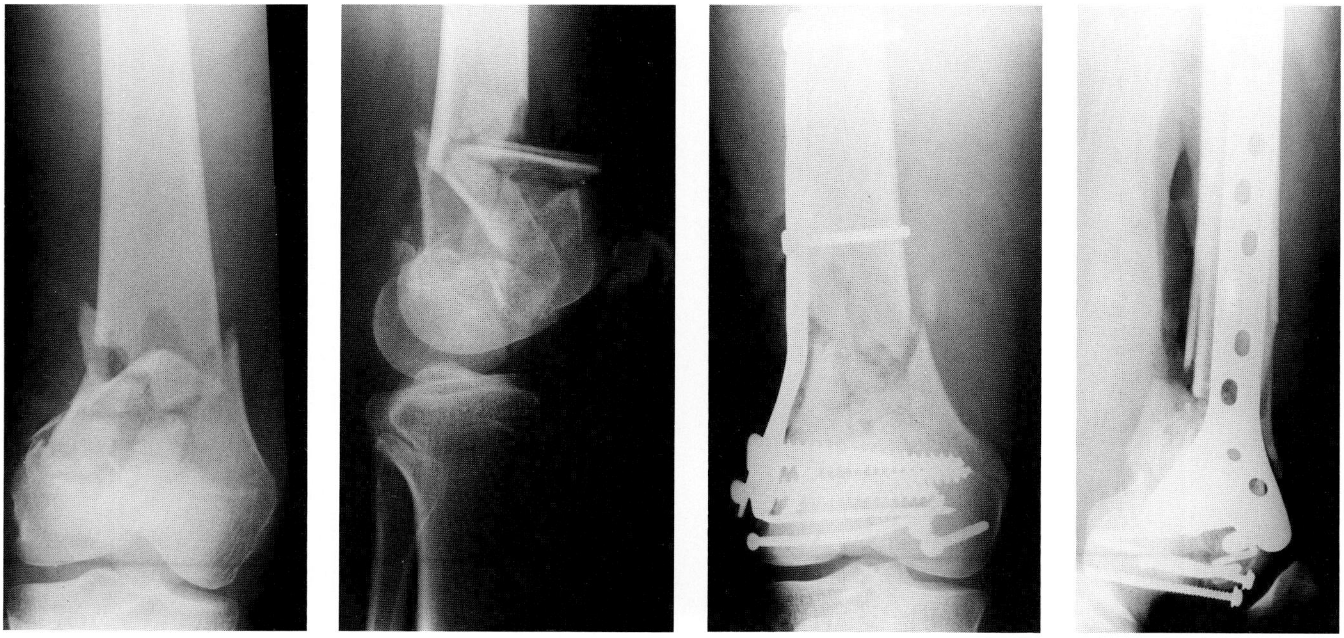

C, D

FIG. 18. AP (**A**) and lateral (**B**) roentgenograms demonstrate medial and lateral Hoffa (coronal plane) fractures of the femoral condyles. Intraoperative AP (**C**) and lateral (**D**) radiographs demonstrate internal fixation of both Hoffa fractures using 3.5-mm screws followed by stabilization of the distal femoral block to the shaft with a condylar buttress plate.

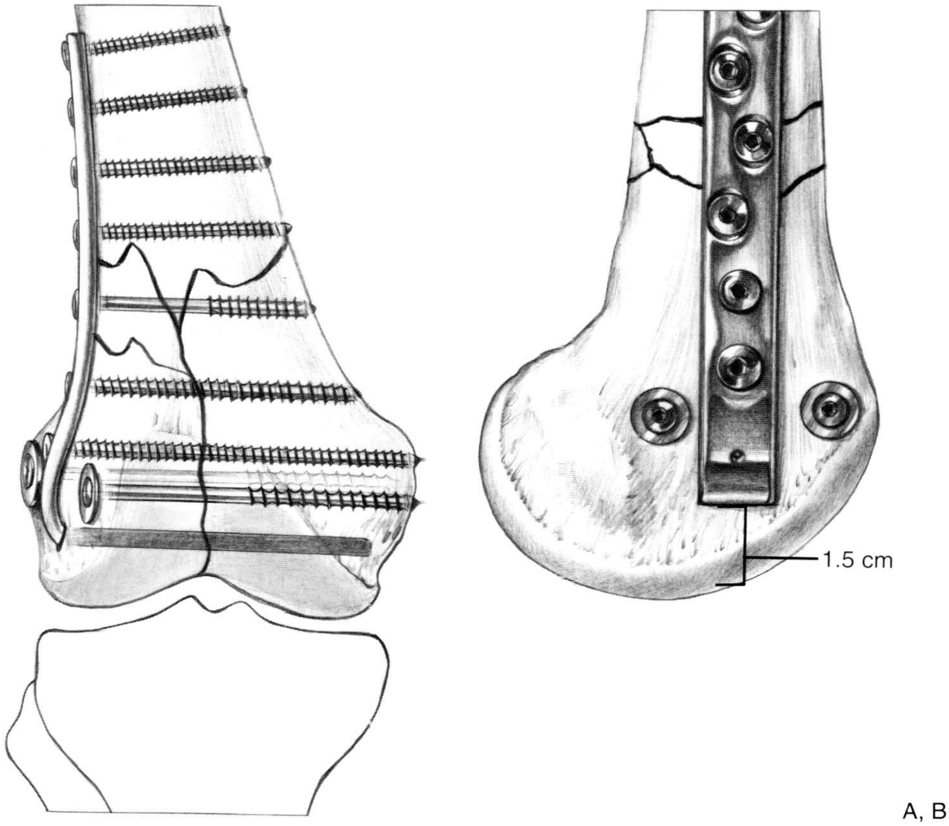

FIG. 19. **A:** AP projection of a type C2 fracture with 95° condylar blade-plate fixation. The blade plate is applied parallel to the knee joint. **B:** Lateral projection. In the sagittal plane, the point of entry of the seating chisel for the blade plate is anterior and in line with the shaft axis 1.5 cm from the joint.

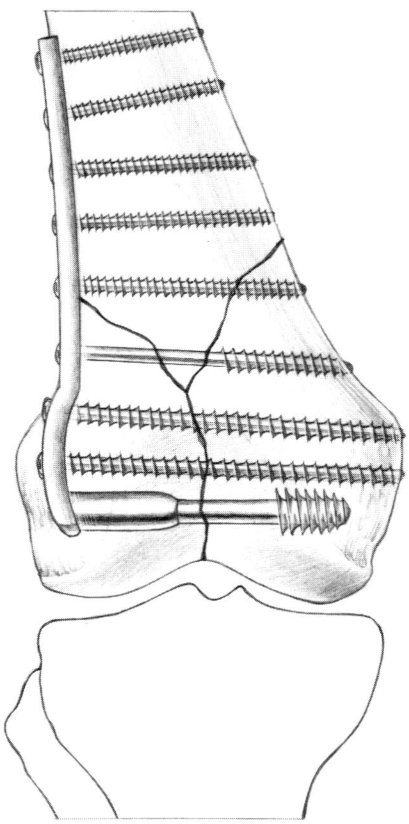

FIG. 20. Internal fixation of a type C2 fracture with a dynamic condylar screw.

ence in treating supracondylar femoral fractures. Because this screw is thick, it must be inserted 5 mm more proximal than a 95° blade plate and positioned correctly in the middle third of the anterior half of the lateral femoral condyle. The large condylar screw is inserted after the intercondylar and coronal plane fracture lines are stabilized with lag screws. Both plates must be slightly recessed into the lateral cortex of the distal femur to prevent medialization of the distal fragment.

In an extremely comminuted intercondylar fractures the articular surface–shaft angle is determined by measurements taken from a radiograph of the opposite femur. Distal and comminuted fractures are stabilized with condylar buttress plates after temporary stabilization with Kirschner wires (see Figs. 14–16). The lag screws (6.5-mm cancellous screws or 7-mm cannulated screws) are inserted through the plate (Fig. 21). Very distal fractures in osteoporotic bone may require application of a second medial T-plates. The VMO is elevated through a straight medial incision and retracted anteriorly. After the superior medial genicular artery is cauterized, a T-plate or a 4.5-mm DCP is inserted. Bone graft from the iliac crest is used to supplement fixation in a comminuted fracture or one that has sustained bone loss (Figs. 22 and 23). Autogenous bone graft is used together with cancellous allograft.

Continuous passive motion may be started immediately in patients with good bone quality and stable fixation but is avoided when bone density or fixation is less than optimal. In both cases, a hinged knee brace is used with the hinges unlocked. The patient must limit ambulation to touch-down weight-bearing for 10 to 12 weeks.

COMPLICATIONS

Infections occur rarely in supracondylar fractures and usually resolve after debridement and a regimen of antibiotics. If the internal fixation device continues to provide stability it should not be removed. Drainage will resolve with debridement and curettage when the plate is removed 18 to 24 months after injury. Malunion can occur after improper application of internal fixation devices. Unless the malposition is severe, the fracture should be allowed to unite. If the malunion limits function, delayed osteotomy and repeat fixation are indicated.

Nonunion is associated with bent or broken implants. When nonunion occurs in a fracture stabilized with a 95° condylar blade plate, the plate is removed and the fixation is repeated with a another blade plate. A more difficult problem arises when a failed 95° condylar screw has produced a large cavity at the bone–screw interface. In this case the fracture might be salvaged by packing the condylar screw cavity with bone graft and applying a 95° condylar blade plate or condylar buttress plate and a medial T-plate or DCP (5). Autogenous bone grafting is indicated for all nonunions.

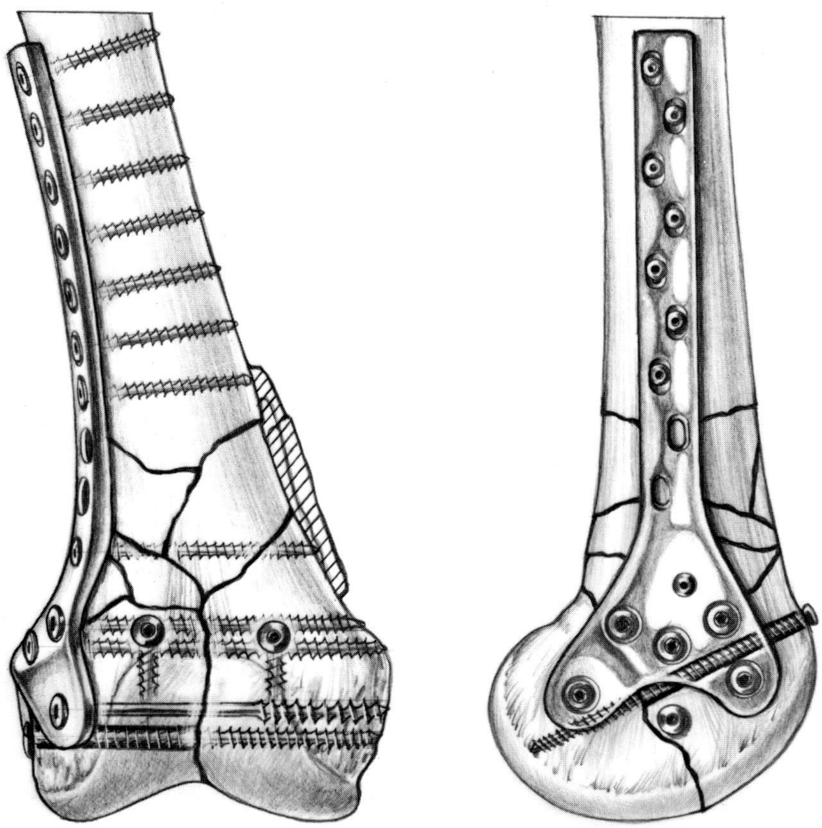

A, B

FIG. 21. AP projection (**A**) and lateral projection (**B**) of internal fixation for a type C3 fracture using a condylar buttress plate.

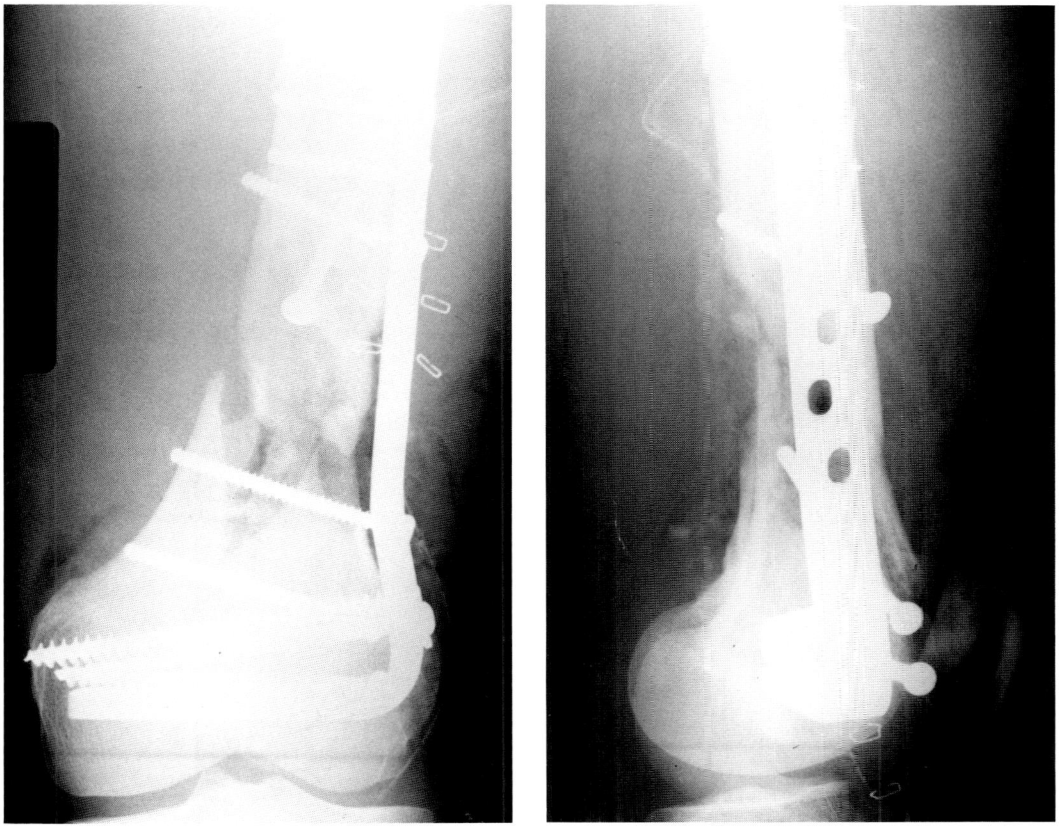

A B

FIG. 22. AP (**A**) and lateral (**B**) roentgenograms demonstrate marked supracondylar bone loss following stabilization of type C2 fracture of the distal femur.

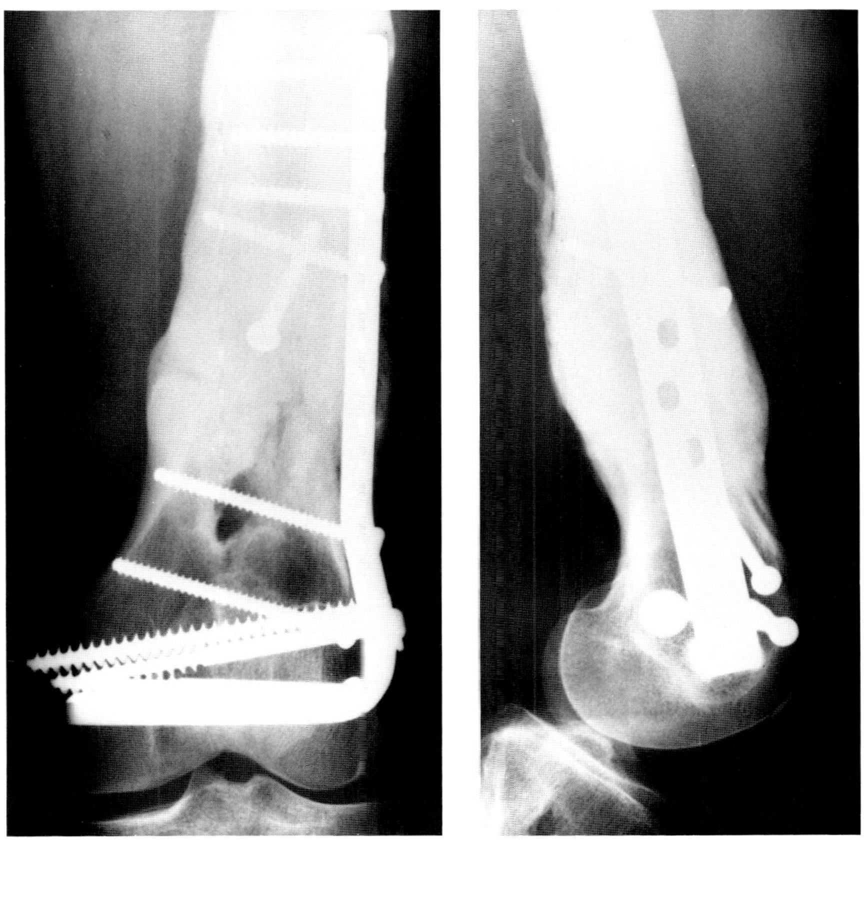

A, B

FIG. 23. AP (**A**) and (**B**) lateral roentgenograms of left femur confirm solid healing following bone grafting of supracondylar region.

SKELETALLY IMMATURE PATIENTS

Distal femoral fractures usually occur as Salter II fractures in adolescents. A large metaphyseal fragment is usually present. A fracture treated by closed reduction is immobilized in a long-leg cast until union occurs, usually between 6 and 8 weeks. However, anatomic reduction rarely can be achieved by closed methods.

Open reduction is performed through a medial or a lateral incision, depending on the location of the metaphyseal fragment. Lag screws are inserted to stabilize the metaphyseal fragment, taking care to avoid the physis. After reduction and stabilization, the limb is immobilized in a cast for 6 to 8 weeks. A high incidence of growth arrest is associated with this injury, and the patient may require bridge resection or an osteotomy in the future.

Intercondylar fractures are rare in children. When they occur these fractures should be treated by anatomic reduction and internal fixation. Kirschner wires are used to fix the articular surface and to stabilize the epiphysis to the metaphysis in young children. In children over the age of 8 years, screws are used to fix the articular surface and to attach small buttress plates. These plates must be removed after fracture union to allow continuing distal femoral growth. The patients must be carefully followed for physeal bony bridges, which may develop and limit longitudinal growth.

REFERENCES

1. Müller ME, Nazarian S, Koch P, Schatzker J. *The comprehensive classification of fractures of long bones.* Berlin: Springer-Verlag; 1990.
2. Gustilo RB, Anderson JT. Prevention of infection in the treatment of one thousand and twenty-five open fractures of the long bones. *J Bone Joint Surg* 1976;58A:453–8.
3. Gustilo RB, Mendoza RM, Williams DN. Problems in the management of type-III (severe) open fractures: a new classification of type-III open fractures. *J Trauma* 1984;24:742–6.
4. Mize RD, Bucholz RQ, Grogan DP. Surgical treatment of displaced, comminuted fractures of the distal end of the femur. *J Bone Joint Surg* 1982;64A:871–9.
5. Sanders RW, Swiontkowski MF, Rosen H, Helfet D. Complex fractures and malunions of the distal femur: results of treatment with double plates. *J Bone Joint Surg* 1991;73A:341–6.

Patellar Fractures

MECHANISMS OF INJURY

Most patellar fractures result from direct trauma associated with falls onto a flexed knee or with impact into an automobile dashboard. Associated injuries include fractures of the ipsilateral femoral shaft, the femoral neck, and the acetabulum. Patellar fractures can also be caused by tension stresses, but this mechanism is associated with sports injuries and usually results in patellar tendon failure with small avulsion fragments.

ANATOMIC CONSIDERATIONS

The patella is covered by the thickest articular cartilage found in the skeletal system and is divided into three facets—the medial, the lateral, and the inferior. The meager anatomic structures surrounding the patella (the periosteum, a single-cell-thick prepatellar bursa, and the skin) provide poor protection from injury.

CLASSIFICATION

Fractures are classified by description and by the severity of the soft-tissue injury.

ASSESSMENT

Physical Examination

The clinical examination is the same as the examination for supracondylar femoral fractures.

Radiographic Evaluation

Useful information about the patella is provided by AP, lateral, and sunrise radiographic views. Because anomalies such as bipartite and tripartite patella (congenital failure of fusion of ossification centers) frequently occur in the superior–lateral area of the patella, the physical examination must correlate with radiographic findings to avoid misdiagnosis.

Special Studies

Tomography is occasionally indicated to delineate fracture patterns. Bone scans, CT scans, and MRI are rarely needed.

EMERGENT MANAGEMENT

The soft-tissue injuries are thoroughly assessed in open injuries. Contusions or abrasions on the skin may warrant a delay in operative reconstruction. After the distal sensory and motor functions and the circulatory status are assessed, the knee is palpated for effusion and ligamentous instability. The limb is then immobilized in a well-padded knee splint until definitive treatment can be carried out. Open patellar fractures are managed urgently by debridement and concurrent internal fixation.

DEFINITIVE MANAGEMENT

The definitive treatment is based on preoperative radiographic findings. Unstable displaced bony fragments smaller than 1 cm^2 are usually excised. Attempts should be made to

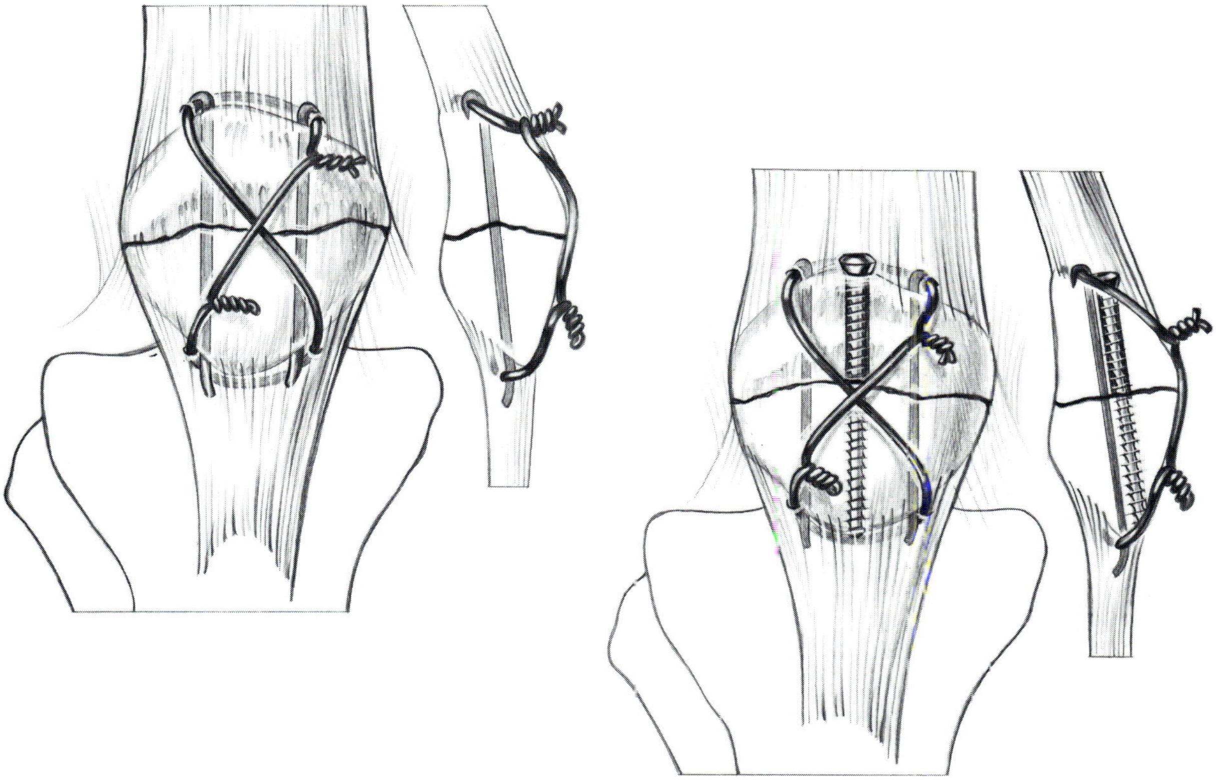

A

B

FIG. 24. **A:** Internal fixation of a transverse patellar fracture using standard tension-band wiring technique. **B:** Internal fixation of a transverse patellar fracture using an additional 3.5-mm lag screw. The superior fragment is overdrilled to 3.5 mm.

salvage larger fragments. Arthroscopy is indicated for diagnostic purposes when the amount of articular incongruity cannot be determined. Open reduction and internal fixation are indicated in active adults when the articular surface is displaced by 2 mm or more. When the patella has sustained a comminuted fracture, salvage procedures are initiated to reconstruct as much of the patella as possible. Total patellectomy is rarely performed at this institution and is reserved for extremely comminuted fractures.

The patella is visualized through a straight anterior linear incision through the mid-patella. Fixation for transverse fractures consists of two parallel 0.062-in Kirschner wires or 3.5-mm cortical lag screws supplemented with an 18-gauge figure-8 wire loop (Figs. 24–27). The parallel wires are inserted centrally into the transverse section of the patella using the tension-band technique (1). Fractures consisting of multiple fragments are reduced and fixed. Small fragments are affixed to larger fragments with 3.5-mm or 2.7-mm lag screws to construct a transverse fracture which is then fixed as noted above (Figs. 28–31).

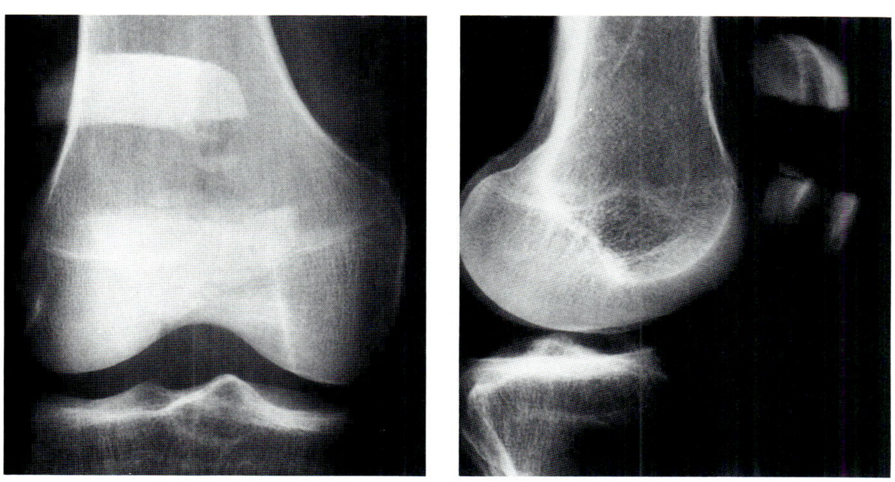

A, B

FIG. 25. AP (**A**) and lateral (**B**) roentgenograms of a displaced transverse fracture of the patella.

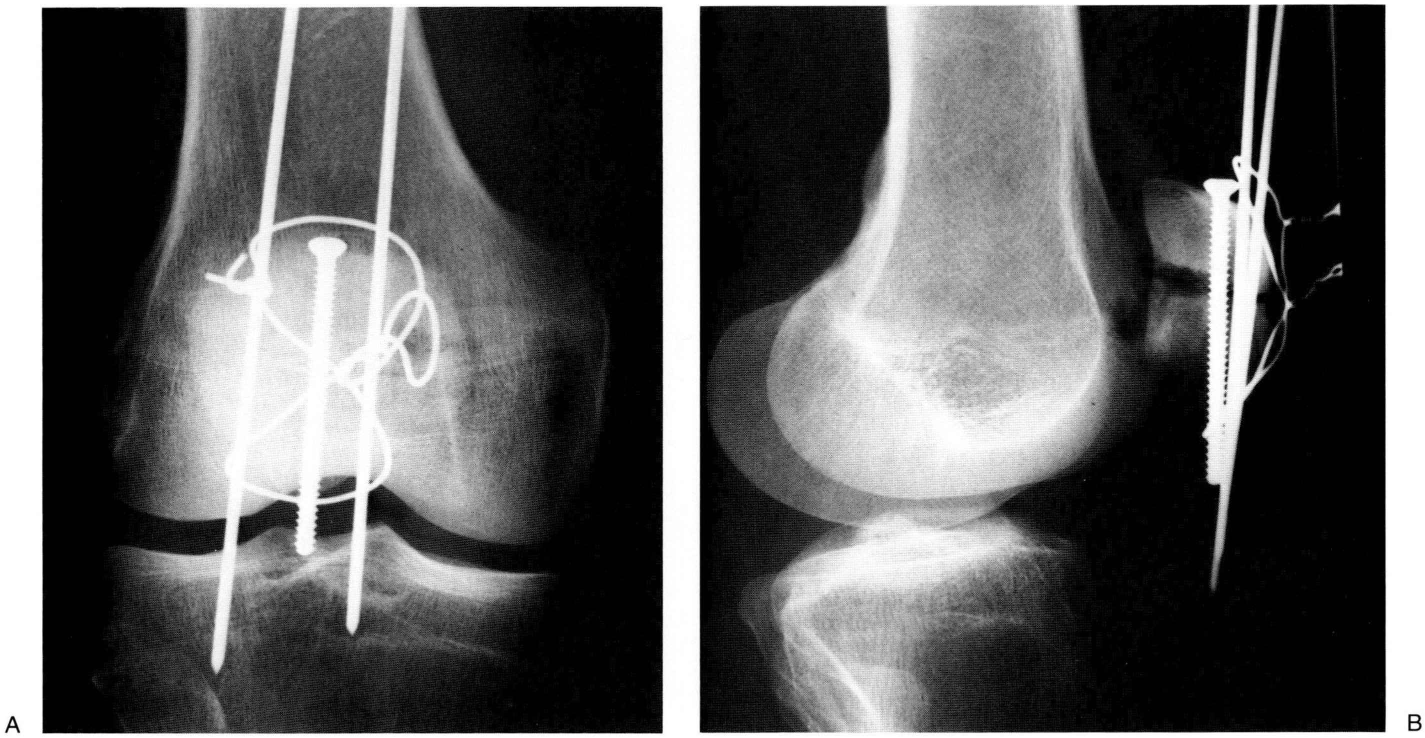

FIG. 26. AP (**A**) and lateral (**B**) roentgenograms (intraoperative views) of fixation of fracture using 3.5-mm lag screws and neutralization using a tension-band wire.

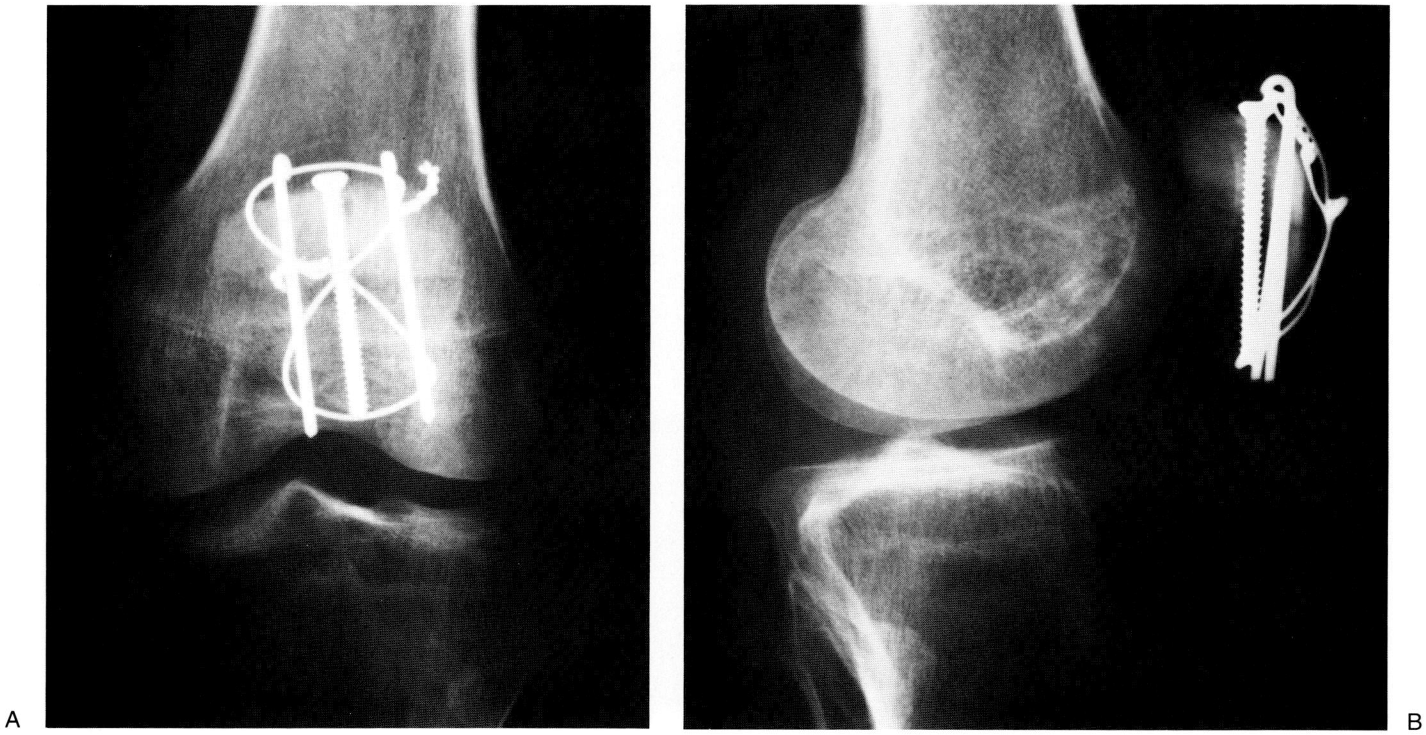

FIG. 27. AP (**A**) and lateral (**B**) roentgenograms show the completed construct with trimmed and impacted wires to avoid quadriceps and patellar tendon impingement.

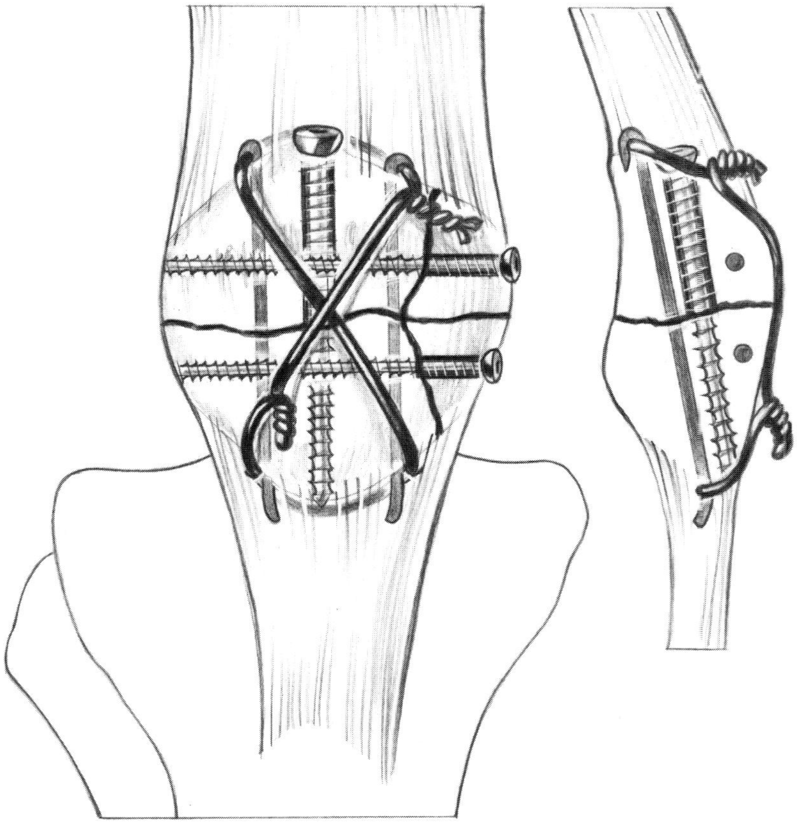

FIG. 28. Internal fixation of a multifragmented patellar fracture using small-fragment lag screws and a tension-band wiring technique.

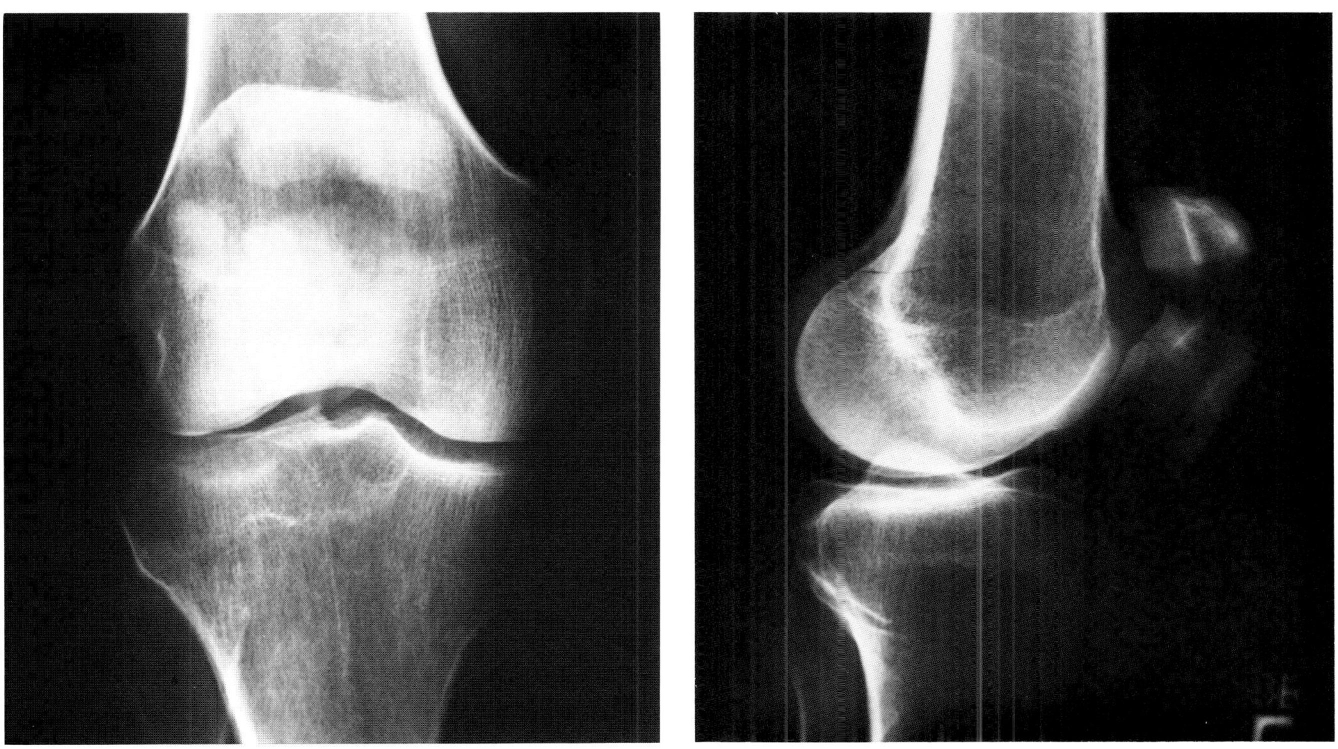

A B

FIG. 29. AP (**A**) and lateral (**B**) roentgenograms of comminuted patellar fracture.

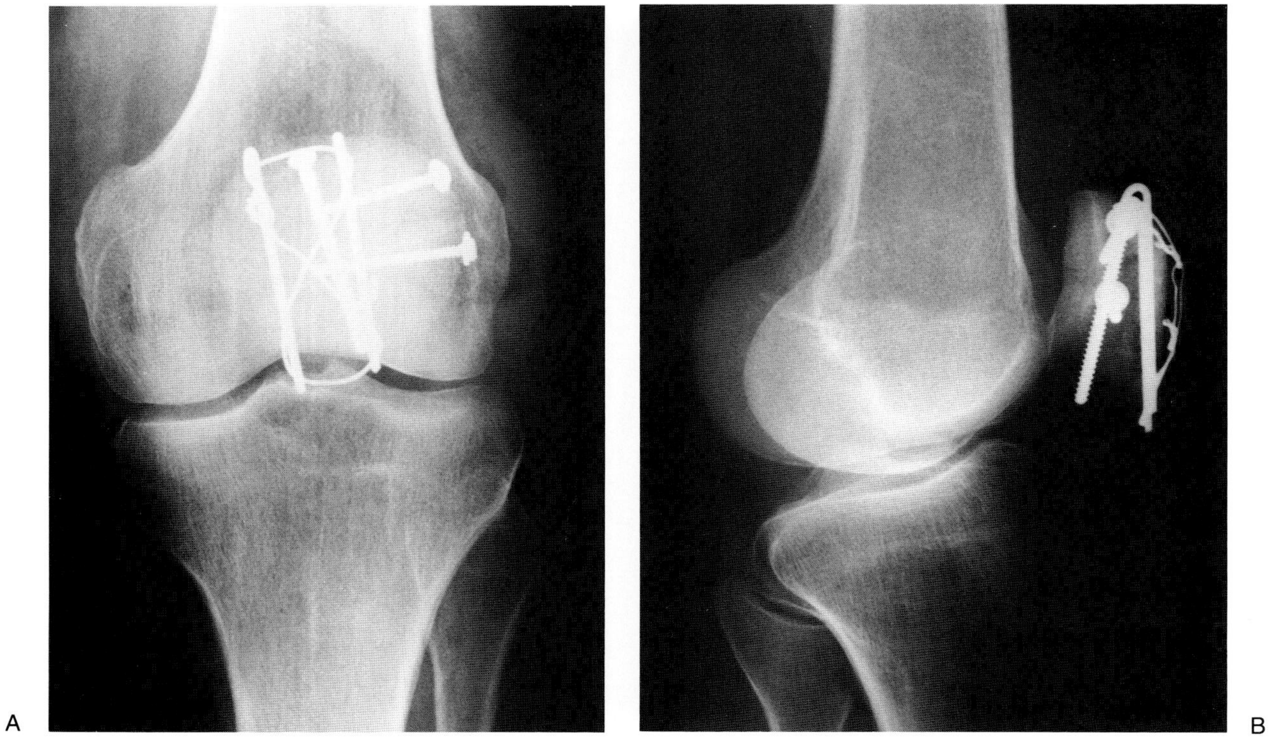

FIG. 30. AP (A) and lateral (B) roentgenograms demonstrate fracture fragments stabilized with small fragment screws (superior and inferior fragments) followed by lag screw fixation of the remaining transverse fracture using a lag screw and tension-band wire.

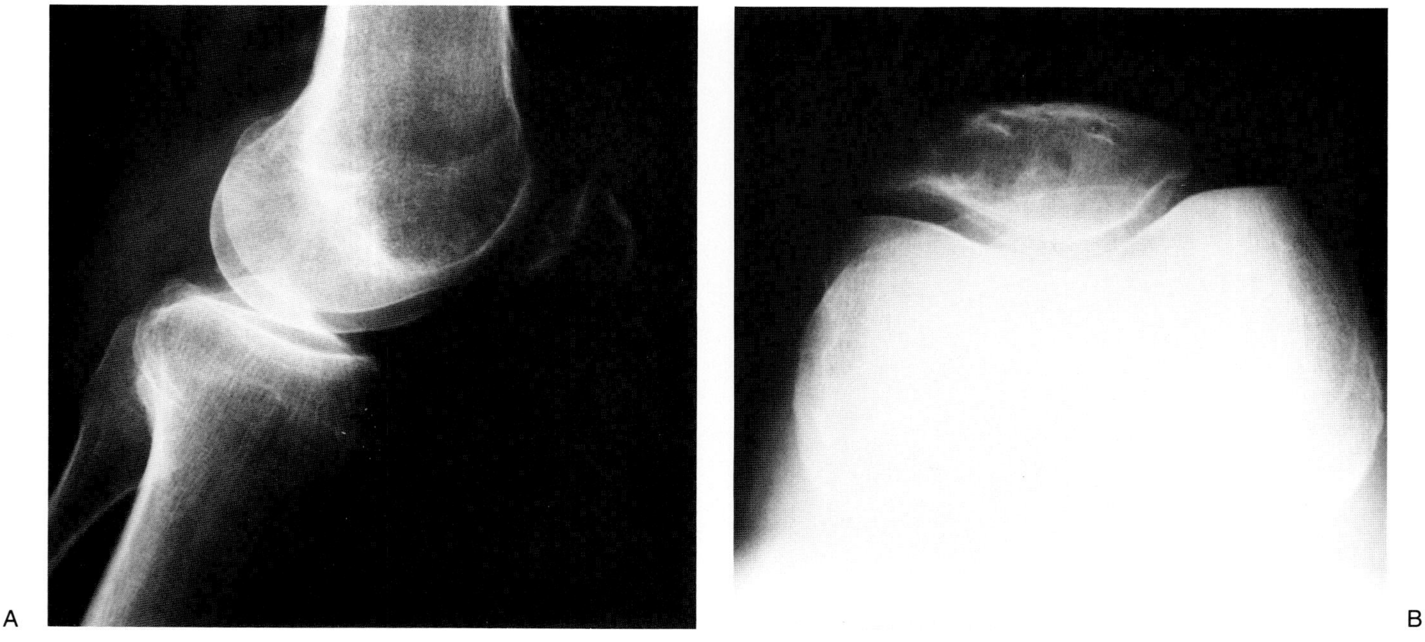

FIG. 31. Lateral (A) and skyline (B) views of patella following hardware removal demonstrate reconstruction of osseous anatomy at 1 year.

Continuous passive motion can be initiated after the wound begins to heal. Active flexion and passive extension exercises are encouraged, and the patient should attain 90° of flexion by the sixth postoperative week. A more rigorous rehabilitation program can achieve almost full ROM by 12 to 16 weeks after injury. Full weight-bearing can be started the first week, but the knee must be supported in a splint for the first 3 to 4 weeks.

COMPLICATIONS

Infection is rare with a patellar fracture but can be treated by wound debridement, primary closure over a drain, and a regimen of intravenous antibiotics. Nonunion is also rare; when it occurs, it is treated by repeat fixation and bone grafting with immobilization in extension for 4 to 6 weeks. Patients often complain of discomfort over the tension-band wires and the wires can be removed in an ambulatory surgical procedure after 4 to 6 months.

SKELETALLY IMMATURE PATIENTS

Patellar fractures in children are treated with the same considerations as fractures in adults.

REFERENCE

1. Weber MJ, Janecki DJ, McLeod P, et al. Efficacy of various forms of fixation of transverse fractures of the patella. *J Bone Joint Surg* 1980;62A:215–20.

Proximal Tibial Fractures

MECHANISMS OF INJURY

Proximal tibial fractures can be caused by a variety of mechanisms. Most commonly, the proximal tibia is fractured by high-energy mechanisms such as a fall from a height onto an extended limb or expulsion from a moving vehicle. Less commonly, proximal metaphyseal injuries may result from direct trauma, e.g., from impact by a car bumper. Injury to the knee joint may be minor or even nonexistent with this mechanism. Proximal tibial injuries also occur from relatively low-energy axial-loading or twisting injuries from skiing, bicycling, and other sports. Lower-extremity injuries that are commonly associated with proximal tibial fractures include fractures of the calcaneus, the femoral shaft, and the femoral neck. The surrounding popliteal vessels, the tibial nerve, and the common peroneal nerve also may be injured.

ANATOMIC CONSIDERATIONS

The proximal tibia slopes approximately 15° in a posterior direction. This contour must be kept in mind when the articular surface is visualized on radiographs (Fig. 32). The articulation of the tibia with the proximal fibula can be dislocated or the fibular head can be fractured as a consequence of a tibial plateau fracture. The medial meniscus, larger than the lateral meniscus, is supported by the meniscotibial ligaments (Fig. 33). Capillary perfusion is excellent in the outer one half to one third of the menisci. The insertion of the knee-joint capsule onto the proximal tibia is located distal to the meniscus. The popliteal artery and vein are tightly constrained by the proximal fascia of the soleus muscle, making the artery vulnerable to injury from a knee dislocation or a significantly displaced proximal tibial fracture.

CLASSIFICATION

The classification of Schatzker (1) is used to grade proximal tibial fractures (Fig. 34). However, for purposes of communication and reporting we commonly refer to the Müller Comprehensive Classification of long-bone fractures adopted by the Orthopaedic Trauma Association (2). For treatment purposes, descriptive terms such as split, split-depression, depression, unicondylar, medial plateau, bicondylar, and metaphyseal extension are used.

ASSESSMENT

Physical Examination

The clinical examination of a patient with a tibial plateau fracture is the same as the examination of a patient with a distal femoral fracture.

Radiographic Evaluation

A tibial plateau fracture can be identified on standard AP and lateral radiographs of the knee. After the fracture is identified, a 15° caudad radiographic view as described by Moore is indicated (3). Two 45° oblique views are used to assess depressions in the articular surface.

Special Studies

When the location of the fracture lines or the amount of depression is uncertain, AP and lateral tomograms or CT

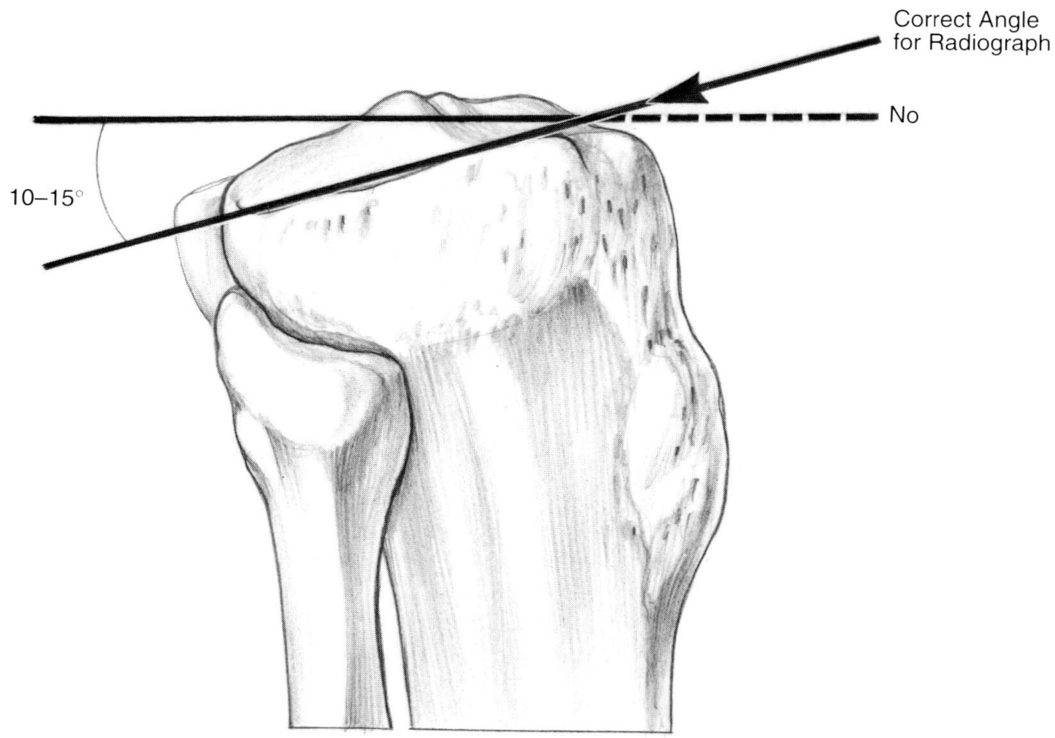

FIG. 32. The articular surface inclines 15° posterior from the axis of the tibial shaft.

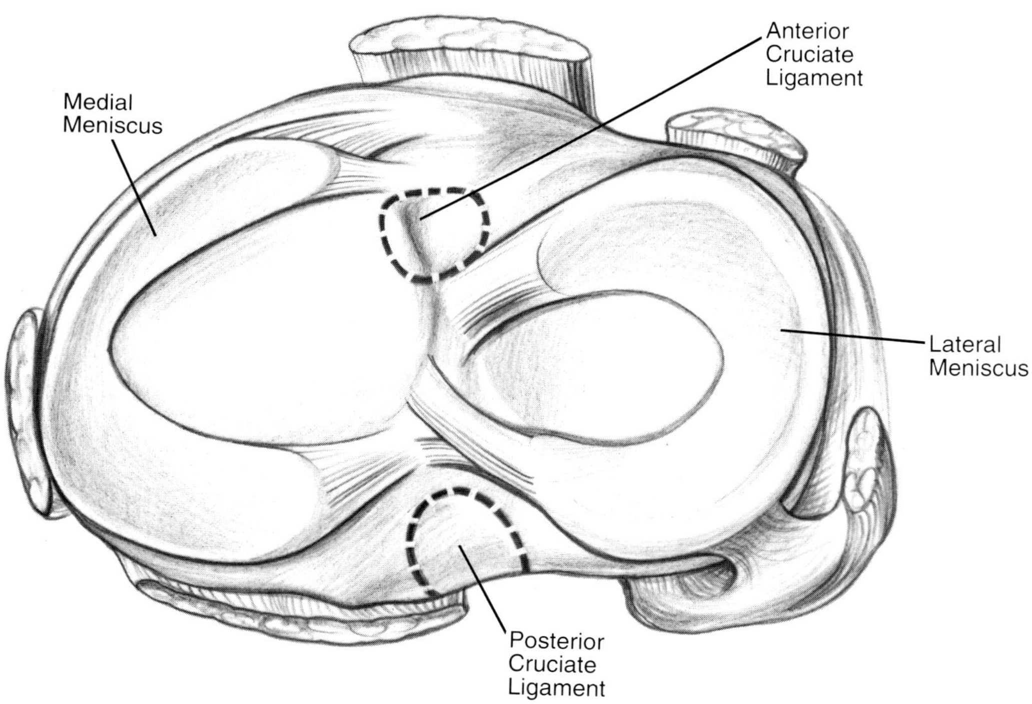

FIG. 33. Superior view of meniscal anatomy.

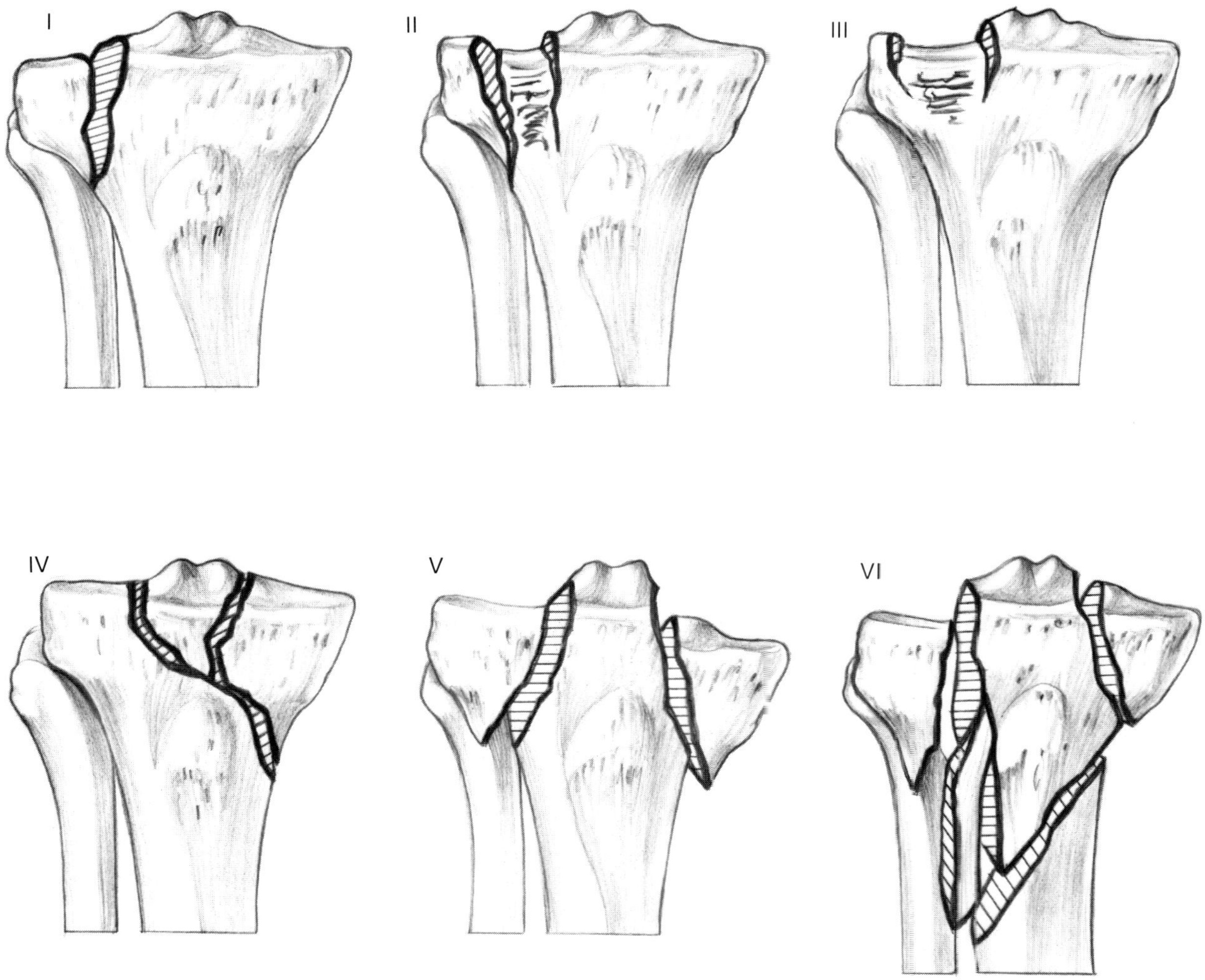

FIG. 34. Schatzker's classification.

scans with lateral reconstructions are invaluable. Angiography is indicated when distal pulses are absent or when the Doppler signal is distorted. Magnetic resonance imaging can provide additional information about soft-tissue injuries and articular pathology but this modality is not used routinely.

EMERGENT MANAGEMENT

The lower extremity must be examined systematically when a tibial plateau fracture is suspected. An estimate must be made of the amount of force that caused the fracture and the force must be determined to be indirect or direct. Direct force is associated with the worst neural, vascular, and soft-tissue devitalization. Open wounds are characterized by contamination and soft-tissue stripping. The distal limb is inspected for disrupted sensory, motor, and circulatory functions. Discovery of a discernible abnormality in the caliber of the pulses or the capillary refill should be followed immediately by duplex scanning and possible arteriography. Finally, the knee is assessed for stability, possibly under anesthesia. After the examination is completed the knee is splinted in extension.

DEFINITIVE MANAGEMENT

Proximal tibial fractures will be discussed according to their radiographic fracture patterns. Factors that influence preoperative planning include age, obesity, the severity of the soft-tissue injury, and the functional requirements of the patient. According to these criteria, an obese patient who is older than 55 and has poor bone quality is a candidate for nonoperative treatment. Radiographic indications for operative treatment include split or depression greater than 3 mm or varus or valgus instability greater than 10°.

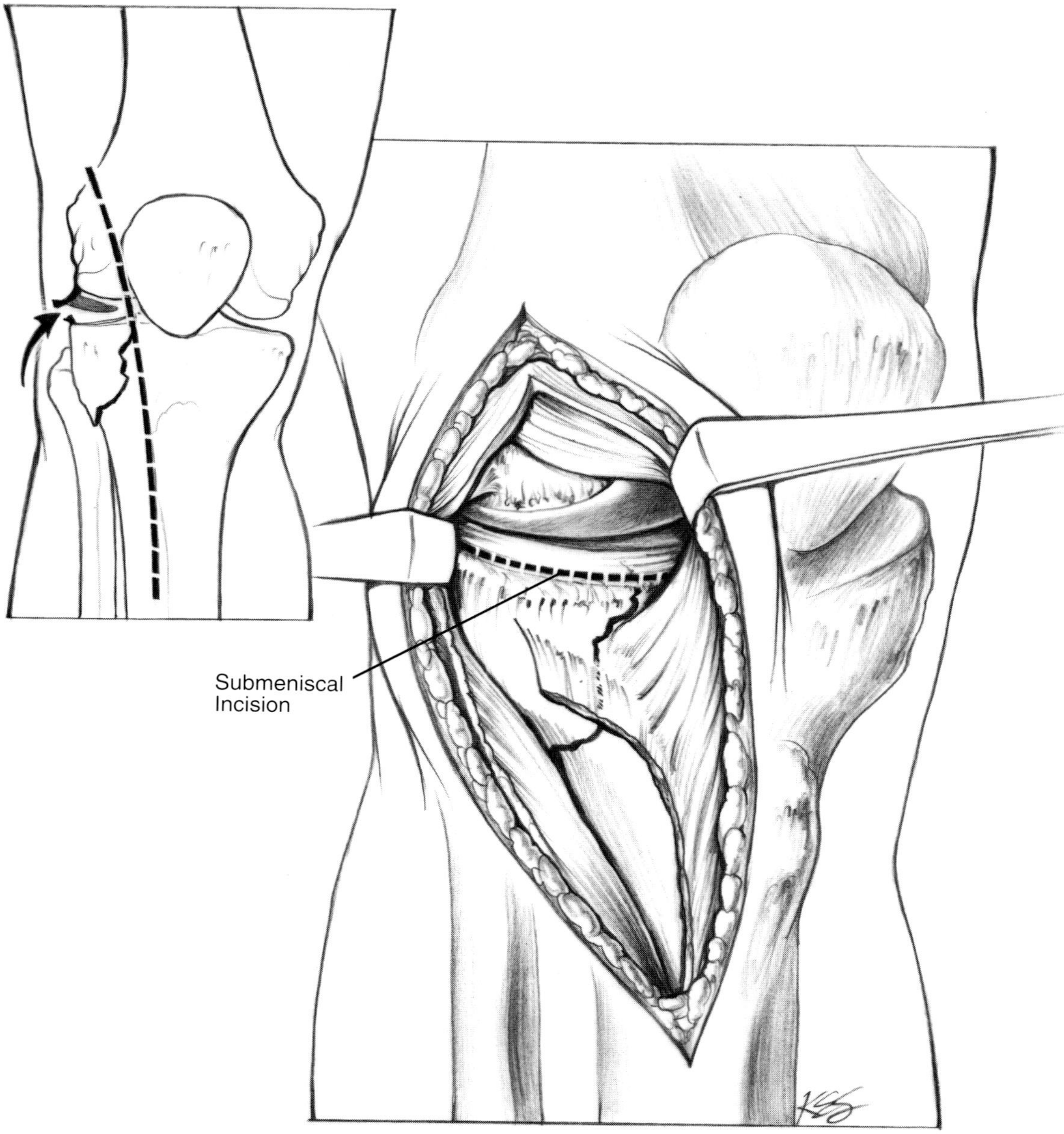

FIG. 35. This variant of the surgical approach for a lateral plateau fracture allows direct visualization via a submeniscal arthrotomy *(inset).*

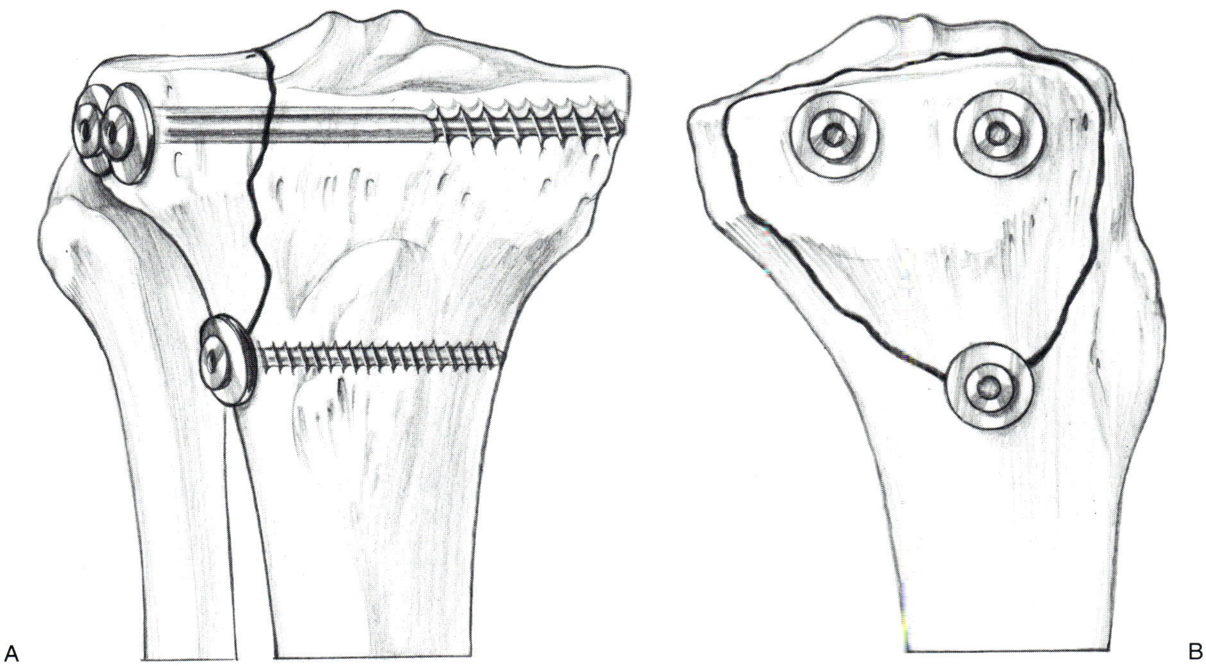

FIG. 36. AP projection (**A**) and lateral projection (**B**) of internal fixation for a type I split fracture of the proximal tibia using two lag screws and an antiglide screw with a washer.

Split Fractures

The patient is positioned supine on the operating table with a roll under the ipsilateral buttock. Prepping the iliac crest is not necessary for this fracture pattern. A tourniquet is applied unless it is contraindicated by severe soft-tissue injuries. If the plateau fragment is nondisplaced, the fracture can be stabilized with cannulated or standard screws placed percutaneously. Arthroscopy may be useful for manipulating small fracture fragments associated with articular displacement. Open reduction is indicated for significantly displaced fractures and for injuries with other associated fractures or ligament injuries.

Fractures in elderly patients with poor bone quality are approached through midline and straight anterior incisions. In younger patients an anterolateral incision is preferred. The iliotibial band is reflected off Gerdy's tubercle, leaving behind enough soft tissue for suture repair. Alternatively, an osteotomy can be performed on the tubercle. The lateral meniscus is mobilized through a submeniscal incision; it can be detached anteriorly for better visualization if necessary, but this is not done routinely. A portion of the coronary ligaments should be left attached to the proximal tibia for suture repair (Fig. 35). The tibial plateau fragment is elevated and provisionally stabilized with Kirschner wires. Fixation in young patients with strong cortical bone consists of two cancellous lag screws and the possible addition of an antiglide screw and washer inserted distally (Fig. 36). Patients with osteoporotic bone require fixation with T- or L-buttress plates. The meniscus is repaired with nonabsorbable suture.

The limb is mobilized by CPM during hospitalization and for 2 to 3 weeks after discharge if the fixation is stable. Touch-down weight-bearing is permitted for 8 to 12 weeks, depending on the quality of the bone and the amount of soft-tissue injury. Hardware removal is indicated only if the knee is symptomatic.

Split Depression Fractures

The positioning of the patient is the same as for split fractures, but in this case the ipsilateral anterior iliac crest is prepared for harvest of bone graft. The surgical approach is determined by the same considerations regarding the patient's age and bone quality that were discussed earlier. The split-fracture component is opened and the depressed segment is elevated with a bone tamp. Bone graft is taken from the iliac crest and packed underneath the elevated segment. The size of the cancellous grafts may be between 1 cm^2 and 3 cm^2 in large depressions. The split fragment is reduced and pinned with Kirschner wires. The choices of suitable hardware are similar to those for split fractures. Buttress plating is indicated for large depressed segments (Figs. 37–39). In young patients, buttress plates are used to stabilize small fragments, and large cannulated screws are used to compress the main fragment and to support the depressed segment. Recently we have been using 3.5-mm small-fragment T-plates to decrease the bulk of the hardware (Figs. 40 and 41). Alternatively, the split fragment can be supported by an antiglide screw and washer or a one-third tubular plate if the depressed segment is small and well supported.

Continuous passive motion and a hinged knee brace that does not limit flexion or extension are warranted if the fragments are well-compressed and stabilized with an antiglide plate or a buttress plate. Like patients with split fractures, patients with split depression fractures are limited to touch-down weight-bearing for 12 weeks.

Depression Fractures

The location and size of the depression must be assessed from tomograms or CT scans. The clinical examination must note whether the knee is stable in extension. The surgical approach is determined by the same criteria as noted earlier and the anterior iliac crest is prepared for harvest of a bone graft.

In skilled hands, depression fractures can be managed arthroscopically. A 1-cm^2 cortical window is made in the metaphyseal flare and the depressed segment is elevated by arthroscopic visualization or by a submeniscal arthrotomy. Placement of a femoral distractor with a 5-mm Schanz screw

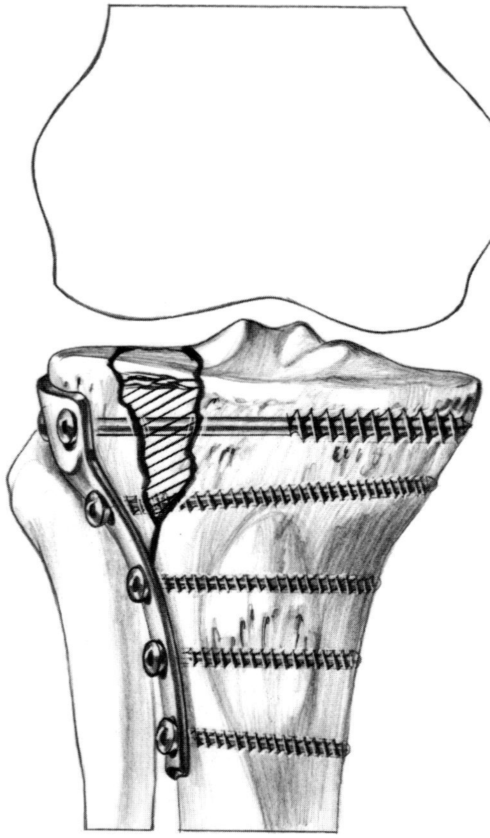

FIG. 37. Internal fixation of a split depression fracture of the tibial plateau using L-buttress plate fixation with bone grafting of the elevated segment.

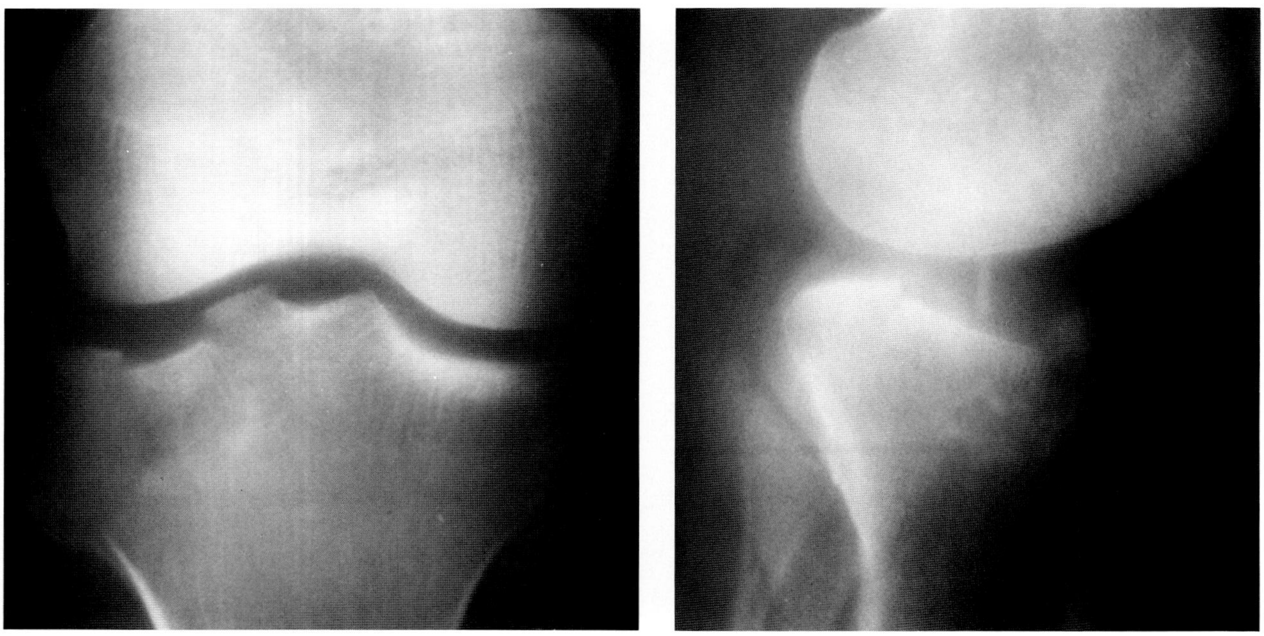

A B

FIG. 38. AP (**A**) and lateral (**B**) tomograms of split depressed lateral plateau fracture (Schatzker II) with three major components.

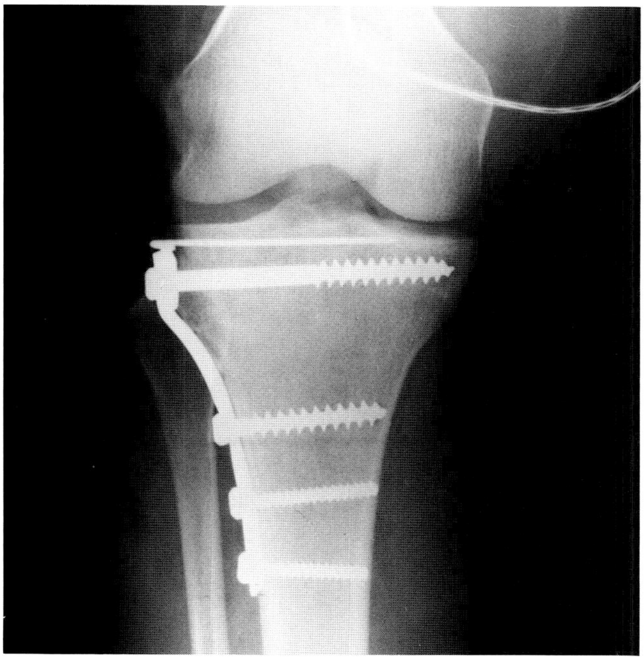

FIG. 39. AP view demonstrates reconstruction of articular surface using subchondral K-wire followed by L-buttress plate fixation of proximal fragment.

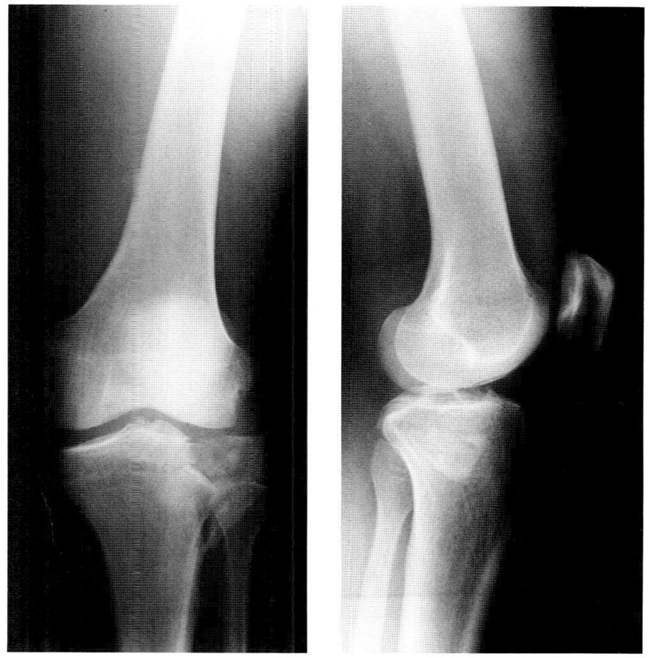

A, B

FIG. 40. AP (**A**) and lateral (**B**) roentgenograms of split depressed (type II) tibial plateau fracture.

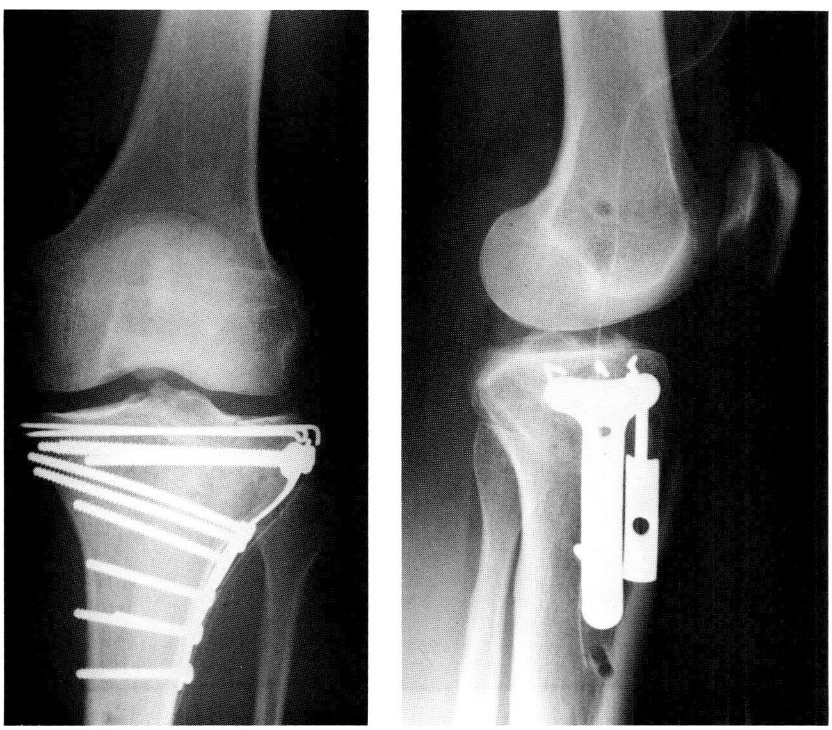

A, B

FIG. 41. AP (**A**) and (**B**) lateral roentgenograms of postoperative montage using a small fragment T-plate and one-third tubular plate for stabilization of split depression fracture with subchondral K-wires to effectively stabilize the articular segment before buttress plate fixation.

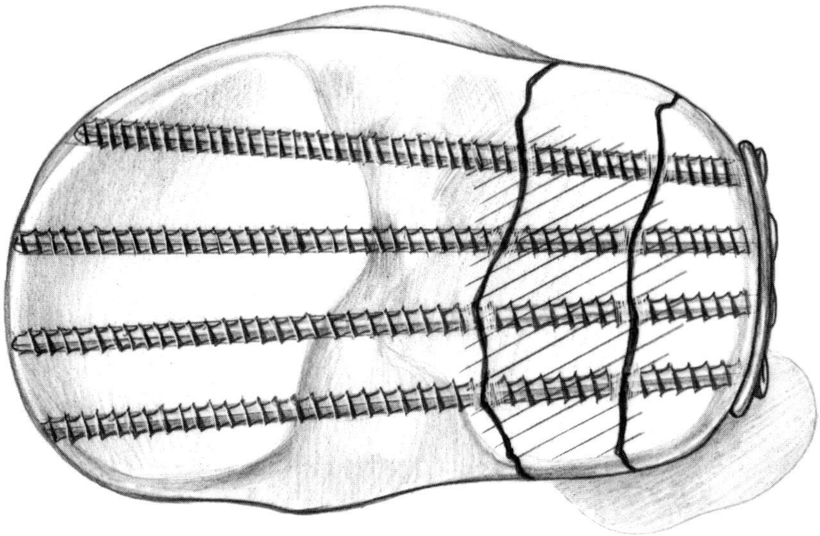

FIG. 42. Orientation of screws in a split depression fracture stabilized with a small-fragment T-plate, seen from superior.

at the center of rotation of the distal femur and distal to the tibial fracture helps to visualize the joint. If more than half the lateral plateau is depressed and the intact portion is supported only by the rim, the depressed segment can be over-reduced by 0.5 mm to 1.0 mm. If the depressed segment is small and well supported, it should be elevated to the level of the intact margins. Once elevated, the segment is supported by the cancellous bone graft, which is inserted with a bone tamp and firmly packed. A large bone graft is held in place by 1 or 2 subchondral screws. Small-fragment T-plates with 3.5-mm screws can also be used to stabilize split depression and depression fractures (Figs. 42–44).

The postoperative management of a depression fracture includes CPM, a hinged knee brace, and ambulation limited to touch-down weight-bearing for 12 weeks. If the depressed area is small (less than 1 cm^2 to 1.5 cm^2) and the rim is intact, the period of touch-down weight-bearing can be shortened to 8 weeks.

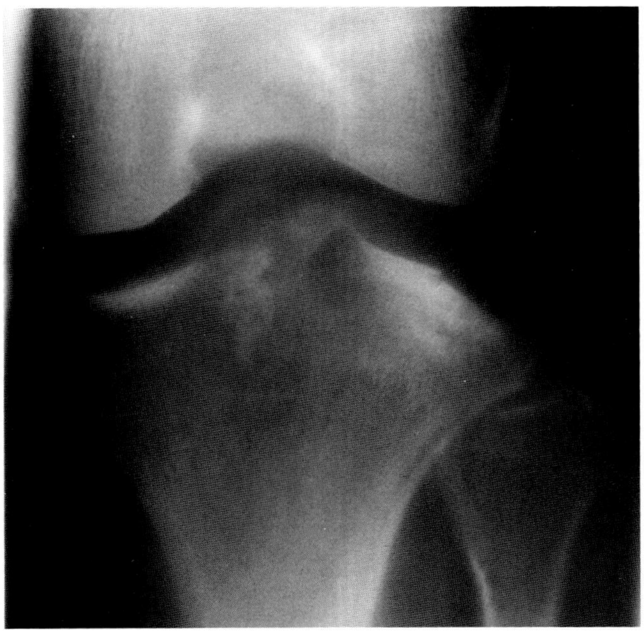

FIG. 43. Management of rim depression fracture (Schatzker type III) of the tibial plateau. AP tomogram demonstrates impaction of cancellous bone with remaining rim of lateral cortex.

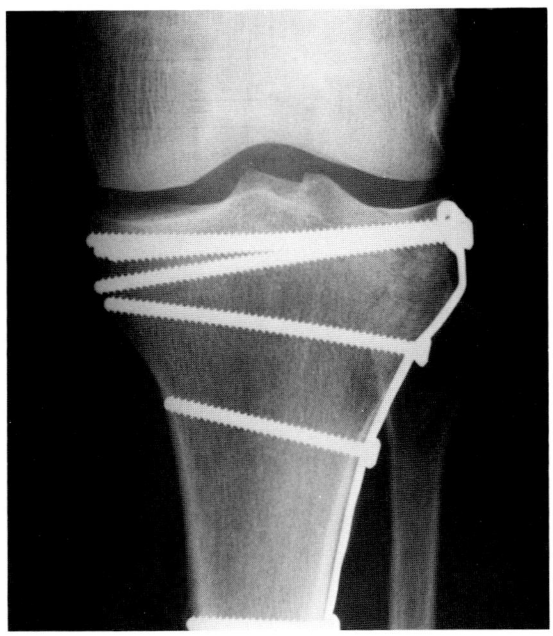

FIG. 44. Postoperative AP roentgenogram demonstrates reconstruction of articular surface using small-fragment T-plate fixation with 3.5-mm cortical screws.

Medial Plateau Fractures

Medial plateau fractures can be very unstable injuries, and the limb must be assessed for varus or valgus instabilities in full flexion. Instability makes the criteria with respect to patients' characteristics and functional demands less important in this type of tibial plateau fracture. A straight anterior approach is used in patients who are older than 50 years, obese, or have moderate functional requirements. In young patients an anteromedial approach is used in conjunction with a submeniscal arthrotomy. The medial fragment is usually a split fracture involving a large portion of the tibial plateau. It must be reduced anatomically and fixed provisionally with Kirschner wires. The meniscus must be preserved when possible. The fracture fragment is fixed with lag screws (6.5-mm cancellous screws in large patients and 3.5-mm cortical screws in smaller patients) and a buttress plate to resist varus forces (Figs. 45–47). Postoperatively these fractures are managed in the same manner as split depression fractures.

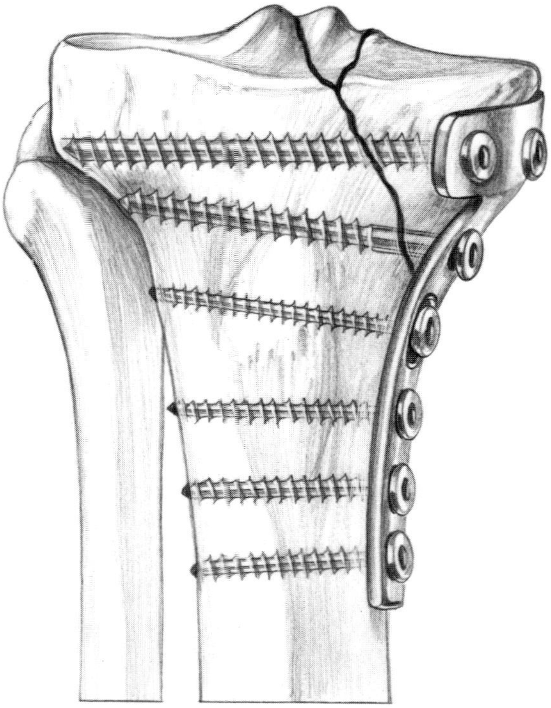

FIG. 45. Internal fixation of a medial plateau fracture using a T-plate.

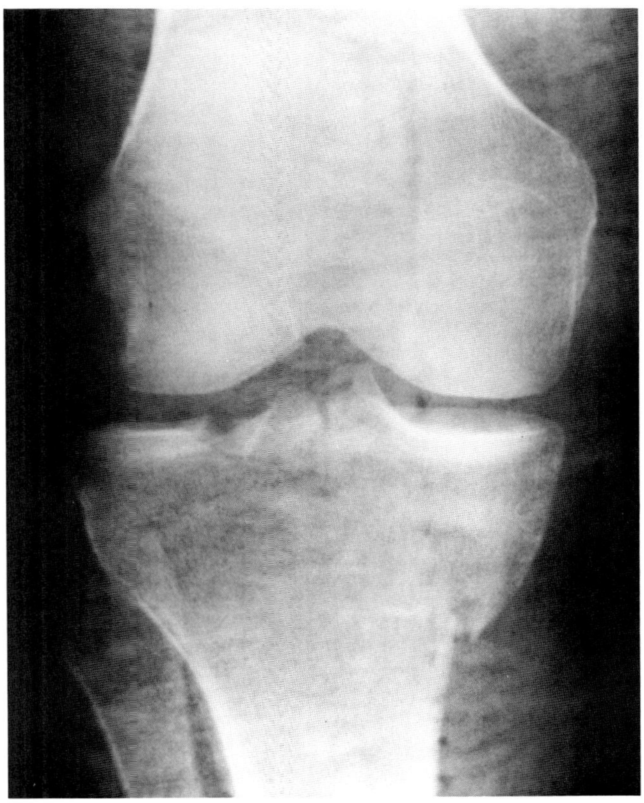

FIG. 46. AP roentgenogram of medial tibial plateau fracture (Schatzker IV).

Bicondylar Fractures

Bicondylar fractures result from significant axial loading and associated injuries must be diligently ruled out. Plain radiographs and tomograms or CT scans must be examined for splitting, gapping, and injury to the tibial eminences. Instability in full extension is indicative of a bicondylar fracture. The tibial plateau with the greatest amount of split or depression must be identified. Until 5 years ago the standard care of patients with these injuries included dual-buttress plating. The "Mercedes" incision was frequently used, but it was accompanied by a very high rate of deep infection (10–20%). Today, neither the approach nor the procedure is recommended.

A straight anterior incision is recommended for elderly or obese patients and for those with limited functional demands. If depression and splitting are worst in the lateral condyle, an anterolateral incision can be substituted. This optional approach is useful when the medial fragment is nondisplaced. The lateral condyle fracture is reduced and fixed provisionally to the intact tibial eminence with Kirschner wires. The medial condyle is then reduced by indirect reduction techniques with Schanz screws and a femoral distractor. The medial condyle can be manipulated further by placing a Schanz screw into the medial tibial condyle and using it to lever the condyle for reduction.

After reduction, Kirschner wires are extended through the medial tibial condyle. Fractures on the lateral side are fixed with cancellous screws and L- or T-buttress plates. The screws are extended into the medial fragment. If the medial fragment is adequately reduced no other fixation is needed. An antiglide one-third tubular plate or a 6.5-mm washer can be added to trap the point of the fragment distally and to pre-

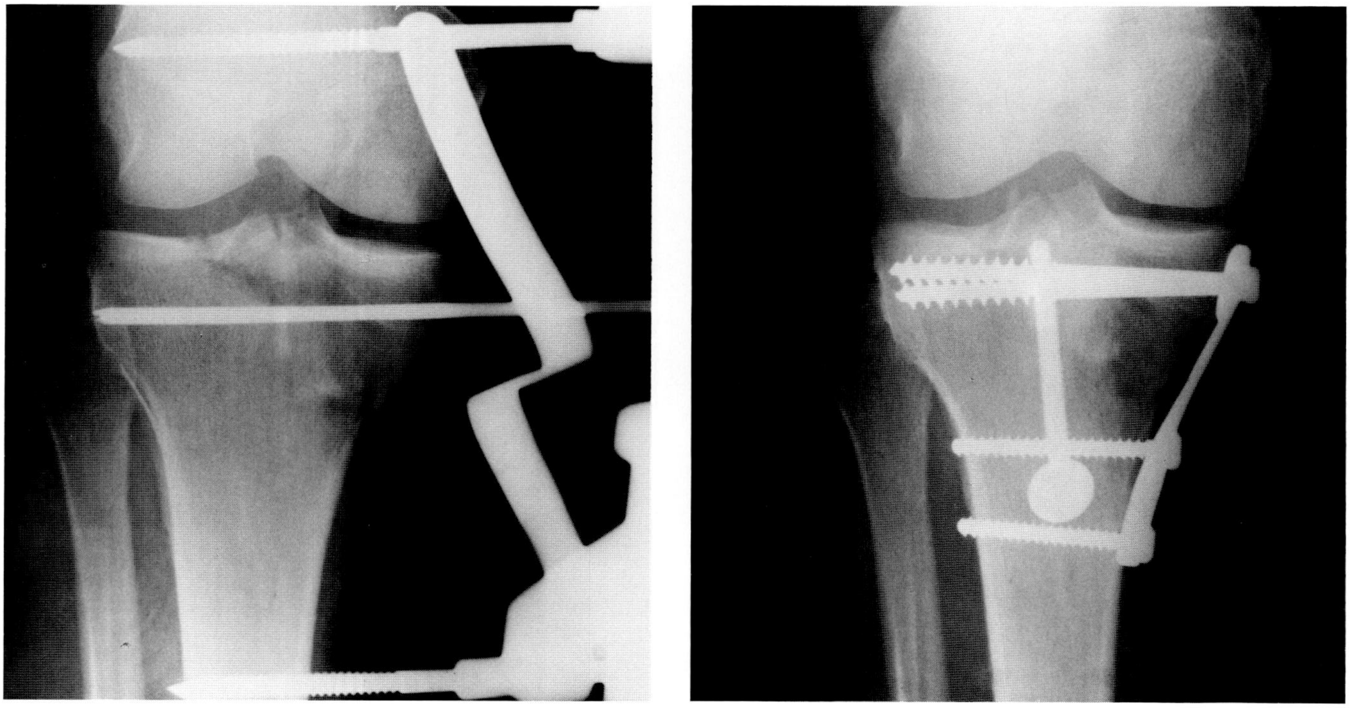

A

B

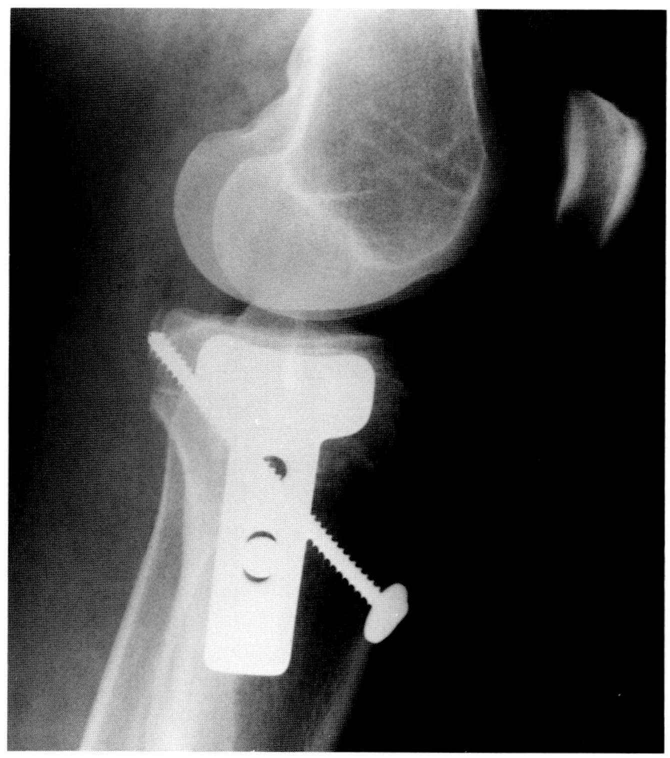

C

FIG. 47. Intraoperative AP roentgenograms demonstrate the articular reconstruction using medial femoral distractor and K-wire fixation (**A**). Postoperative montage (**B,C**) using medial T-plate and anterior-to-posterior lag screw.

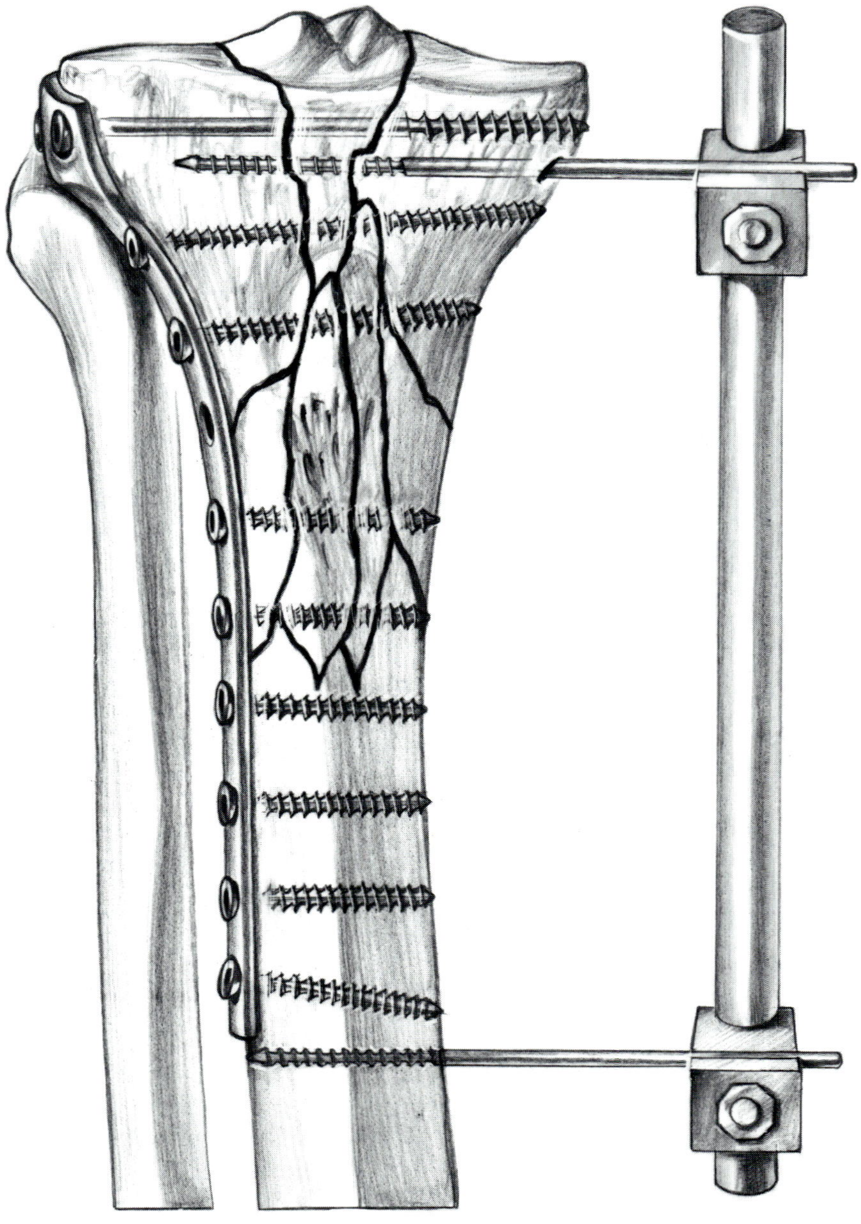

FIG. 48. Internal fixation of a type VI fracture using a medial two-pin external fixator to neutralize varus malalignment.

vent shearing from axial loads. The screws can be inserted percutaneously to reduce the amount of soft-tissue stripping. The medial fragment is compressed further with 7-mm cannulated screws or the antiglide washers inserted percutaneously.

Alternatively, a medial two-pin external fixator can be used to buttress the fracture without stripping the soft tissues further (Fig. 48). The two-pin external fixator is left in place for 6 to 12 weeks until the fracture has united and can be used concurrently with CPM. Early active ROM exercises in a hinged knee brace should be initiated. Ambulation is limited to partial weight-bearing for 12 weeks.

Bicondylar Fractures with Metaphyseal Extensions

These injuries are caused by the highest amounts of energy. Although the degree of articular damage in a bicondylar fracture may vary, injury to the metaphyseal component is usually severe. Radiographs, tomograms, or CT scans of the tibial tubercle must be assessed for avulsion fractures. The timing of surgery is dependent on two criteria: the amount of soft-tissue injury and the circulatory integrity of the limb. Long L- and T-plates and tibial-head plates are used to stabilize these injuries (Figs. 49 and 50). The lateral plateau is usually the most severely damaged structure. Deep dissection is limited

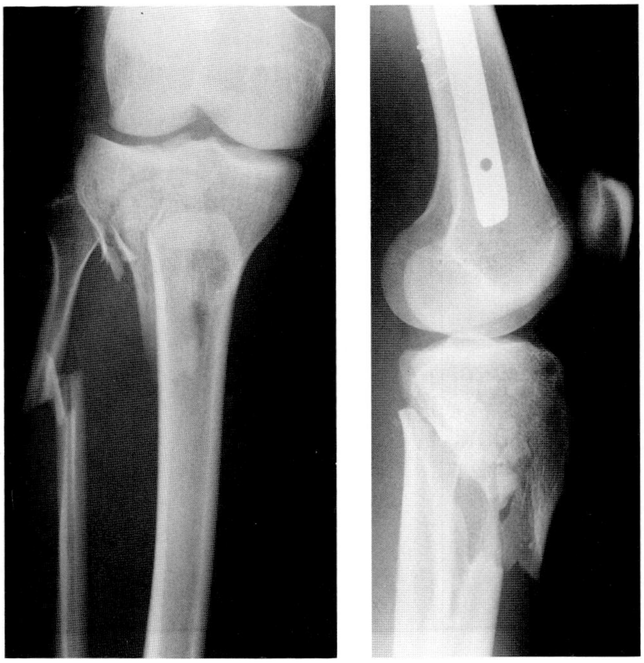

A, B

FIG. 49. AP (**A**) and lateral (**B**) roentgenograms of Schatzker VI tibial plateau fracture. Note complete metaphyseal–diaphyseal separation.

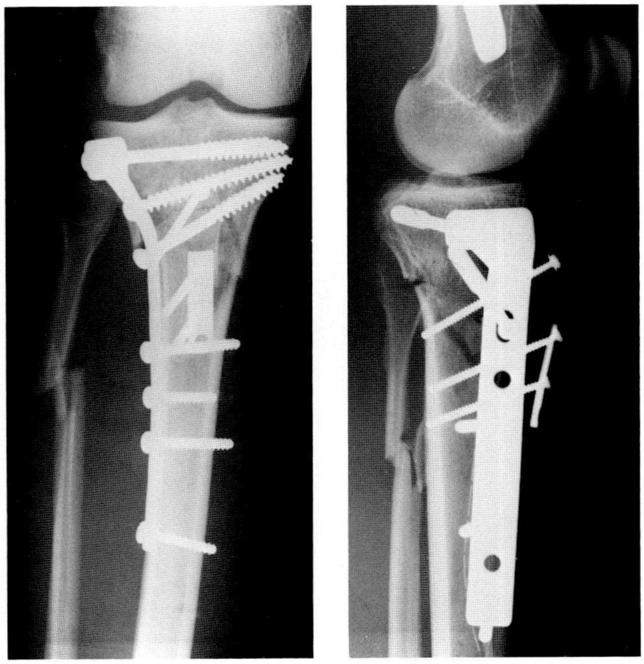

A, B

FIG. 50. Postoperative AP (**A**) and lateral (**B**) radiographs of the reconstruction. A lateral L-plate, an anterior one-third tubular plate, and lag screw fixation were used for fixation of the tubercle component.

to the lateral compartment. If a fracture component is depressed, it is elevated and supported by bone graft. The lateral split component is fixed with cancellous screws. The fractured metaphyseal segments are bridged with a long plate. More severely comminuted fractures at the metaphyseal–diaphyseal junction warrant use of a tibial-head plate, which is thicker and more rigid than standard large-fragment T- and L-plates (Figs. 51 and 52). The tibial tubercle is fixed with anteroposterior lag screws when possible. Finally, the medial fragment is fixed with antiglide percutaneous screws, one-third tubular plates, or a two-pin external fixator. Medial dissection must be kept to the minimum to reduce the risk of deep infection.

Continuous passive motion is used when the stability of the fixation is adequate. If a two-pin external fixator was used it is left in place from 6 to 12 weeks. Full weight-bearing is delayed from 12 to 16 weeks. Active ROM exercises must be delayed when the tibial tubercle is a free or poorly stabilized fragment.

COMPLICATIONS

Infection is the most common complication associated with bicondylar injuries but can often be avoided by using internal fixation devices that do not require stripping the soft tissues off the condyles. When stripping is unavoidable, aggressive management by debridement, irrigation, and closure over drains is required. Antibiotic-impregnated methylmethacrylate beads can be inserted temporarily. Administration of intravenous antibiotics is indicated for 7 to 10 days, followed by long-term suppression of the infection with specific antibiotics that are indicated by a culture. Finally, the medial head of the gastrocnemius can be transferred to solve associated soft-tissue coverage problems. Plates should not be removed until the fracture has healed, usually 12 to 18 months after injury.

Arterial injuries must be diagnosed and repaired early. Early repair correlates with a lower incidence of compartmental syndrome and limb loss. Posttraumatic degenerative arthritis is often associated with delayed mobilization and angular malunions. Angulation in younger patients is managed by osteotomy, and in older patients by arthroplasty. Patients usually tolerate valgus deformities better than varus deformities. Nonunion is rare with these injuries.

SKELETALLY IMMATURE PATIENTS

Tibial metaphyseal injuries are common in children, although articular involvement of the plateau surfaces is rare. When articular displacement in young children is greater than 2 mm, the tibial articular surface is reduced and fixed with Kirschner wires. Adolescents in whom the physis is nearly closed or already closed are treated like adults. Bone grafting may be required and both CPM and early active ROM exercises are mandatory.

Proximal metaphyseal injuries in children between the ages of 6 and 8 years are treated by closed reduction. If a gap remains after closed reduction, open reduction may be indi-

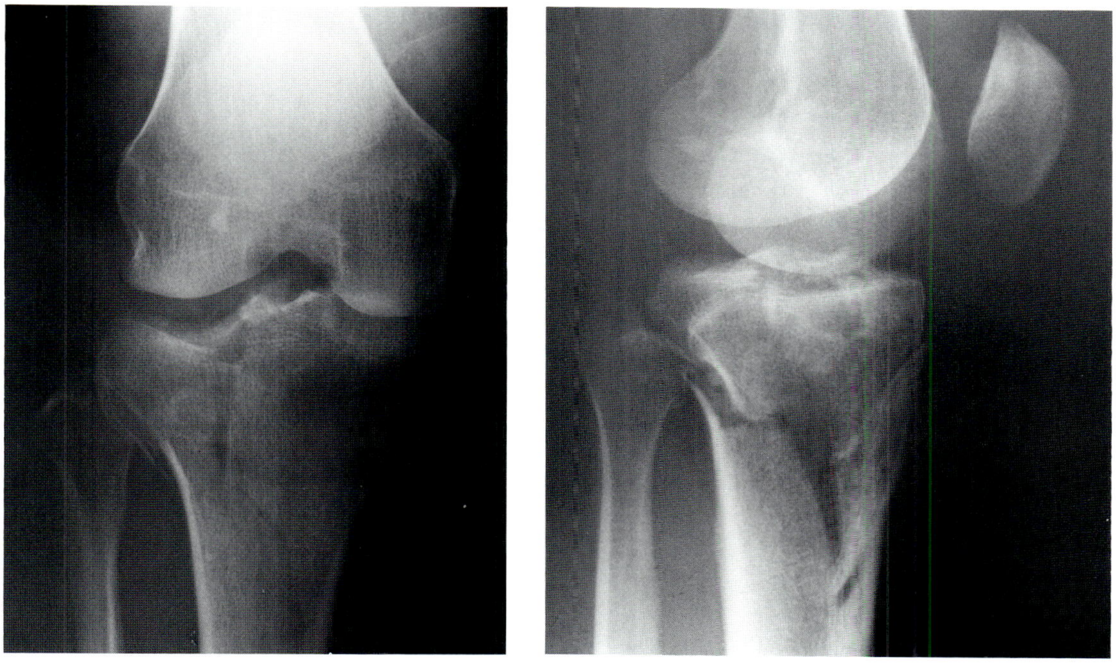

A B

FIG. 51. AP (**A**) and lateral (**B**) roentgenograms exhibit Schatzker VI tibial plateau fracture with depression of lateral plateau.

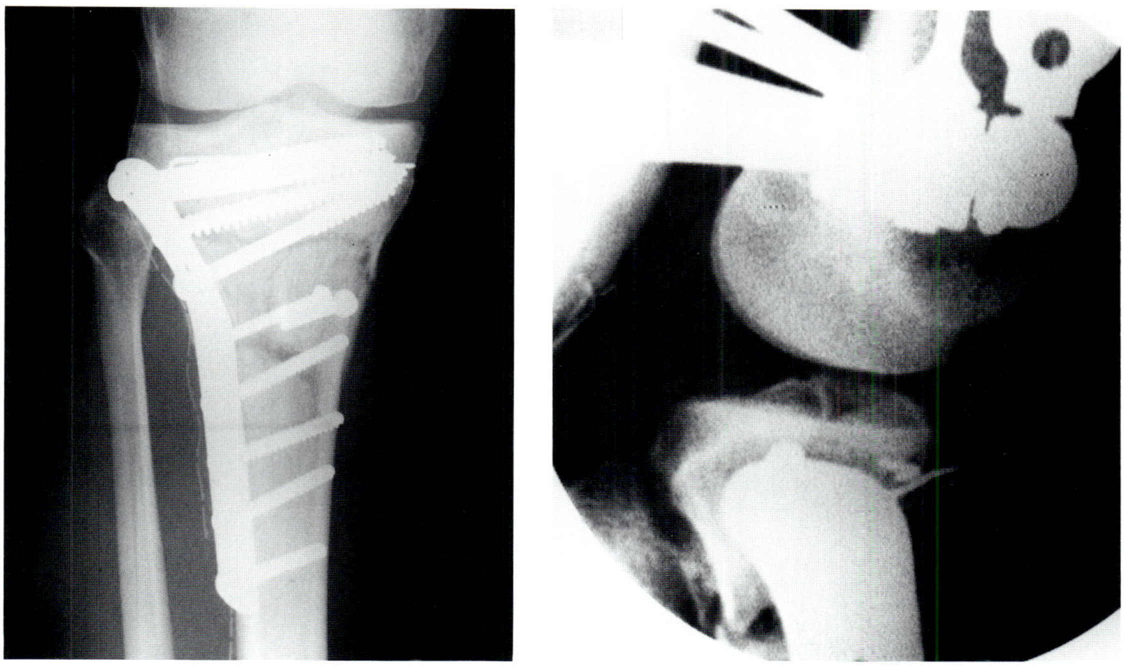

A B

FIG. 52. A: AP roentgenogram of fixation using lateral tibial head plate with lag screw fixation. **B:** Lateral intraoperative view demonstrates reconstruction of joint surface.

cated to remove the pes anserinus or the periosteum. Proximal metaphyseal injuries may be associated with recurrent valgus deformities, which can sometimes be treated by bracing but usually require a corrective osteotomy. To prevent valgus deformities, a straight-leg cast should be used and osteotomy should be delayed for as long as possible.

REFERENCES

1. Schatzker J, McBroom R. Tibial plateau fracture: the Toronto experience 1968-1975. *Clin Orthop* 1979;138:94–104.
2. Müller ME, Nazarian S, Koch P, Schatzker J. *The classification of fractures of long bones.* Berlin: Springer-Verlag; 1990.
3. Moore TM, Harvey JP. Roentgenographic measurement of tibial-plateau depression due to fracture. *J Bone Joint Surg* 1974;56A:155–60.

Tibial Eminence Fractures

MECHANISMS OF INJURY

Tibial eminence fractures are caused by direct blows to the upper tibia from anterior to posterior or by a combination of torsional and angulatory loading. Direct blows usually fracture the medial tibial eminence by avulsion of the PCL. Femoral shaft fractures are a common associated injury (Fig. 53). Fractures caused by axial loading are associated with posterior wall acetabular fractures and hip dislocations. The force is applied through a flexed knee and directed along the femur. This injury commonly occurs in passengers riding in the front seat of a car during a motor vehicle accident.

Avulsions of the lateral tibial spine result from more complex injuries that may include torsional or angulatory stresses or combined loads. Athletes and pedestrians struck by vehicles frequently sustain these injuries. Fractures of the lateral tibial spine are seen often in young patients and are associated with capsular avulsions, tibial rim avulsions, collateral ligament ruptures, and knee dislocations. Vascular damage commonly accompanies these injuries.

ANATOMIC CONSIDERATIONS

The PCL inserts onto the medial tibial spine and the posterior aspect of the tibial plateau. This insertion lies posterior to the ligaments of Humphrey and Wrisberg, which run between the posterior meniscus and the PCL. The ACL inserts onto the lateral tibial spine (see Fig. 33). The area of insertion is less broad than that of the PCL and, except for injuries in skeletally immature patients, avulsion fractures of the ACL are usually smaller and more comminuted. The collateral ligaments and the popliteal vessels lie immediately adjacent to the capsule.

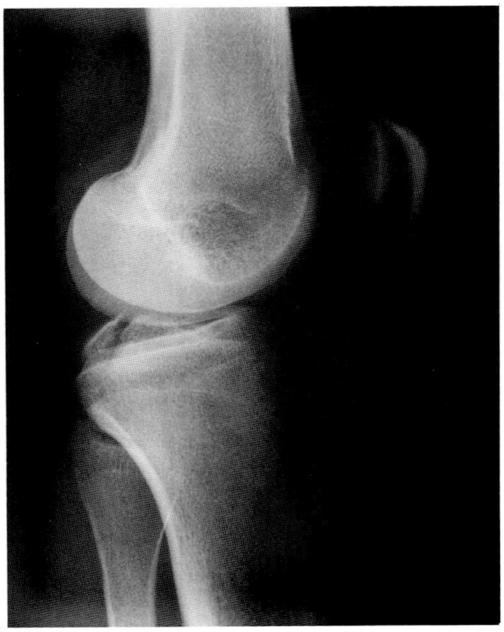

FIG. 53. Lateral view of knee following reconstruction of femoral shaft fracture demonstrates PCL avulsion from left proximal tibia.

CLASSIFICATION

Tibial spine fractures are classified as medial (posterior) and lateral (anterior) avulsion fractures. Although more detailed classifications have been published, these fractures are best classified by the location of the tibial spine and the size and displacement of the fragment.

ASSESSMENT

Physical Examination

After a history of the injury is obtained, the limb is examined for soft-tissue injury. Open wounds are uncommon and the timing of surgery and method of management are determined by the amount of contusion, abrasion, and swelling. Motor, sensory, and circulatory functions of the distal limb must be assessed. Because a suspected lateral spine avulsion fragment may in fact be a knee dislocation, circulatory integrity must be noted. The knee is assessed for effusion, for anteroposterior instability by the Lachman test and a positive drawer sign, and for medial and lateral instability.

Radiographic Evaluation

Tibial spine injuries are evaluated from AP, lateral, and tibial plateau radiographic views (Fig. 54).

Special Studies

Plane tomography or CT scans may be used as supplemental diagnostic tools to delineate fracture detail. Computerized tomography scans with lateral or three-dimensional reconstructions can be substituted for plane tomography. Magnetic resonance imaging may delineate ligamentous or meniscal injuries in small lateral tibial spine fractures.

EMERGENT MANAGEMENT

After physical and radiographic evaluations are completed, the knee is splinted and the limb is assessed frequently

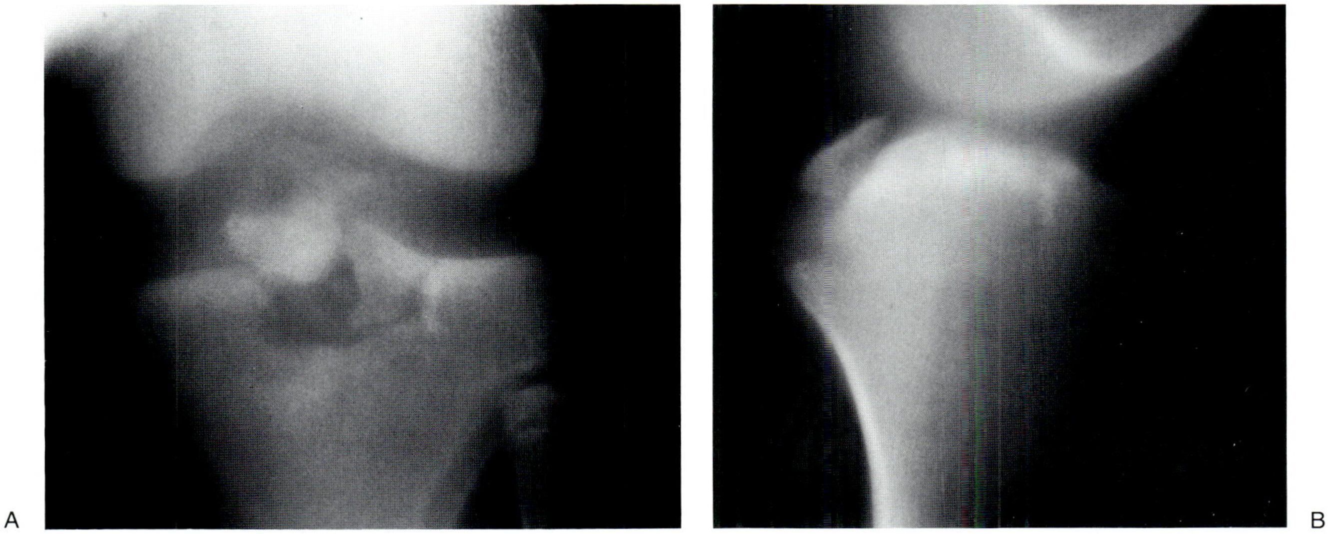

FIG. 54. AP (**A**) and lateral (**B**) tomograms show the extent of tibial PCL avulsion with extension into eminence.

for the next 12 to 24 h. Arteriography is indicated in the presence of severe soft-tissue injury, abnormal distal pulses, or questionable findings on duplex scans.

DEFINITIVE MANAGEMENT

The amount of displacement of a medial spine avulsion is determined by reviewing the preoperative radiographs and tomograms or CT scan. This information must be combined with the results of a posterior sag test or a positive posterior drawer sign. Instability with 3 mm to 5 mm of displacement of the medial spine fragment is managed by ORIF. The surgical approach for lateral spine avulsions is determined by evaluating the ligamentous and capsular integrity of the contralateral knee. Radiographs and CT scans are obtained to determine the size of the bone fragment and to assess the technical possibility of spine-fragment fixation. Magnetic resonance imaging may be useful to determine the status of other ligaments as well. The need for meniscal repair or partial resection may be determined by arthroscopy.

The decision to stabilize a PCL avulsion fragment operatively is based on the amount of displacement, the instability of the knee, and the age and functional requirements of the patient. Significant posterior knee instability usually warrants operative stabilization in all but the most debilitated patients. Tomograms or CT reconstructions are scrutinized to determine the location of the fragment in relation to the posterior tibial plateau landmarks. A tourniquet should be applied during surgery unless an arterial injury is known to exist. The patient is positioned prone and the leg is draped free. A posterior approach to the proximal tibia is made with careful blunt retraction (Fig. 55). One or more genicular

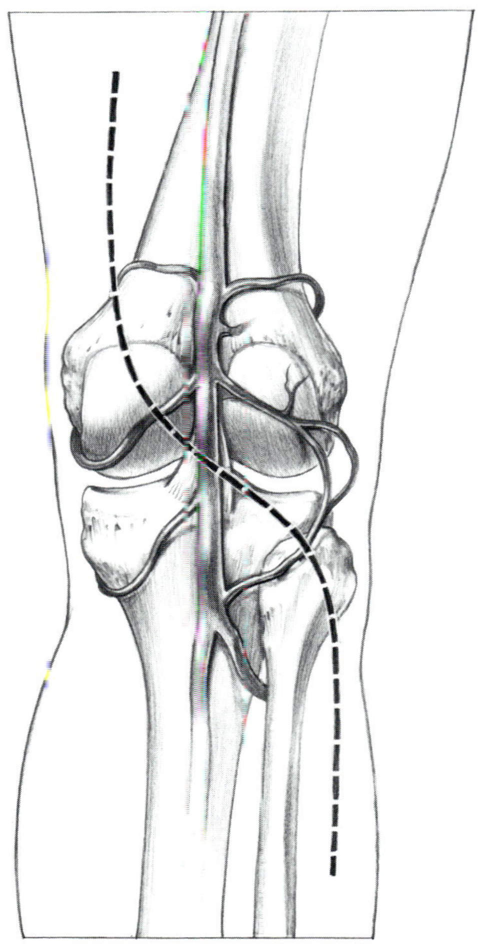

FIG. 55. The Trickey approach to a posterior knee joint. A lazy-S incision avoids tendency to skin contracture.

veins or arteries may require clipping and division and those areas should be observed carefully when the tourniquet is deflated. No clamping should be done with this popliteal approach unless the area to be clamped can be visualized clearly and bleeding can be controlled proximally and distally. Large fracture fragments are stabilized with two 3.5-mm or 4-mm cortical lag screws or cancellous screws placed in line with the PCL (Figs. 56 and 57; see also Figs. 53 and 54). Spiked washers (2.7 mm) can be added to trap small comminuted fracture fragments. Except for posterior instability or severe combined instabilities, PCL midsubstance tears are treated nonoperatively or by the bone–patellar tendon–bone reconstruction technique.

Preoperative planning for lateral tibial spine injuries is influenced by the age and functional requirements of the patient, associated ligament instabilities, and the findings on the arthroscopic examination or MRI. Patients with minor injuries and combined medial collateral ligament and capsular avulsion injuries require operative repair. Young patients with tibial spine fragments larger than 8 mm or those with demanding functional requirements warrant screw fixation with 3.5-mm cortical lag screws or 4.0-mm cancellous screws. If repair is necessary, open repair through a medial arthrotomy is preferred to arthroscopy. The capsular avulsion fragments can be fixed with lag screws with spike washers. Medial collateral ligament lesions are not repaired when they occur as isolated injuries. Lesions that occur concurrently with capsular avulsion injuries are repaired with screws and washers or with spiked staples. The flap tears are resected. Resections in the posterior horn are done arthroscopically.

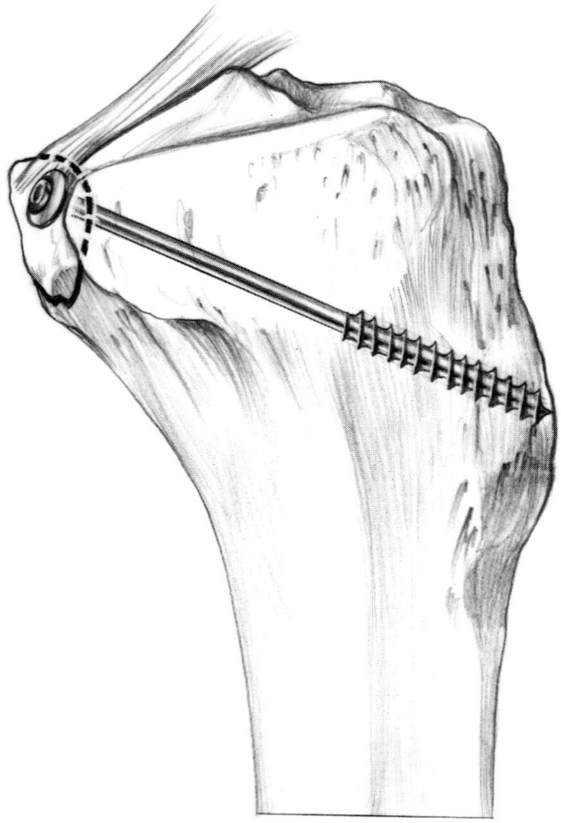

FIG. 56. Lateral view of a PCL avulsion stabilized with two 4-mm lag screws and washers.

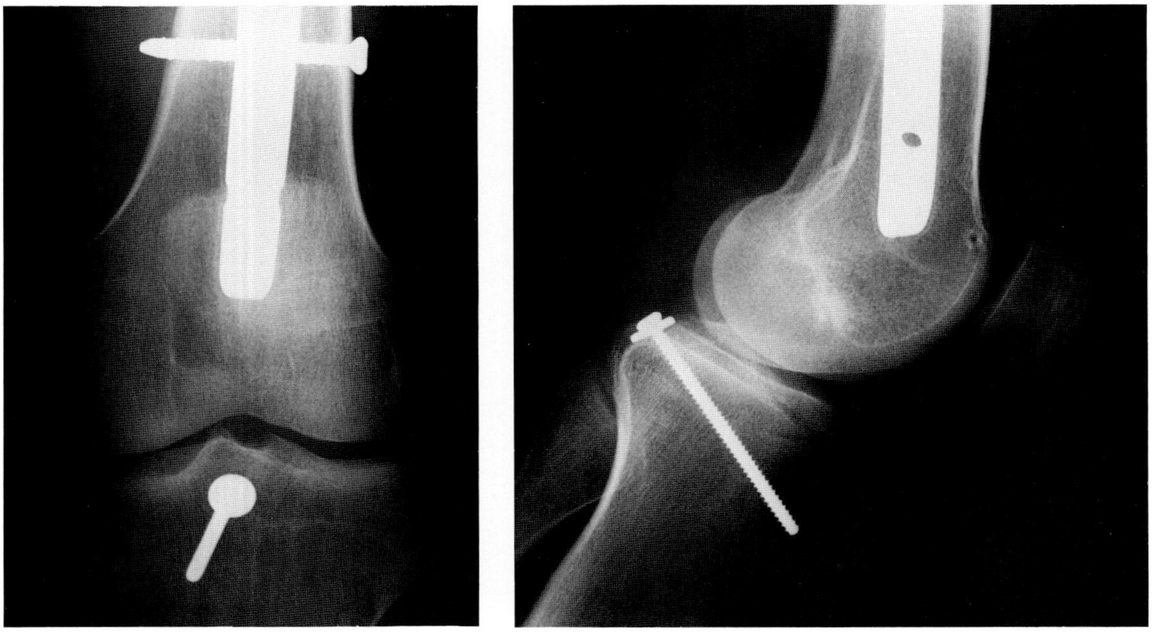

A B

FIG. 57. AP (**A**) and lateral (**B**) roentgenograms following open reduction with 3.5-mm lag screw fixation of PCL avulsion with washer.

The postoperative management of medial tibial spine avulsions with associated PCL injuries includes CPM and hinged knee-brace support. Full extension is achieved slowly over 3 to 4 weeks. The knee brace, which applies varus and valgus stresses in full extension, is used concurrently with touch-down weight-bearing for 8 weeks. Rehabilitation of lateral tibial spine repairs depends on the presence of associated ligament injuries and other repairs. Most injuries are treated with CPM, knee-bracing, and touch-down weight-bearing. A meniscal repair may restrict ROM in the brace.

COMPLICATIONS

Malunion or nonunion may result in blocked extension. This complication is usually associated with injuries to the lateral spine and can be avoided by confirming full extension intraoperatively. Depending on when the injury occurred, extension may be restored by reduction and fixation or by resection and possible reconstruction. Severely disabling chronic instability may be improved by ligamentous reconstruction.

SKELETALLY IMMATURE PATIENTS

Tibial spine avulsion fractures, especially lateral spine avulsions, are common in children. Closed reduction under anesthesia is usually appropriate when the fragment is elevated more than 5 mm; extending the limb fully usually reduces this fracture. Medial spine avulsions may also reduce spontaneously in full extension. When the fracture is reduced in this manner, the leg is casted in extension for 6 weeks and rehabilitated gradually. If the fracture cannot be reduced by extension and displacement is greater than 5 mm, the preoperative evaluation and operative approach are identical to those for adults.

Orthopaedic Trauma Protocols, edited by
Sigvard T. Hansen, Jr., and Marc F. Swiontkowski,
Raven Press, Ltd., New York, © 1993.

CHAPTER 27

Tibial Shaft Fractures

Marc F. Swiontkowski

MECHANISMS OF INJURY

Tibial shaft fractures caused by high-energy trauma usually occur in young active adults. The mechanisms of most high-energy fractures are automobile, motorcycle, or car–pedestrian accidents. Most commonly, high-energy fractures result from bumper injuries and are associated with other injuries in the ipsilateral limb and the contralateral tibia. Low-energy fractures may occur secondary to athletic injuries or twisting falls. The amount of energy absorbed by a fracture, which can be estimated from the history of injury, strongly influences the timing and the type of treatment.

ANATOMIC CONSIDERATIONS

Because the medial border of the tibia is subcutaneous, it is particularly vulnerable to open wounds from bony displacement. On the posterior aspect, the tibia is covered by muscle contained within the deep and superficial posterior compartments (Fig. 1). The structures most vulnerable to injury in widely displaced tibial midshaft fractures are the tibial artery and nerve. The lateral compartment of the peroneal muscles encases the middle third of the fibula. The ankle and toe dorsiflexors of the anterior compartment protect the anterolateral surface of the tibia. The deep peroneal nerve is most vulnerable to stretch injury and direct injury in the area where it crosses the neck of the fibula.

CLASSIFICATION

For management purposes, tibial shaft fractures are classified first by the degree of soft-tissue injury and next by the level of fracture, the presence of an associated fibular fracture, and the degree of comminution. The AO Comprehensive Classification of Long Bone Fractures is recommended for reporting purposes (Fig. 2) (1).

Department of Orthopaedics. Harborview Medical Center, University of Washington, Seattle, Washington 98104

ASSESSMENT

Physical Examination

A baseline neurovascular assessment must be conducted in an alert and cooperative patient after evaluation of head, chest, abdominal, pelvic, and spinal injuries. The neurologic assessment includes the status of motor function, sensory response to light touch and pinprick, and pain response to passive stretch. Whenever possible, the same examiner should perform all the serial evaluations for the first 12–24 h after admission. If the patient is unresponsive or has sustained a head injury, the anterior and deep posterior compartments are palpated for tenseness, and repeated or continuous monitoring of these compartmental pressures should be strongly considered. The dorsalis pedis and the posterior tibial pulses are palpated and an ultrasound Doppler examination should be performed if necessary. The size of the open wound and the degree of contamination are assessed and recorded and a Betadine dressing is placed over the wound. Repeated examinations of the wounds in the emergency department exposes the patient to infection and is discouraged. The knee and the ipsilateral femur are assessed for effusion, local tenderness, and contusions.

Radiographic Evaluation

When operative management is planned, high-quality AP and lateral radiographic views are supplemented with AP and lateral views of the uninjured side for thorough preoperative planning. The radiograph of the injured tibia must include the knee and the ankle and, when injury to either

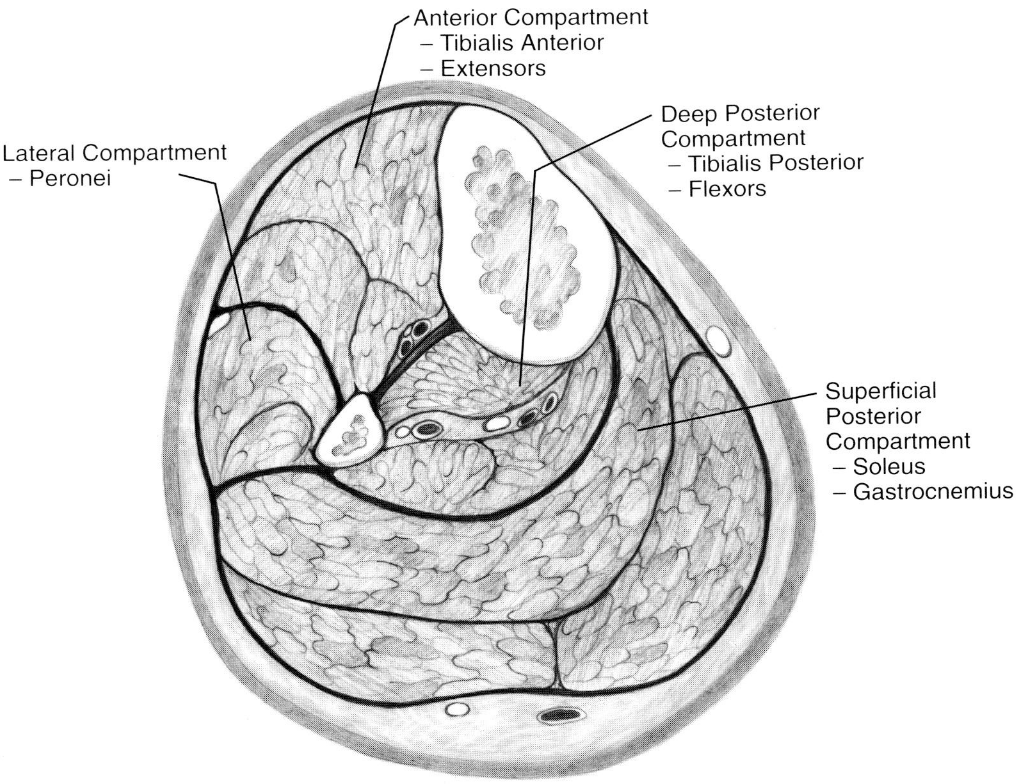

FIG. 1. Cross-section of the upper third of the lower leg.

structure is suspected, separate films of these joints must be obtained.

Special Studies

Arteriography is indicated in a well-aligned tibial fracture when pulses are absent or abnormal findings are revealed on the Doppler examination. The decision to order an arteriogram should be made in consultation with a vascular surgeon. Plane tomography and CT scanning are usually not indicated for tibial shaft fractures.

EMERGENT MANAGEMENT

The injured leg should be aligned, splinted, and examined at the site of the accident, and open wounds should be covered with sterile dressings. On arrival in the emergency department, the patient undergoes examination of the distal limb and the knee. A thorough evaluation of other injuries is critical for planning treatment of a tibial fracture. The most crucial aspect of the examination of the injured limb is assessment of compartmental function. When a tibial fracture occurs as an isolated injury, the patient should be hospitalized for serial examinations and limb elevation. Treatment options are discussed with the patient and the family. However, when a fracture occurs in association with other injuries, admission for evaluation becomes mandatory. When a patient is unable to cooperate with serial examinations conducted 1 to 2 hours apart, serial or continuous compartmental pressure measurements should be performed.

DEFINITIVE MANAGEMENT

The most important factor influencing treatment selection is the amount of soft-tissue injury (see Chapter 30). The second most important consideration is the extent of a patient's visceral injuries and other skeletal injuries. The method of stabilization must be chosen as soon as possible to allow time for adequate preoperative planning. Treatment methods for tibial shaft fractures include reduction and casting, external skeletal fixation, plate fixation, and reamed or unreamed intramedullary nailing. The indications and benefits of each method are discussed separately.

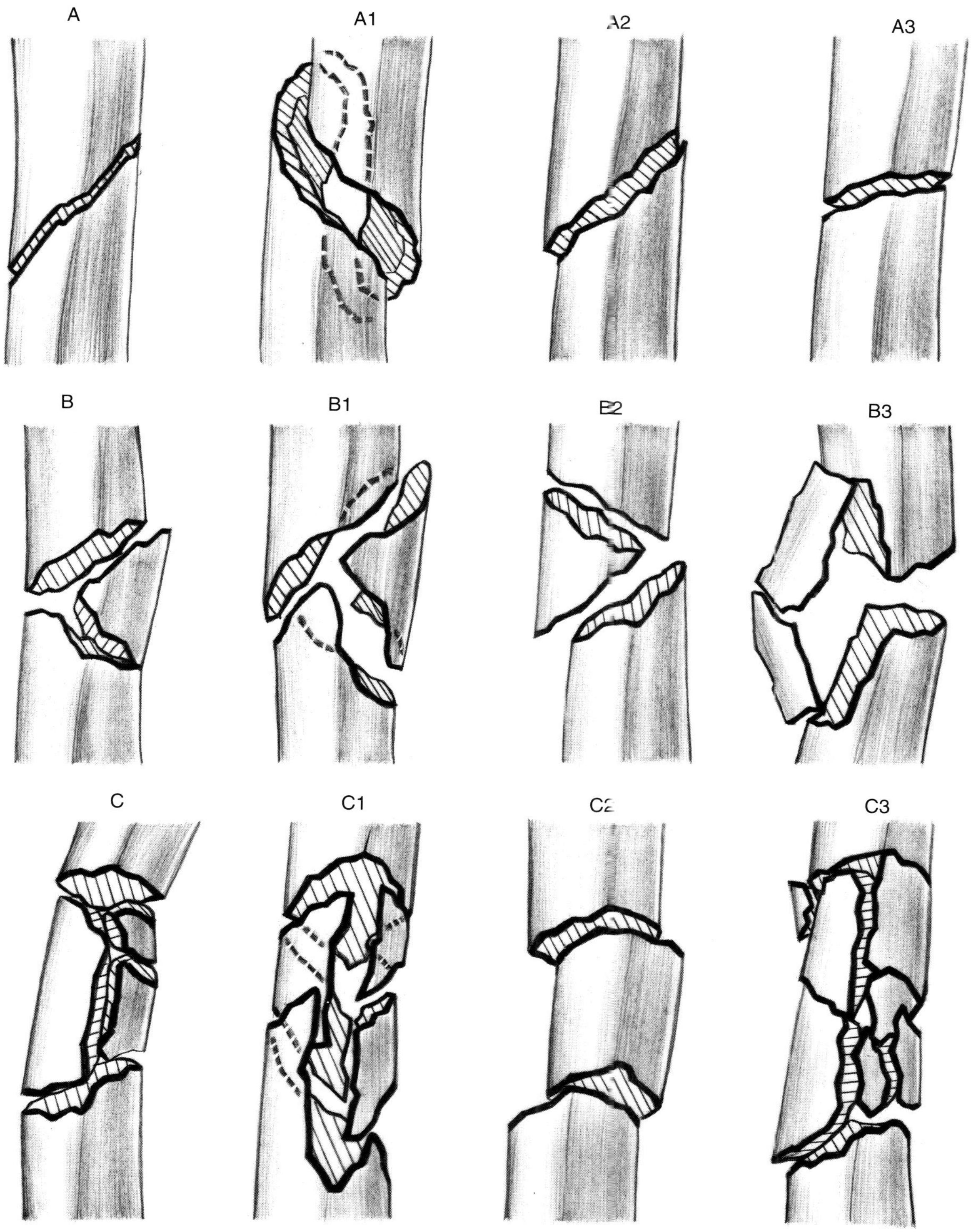

FIG. 2. AO classification of tibial fractures. (Adapted from Müller ME, Algöwer M, Schneider R, Willenegger H. *Manual of Internal Fixation,* 3rd ed. Berlin: Springer-Verlag, 1991. Müller ME, Nazarian S, Koch P, Schatzker J. *Comprehensive Classification of Fractures of Long Bones.* Berlin: Springer-Verlag, 1990. Used with permission.)

Reduction and Casting

Closed reduction and casting are a viable consideration only in closed, low-energy fractures in young patients. The periosteum of young patients is biologically active and fractures in these patients require shorter healing times. The long-term effects of joint immobilization in young patients are inconsequential. Fracture patterns that are stable in length (transverse, short oblique, or minimally displaced fractures) are best suited to this treatment. Good anatomic results are achieved only when the fibula has also been fractured. Closed treatment of the tibia is usually contraindicated when the fibula is intact because the tibia has a tendency to heal in varus (2). Patients with tibial fractures graded higher than C-0 should be hospitalized for observation and serial examinations for compartmental syndrome.

Closed reduction may be accomplished after administration of spinal anesthesia or brief general anesthesia. General anesthesia is preferred to allow accurate early evaluation of compartmental function. The patient lies supine and the fractured limb is allowed to hang over the edge of the operating table. The fracture is reduced by plantarflexing the ankle and applying linear traction. For reduction of a transverse fracture pattern, the deformity can be recreated to "lock on" the distal fragment. After the reduction maneuver is performed, a plaster cast is applied to the leg. While the surgeon controls the reduction, cool-water-dipped plaster is applied over a thin layer of Webril connecting the foot section to the lower leg section. The reduction is evaluated by fluoroscopy with the knee in flexion after the short-leg section of the cast has been applied. Full-length radiographs are obtained to confirm the fracture alignment after the above-knee section of the cast has been applied. Angulation must not exceed 5° in any plane.

After reduction, patients are hospitalized for 24 to 36 h for serial examinations to rule out compartmental syndrome. If a patient experiences any abnormal sensations or motor function or has significant discomfort, the cast should be split anteriorly to the skin. Radiographs should be obtained on a weekly basis and wedges are made in the cast as necessary. The original plaster cast can be replaced with a fracture brace in less than 6 weeks or with a short-leg patellar tendon-bearing cast 6 to 8 weeks after injury.

External Skeletal Fixation

Although other fixation devices, such as unreamed tibial nails, are widely used in tibial fractures with significant soft-tissue injuries, external skeletal fixation continues to be the principal treatment method for open grade III tibial fractures and fractures in children (3). The greatest advantage of using external skeletal fixation in high-grade injuries lies in preventing further disruption of the osseous circulation by placing the half-pins far from the fracture site. The most important aspects of preoperative care are accurate evaluation of the wound and grading of the soft-tissue injuries. Radiographs are examined for the presence of foreign material and for grading according to displacement, comminution, and the level of the fracture. The need for careful debridement increases with greater amounts of contamination, displacement, and comminution. Radical resection of free bone fragments results in lower rates of deep infection. In general, debridement should take as long to accomplish as the time anticipated to place the external fixator.

In unstable fractures, the more experienced surgeon should hold the reduction in place while an assistant applies the frame. Pointed reduction forceps or a short DCP may be used to hold the reduction temporarily, but these devices should not be used if they will further strip the bone. Fixation is provided by 5-mm Schanz screws used as half-pins. In general, the most proximal pin is applied distal to the tibial tubercle. The holes for the Schanz screws should be predrilled with a water-cooled 3.5-mm drill bit. Paying special attention to correct rotation, the fracture is then reduced and the distal half-pin is applied, making sure that the connecting rod overlies the tibia. Radiographic visualization can be enhanced by using 300-mm or 350-mm carbon-fiber rods. Fluoroscopy is useful during this phase of stabilization. When stacked rods are to be used, they must be applied before the second pin is placed because the clamps must be aligned perfectly over the tibial crest for accurate placement of all four pins. Four fixator pins are inserted through intact skin as close to the fracture site as the soft tissues allow and are spread as widely as possible through the fracture segments (Fig. 3). Pins placed distally near the tibialis anterior tendon loosen rapidly and pin placement in this area should be avoided if possible. When two bony segments maintain only limited contact or when a segmental defect exists, a second medial row of pins should be applied at 90° to the anterior row and the two bars should be interconnected. Pin placement, length, and reduction must be confirmed radiographically before the patient leaves the operating room.

The pin tracts are cleansed 2 or 3 times daily with cotton swabs soaked in peroxide. No ointments are applied. The presence of soft-tissue injury around the tibia requires immobilization of the ankle joint, and weight-bearing must be delayed until 6 weeks after injury. Dynamization, changing the arrangement of bars and locking nuts to compress the fracture fragments, should be done sequentially over 2 to 3 months. With fastidious pin care, the fixator frame can be maintained until the fracture has united. Premature conversion to a walking cast is the primary cause of malunion and nonunion. If conversion from external skeletal fixation to intramedullary nailing is being considered, it should be accomplished as soon as the soft tissues have healed. Conversion to reamed nails can be done safely within 2 to 3 weeks after injury but should not be done in the presence of a pin-tract infection. Patients must be informed that reamed nailing after external skeletal fixation is associated with a 20% to 40% rate of deep infection (3).

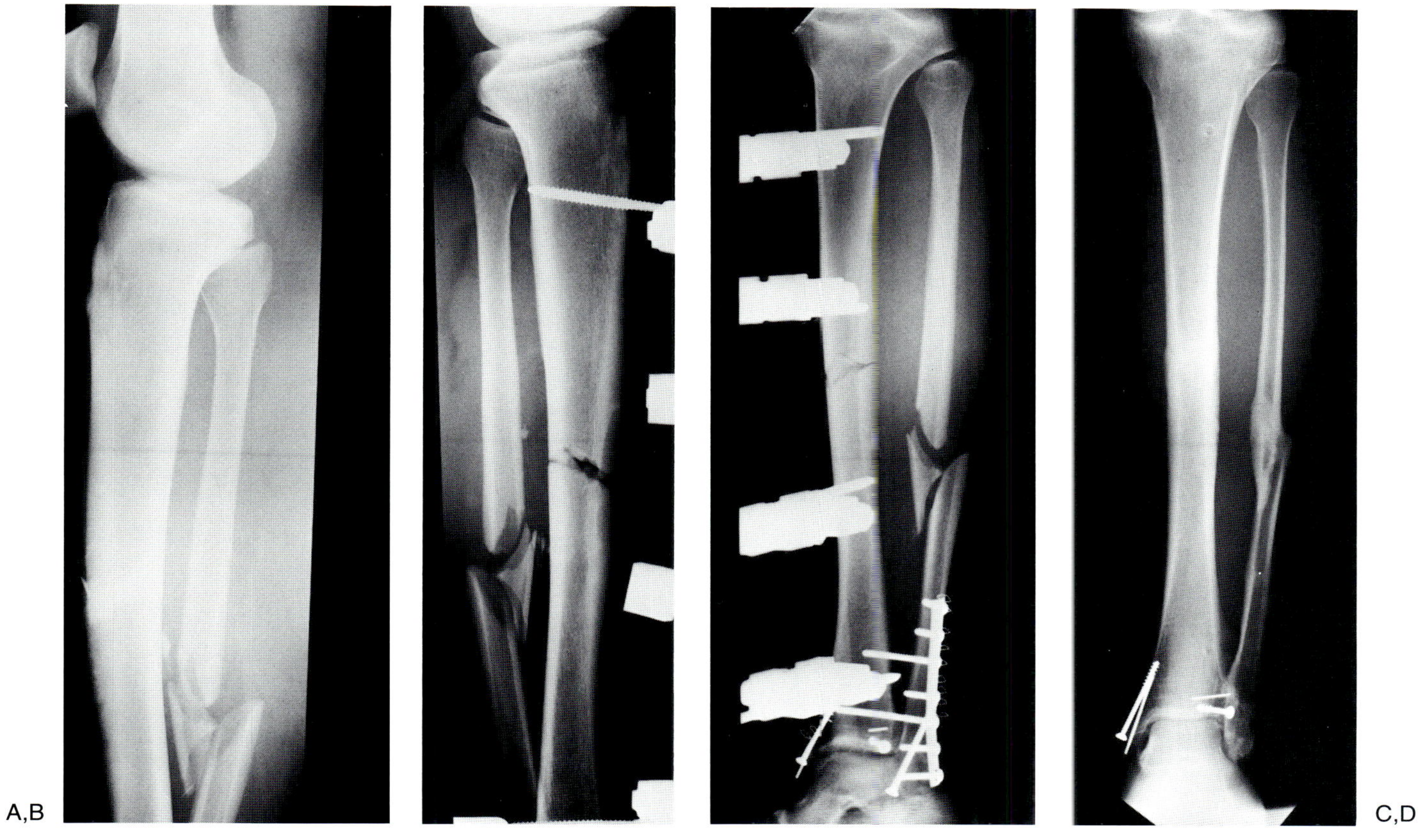

FIG. 3. **A:** A 22-year-old man with a grade IIIA open tibial shaft fracture and a IIIB open ankle fracture. **B:** Intraoperative radiograph with provisional stabilization. **C:** Postoperative AP view of tibia and ankle fixation. **D:** Follow-up view at 2 years. There is no sign of osteomyelitis at either site. The patient has significant ankle discomfort with activity.

Plate Fixation

Open reduction and internal fixation with plating may be indicated in the management of tibial fractures. Plates can be applied to fractures with joint involvement or to displaced or angulated fractures that are located too proximally or too distally to be treated with intramedullary fixation. The length and the type of plate to be used, the position of the lag screws, and the surgical approach should be determined during preoperative planning. When fractures enter a joint, L-, T-, or tibial head buttress plates are generally used proximally and cloverleaf or modified semitubular plates are used distally. Compression plating with lag screws is usually indicated for closed fractures after a fasciotomy has been performed to decompress a compartmental syndrome. Plate fixation is rarely indicated for closed displaced fractures or open fractures (4). New "low-contact" plates are associated with less bone atrophy, and for this reason may be used more widely in the future for tibial diaphyseal fractures (Fig. 4). Useful reduction aids for tibial plate fixation include femoral distractors, articulated tensioning devices, and pointed bone clamps.

Several other considerations must be kept in mind when plating is planned. Soft-tissue stripping and tourniquet inflation must be kept to a minimum. Fully threaded cancellous screws are ordinarily used in the tibial metaphysis, whereas cortical screws are used in the tibial diaphysis. Active range-of-motion exercises can be started in compliant patients soon after fracture stabilization, although full weight-bearing should be delayed until fracture consolidation can be seen on radiographs, usually between 8 and 12 weeks.

Intramedullary Nailing

Intramedullary nailing is gaining wider acceptance in the treatment of closed tibial shaft fractures. Patients with closed isolated fractures that are amenable to closed management are fully informed of the risks and benefits associated with each management technique and are allowed to choose the procedure that will be performed. However, fractures in multiply injured patients are stabilized by the most optimal procedure established for each fracture grade. Reamed intramedullary nailing is the procedure of choice for grades 0

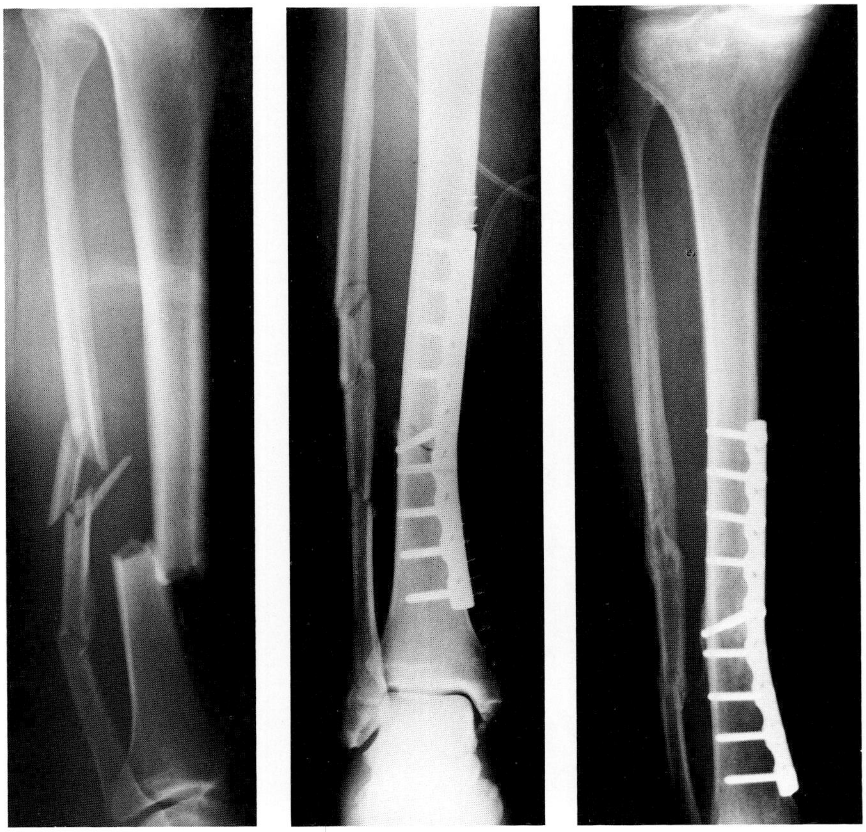

A,B,C

FIG. 4. Closed tibia and fibular fracture in a 60-year-old man with a grade IIIB open ipsilateral distal femur fracture. **A:** Preoperative view. **B:** Immediate postoperative view. **C:** Eighteen-month follow-up x-ray revealing uneventful union.

through II closed fractures. Unreamed interlocked nailing is preferred for grade I and II open fractures and is sometimes the best choice for grade IIIA and IIIB open fractures (3). Prospective comparative data must be published before external skeletal fixation is abandoned for the treatment of open grade III fractures.

A preoperative radiograph of the contralateral tibia is obtained to determine the appropriate length and diameter of the implant to be used. Radiographs of the injured side are examined to confirm a fracture's suitability for intramedullary fixation, a particularly important decision in very proximal or distal fractures. In both closed and open fractures, the size of the nail must correspond to the degree of soft-tissue injury: the greater the soft-tissue injury, the smaller the diameter of the nail. Reaming the tibial diaphysis results in necrosis of the endosteal surface and extensive reaming increases the incidence of complications. Reaming is begun with a reamer that is no larger in diameter than the narrowest portion of the tibial medullary canal on preoperative radiographs (usually around 8 mm). A tourniquet should never be used during reaming because it undermines the cooling effect of blood on the endosteal surface. Moreover, tourniquets should be avoided in all open fractures unless they serve a particular purpose (e.g., to assist dissection around a nerve).

Closed fractures are reduced on a fracture table with the foot on the injured side taped to the traction footplate. Alternatively, a calcaneal pin with a traction bow can be used. Minimal traction is usually required for reduction. The transverse post must not contact the popliteal fossae. The patellar tendon is retracted laterally through a linear midline incision. The tibial canal is reamed 0.5 mm to 1 mm wider than the diameter of the selected nail and the proximal end of the nail is buried within the bone. Distal interlocking is done freehand, the same as for femoral fractures, but this technique is easier to perform in the tibia because the soft-tissue coverage on the medial surface of the distal tibia is minimal (Fig. 5).

In open fractures, debridement remains the most critical aspect of the operation. The diameter of the tibial canal is determined by sizing nails or sounds to determine the size of the unreamed nail that may be used. A tibia diameter of 8 mm or 9 mm is required for internal fixation with unreamed nails. Fluoroscopy is useful for maneuvers in this area to ensure that the posterior cortex of the proximal tibia is not perforated by the nail. Proximal and distal locking procedures are identical. To prevent splitting the anterior cortex of the upper tibia, 9-mm and 10-mm reamers must occasionally be passed in the metaphysis only to allow the unreamed nail entry to the diaphysis (Fig. 6).

Active range of motion exercise in the knee and the ankle is begun immediately after internal fixation of closed tibial fractures. In open tibial fractures, the range of active knee and ankle motion is limited by the soft-tissue wounds. Casting is unnecessary in compliant patients. However, a night

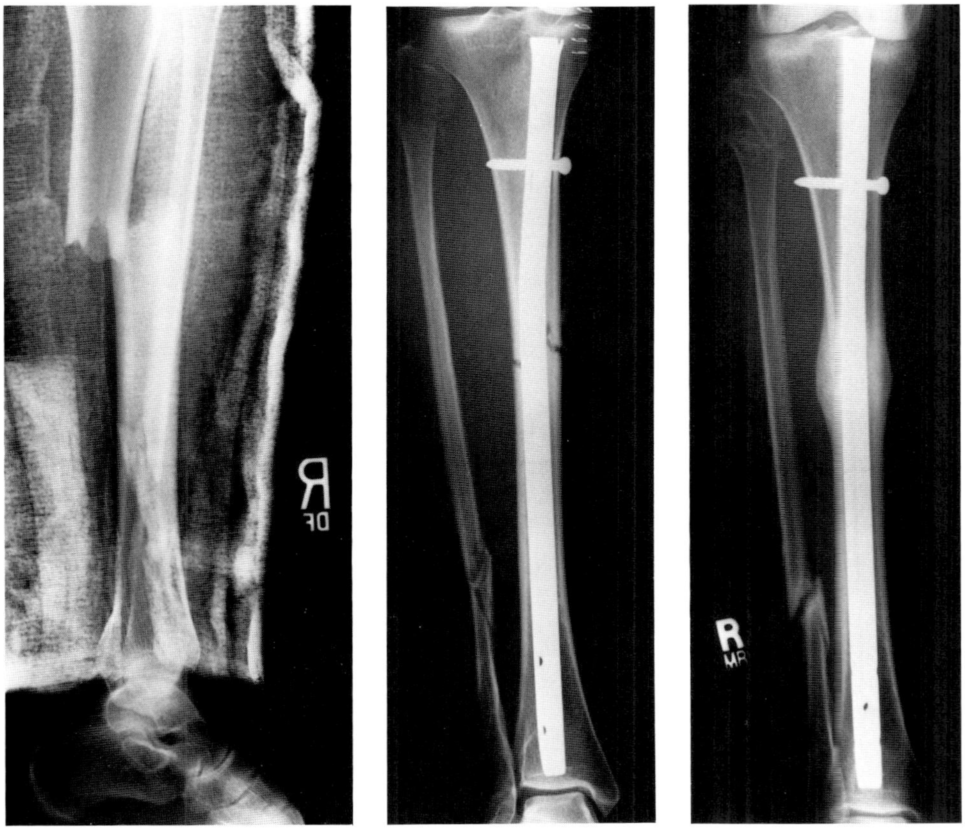

A,B,C

FIG. 5. A 29-year-old woman sustained this closed tibia–fibular fracture. In her opposite limb she sustained a grade IIIB open segmental tib-fib fracture. To facilitate an early return to function, this tibia was treated with closed, reamed nailing on the date of admission. **A:** Preoperative lateral view. **B:** Postoperative view showing dynamic interlocking nail. **C:** Follow-up at 1 year.

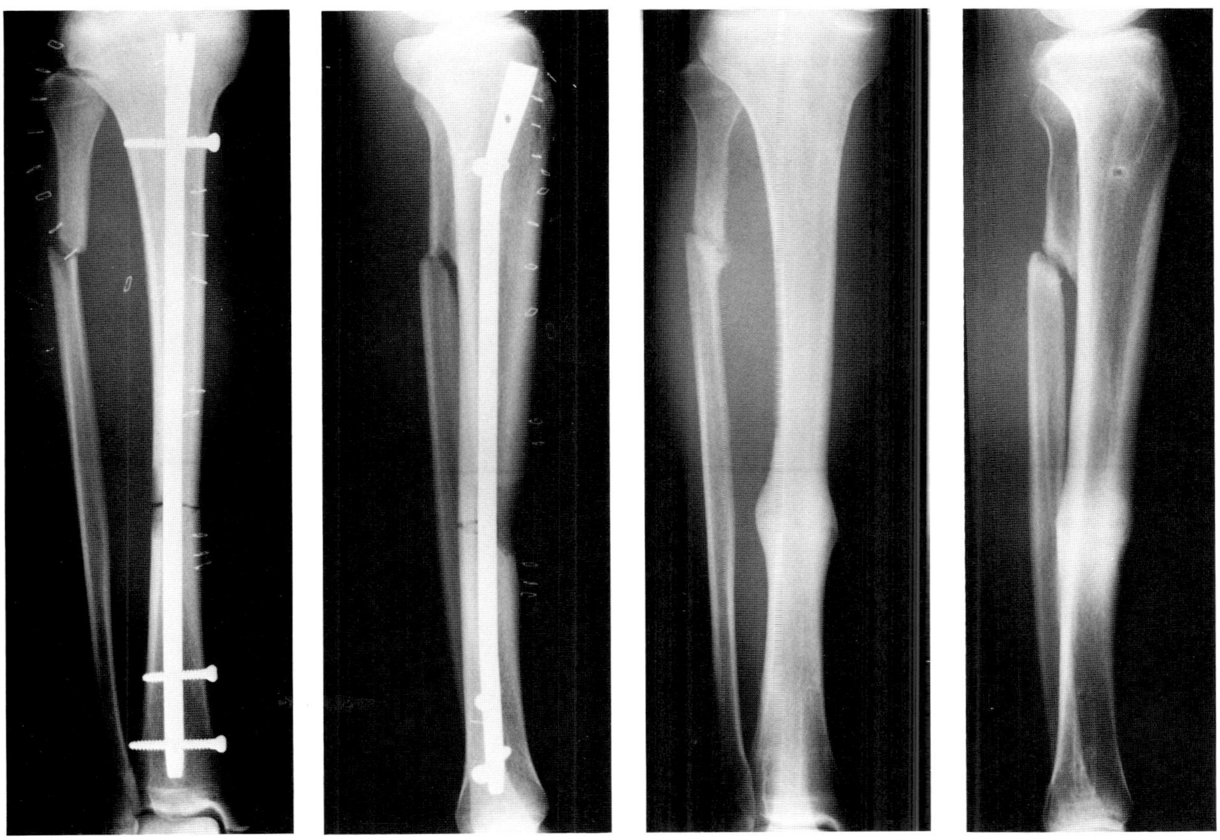

A,B

C,D

FIG. 6. A 25-year-old man sustained a grade IIIA open tib-fib fracture in a motorcycle accident. This was treated with debridement and unreamed interlocking nailing (8 mm). **A,B:** AP and lateral radiographs immediately post-op. **C,D:** Eighteen-month follow-up radiographs.

splint in a neutral position or a bivalved cast may be useful to prevent equinus deformity. Weight-bearing is restricted to touch-down weight until callus formation is evident on radiographs. After callus formation is evident, weight-bearing is permitted without dynamization (removal of a cross-screw) with reamed or unreamed nailing. Closed fractures treated by reamed nailing heal within 4 to 6 months; open fractures treated by unreamed nailing heal within 6 to 12 months. When unreamed nails have been used, the locking screws, and occasionally the nail itself, can break with full weight-bearing. Failure of a fixation device may be attributed to the prolonged healing time required for an open fracture.

COMPLICATIONS

Compartmental syndromes can occur in both closed and open fractures and must be treated by four-compartment fasciotomy and stabilization of the fracture. When the tibia is exposed for fasciotomy, plate fixation becomes a viable option for stabilization (Fig. 7). Alternatively, unreamed nailing may be performed, but casting and external skeletal fixation are to be avoided in this setting. Deep infection can develop with open treatment of closed fractures but occurs more commonly after open fractures. Infection is managed by debridement, intravenous antibiotics, and muscle-flap coverage if soft-tissue coverage is a problem, but the implant should be left in place if it continues to provide fracture stability. Deep infections following intramedullary nailing can be treated in the same way provided that the patient is not septic. Fractures that develop infection after the intramedullary nail is already in place usually heal, and the drainage resolves after the nail is removed and the tibial canal is overreamed by 1 mm to 2 mm.

Nonunion can be treated by intramedullary nailing if no infection is present. Caution must be observed if external skeletal fixation was applied during the acute phase of treatment. When an injury contraindicates nailing or when translation at the nonunion site requires extensive stripping of the soft tissues, a plate can be applied. Bone graft from the iliac crest is orinarily used to supplement the fixation under these circumstances. Malunion may occur after any type of treatment. Angulatory deformities of less than 10° are usually managed conservatively. Shortening that exceeds 2 cm may warrant operative intervention. Closed femoral shortening of the longer leg is the safest and the most predictably successful procedure to treat limb-length inequality.

SKELETALLY IMMATURE PATIENTS

Pediatric tibial fractures are almost always managed in closed fashion. External skeletal fixation is usually used to stabilize open or closed fractures with significant shortening in multiply injured children. Intramedullary nailing is contraindicated in the presence of an open upper tibial physis. A rare indication for plating is a closed fracture in a multiply injured child; the plate should be removed after 9 to 12 months to prevent its encasement in bone. Obviously, this precaution is most important in children under the age of 10 years. In isolated fractures, a long-leg cast can be converted to a patellar tendon-bearing cast or a brace after 4 weeks.

Senior Editor's Note: The new 3.5-mm LC-DCP may prove useful in both closed and open tibial fractures in multiply injured children when it is applied according to good surgical principles, including indirect reduction. The infection rate associated with this plate promises to be very low because its effect on bone circulation is minimal and removal is simple. The shape of the plate and the site of application over the periosteum suggest that it is less likely to become encased in bone.

REFERENCES

1. Müller ME, Nazarian S, Koch P. *The classification of fractures.* Translated by J. Schatzker, Toronto. Berlin: Springer-Verlag; 1988.
2. Teitz CC, Carter DR, Frankel VH. Problems associated with tibial fractures with intact fibulae. *J Bone Joint Surg* 1980;62A:77–776.
3. Holbrook JL, Swiontkowski MF, Sanders R. Treatment of open fractures of the tibial shaft: Ender nailing vs. external fixation. A randomized, prospective comparison. *J Bone Joint Surg* 1989;71A:1231–1238.
4. Bach AW, Hansen ST. Plates versus external fixation in severe open tibial shaft fractures: A randomized trial. *Clin Orthop* 1989;241:89-94.

Orthopaedic Trauma Protocols, edited by
Sigvard T. Hansen, Jr., and Marc F. Swiontkowski,
Raven Press, Ltd., New York, © 1993.

CHAPTER 28

Foot and Ankle Joint

Bruce J. Sangeorzan, M.D.

Ankle Fractures and Dislocations

MECHANISMS OF INJURY

Most ankle fractures are caused by indirect rotatory forces or by forced abduction or adduction. Dislocations usually occur on the posteromedial aspect of the ankle in young people who are predisposed to generalized ligament laxity (1). Syndesmosis rupture is uncommon but should be ruled out.

Tibial plafond fractures also involve the ankle joint but are distinct injuries. This fracture usually results from direct force applied to the weight-bearing surface of the distal tibial plafond and results in extensive damage to the articular surface. Dislocation of the ankle in the absence of a fracture is uncommon. However, this injury may be caused by forced inversion and axial loading on a foot in maximal plantar flexion. The injury is usually posteromedial and occurs in young people; generalized ligament laxity seems to be a predisposing condition. In a closed injury, closed reduction and casting usually produce a satisfactory result. In an open injury, open reduction and primary repair of the lateral ligaments are indicated. Syndesmosis rupture is uncommon but should be ruled out.

ANATOMIC CONSIDERATIONS

For the ankle joint to function normally, the distal fibula must be realigned to the distal tibia by stabilizing the talar mortise and restoring the rotation and the length of the fibula. The clear space between the injured distal tibia and fibula must be reduced to less than 5 mm, and the talocrural angle must be reduced to within 3° of the normal angle on the contralateral side.

Department of Orthopaedics, Harborview Medical Center, University of Washington, Seattle, Washington 98104

CLASSIFICATION

Two classification systems are used to describe ankle fractures. The first, proposed by Lauge–Hansen (2), describes ankle fractures in terms of the position of the foot and the direction of the deforming force at the moment of injury. This classification consists of four categories: supination–adduction, supination–eversion, pronation–abduction, and pronation–eversion. The severity of each type of fracture is further subdivided into stages of injury. The Danis–Weber classification (1) categorizes ankle fractures by the location of the fibular fracture in relation to the syndesmosis and the interosseous ligament (Fig. 1).

Class A: Fractures located distal to the interosseous ligament and the syndesmosis.

Class B: Fractures involving part or all of the syndesmosis (syndesmotic instability is seen approximately 50% of the time).

Class C: Unstable fractures located above the syndesmosis with syndesmotic ligament and interosseous membrane involvement.

ASSESSMENT

Physical Examination

The ankle is examined for skin integrity, the presence of posterior tibial and dorsalis pedis pulses, and hindfoot and forefoot deformities. A flexion or extension deformity in the toes may be indicative of an entrapped tendon. Excessive skin tension over the pretibial area should be corrected immediately by distraction before the radiographic evaluation is performed.

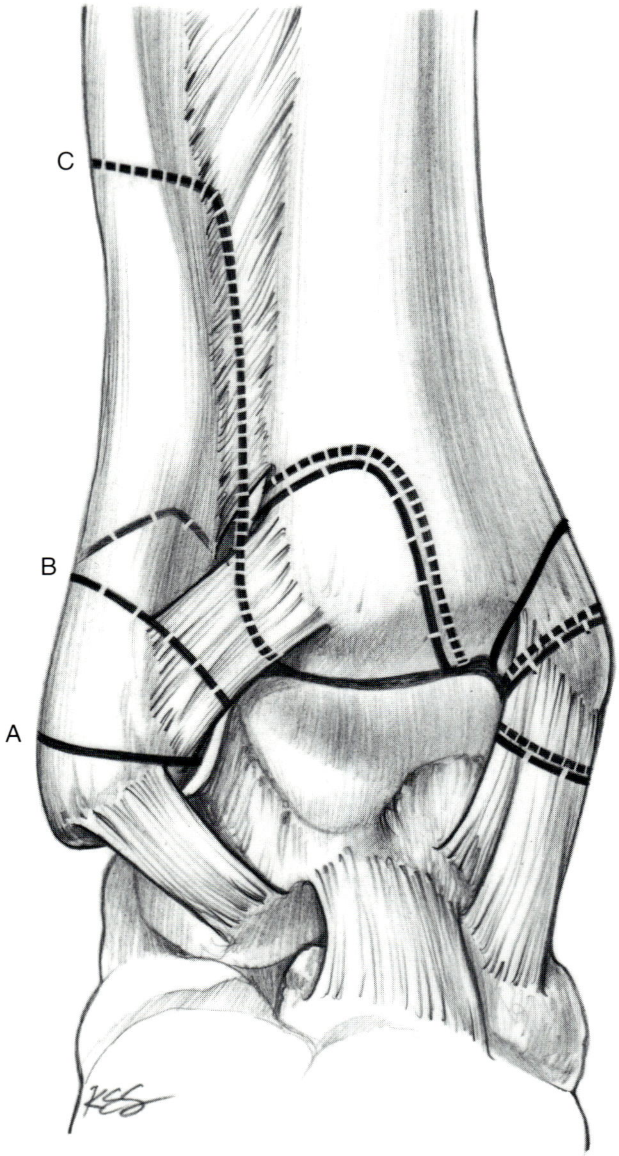

FIG. 1. Diagrammatic representation of the Danis–Weber classification system.

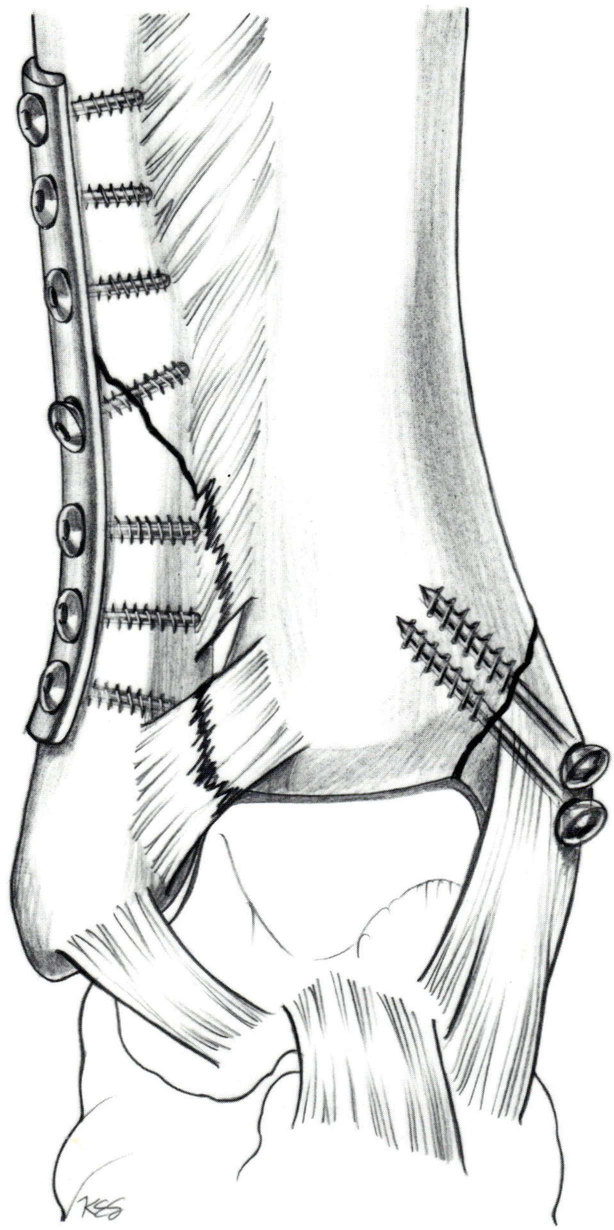

FIG. 2. Standard fixation for an unstable ankle fracture.

Radiographic Evaluation

Mortise and lateral radiographic views are taken with the foot in a plantigrade position. Fractures, diastasis of the distal tibiofibular joint, and osteochondral lesions can be seen on radiographs. When a fracture is not evident but a medial injury and widening of the ankle are noted, the anteroposterior and lateral radiographs of the entire tibia and fibula should be examined for a proximal fibular fracture.

Special Studies

Tomograms of tibial plafond fractures are frequently required to assess displacement of the articular surface.

EMERGENT MANAGEMENT

Severely displaced ankle fractures should be reduced closed and splinted without delay to limit swelling and prevent skin necrosis. Delaying treatment for as long as 12 hours is associated with a high incidence of morbidity and skin slough. Open fractures are treated by debridement and internal fixation within 4 to 6 hours after injury (3).

DEFINITIVE MANAGEMENT

Most ankle dislocations and some fractures can be reduced closed by reversing the force of the injury after the patient is sedated with a hematoma block. With this technique the talus is replaced in its normal anatomic position within the mortise, and the length of the fibula is restored by appropriate rotation. Ankle injuries that are reduced closed are immobilized in a cast for 6 weeks. Nonoperative treatment is usually inappropriate in multiply injured patients because the presence of associated wounds or the need for mobility may contraindicate casting.

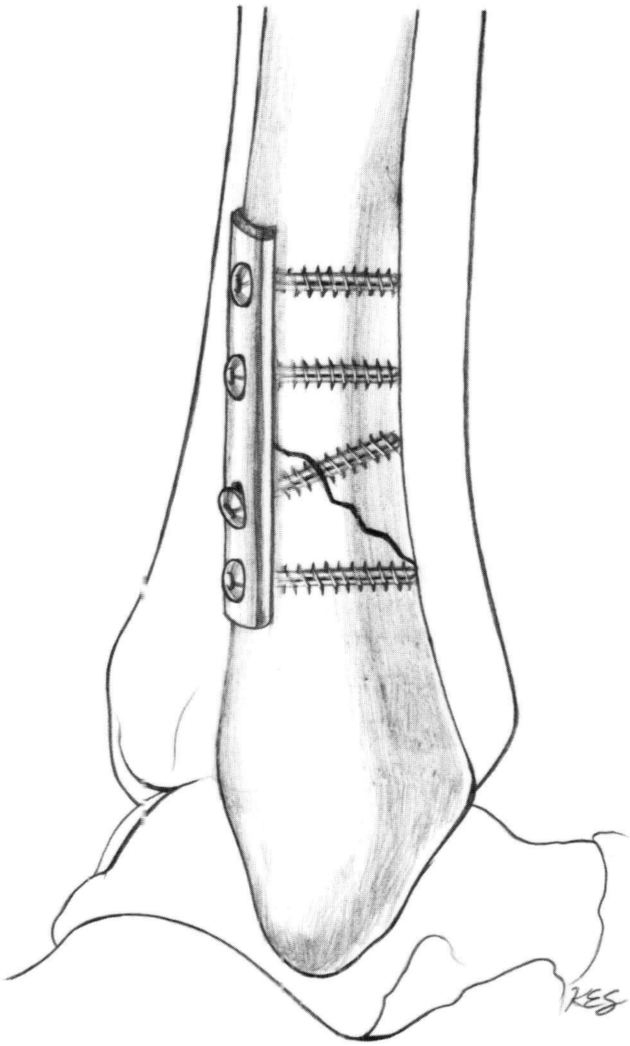

FIG. 3. The lateral view of an ankle fracture fixed by the anti-glide technique. Placement of the two distal screws is optional.

Ankle Fractures

Operative stabilization of a bimalleolar ankle fracture is done through a double incision. The first incision is made laterally over the fibula and the second is made anteromedially, curving gradually along the medial malleolus. The joint is visualized and inspected for loose debris and osteochondral fragments through the medial incision.

The fibula is reduced first and is stabilized with a lateral plate; next, the medial malleolus is fixed with screws (Fig. 2) (4). The anti-glide plating technique (Fig. 3) is used on oblique fibular fractures to inhibit the distal oblique fragment from gliding along the fracture when load is applied (5). The most important part of this technique is to apply the plate at the apex of the fracture so that the direction of displacement is converted to a compression force at the fracture line. The plate is usually applied posteriorly to the apex of the fracture, where it wedges the distal fragment between the plate and the proximal fragment (see Fig. 3).

An ankle fracture stabilized with rigid plate-and-screw fixation is immobilized in a restricted weight-bearing cast or splint until evidence of healing is demonstrated on radiographs. After the cast is removed, early motion is begun in a removable brace. In a cooperative patient in whom rigid fixation has been achieved, motion can be initiated after wound healing is ensured. A short-leg nonweight-bearing cast may be used for 8 weeks on noncompliant patients, and unrestricted weight-bearing should be postponed until the fracture has healed. Isometric exercises in the cast are encouraged.

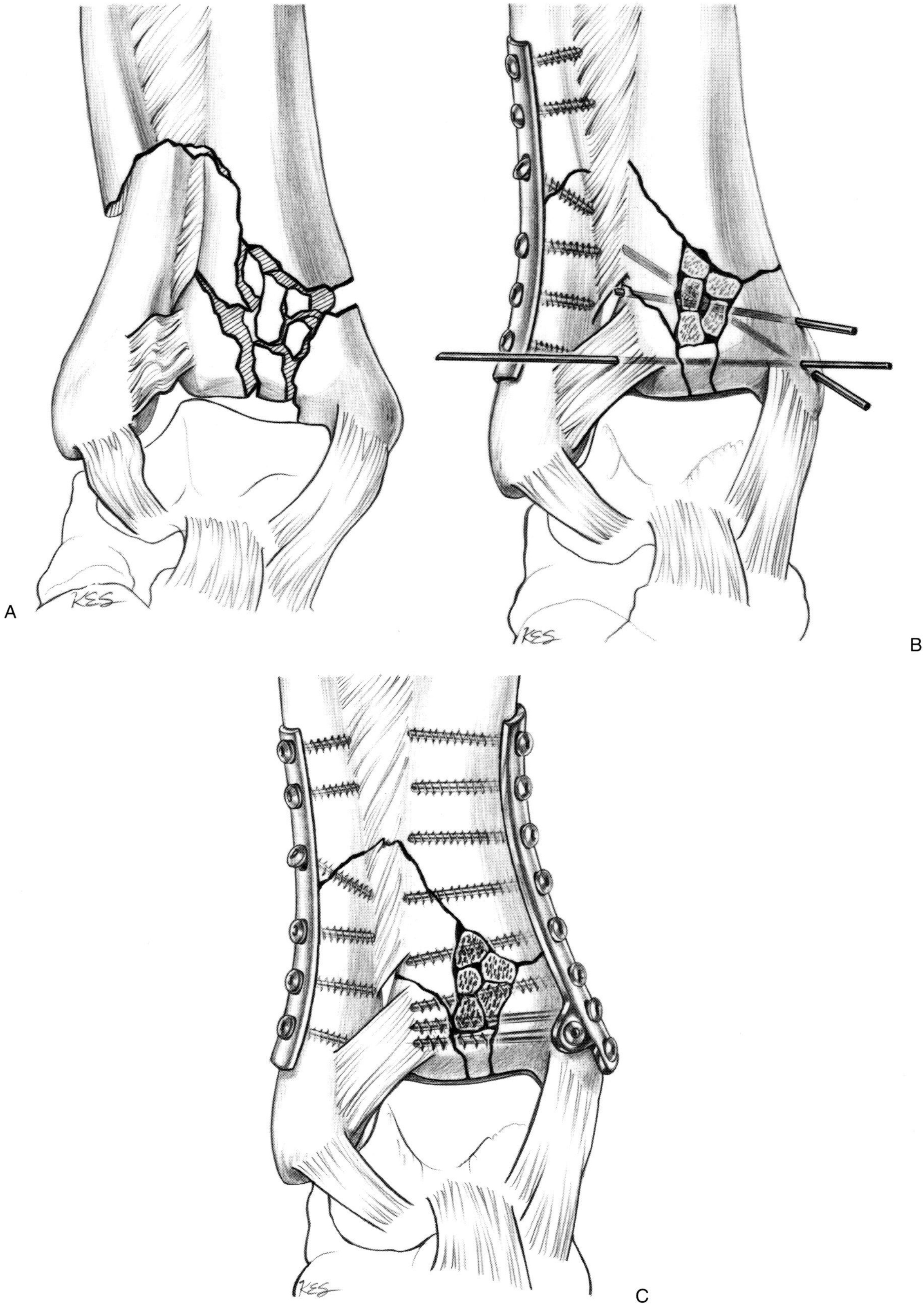

FIG. 4. A: A typical type III tibial plafond fracture. **B:** The length of the fibula has been restored and is held securely by a plate. The articular surface of the tibia has been provisionally fixed with Kirschner wires. **C:** A cloverleaf buttress plate is applied medially and the defect is filled with bone graft.

Tibial Plafond Fractures

Tibial plafond fractures are caused by axial loading and result in comminution of the weight-bearing surface (Fig. 4A). These fractures are more difficult to treat and the operation is accomplished step by step:

1. The length of the fibula is restored and the fibula is plated.
2. The articular surface of the tibia is reconstructed to the stable fibula and the attached tibial fragment.
3. The articular surface first is fixed provisionally with Kirschner wires, then definitively with screws (Fig. 4B).
4. The defect is filled with bone graft.
5. A buttress plate is applied (Fig. 4C).

A cloverleaf plate, applied anteromedially along the distal tibia, is the most widely accepted fixation for a tibial plafond fracture. Incisions advocated by the AO group are used—a lateral incision is made over the fibula and an anterior incision is made parallel to the anterior tibial tendon. A skin bridge at least 7 cm wide should be maintained between these two incisions.

The soft-tissue envelope around the distal fibula and the tibia is tenuous and is easily injured by a high-energy injury, a direct blow, or delayed reduction. The injury is usually located too distal to allow local rotational skin flaps, and soft-tissue loss is therefore treated aggressively by early free-flap coverage. Because the weight-bearing surface of the distal tibia is disrupted with this injury, weight-bearing is postponed until the fracture shows evidence of solid consolidation, in some cases longer than 6 months. In general, ROM exercises can be instituted early. Healing is monitored by radiographs obtained at 2, 6, and 12 weeks, then at monthly intervals until the fracture has united.

COMPLICATIONS

The appearance of a large metaphyseal defect after reduction may be indicative of delayed union. If the fracture does not show significant callus formation by 12 postoperative weeks, bone grafting is recommended.

SKELETALLY IMMATURE PATIENTS

Minimally displaced ankle fractures in children are immobilized in cast without reduction. Fractures involving the joint and physeal injuries warrant the same detailed open reduction and internal fixation as adult injuries. Complex distal tibial fractures, including triplane injuries, may require a thorough evaluation of CT scans or tomograms. Anatomic reduction of these fractures can be maintained by a screw placed through the epiphysis parallel to the physeal cartilage.

REFERENCES

1. Colville MR, Colville JM, Manoli A II. Posteromedial dislocation of the ankle without fracture. *J Bone Joint Surg* 1987;69A:706–11.
2. Lindsjö U. Classification of ankle fractures: the Lauge-Hansen or AO system? *Clin Orthop* 1985;199:12–16.
3. Franklin JL, Johnson KD, Hansen ST Jr. Immediate internal fixation of open ankle fractures. Report of thirty-eight cases treated with a standard protocol. *J Bone Joint Surg* 1984;66A 1349–56.
4. Müller ME, Allgöwer M, Schneider R, Willenegger H. *Manual of internal fixation.* Berlin: Springer-Verlag; 1990.
5. Schaffer JJ, Manoli A II. The anti-glide plate for distal fibular fixation: a biomechanical comparison with fixation with a lateral plate. *J Bone Joint Surg* 1987;69A:596–604.

Subtalar Dislocations

MECHANISMS OF INJURY

Forced inversion of a plantarflexed forefoot produces medial subtalar dislocations. Lateral subtalar dislocations occur when the foot is forced into eversion. The force required to dislocate the subtalar joint can be mild (a basketball inversion injury) or severe (an open lateral fracture–dislocation) (1–3). A subtalar dislocation is often associated with a facet fracture of the talocalcaneal joint. The edge of the lateral process or the posterior aspect of the posterior facet can fracture as the calcaneus glides out from underneath the talus. Lateral subtalar dislocations are associated with distal fibular fractures (3).

ANATOMIC CONSIDERATIONS

The talus and the calcaneus are joined by a strong talocalcaneal interosseous ligament that originates at the tarsal canal and courses through the tarsal sinus. The longest and strongest portion of this fibrous connection is the cervical ligament, which is found on the far lateral side of the talocalcaneal interosseous ligament. A fibrous capsule also surrounds the articular margins of the facets, but it is considerably weaker. The deltoid ligament bridges the dorsomedial side of the talonavicular joint. In medial dislocations, the head of the talus may be buttonholed between the extensor hallucis longus and the extensor digitorum longus.

CLASSIFICATION

Subtalar dislocations are usually described as medial or lateral. In both injuries the talocalcaneal joint is dislocated and the talonavicular and the calcaneocuboid joints remain reduced.

ASSESSMENT

Physical Examination

A subtalar dislocation is characterized by significant displacement of the hindfoot and possible tenting of neurovascular structures over bony prominences. The status of motor function and sensation and the position of the ankle are noted during examination. The soft-tissue coverage in this area is meager and the skin may be stretched taut over a bony prominence in a significant dislocation. Crepitus along the joint line may be indicative of a lateral process fracture or a minor facet fracture of the subtalar joint. The functions of the extensor hallucis longus and the other toe extensors are noted to rule out their entrapment under the head of the talus.

Radiographic Evaluation

Routine diagnostic radiographs include standard AP, lateral, and oblique views of the foot. After reduction, these radiographic views and Brodén's hindfoot oblique view are taken to assess the integrity of the subtalar joint.

Special Studies

If the integrity of the subtalar joint is in question or the presence of loose intraarticular bodies is suspected, a two-plane CT scan should be obtained.

EMERGENT MANAGEMENT

The significant deformity that accompanies a subtalar dislocation may threaten the blood supply to the soft tissues if reduction is delayed. For this reason, and to reduce the pressure on the tented neurovascular structures, immediate closed reduction should be attempted in the emergency department. Unless radiographs can be obtained immediately to diagnose a fracture and to delineate any occult fractures, reduction should be attempted without radiographic evaluation.

DEFINITIVE MANAGEMENT

Closed reduction is performed after an intraarticular injection of lidocaine. The reduction maneuver is performed gently with the knee bent to relax the gastrocsoleus musculature, and traction is applied to the heel and the midfoot until the hindfoot is pulled out to length. Postoperatively, the leg is immobilized in a short-leg nonweight-bearing cast for 3 weeks and then protected in a removable walking brace.

The criteria for open reduction in the operating room are significant displacement and failure of closed reduction (particularly of a laterally displaced dislocation with associated fracture). Operative management of a closed subtalar dislocation begins with a second attempt at closed reduction under anesthesia. The patient is positioned supine on the operating table, and the hip and knee are flexed past 90° to relax the gastrocnemius and soleus muscles. If the second attempt at closed reduction is unsuccessful, open reduction is warranted.

Medial dislocations usually can be reduced closed. When open reduction is necessary, an incision is tailored to fit the individual circumstances. A lateral longitudinal incision can be made parallel to the subtalar joint above the sural nerve, a medial incision can be made on the medial side of the joint, or both incisions may be required.

Lateral dislocations can be reduced through a medial incision that exposes the medial surfaces of the talar head and neck. The location of the tibialis posterior tendon and the flexor digitorum longus may impede reduction of the dislocation. A Freer elevator is applied to any soft tissues that are bow-strung around the talar head and neck.

Patients with closed dislocations that require open reduction are restricted to minimal weight-bearing for the first 2 weeks. The leg is immobilized in a short-leg walking cast for an additional 4 weeks. After ORIF of a facet fracture, patients remain nonweight-bearing for 6 to 8 weeks and ROM exercises are instituted after 3 weeks.

COMPLICATIONS

Restricted subtalar motion is a common sequella of this injury and is associated with immobilization lasting longer than 6 weeks. Recurrent dislocations are rare. A careful neurovascular examination should be performed after reduction to document the integrity of the neurovascular bundle. Avascular necrosis of the talus is rare.

SKELETALLY IMMATURE PATIENTS

Subtalar dislocations in children are treated in the same manner as dislocations in adults.

REFERENCES

1. Buckingham WW Jr. Subtalar dislocation of the foot. *J Trauma* 1973;13:753–65.
2. DeLee JC, Curtis R. Subtalar dislocation of foot. *J Bone Joint Surg* 1982;64A:433–37.
3. Monson ST, Ryan JR. Subtalar dislocation. *J Bone Joint Surg* 1981;63A:1156–58.

Chopart's Dislocations

MECHANISMS OF INJURY

Isolated Chopart's dislocations are rare and the exact mechanisms of injury have not been clearly established, although evidence exists that medial, lateral, or rotatory forces applied to a plantarflexed foot can produce this injury. A Chopart's dislocation is commonly associated with a crushing injury and with significantly comminuted fractures of other tarsal bones, especially of the calcaneocuboid joint. Mobility in the Chopart's joint during eversion may make the joint more susceptible to injury in this position.

ANATOMIC CONSIDERATIONS

The Chopart's joint is a complex articulation that includes the calcaneocuboid and the talonavicular joints. In a small number of patients a true articulation also exists between the navicular and the cuboid. Complete range of motion of this joint is needed for normal gait.

CLASSIFICATION

No formal classification system exists for Chopart's dislocations because this injury is rare. Dislocations are described in terms of the relationships between the navicular and the cuboid to the calcaneus and the talus after injury. For example, when the navicular is displaced plantar to the talus, the dislocation is described as a plantar dislocation. Main and Jowett (1) have described several midfoot injuries that involve Chopart's joint, but their descriptions are complex and are not useful in a clinical setting.

ASSESSMENT

Physical Examination

The forefoot is examined for discoloration and deformity as well as for sensory, motor, and vascular deficits. Significant swelling may be indicative of an occult midfoot disruption.

Radiographic Evaluation

Anteroposterior, lateral, and oblique radiographic views are taken with simulated weight-bearing and are carefully examined for intraarticular fractures in the talonavicular and the calcaneocuboid joints. An oblique radiographic view is particularly useful in assessing the calcaneocuboid joint.

Special Studies

No special studies are required.

EMERGENT MANAGEMENT

True dislocations, in which the forefoot is displaced plantar to the talus and the calcaneus, may involve an injury to the dorsal neurologic structures. Urgent reduction is indicated for all dislocations that place neurologic structures at risk. Reduction can be performed in the emergency room after administration of an ankle block or a hematoma block with lidocaine.

DEFINITIVE MANAGEMENT

Open reduction and internal fixation of a Chopart's dislocation are accomplished through a longitudinal medial incision, which can be combined with a lateral incision. Although clear indications for internal fixation of a Chopart's dislocation do not exist, internal fixation with smooth pins provides stability and facilitates rehabilitation. After ORIF the patient is restricted to minimal weight-bearing for 4 weeks and can then begin ambulation in a short-leg walking cast for 2 weeks. The pins are removed after this regimen has been completed.

COMPLICATIONS

Stiffness is a common sequela after an intraarticular fracture.

SKELETALLY IMMATURE PATIENTS

Chopart's dislocations in children are treated in the same manner as injuries in adults.

REFERENCE

1. Main BJ, Jowett RL. Injuries of the midtarsal joint. *J Bone Joint Surg* 1975;57B:89–97.

Lisfranc's Fracture–Dislocations

MECHANISMS OF INJURY

Lisfranc's fracture–dislocations can be caused by indirect or direct forces. Indirect injuries are the most common and usually occur after axial load is applied to a plantarflexed foot. In this mechanism, the forefoot is displaced medially or laterally by secondary forces (1). Injuries caused by direct force usually involve crushing or a direct blow. Secondary injuries associated with Lisfranc's fracture–dislocations include intercuneiform disruptions, calcaneocuboid joint fractures, navicular fractures, and forefoot injuries, particularly metatarsal neck fractures.

ANATOMIC CONSIDERATIONS

The Lisfranc's tarsometatarsal (TMT) joint comprises articulations among the five metatarsals, the three cuneiforms, and the cuboid. The TMT joint is shaped like a Roman arch: each plantar component is narrower than its adjacent dorsal component. Displacement usually occurs on the dorsal side. The second metatarsal (the keystone) articulates with the intermediate cuneiform. It is locked into place between the medial and lateral cuneiforms, which extend further distally than the intermediate cuneiform. This articulation stabilizes the midfoot but also inhibits motion in the second TMT joint, which is often fractured in a Lisfranc's fracture–dislocation.

CLASSIFICATION

The classification of Lisfranc's fracture–dislocations includes three types of injuries (Fig. 5).

Type A: Complete dislocation. The entire forefoot is displaced medially or laterally through the TMT joint.

Type B: Partial dislocation. The medial or lateral portion of the foot is displaced.

Type C: Divergent dislocation. The medial ray is dislocated medially and the lesser rays are dislocated laterally.

In addition to this classification, Lisfranc's injuries may involve intercuneiform dislocations.

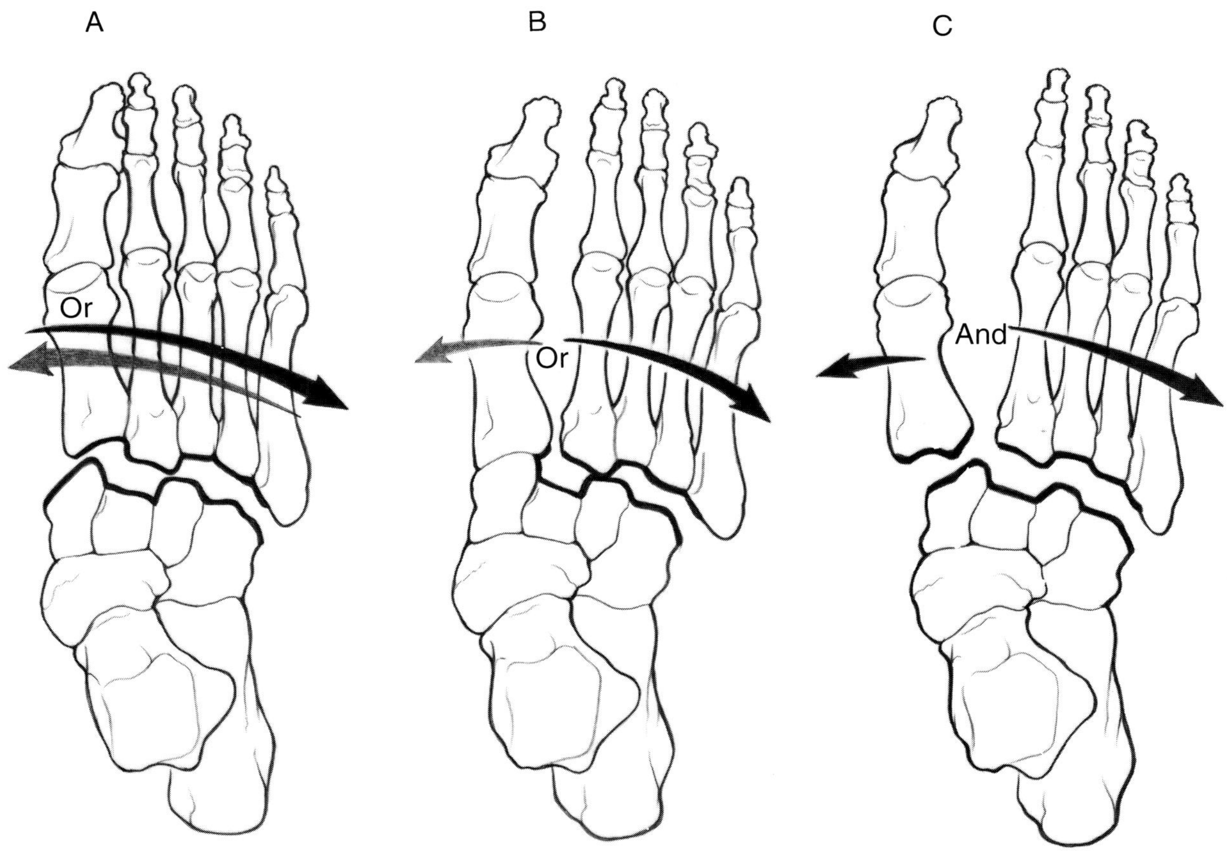

FIG. 5. Diagrammatic representation of the three types of Lisfranc's fractures.

ASSESSMENT

Physical Examination

Physical examination includes an assessment of skin and vascular integrity, neuromuscular function, and pain with passive stretch. Compartmental syndrome often occurs in midfoot injuries.

Radiographic Evaluation

Anteroposterior, lateral, and oblique radiographic views are taken with simulated weight-bearing. Stress films are useful to confirm an uncertain diagnosis but are too painful to obtain acutely without analgesia or sedation (Fig. 6).

Special Studies

No special studies are required.

EMERGENT MANAGEMENT

Emergent management consists of elevation and splinting. When a compartmental syndrome is suspected, a catheter is extended deep into the abductor muscle belly of the calcaneal compartment to measure compartmental pressures. The compartment is decompressed through dorsal and medial incisions. By making an incision in the foot to decompress a compartmental syndrome, a closed injury is transformed into an open injury, and operative stabilization of the Lisfranc's dislocation must be done at the same time.

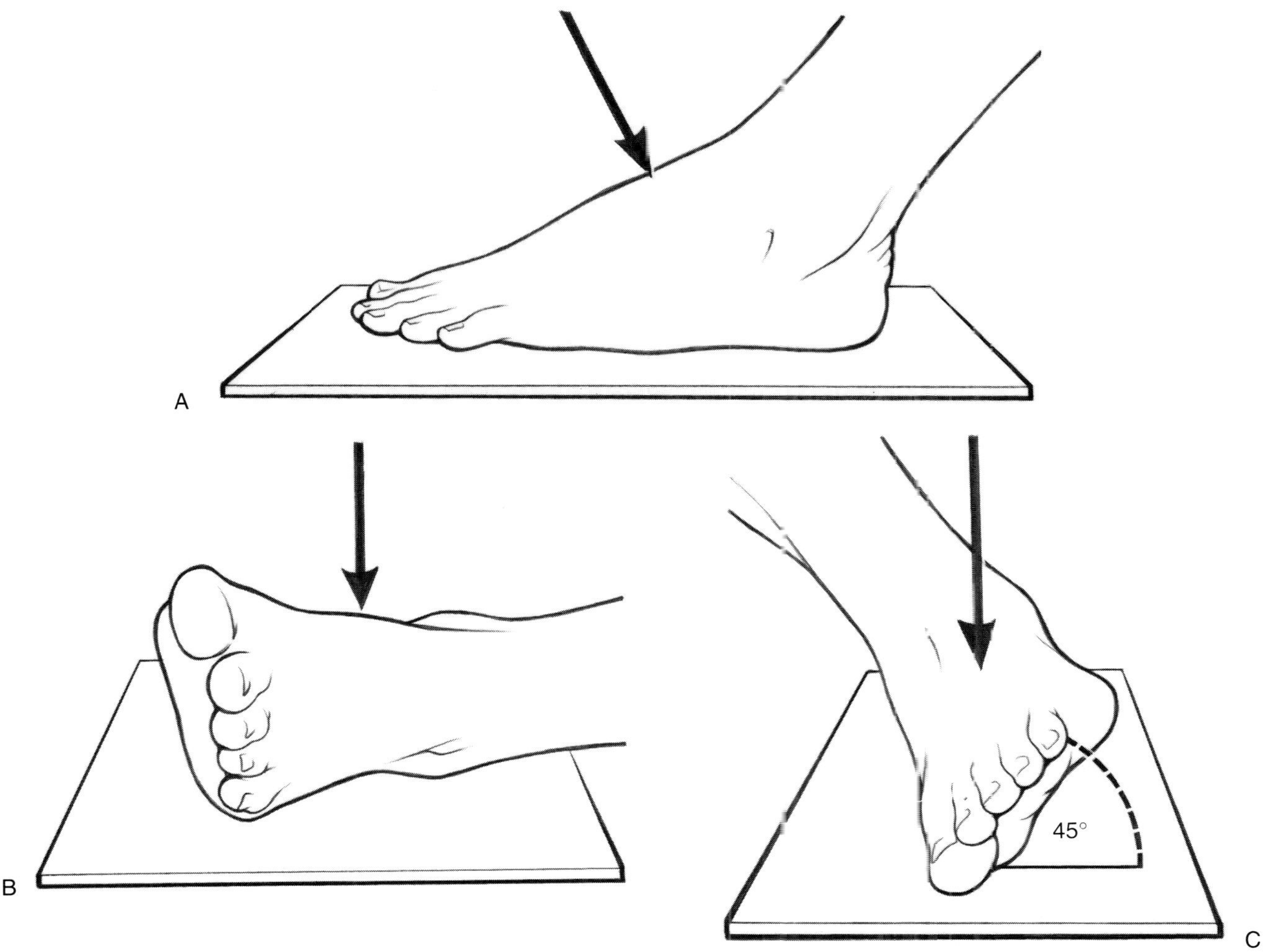

A B C

FIG. 6. A: The positioning for a simulated weight-bearing AP radiographic view of the foot. **B:** The positioning for a simulated weight-bearing lateral radiographic view of the foot. **C:** The positioning for an oblique radiographic view of the foot.

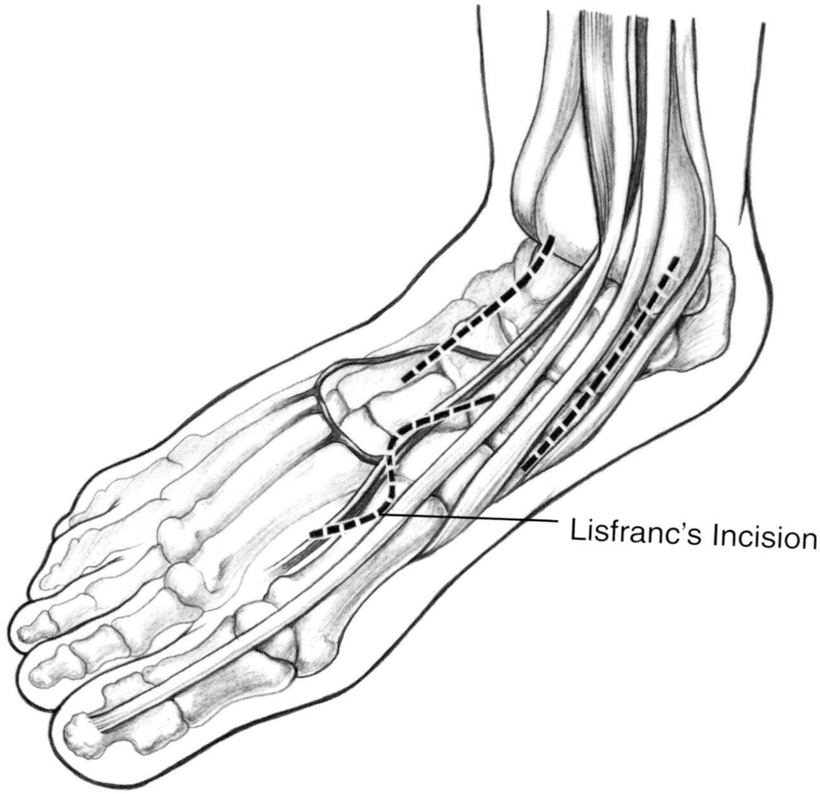

FIG. 7. The incision courses first over the second TMT joint, then over the first TMT joint.

DEFINITIVE MANAGEMENT

The preoperative plan is made after the radiographs are evaluated to identify which joints are involved in the dislocation. Fractures in the first and second TMT joints are approached through a lazy-S incision that follows the interval between the joints (Fig. 7). One screw is placed from the first metatarsal into the first cuneiform and another screw is placed from the second metatarsal into the second cuneiform (Fig. 8). In the presence of an intercuneiform dislocation, the incision is enlarged proximally and a screw is placed percutaneously from the medial to the intermediate or lateral cuneiform. Intraoperative radiographs are obtained to confirm reduction (Figs. 9 and 10).

Fractures in the third and fourth metatarsals are exposed through a longitudinal incision made between the third and fourth TMT joints. These joints are very mobile and require fixation with Kirschner wires. When the fifth ray is unstable it is fixed with a Kirschner wire through an incision over the proximal fifth metatarsal. If screws are placed in these metatarsals they must be removed before significant weight-bearing activities are begun. Postoperatively the foot is protected in a short-leg posterior splint. A short-leg cast is applied after 6 weeks and the patient is allowed to ambulate in cast for between 2 and 3 weeks. After this the cast is removed and replaced with a removable brace until the

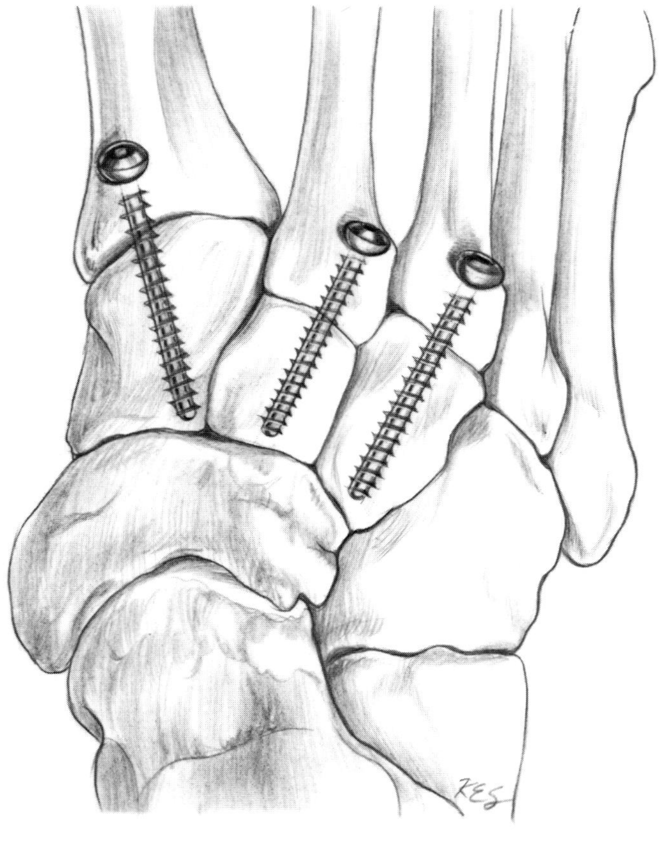

FIG. 8. The idealized fixation for a Lisfranc's fracture–dislocation.

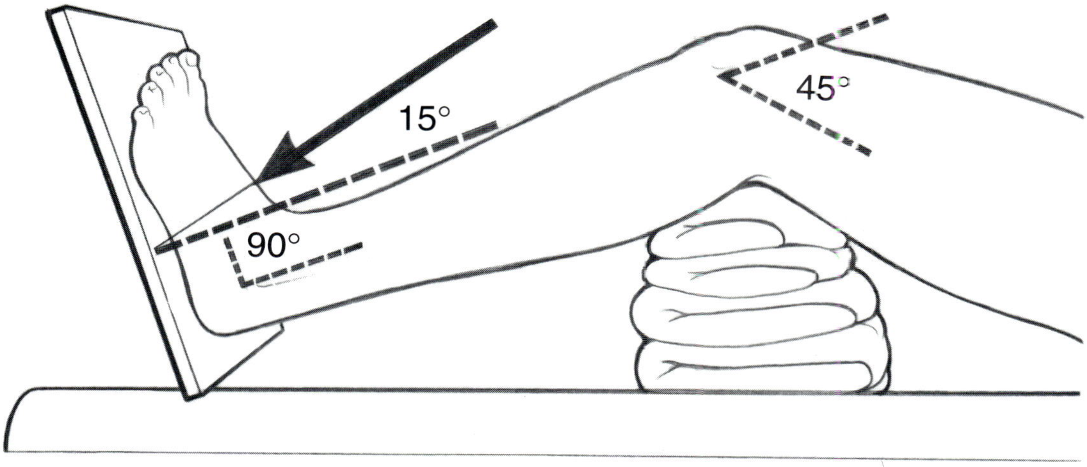

FIG. 9. The positioning for a simulated weight-bearing AP radiograph.

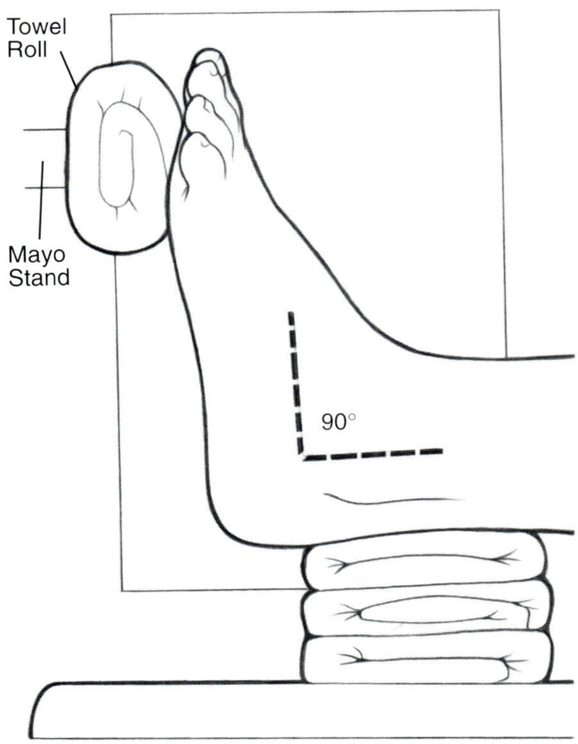

FIG. 10. The positioning for a simulated weight-bearing lateral radiograph.

patient can ambulate comfortably. If necessary, a custom-molded total-contact insole is inserted into the patient's shoe.

In an isolated dislocation that has been treated with rigid internal fixation, the cast can be removed after 2 weeks. Early ROM exercises of the foot can be instituted at that time if the reduction is stable. These exercises include active plantarflexion and dorsiflexion of the ankle, inversion and eversion of the subtalar joint, and forefoot motion.

COMPLICATIONS

A Lisfranc's fracture–dislocation is a severe injury and some residual stiffness and pain are expected after rehabilitation. Compartmental syndrome often accompanies a severe displacement. Narrowing of the articular surfaces is commonly seen on radiographs but this finding may be clinically insignificant. The dorsal neurovascular structures may be injured. Planovalgus deformity in the foot is a late complication associated with a missed diagnosis or an isolated dislocation.

SKELETALLY IMMATURE PATIENTS

Lisfranc's fracture–dislocations in children are treated in the same manner as injuries in adults. Fixation may be provided by smooth Kirschner wires.

REFERENCE

Arntz CT, Veith RG, Hansen ST Jr. Fractures and fracture–dislocations of the tarsometatarsal joint. *J Bone Joint Surg* 1988;70A:173–81.

Talar Fractures

MECHANISMS OF INJURY

Talar fracture patterns vary according to the mechanism of injury. Vertical fractures, including those of the talar neck, are usually the result of acute dorsiflexion injuries. The talar neck is forced across the anterior aspect of the distal tibia until fracture occurs. Fractures of the head, body, and inferior facets are usually caused by high-energy injuries. Fractures of the talar head involve applications of indirect medial or lateral forces to the forefoot. Fractures of the body are usually caused by high-energy force applied to a foot positioned in plantarflexion, when the talus is unstable in the ankle joint. Facet fractures are frequently caused by inversion or eversion injuries and may be associated with subtalar dislocations.

ANATOMIC CONSIDERATIONS

Two anatomic factors increase the likelihood of a poor outcome after an injury to the talus: extensive articular cartilage that covers 60% of the talar surface and limited blood supply.

The talus has seven articulations. The normal function of each articulation is dependent on that of the others by way of complex structural relationships. The talonavicular joint is the definitive joint for midfoot motion. The talar dome and its lateral articulation with the fibula are weight-bearing joints and three weight-bearing articular facets are found in the subtalar joint. Displacement of the talar body or neck can significantly disrupt these articular structures and threaten the blood supply to the talus.

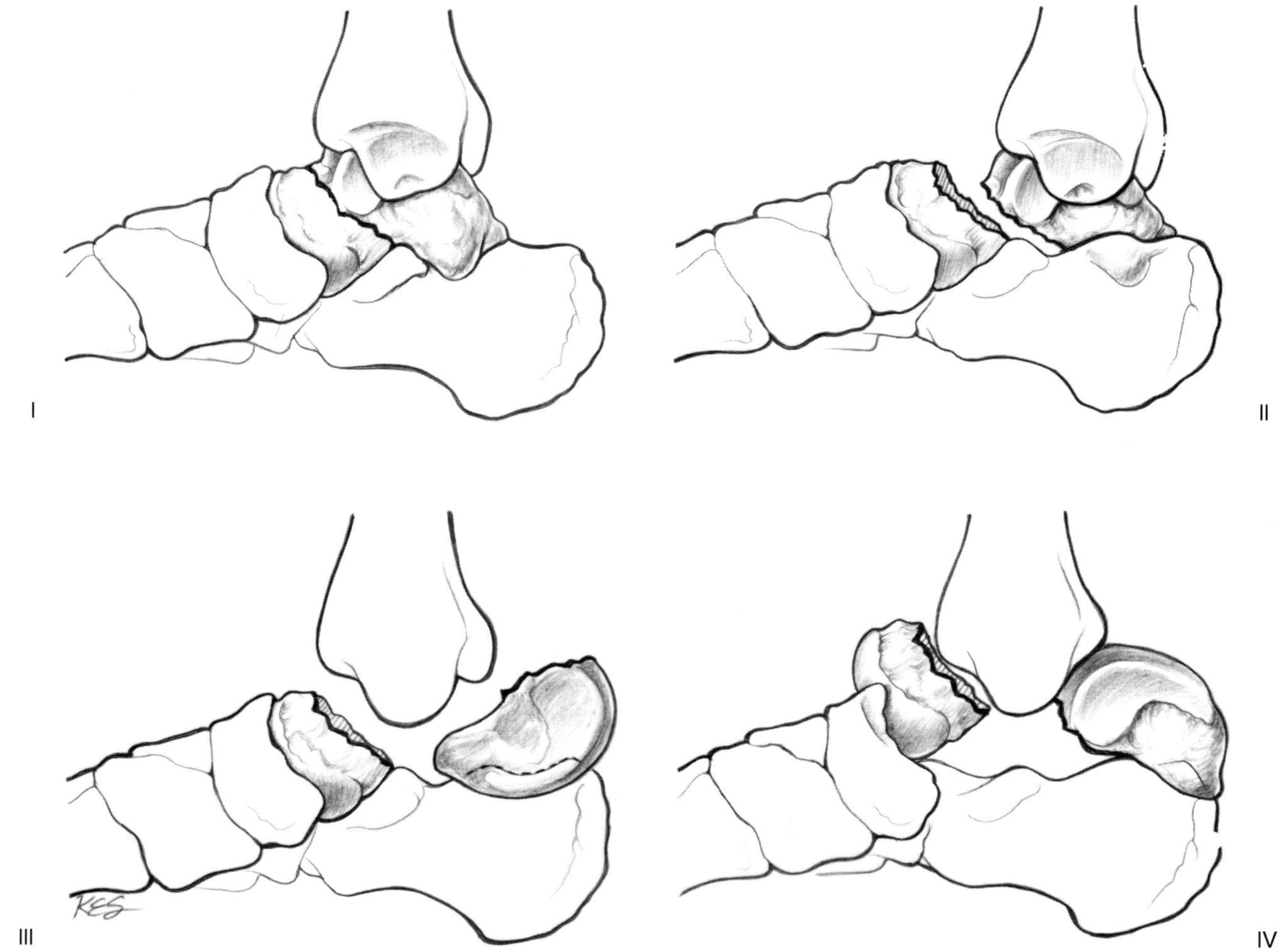

FIG. 11. Diagrammatic representation of Hawkins' classification of talar neck fractures.

CLASSIFICATION

Fractures of the lateral and posterior processes and those involving the talar head are associated with the best functional outcomes. The worst prognoses are associated with fractures of the talar neck and the talar body. Talar neck fractures were classified by Hawkins (1) according to the amount of displacement in the subtalar and the ankle joints (Fig. 11).

Hawkins type I: No displacement.

Hawkins type II: Subluxation of the subtalar joint without involvement of the ankle joint.

Hawkins type III: Subluxation of the subtalar and the ankle joints.

Hawkins type IV: Hawkins type III injury with a talonavicular joint dislocation (2).

ASSESSMENT

Physical Examination

Talar fractures are assessed by the same parameters that are used to evaluate other injuries in the foot. Particular attention is directed to the ankle and the subtalar joints.

Radiographic Evaluation

The radiographic series that is used routinely for evaluating foot injuries (AP, lateral, and oblique views with simulated weight-bearing) is obtained for the evaluation of talar fractures. In addition, a modified AP radiographic view described by Canale (2), in which the foot is pronated 15° and tilted 15° cephalad to the x-ray beam, is obtained to outline the talar neck. Mortise views are taken of all talar fractures to rule out subluxation.

Special Studies

Special studies are seldom required. Computerized tomography scans are obtained in the event of incomplete intraarticular congruity after reduction. For lateral process fractures, CT scans may be useful for assessing the size of the fragment and the advisability of fixation over excision.

EMERGENT MANAGEMENT

Nondisplaced fractures or fractures that involve the facets or the talar dome are managed by early splinting and elevation. Nondisplaced fractures are immobilized in a short-leg cast for 6 to 8 weeks.

DEFINITIVE MANAGEMENT

Displaced fractures of the talar neck involving an articular surface are considered to be surgical emergencies and require immediate ORIF to avoid significant morbidity associated with avascular necrosis (Figs. 12–15). The talar neck is

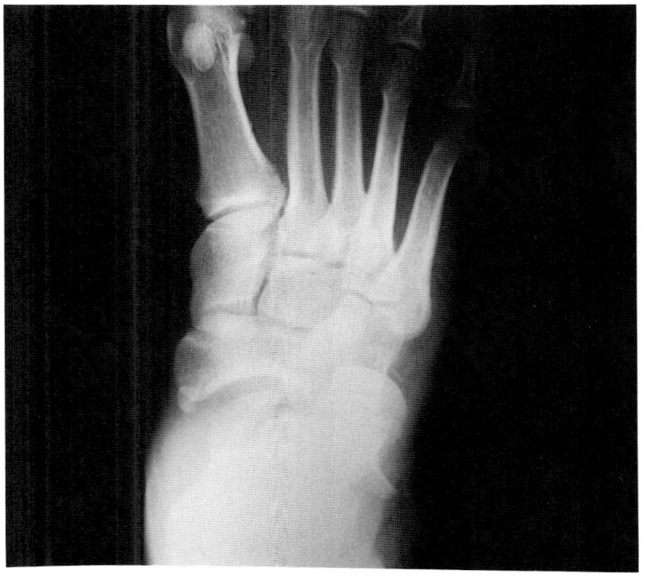

FIG. 12. This is an AP view of the foot of a patient with a Hawkins type IV fracture. The neck and head are extruded laterally from the talonavicular joint and dorsally from the subtalar joint. One-third of the head is displaced plantarly.

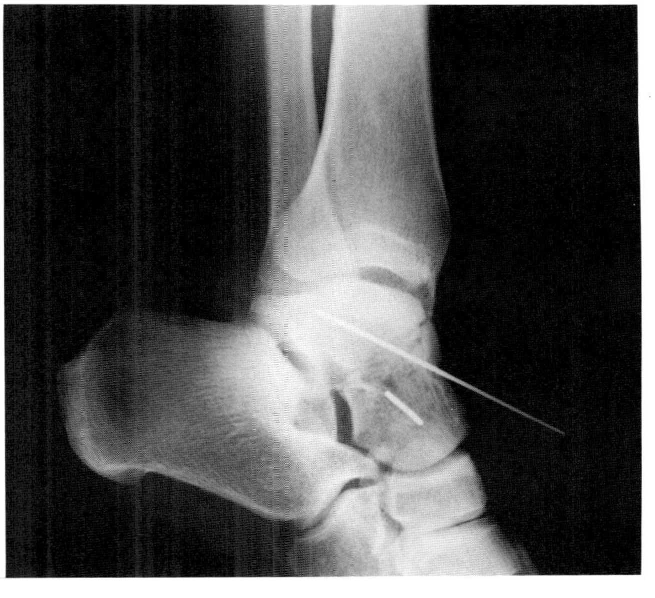

FIG. 13. A lateral intraoperative view after provisional stabilization of the three main fragments.

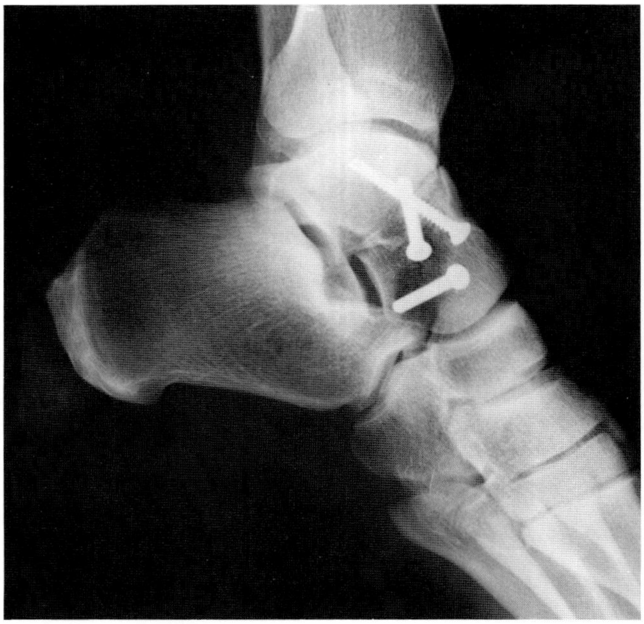

FIG. 14. A lateral view following stabilization with three screws. Note that the posterior and middle facets are congruent.

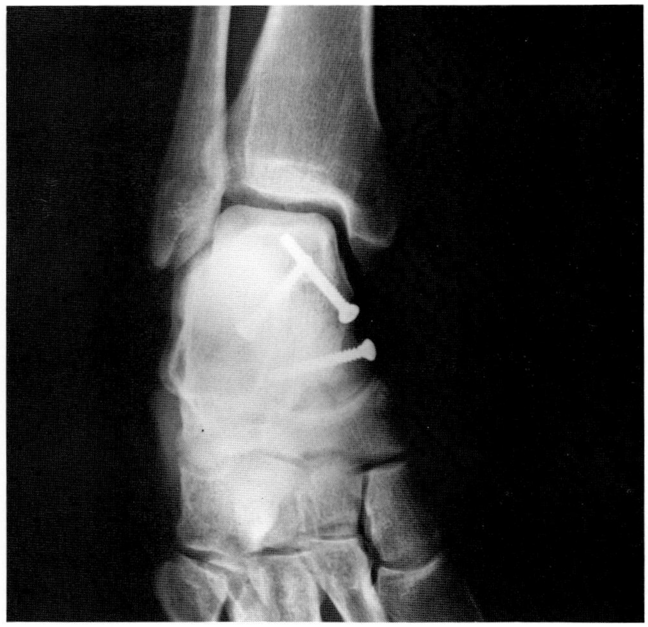

FIG. 15. An AP view of the ankle of the same patient with the foot plantarflexed showing both the talonavicular joint and the tibiotalar joint.

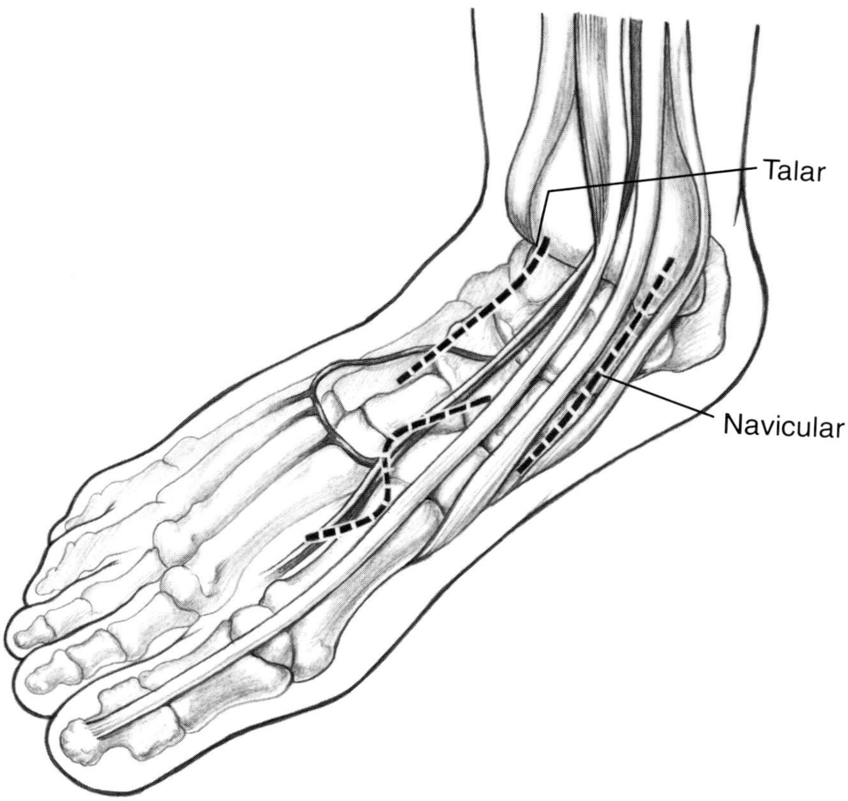

FIG. 16. The surgical approach used for a talar neck fracture.

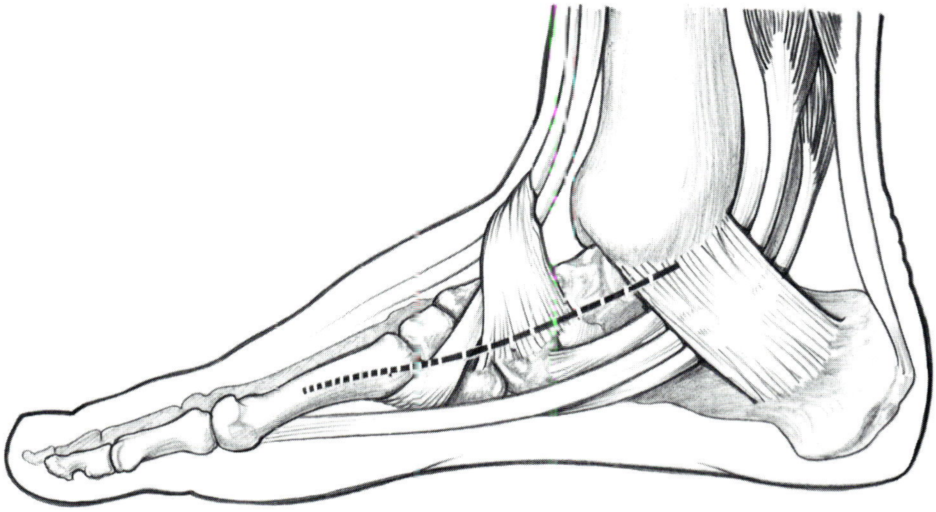

FIG. 17. The medial incision is placed between the anterior and posterior tibial tendons and may be extended proximally to perform a medial malleolar osteotomy.

approached by combined medial and lateral incisions (Fig. 16) (3). The medial incision is started at the level of the medial malleolus and is enlarged to bisect the interval between the anterior and the posterior tibial tendons (Fig. 17). An anterolateral incision is made to supplement the medial incision and to better visualize the reduction and placement of the crossed 3.5-mm cortical lag screws (Fig. 18). Postoperatively, talar fractures are managed with partial weight-bearing until the fracture has united. Fractures of the talar body or the talar neck usually unite in approximately 8 weeks. After 2 weeks, the amount of weight-bearing that is allowed and possible mobilization out of cast are dependent on bone quality and the strength of fixation.

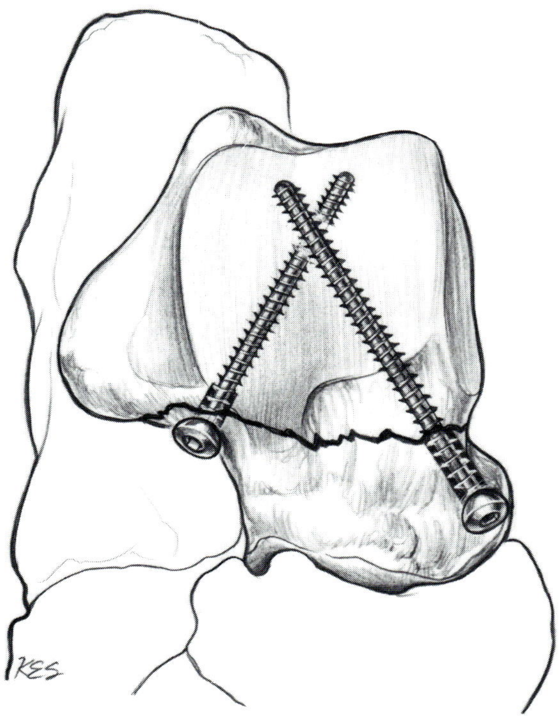

FIG. 18. Standard fixation for a talar fracture.

COMPLICATIONS

Degenerative arthritis is often a sequela of displaced intraarticular fractures. Avascular necrosis is a widely discussed complication of talar neck fractures but the exact cause of this problem is unknown. Many talar fractures that heal in an anatomic position and develop avascular necrosis are asymptomatic.

SKELETALLY IMMATURE PATIENTS

Talar fractures in children are treated in the same manner as fractures in adults.

REFERENCES

1. Hawkins LG. Fractures of the neck of the talus. *J Bone Joint Surg* 1990;52A:991–1002.
2. Canale ST, Kelly FB Jr. Fractures of the neck of the talus. Long-term evaluation of seventy-one cases. *J Bone Joint Surg* 1978:60A:143–56.
3. Mayo KA: Fractures of the talus: principles of management and techniques of treatment. *Tech Orthop* 1987;2:42–54.

Calcaneal Fractures

MECHANISMS OF INJURY

Calcaneal fractures are usually caused by axial loading, e.g., by a fall from a height onto the heel. Avulsion fractures can result from indirect force. For example, a portion of the dorsal tuberosity can be avulsed by the Achilles tendon insertion from contractions of the gastrocnemius and soleus muscles, or the anterior process of the calcaneus can be avulsed by the calcaneonavicular ligament from rapid inversion of the foot (1). Because these are predominantly loading injuries, the incidence of associated injuries is high. The most common associated injuries are compression fractures of the lumbar spine, associated fractures in the lower extremity, and fractures of the contralateral calcaneus. Patients with calcaneal fractures should always be screened for fractures of the lumbar spine.

ANATOMIC CONSIDERATIONS

The calcaneus consists of a cortical shell which is filled with cancellous bone and reinforced with trabeculae that support tension and compression loads. These trabecular supports are concentrated beneath the posterior facet and are known as the thalamic segment of the calcaneus. The bone beneath the tarsal sinus is also dense. These two areas of dense bone form a radiographic angle known as the angle of Gissane, which represents the normal relationships among the three facets (Fig. 19).

The medial wall of the calcaneus lies in close proximity to the tibial nerve, the tibial artery, and the flexor tendons. The wall slopes sharply away from the sustentaculum, the most prominent structure on the medial side of the calcaneus. In comparison, the lateral wall is relatively flat but usually exhibits a pronounced peroneal trochlea. The peroneal tendons and the sural nerve course along the lateral aspect of the calcaneus. Three facets are located on the superior surface of the calcaneus. Anteriorly, the calcaneus articulates with the cuboid. Operative treatment of calcaneal fractures is complicated by the complexity of these articular surfaces.

CLASSIFICATION

Many classification systems have been devised to grade calcaneal fractures but none has any prognostic significance. Fractures of the calcaneus are described as extraarticular or intraarticular injuries. Extraarticular fractures consist of avulsions by the tuberosity and usually include fractures of the anterior process. However, because a large anterior process fragment may contain an articular fragment, extraarticular calcaneal fractures should not routinely be assumed to be low-priority injuries.

Intraarticular fractures are further divided into tongue-type fractures and depressed fractures. The posterior facet remains attached to the dorsal surface of the tuberosity in a tongue-type fracture; in a depressed fracture, the posterior facet is impacted into the body and is separated from the tuberosity (Fig. 20).

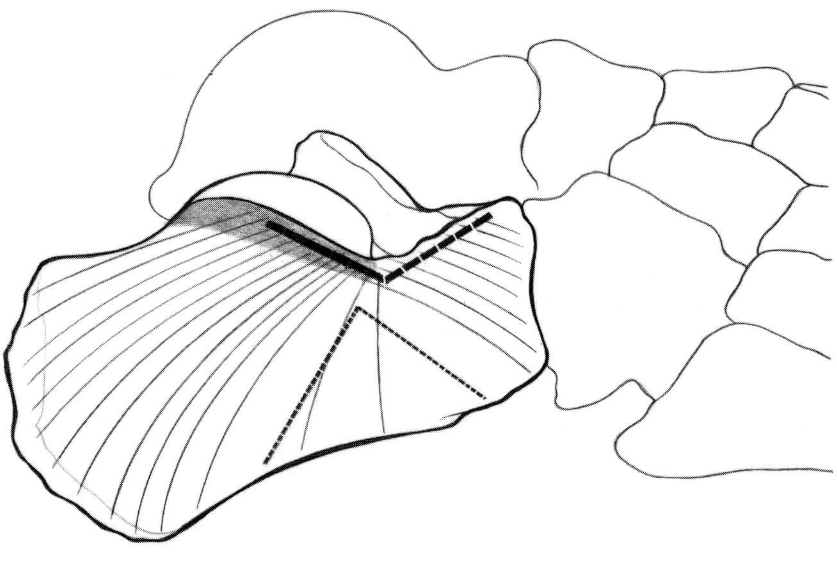

FIG. 19. The angle of Gissane. The condensed trabeculae beneath the posterior facet *(solid line)* form the thalamic segment. Dense bone beneath the tarsal sinus is represented by a *dotted line.*

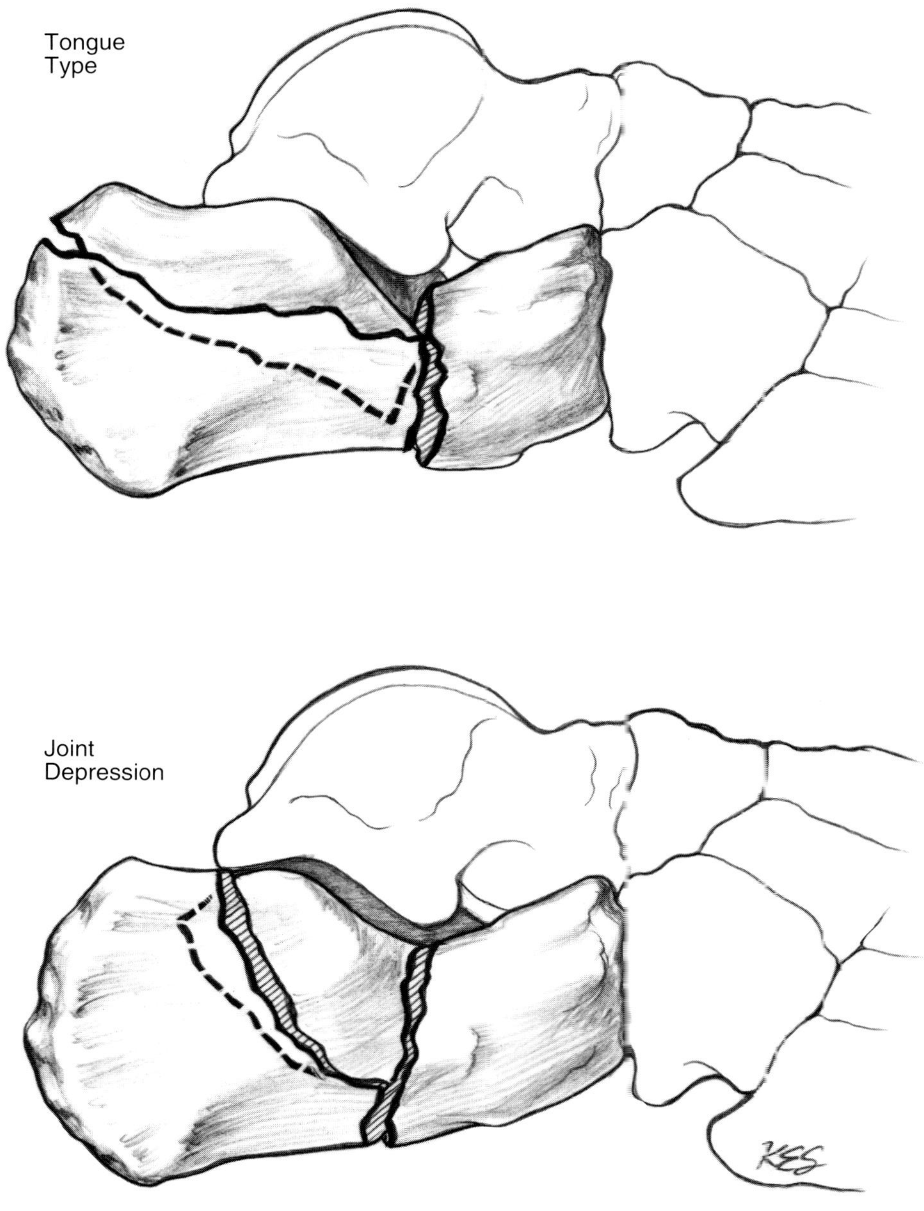

FIG. 20. Diagrammatic representation of tongue-type and joint-depression-type calcaneal fractures.

ASSESSMENT

Physical Examination

The entire affected lower limb and the lumbar spine are examined for associated injuries. Examination of the foot includes an assessment of the tibial and sural nerves and of the flexor tendons, which may be entrapped in the fracture. Intracompartmental pressures are monitored for compartmental syndrome when pain is out of proportion to the injury.

Radiographic Evaluation

Routine radiographic evaluation includes an axial view, an oblique view, and AP and lateral views taken with simulated weight-bearing. The relationships of the midfoot structures in the calcaneocuboid joint are best seen on AP radiographs; the type of fracture and the amount of displacement in the posterior facet are revealed on the lateral view; the position of the tuberosity, shortening, and lateral translation are demonstrated on an axial radiograph; associated midfoot injuries are seen on an oblique radiographic view. Brodén's views assess the congruity of the subtalar joint (Fig. 21) (2).

Special Studies

A fracture that may require operative reduction is evaluated further by CT scans taken in semicoronal and transverse planes (Fig. 22). The view in the transverse plane, taken parallel to the plantar surface of the foot, delineates the relationship between the calcaneal tuberosity and the sustentaculum

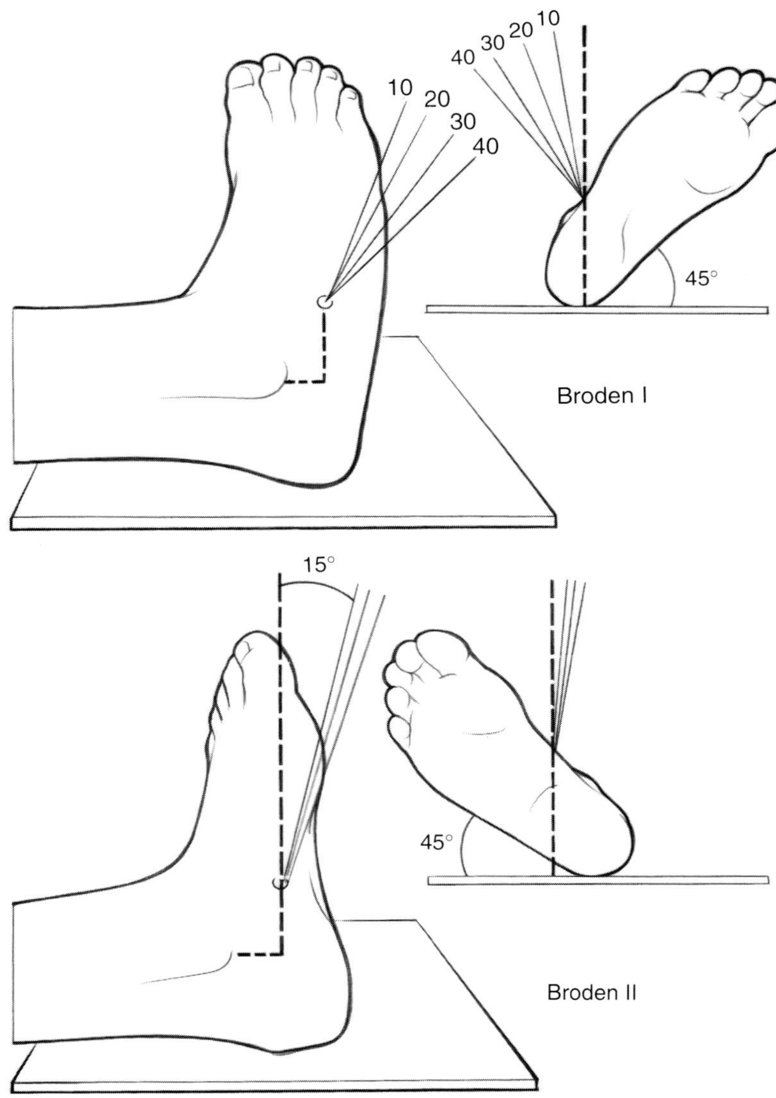

FIG. 21. The positioning required for a hindfoot oblique (Brodén's radiographic view).

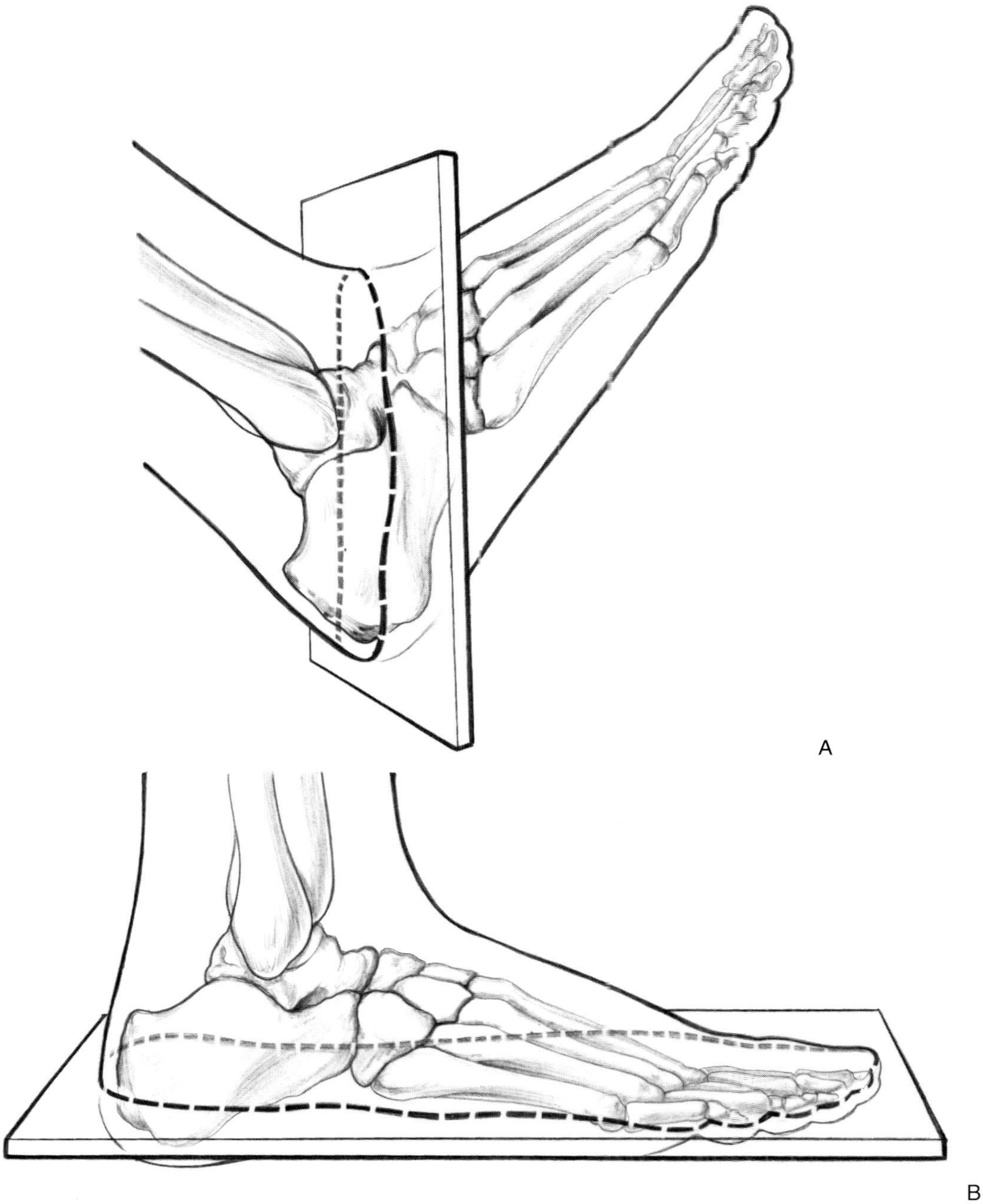

FIG. 22. A: Positioning required for a CT scan in the semicoronal plane. The foot is angled at 45° so that the plane of the CT scan is perpendicular to the posterior facet. **B:** Positioning required for a CT scan in the transverse plane. The patient lies supine with the foot plantigrade. The plane of the CT is parallel to the plantar surface of the foot.

and confirms displacement within the calcaneocuboid joint. The view in the semicoronal plane is used to assess the amount of displacement within the posterior facet and the lateral wall. To obtain this view the foot is fixed in a plantigrade or neutral position and the knee is bent 45° on pillows. In this position the posterior facet lies perpendicular to the beam of the CT scanner.

EMERGENT MANAGEMENT

In general, management of a calcaneal fracture is not considered to be an emergency because it is not life-threatening and does not prevent mobility. Therefore, initial treatment consists of elevation and application of a bulky dressing. Appropriate imaging modalities are obtained, and the patient

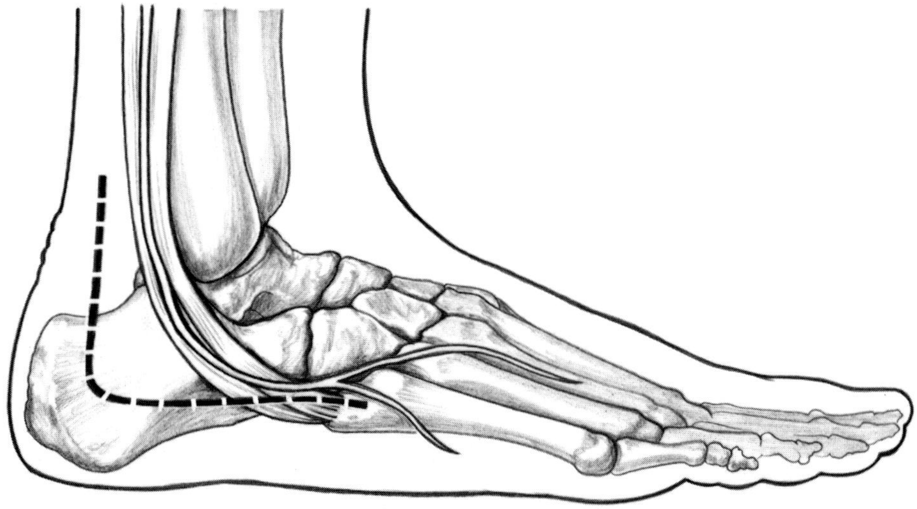

FIG. 23. The skin incision for the extensile–lateral (Benirschke) approach.

is observed for signs and symptoms of compartmental syndrome.

DEFINITIVE MANAGEMENT

Closed calcaneal fractures are managed by bulky dressings and elevation. Operative treatment is planned when the swelling has receded, usually 5 to 10 days after injury. Conversely, open calcaneal fractures are managed acutely by ORIF using appropriate soft-tissue techniques. The patient is placed in the lateral position on the operating table. A modified lateral approach is made to visualize the entire lateral wall, the calcaneus, and the calcaneocuboid joint without exposing the peroneal tendons (Fig. 23). The anatomic relationship of the calcaneal tuberosity to the sustentaculum is restored by distraction with a Schanz pin and fixed provisionally with a Kirschner wire (Fig. 24).

Next, the anatomic relationship between the anterior process and the sustentaculum is restored in a similar manner, and provisional fixation is applied to hold this segment in the appropriate position. The articular surface of the posterior facet is restored and provisionally stabilized with Kirschner wires. The joint surface is then stabilized definitively with two 3.5-mm cortical lag screws. The anatomic position of all the involved structures is maintained by a 3.5-mm lateral reconstruction plate (Fig. 25). Fixation occasionally is supplemented with an H- or L-shaped plate.

After surgery, touch-down weight-bearing is allowed for 12 weeks. The surgical dressing is changed between the third and fifth postoperative days, and ankle and subtalar ROM exercises are begun at that time. These activities are supervised by a physical therapist until the patient is able to do the

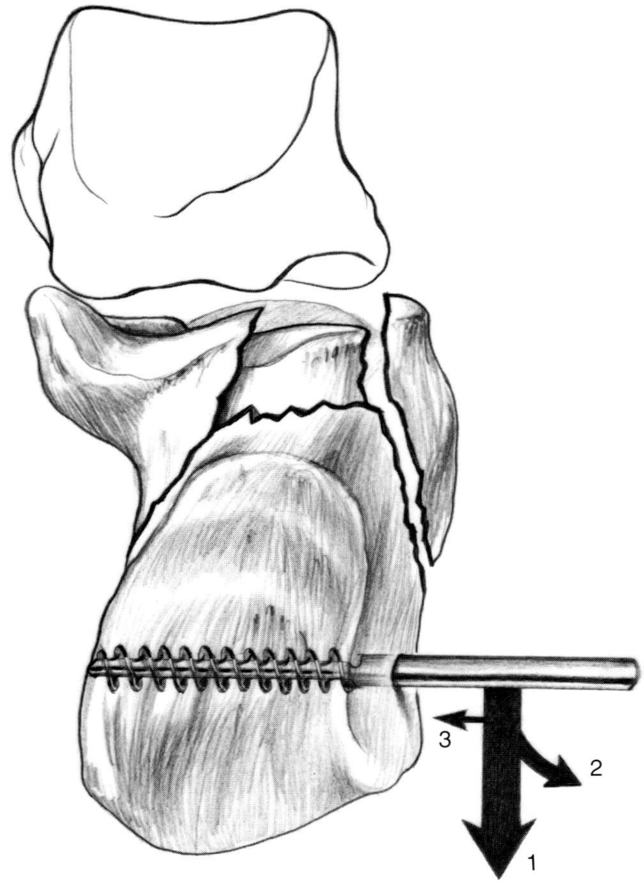

FIG. 24. In a posterior facet depressed-type injury, the tuberosity segment is pulled (1) distally, (2) out of varus, and (3) medially with a Schanz pin. The relative sizes of the arrows suggest the amounts of force used in each direction.

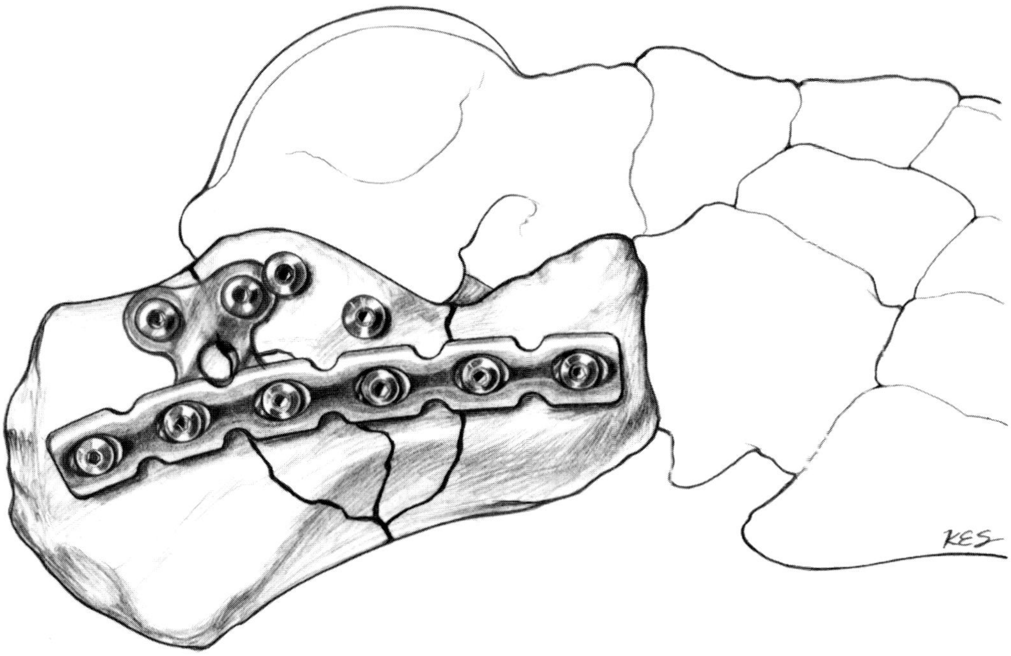

FIG. 25. Postoperative view of standard traction for a joint depression fracture.

exercises independently (3). This fracture is restricted to minimal weight-bearing longer than most other fractures, but early motion must be initiated as soon as the fixation allows.

Approximately 7 days postoperatively the patient is discharged from the hospital and is seen again 2 weeks later for suture removal and wound examination. Six weeks postoperatively, radiographs are taken in lateral, axial, and Brodén's views to monitor anatomic alignment and bone healing. These radiographs are repeated at 10 weeks and partial weight-bearing (20–50 lb) can be initiated at that time. Progression to full weight-bearing is begun 12 weeks postoperatively, and the radiographic series is repeated once again at 16 weeks. The heel is often hypersensitive after a long period of nonweight-bearing, and a soft heel orthosis can be inserted into the patient's shoe during early ambulation.

COMPLICATIONS

Complications after a calcaneal fracture include failure of fixation, posttraumatic arthritis, delayed wound healing, infection, and sural nerve transection. Patients are advised of the possibility of these complications preoperatively and are told that if the sural nerve obstructs the operative approach it will be transsected and the lateral border of the foot will be permanently insensate. Delayed wound healing, which is defined as a wound that continues to drain for longer than 5 days, occurs in approximately 10% of patients. Wounds that are severe enough to require skin grafting or skin-flap coverage are uncommon.

SKELETALLY IMMATURE PATIENTS

Calcaneal fractures are rare in children but are managed in the same manner as fractures in adults. The implants selected are based on the size of the fragments. Small plates and screws or, occasionally, Kirschner wires may be more appropriate.

REFERENCES

1. Böhler L. Diagnosis, pathology, treatment of fractures of the os calcis. *Bone Joint Surg* 1931;13A:75–89.
2. Brodén B. Roentgen examination of the subtaloid joint in fractures of the calcaneus. *Acta Radiol* 1949;31:85–91.
3. Stephenson JR. Treatment of displaced intraarticular fractures of the calcaneus using medial and lateral approaches, internal fixation, and early motion. *Bone Joint Surg* 1987;69A:115–30.

Navicular Fractures

Mechanisms of Injury

Navicular fractures are usually caused by axial loading directed through the metatarsals along the plantarflexed foot. The navicular is thus compressed between the talus and the base of the second metatarsal. The resulting fracture pattern is determined by the position of the foot at the time of injury. Avulsion fractures, tuberosity fractures, and dorsal-lip fractures can occur from indirect forces. Because most navicular fractures are caused by high-energy injuries, associated tarsal and metatarsal fractures often occur in the same limb and multiple-system injuries are common (1,2).

ANATOMIC CONSIDERATIONS

The navicular lies between the talus and the three cuneiforms. Its articulation with the talus forms a mobile joint but it shares little motion with the cuneiforms. The navicular holds the key position in the medial longitudinal arch of the foot, and any disruption in its anatomy changes the overall alignment of the foot (1,2).

Blood supply to the navicular is provided by dorsal and plantar vessels that surround the navicular like a tire around a wheel, sending in 6 to 10 spokes of radial blood vessels. However, the central third of the navicular is relatively avascular and the number of vessels that supply the bone with blood decreases with age.

CLASSIFICATION

Navicular fractures are classified into three categories:

1. Fractures of the tuberosity. A fracture of the tuberosity can result from a direct blow to the medial side of the foot or from avulsion by the posterior tibial tendon.
2. Chip fractures of the dorsal lip. A fracture of the dorsal lip is usually associated with an injury to Chopart's joint and can jeopardize the stability of the midfoot and the calcaneocuboid joint.
3. Fractures of the body. A fracture of the body is caused by a high-energy injury and often results in displacement of the hindfoot, the midfoot, and the forefoot. Of the three categories of navicular fractures, this injury has the worst prognosis. Fractures of the body are classified as nondisplaced or displaced; displaced fractures are divided further into three subgroups based on the severity of the injury and the resulting fracture pattern (Fig. 26) (1).

ASSESSMENT

Physical Examination

The foot is examined for disruption of the blood supply and for sensory deficits. A compartmental syndrome should be suspected in all midfoot injuries and must be ruled out by clinical examination or confirmed by direct measurement of compartmental pressures.

Radiographic Evaluation

Anteroposterior and lateral radiographic views are taken with simulated weight-bearing. A navicular fracture frequently occurs in a relatively obscure plane and is usually best evaluated from an oblique view.

Special Studies

A CT scan is usually not required but can be performed if the fracture is not clearly defined on plain films.

EMERGENT MANAGEMENT

Emergent management consists of splinting and elevation until the swelling subsides. If a compartmental syndrome is present, ORIF is not delayed but is done concurrently with the compartmental release.

DEFINITIVE MANAGEMENT

Nondisplaced fractures and fractures of the dorsal lip are treated in a short-leg nonweight-bearing walking cast for 4 weeks. If the shape of the foot is grossly distorted, closed reduction should be attempted after a local anesthetic block is administered to relax the soft tissues. Strengthening and ROM exercises are initiated after the cast is removed.

Open reduction and internal fixation are performed with the patient lying supine on the operating table. Two incisions are frequently employed: the first is made on the medial aspect of the foot over the posterior tibial tendon, and the second is made on the dorsal side lateral to the navicular (see Fig. 16). A small medial distractor is used to lengthen the medial border of the foot. Distraction allows visualization of the talonav-

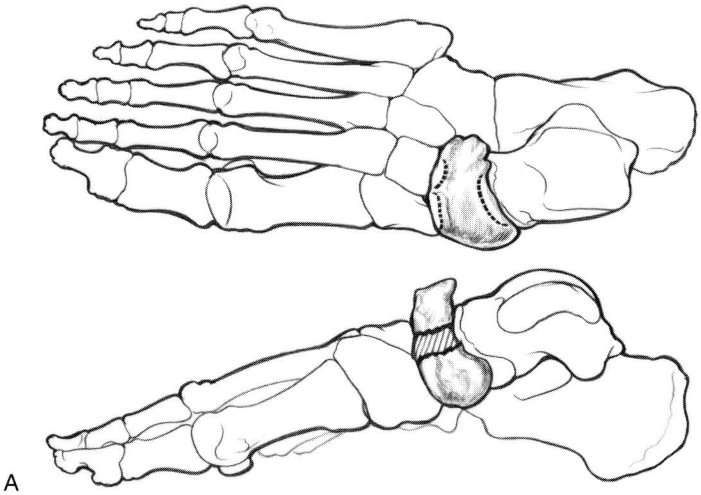

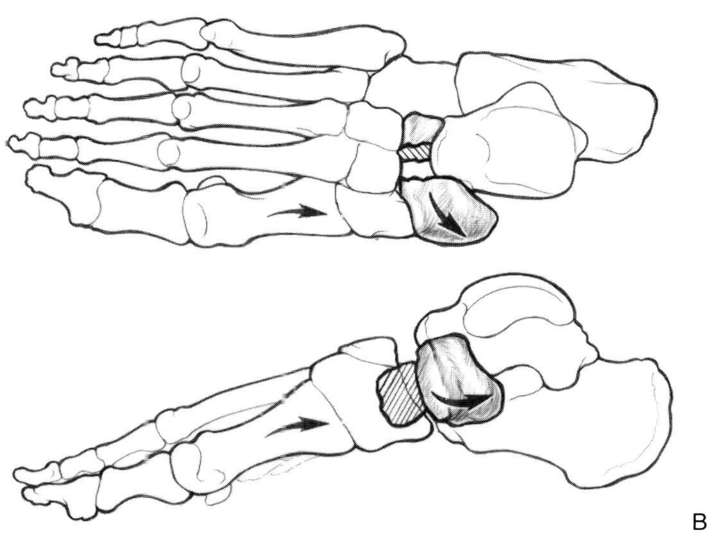

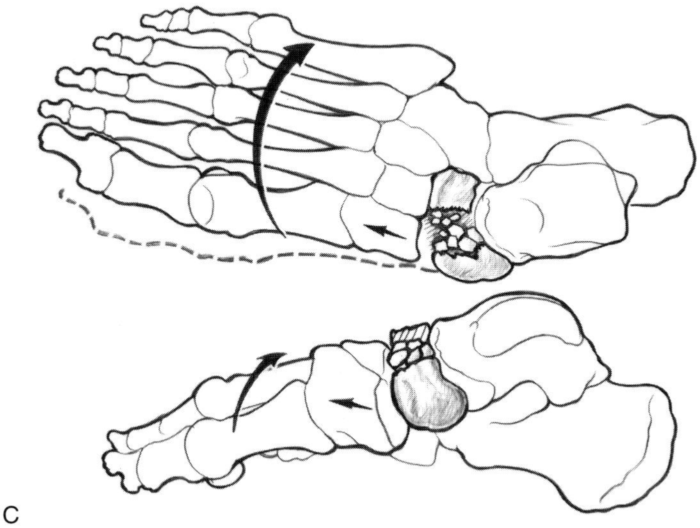

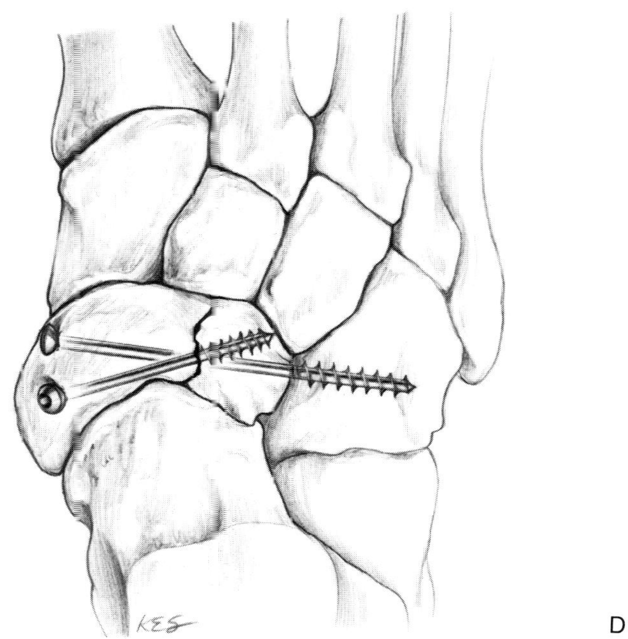

FIG. 26. A: Diagrammatic representation of a type I navicular fracture. The body is split and the dorsal half is displaced dorsally. **B:** A type II injury. The navicular is split in the sagittal plane. The body and the medial ray migrate proximally. **C:** The reduction maneuver for a type III fracture; linear traction and supination of the forefoot and the midfoot. **D:** One fixation option for a type II navicular fracture.

icular and the naviculocuneiform joints while the fracture is reduced and fixed securely with one or two 3.5-mm cortical lag screws (Fig. 26). A large avulsion fracture of the tuberosity may include a portion of the articular surface. An alternative approach is through a dorsal longitudinal incision made directly over the dorsal fracture line. This approach allows visualization of the fracture and the involved joint with minimal dissection. Screws are then placed with Weber forceps maintaining the reduction through medial and lateral stab wounds (Figs. 27–29).

Postoperatively the foot is immobilized in a nonweight-bearing cast for 6 to 8 weeks. After this, weight-bearing is begun in a commercially manufactured removable brace. Ultimately, the patient's shoe is fitted with a medical arch support.

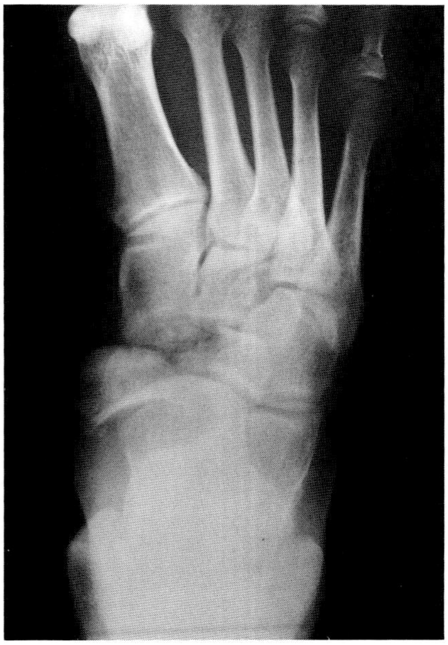

FIG. 27. An AP view of a foot with type II navicular body fracture.

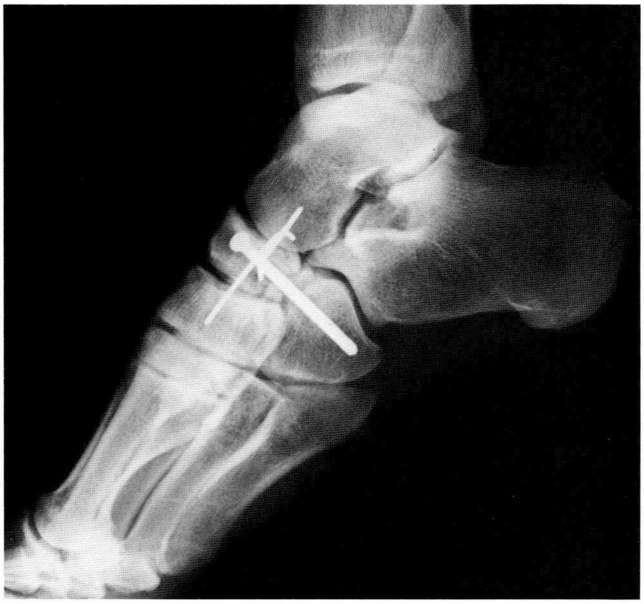

FIG. 29. A lateral view of the same patient showing the restored length of the medial column. Note that a straight line could be drawn along the top of the talus navicular and the cuneiforms.

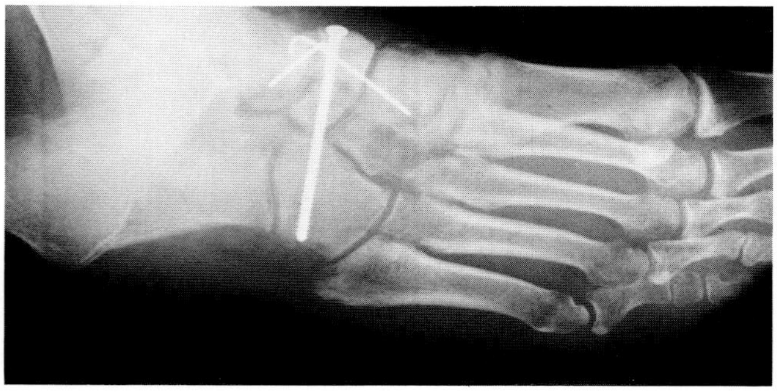

FIG. 28. An oblique intraoperative of the same patient following stabilization of the long screw into the cuboid and K-wire into the talus and cuneiforms.

COMPLICATIONS

Complications from a navicular fracture can include malunion, posttraumatic arthritis, and avascular necrosis. If the navicular collapses, the talus can be fused to the cuneiforms with tricortical bone grafting to maintain the length and plantar orientation of the medial column of the foot.

SKELETALLY IMMATURE PATIENTS

Navicular fractures are rare in children but are treated in the same manner as fractures in adults. Kirschner wires are usually used for fixation.

REFERENCES

1. Sangeorzan BJ, Benirschke SK, Mosca V, Mayo KA, Hansen ST Jr. Displaced intraarticular fractures of the tarsal navicular. *J Bone Joint Surg* 1989;71A:1504–10.
2. Eichenholtz SN, Levine DB. Fractures of the tarsal navicular bone. *Clin Orthrop* 1964;34:142–57.

Cuboid Fractures

MECHANISMS OF INJURY

Cuboid fractures usually occur in combination with other midfoot injuries, such as fractures of the talonavicular joint, the anterior calcaneus, or the base of a metatarsal. A direct blow to the lateral side of the foot often results in a nondisplaced fracture, whereas an indirect force usually compresses the cuboid between the bases of the fourth and fifth metatarsals on the anterior side of the calcaneus (1).

ANATOMIC CONSIDERATIONS

The cuboid articulates with the calcaneus, the lateral cuneiform, the fourth and fifth metatarsal bases, and, at times, with the navicular. The complex arrangement of these structures makes the occurrence of an isolated injury unlikely. The cuboid's articulations with the fourth and fifth metatarsals allow significantly greater motion in the lateral border of the foot than in the medial border. Malunion of the cuboid may make these articulations painful.

CLASSIFICATION

A meaningful classification system for cuboid fractures is precluded by their infrequent occurrence. Injuries of the cuboid are defined as nondisplaced or displaced, although minor avulsion fractures can also occur.

ASSESSMENT

Physical Examination

The clinical examination of a cuboid fracture is similar to that of other midfoot injuries. The foot is examined for tendon lacerations, vascular disruptions, neuromuscular deficits, and for signs and symptoms of compartmental syndrome. Because the incidence of associated injuries is high, the entire musculoskeletal system is carefully examined for other fractures.

Radiographic Evaluation

Standard radiographic evaluation includes AP, lateral, and oblique views of the foot (see Fig. 6). An oblique radiographic view is particularly important for evaluating a cuboid fracture and is the ideal view for assessing subluxation elsewhere in the midfoot (2).

Special Studies

No special studies are required.

EMERGENT MANAGEMENT

The foot is splinted in a neutral position and wrapped in a bulky dressing. Operative reduction is planned after the swelling subsides.

DEFINITIVE MANAGEMENT

Operative reduction and stabilization are performed with the patient lying supine with a large roll placed under the ipsilateral hip. A longitudinal incision is made dorsal to the peroneal tendons while the sural nerve is protected. A small distractor is placed laterally from the calcaneus to the metatarsals to lengthen the lateral border of the foot, which is usually shortened by the injury. Distraction allows reduction of the proximal and distal articular surfaces of the cuboid and usually creates a large defect for bone grafting and buttressing. A buttress plate is applied over the bone graft (Fig. 30).

Postoperatively, the foot is immobilized in a cast for 6 to 8 weeks. Weight-bearing is restricted to 15 pounds for the first month and then progresses to full weight-bearing. A heel orthosis or an insole can be inserted into the shoe for the patient's comfort during ambulation.

COMPLICATIONS

Like any articular injury, a cuboid fracture is susceptible to degenerative arthritis. Malalignment of the foot can result from compression of the fracture line or from malunion.

SKELETALLY IMMATURE PATIENTS

Cuboid fractures are rare in children but are treated in the same manner as fractures in adults.

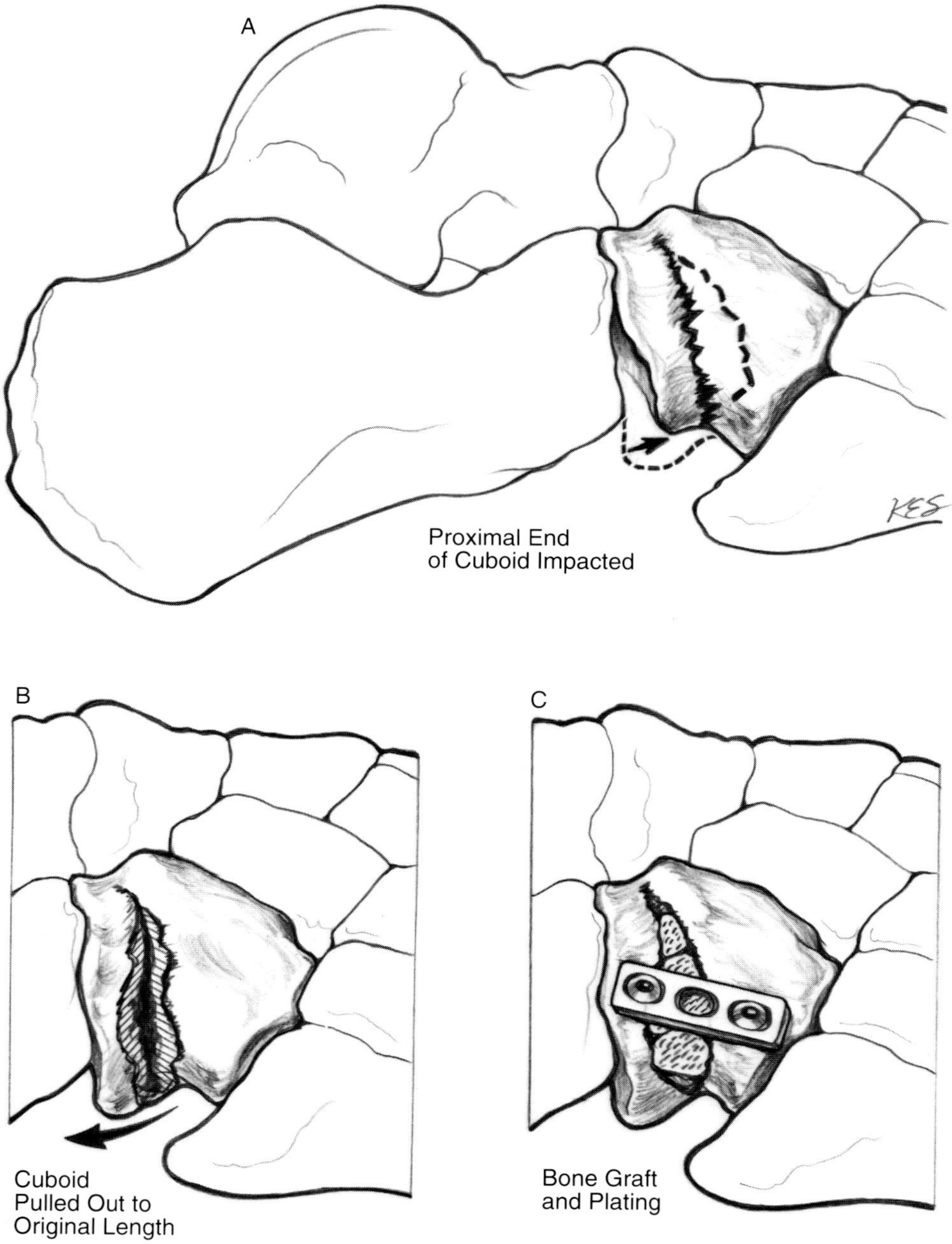

FIG. 30. A: The proximal end of the cuboid is impacted. **B:** The cuboid is pulled out to its original length. **C:** Bone graft and a plate are applied.

REFERENCES

1. Hermel MB, Gershon–Cohen J. The nutcracker fracture of the cuboid by indirect violence. *Radiol* 1953;60:850–54.
2. Sangeorzan BJ, Swiontkowski MF. Displaced fractures of the cuboid. *J Bone Joint Surg* 1990;72B:376–78.

Cuneiform Fractures

MECHANISMS OF INJURY

Cuneiform fractures usually result from direct trauma but can also occur indirectly by way of injury to the metatarsals. A cuneiform fracture can occur as an isolated injury or it can be associated with a Lisfranc's fracture–dislocation or a metatarsal fracture.

ANATOMIC CONSIDERATIONS

Despite its name, the shape of the first cuneiform is long and rectangular. A relatively mobile articulation exists between the first cuneiform and the intermediate cuneiform, but mobility is variable in the articulation between the first cuneiform, the navicular, and the first metatarsal. The first cuneiform maintains the shape of the medial ray of the foot, including the length and the position of the first metatarsal. The distal lateral side of the first cuneiform helps to lock the base of the second metatarsal into the keystone position in the midfoot. The distal base of the cuneiform accepts the insertion of the anterior tibial tendon, the major dorsiflexor of the foot. The midfoot assumes a cavus position when the cuneiform is shortened. Avulsion fractures usually occur at the metatarsal–cuneiform joint and are treated like Lisfranc's fracture–dislocations. Plantar avulsions injuries may involve the Lisfranc's ligament, which connects the base of the second cuneiform and the medial cuneiform.

CLASSIFICATION

No formal classification system exists for cuneiform fractures. Fractures of the body of the cuneiform are described as nondisplaced or displaced.

ASSESSMENT

Physical Examination

The entire foot is palpated for an occult tarsal fracture or joint disruption. Attention is directed to the TMT joint of the second ray and to the intercuneiform articulation, which may be injured concurrently.

Radiographic Evaluation

Anteroposterior, lateral, and oblique radiographic views of the foot are taken with the foot in a neutral position (see Fig. 6).

Special Studies

No special studies are required.

EMERGENT MANAGEMENT

Emergent management consists of elevation and splinting. In the presence of a compartmental syndrome, operative stabilization of the injury is done simultaneously with the compartmental release.

DEFINITIVE MANAGEMENT

Operative treatment is performed with the patient lying supine on the operating table after swelling subsides. The cuneiforms are visualized through two incisions: a medial longitudinal incision between the tibial tendons and a dorsal incision over the base of the second metatarsal. The reduction is stabilized with lag screws or with a small plate (Fig. 31) (1). Postoperatively, the leg is immobilized in a short-leg nonweight-bearing cast for 4 weeks. After this, partial to complete weight-bearing is allowed in cast for approximately 8 weeks until the fracture has united (Figs. 32–34).

COMPLICATIONS

Complications after cuneiform fractures arise from failure to diagnose the injury, a missed compartmental syndrome, or failure to maintain reduction. Like other midfoot injuries, cuneiform fractures are associated with a high incidence of compartmental syndrome. All these complications can be avoided by a thorough examination of the midfoot and by appropriate operative treatment.

SKELETALLY IMMATURE PATIENTS

Displaced cuneiform fractures in children are rare, but when they occur are treated in the same manner as injuries in adults. Kirschner wires are usually used for fixation.

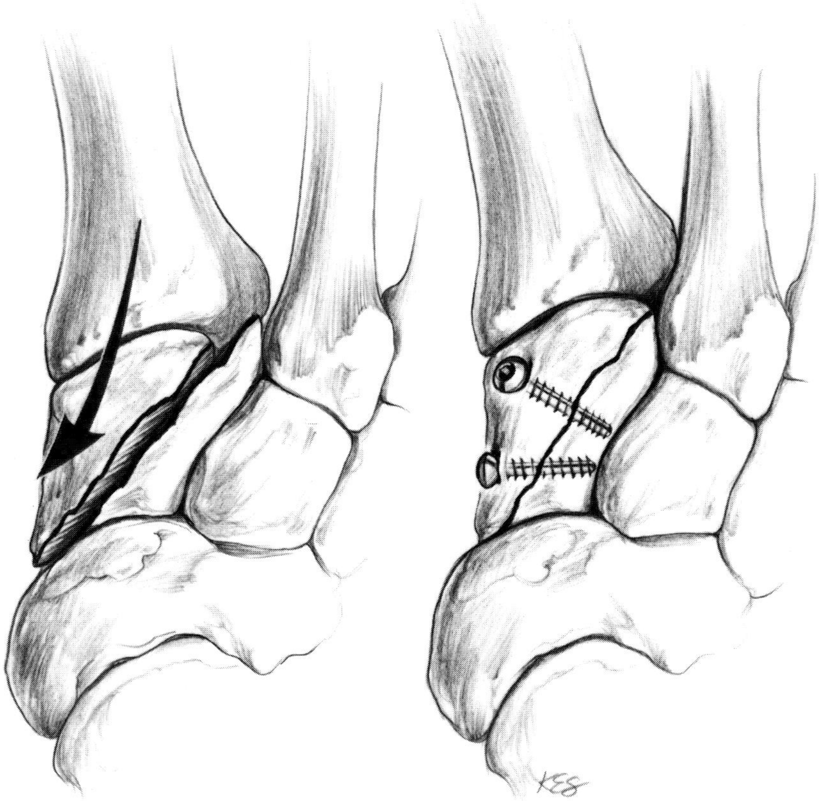

A, B

FIG. 31. **A:** The mechanism of injury of a cuneiform fracture is probably axial load applied through the first ray *(arrow).* The oblique fracture line can extend from proximal–medial to distal–lateral or from distal–medial to proximal–lateral. **B:** Fixation of a cuneiform fracture.

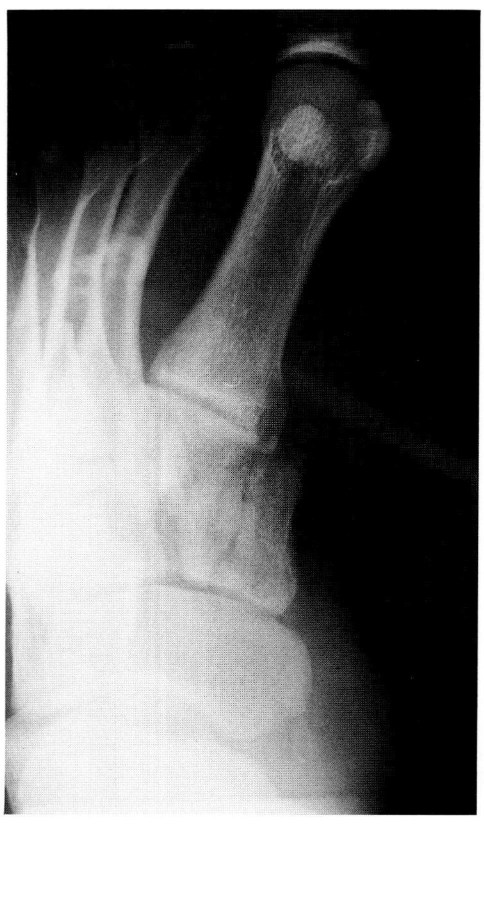

FIG. 32. Displaced cuneiform fracture. It appears that the entire first ray has been shortened into the substance of the navicular.

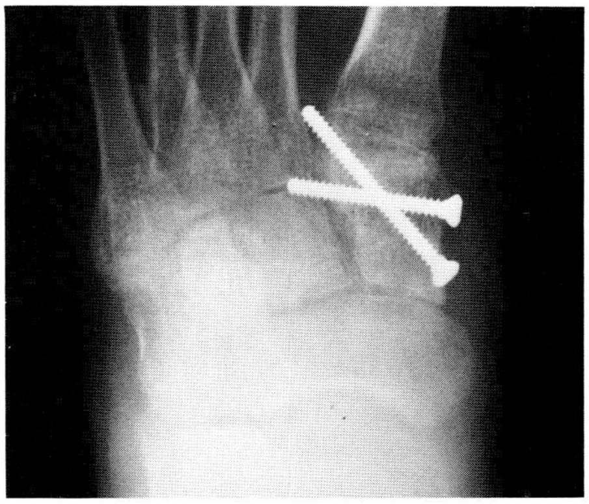

FIG. 33. An AP view at 8 weeks showing relatively normal anatomy and healed cuneiform.

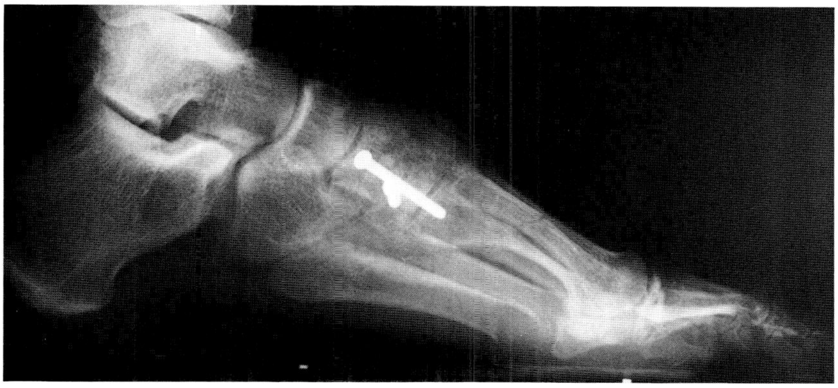

FIG. 34. A lateral view of the same patient.

REFERENCE

1. Sangeorzan ES, Mayo KA, Hansen ST. Intraarticular fractures of the tarsal bones. Part II: Talus and lesser tarsals. *Clin Orthop* [in press].

Metatarsal Fractures

MECHANISM OF INJURY

The most common cause of metatarsal fractures are crush injuries and motor vehicle accidents.

ANATOMIC CONSIDERATIONS

The metatarsals are fixed to the tarsals by a dense network of ligaments. The metatarsals provide length and shape to the foot and act as levers during the toe-off phase of gait.

CLASSIFICATION

No formal system exists for classifying metatarsal fractures. General guidelines for classification consist of the pattern of the fracture and the location of the injury. Fracture may occur at the base of a metatarsal (e.g., a Lisfranc's fracture–dislocation), in the diaphysis, or in the neck. A Jones fracture, located at the metaphyseal–diaphyseal junction of the fifth metatarsal, results from cumulative trauma.

ASSESSMENT

Physical Examination

The metatarsals are palpated for disruption of normal anatomic relationships and the integrity of the various extrinsic tendon insertions is assessed. The presence of pulses is documented for possible compartmental syndrome.

Radiographic Evaluation

Standard radiographic evaluation consists of AP, lateral, and oblique radiographic views of the foot.

Special Studies

No special studies are required.

EMERGENT MANAGEMENT

In general, no emergent management is required.

DEFINITIVE MANAGEMENT

Most metatarsal fractures, including nondisplaced fractures and those involving a step-off in a nonarticular plane, are treated in a cast with weight-bearing allowed as tolerated. Operative intervention is required for fractures involving the TMT joint or an intraarticular segment and for displaced fractures that alter the weight-bearing surface or the alignment of the foot. In addition, operative stabilization is

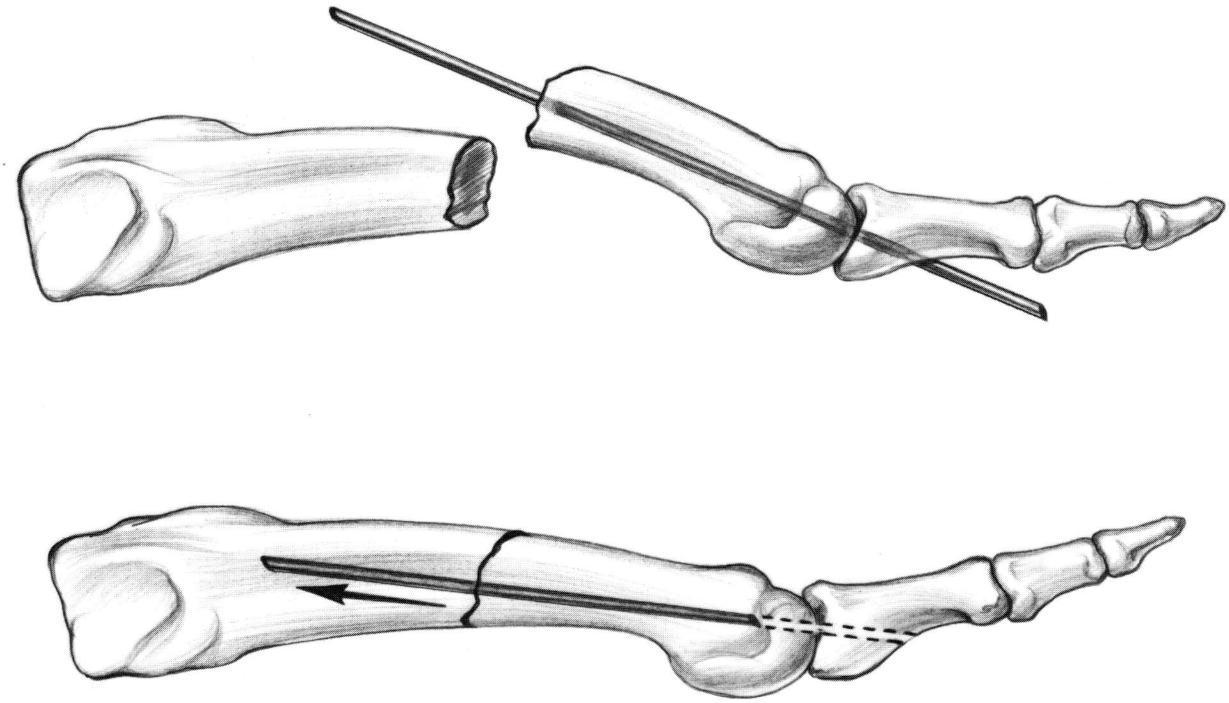

FIG. 35. Schematic representation of intramedullary fixation of a metatarsal fracture.

advised for all metatarsal fractures that occur as components of polytrauma when their presence impedes mobilization (22).

Operative treatment is usually carried out with the patient lying in a supine position on the operating table. Two or three longitudinal incisions are usually required to visualize all the metatarsal shafts. Diaphyseal injuries and fractures of the metatarsal neck are usually managed by intramedullary fixation with smooth pins. Fractures with joint involvement are stabilized by rigid internal fixation with screws, plates, or a combination of these devices. Metatarsal shaft fractures are managed by plating or by intramedullary fixation (Fig. 35). Postoperatively, the foot is immobilized in a nonweight-bearing cast for 4 weeks, followed by a weight-bearing cast for 2 to 4 more weeks.

COMPLICATIONS

Metatarsalgia or changes in the weight-bearing alignment of the foot may occur as consequences of malunion. If the weight-bearing distribution is disturbed, a corrective osteotomy may be required.

SKELETALLY IMMATURE PATIENTS

Metatarsal fractures in children are treated in the same manner as fractures in adults.

REFERENCE

1. Shereff M. Complex fractures of the metatarsals. *Orthopedics* 1990;13:8.

Orthopaedic Trauma Protocols, edited by
Sigvard T. Hansen, Jr., and Marc F. Swiontkowski.
Raven Press, Ltd., New York, © 1993.

CHAPTER 29

Associated Fractures

Marc F. Swiontkowski

Ipsilateral Fractures of the Femur and the Tibia

MECHANISMS OF INJURY

Ipsilateral fractures of the femur and the tibia (floating knee injuries) occur more commonly than double-level fractures in the femur. This combination of fractures occurs in the mid-shaft of both bones when axial load is applied to an extended knee. A tibial plateau or a proximal metaphyseal fracture occurs in association with the femoral shaft fracture when a direct blow is applied to the tibia.

ANATOMIC CONSIDERATIONS

A floating knee injury is associated with a high incidence of arterial injuries because of the proximity of the popliteal artery to the proximal tibia and knee.

CLASSIFICATION

Femoral and tibial fracture components are classified as individual fractures.

ASSESSMENT

Physical Examination

The physical examination for each component is the same as that for an isolated injury.

Radiographic Evaluation

The radiographic examination is the same as that for an isolated injury.

Special Studies

The status of the distal arterial circulation must be carefully assessed. Arterial injuries should be ruled out by ultrasound Doppler, and if any asymmetry is noted, arteriography is indicated. The preoperative evaluation of an intraarticular tibial fracture may include tomography or CT.

EMERGENT MANAGEMENT

The tibial fracture component should be aligned and splinted and the femoral fracture component should be immobilized in a portable Thomas splint or in roller traction. When diagnosis of an arterial injury is made, emergent repair must be performed by a consulting vascular surgeon.

DEFINITIVE MANAGEMENT

Operative stabilization of both fractures yields more normal knee motion than stabilization of only one fracture or of neither fracture (1). The femoral fracture component assumes priority and should always be fixed first. In this way, the patient can be mobilized out of traction with the tibia splinted if operative stabilization of the tibial fracture must be delayed (Fig. 1; see Chapter 25).

When both fractures are diaphyseal and closed, both are managed by closed interlocked nailing. The femoral fracture component should always be treated by this method except

Department of Orthopaedics, Harborview Medical Center, University of Washington, Seattle, Washington 98104

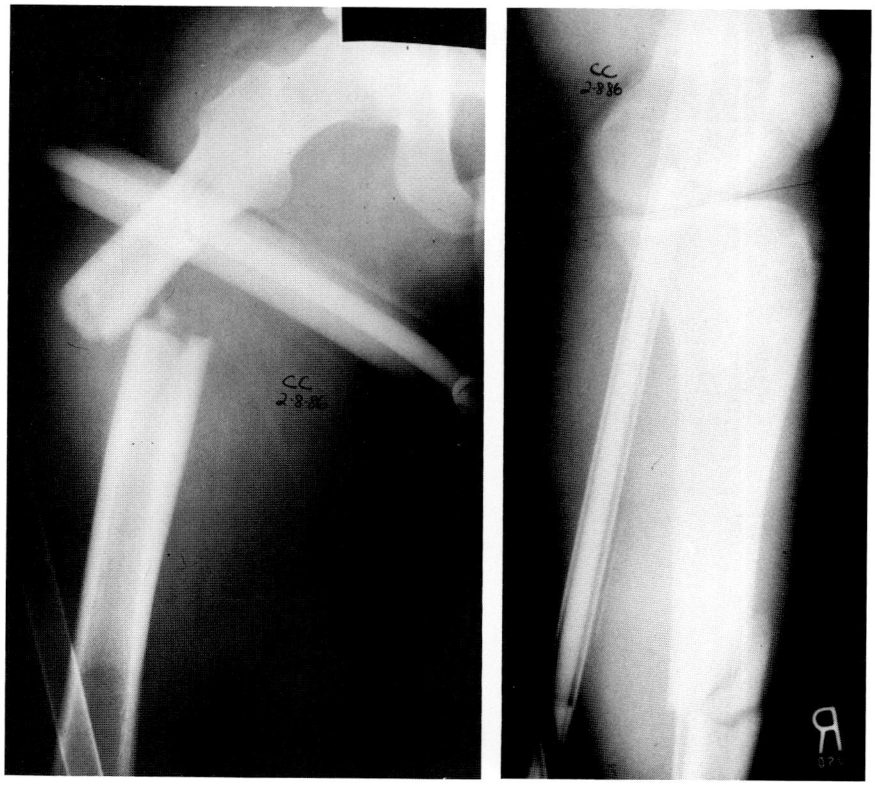

A,B

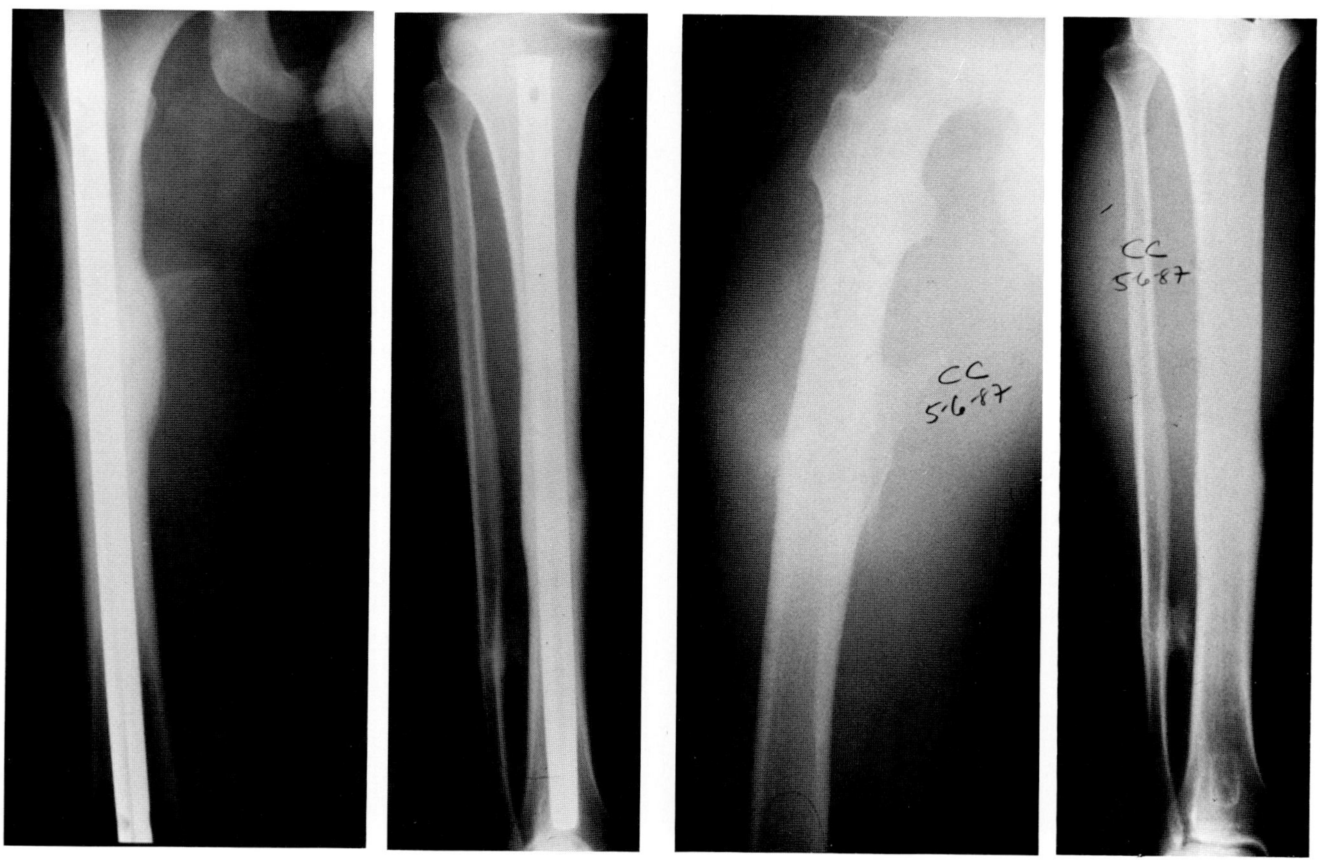

C,D

E,F

FIG. 1. A,B: A 19-year-old man sustained ipsilateral, closed fractures of the tibial and femoral shaft. **C,D:** These were managed with closed nailing techniques. **E,F:** Eighteen-month postinjury radiographs after nail removal reveal complete union. The patient had a full, functional recovery with 140° knee flexion.

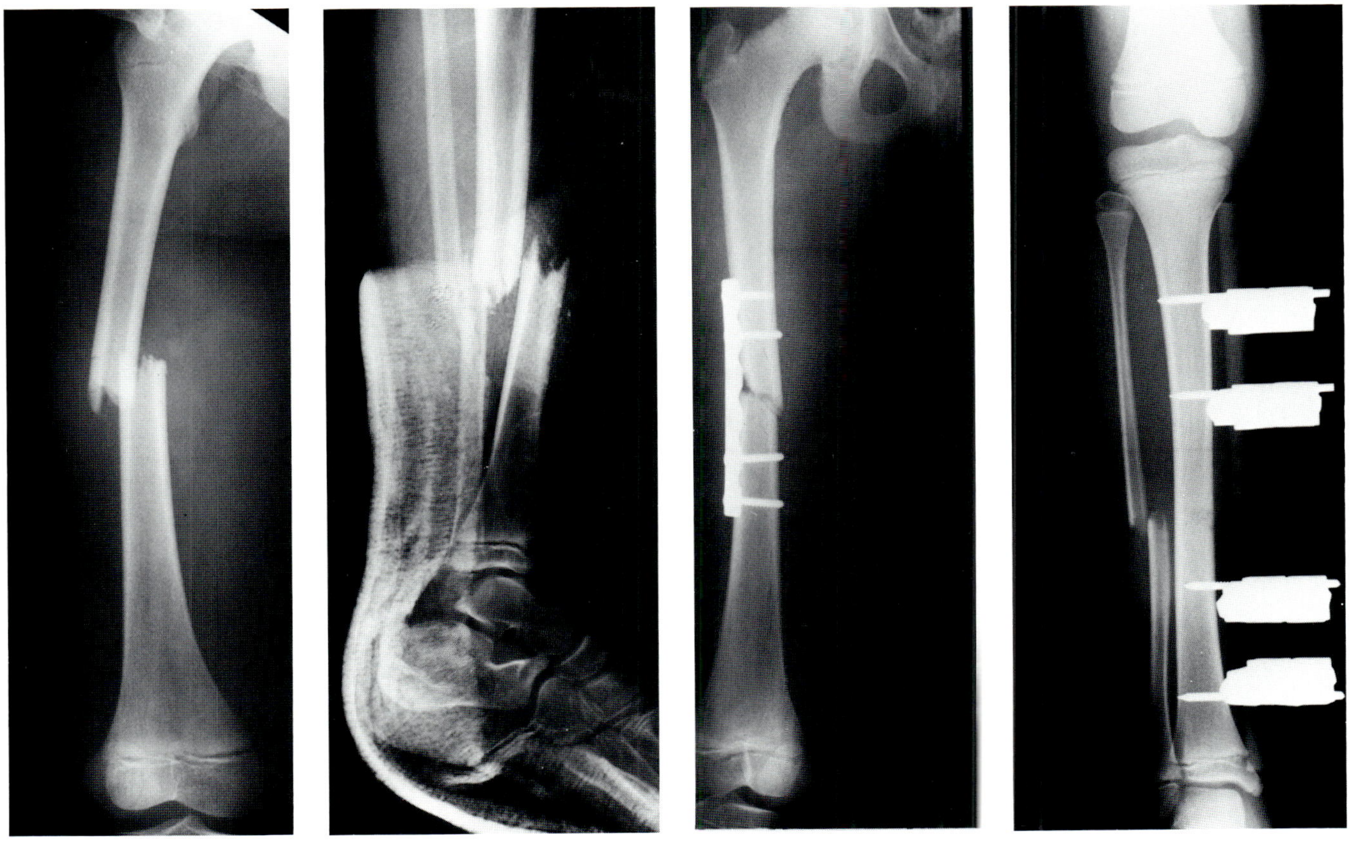

A,B C,D

FIG. 2. A 9-year-old girl was injured in a motor vehicle accident as an unrestrained passenger. In addition to a moderately severe closed head injury, she sustained a closed femoral shaft fracture (**A**) and a grade IIIA open tib-fib fracture (**B**). These were treated by limited exposure and plating for the femur (**C**) and by debridement and external fixation for the tibia (**D**). These fractures have gone on to uneventful union.

in very unusual circumstances. Unreamed interlocked nailing is used for grade I, grade II, and minimally contaminated grade IIIA open injuries. External skeletal fixation is used for extremely severe open injuries. Plate fixation is indicated for intraarticular fractures, metaphyseal fractures, and closed tibial fractures with simple fracture patterns that require fasciotomies.

COMPLICATIONS

Management of nonunion and deep infection in the tibia is discussed in Chapter 27. These complications are rare in femoral fractures. Compartmental syndromes are identified by vigilant serial examinations. In children, the proximal tibial epiphysis can slip, resulting in spontaneous reduction and in trapping of part or all of the popliteal artery.

SKELETALLY IMMATURE PATIENTS

Isolated floating knee injuries in children under the age of 8 years can be managed by a brief time in traction (for the femoral fracture), followed by spica casting. Open fractures of either bone or closed fractures with associated head, chest, or abdominal trauma are managed by external skeletal fixation or plating (Fig. 2). In children over the age of 10 years, femoral fractures can be treated by closed femoral nailing. Tibial fractures can be treated by casting, plating, or external skeletal fixation to shorten the hospital stay and promote the rapid return of knee function. Articular fractures of the tibia are rare in children, but when they occur they should be managed by open reduction, lag screw fixation, and buttressing with casting or plating.

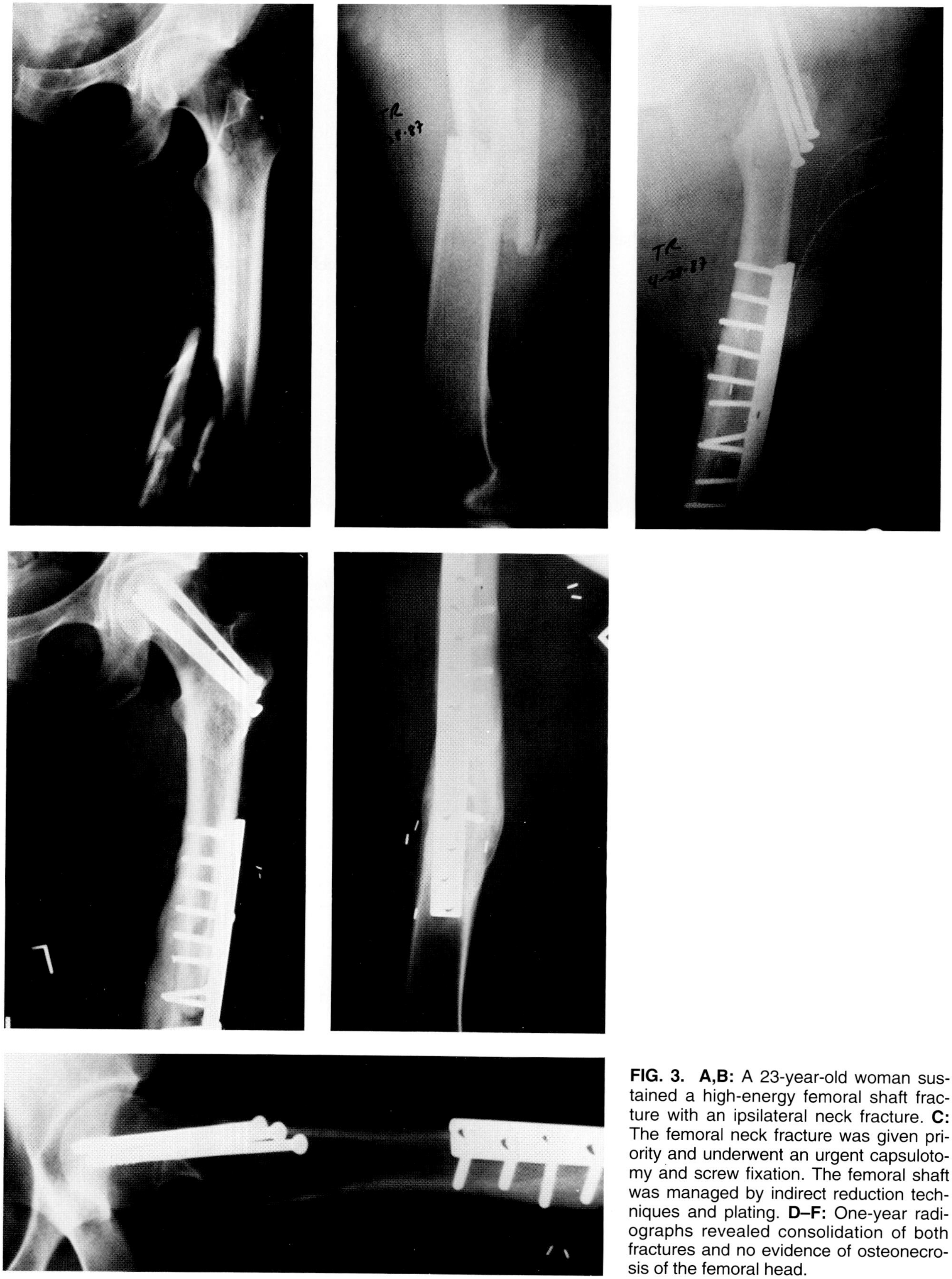

FIG. 3. A,B: A 23-year-old woman sustained a high-energy femoral shaft fracture with an ipsilateral neck fracture. **C:** The femoral neck fracture was given priority and underwent an urgent capsulotomy and screw fixation. The femoral shaft was managed by indirect reduction techniques and plating. **D–F:** One-year radiographs revealed consolidation of both fractures and no evidence of osteonecrosis of the femoral head.

Ipsilateral Fractures of the Hip and the Femoral Shaft

MECHANISMS OF INJURY

The most common mechanism of these double-level fractures is axial loading, an injury that can occur, for example, from striking the dashboard during a high-energy automobile collision. Ipsilateral intertrochanteric and femoral shaft fractures are less common than ipsilateral femoral neck and shaft fractures.

ANATOMIC CONSIDERATIONS

When the femoral neck fracture is the more proximal component of the two fractures, significant concerns are raised regarding the effects of operative stabilization on femoral head vascularity and potential osteonecrosis. These concerns are less important when the proximal fracture is extracapsular.

CLASSIFICATION

When ipsilateral fractures are graded, the most important consideration is whether the proximal fracture is intracapsular or extracapsular. Individual fractures are classified separately, but when they occur in combination they demand unique treatment considerations. Most femoral neck fractures are vertical and are frequently nondisplaced.

ASSESSMENT

Physical Examination

The physical examination is the same as that of a patient with an isolated femoral shaft fracture.

Radiographic Evaluation

The radiographic evaluation is the same as the evaluation of an isolated femoral shaft fracture.

Special Studies

Angiography is usually not required.

EMERGENT MANAGEMENT

Approximately 2.5% of femoral shaft fractures occur concurrently with femoral neck fractures (2). The stability of the femoral neck fracture component can be compromised during treatment of the femoral shaft fracture if the femoral neck fracture was not diagnosed during the initial evaluation (3). Missed diagnoses occur in approximately 30% of ipsilateral femoral neck fractures. To avoid this scenario, the admitting AP pelvic radiograph should be supplemented by an AP hip radiograph, and both must be evaluated carefully. After a femoral neck fracture is recognized, treatment should not be delayed.

DEFINITIVE MANAGEMENT

Ipsilateral Intertrochanteric–Femoral Shaft Fractures

Operative stabilization is indicated for combined ipsilateral intertrochanteric–femoral shaft fractures. A second-generation interlocking nail can be used for stabilization if the intertrochanteric fracture component is reduced and provisionally stabilized before the starting point is developed. Alternatively, a hip screw can be used with retrograde Ender nails, but in this case the femoral shaft fixation must be supplemented with a fracture brace or a spica cast during the early postoperative phase.

Ipsilateral Femoral Neck and Shaft Fractures

The femoral neck fracture component of ipsilateral femoral neck and shaft fractures is susceptible to posttraumatic osteonecrosis and must receive treatment priority. Although second-generation nails are promoted for use in this situation, they must be used with caution. Their use should be restricted to nondisplaced femoral neck fractures located above femoral shaft fractures. The femoral neck fracture must be stabilized provisionally with either Kirschner wires or screws placed anterior to the starting point of the nail. Management of the femoral neck fracture component includes urgent reduction, capsulotomy, and fixation with three cannulated screws. The femoral shaft can then be stabilized by plating (see Fig. 2) or by retrograde femoral nailing (Fig. 3). This situation is one of the few remaining standard indications for plate fixation in femoral shaft fractures.

Retrograde nailing is performed with the patient positioned supine on the fracture table. The starting point of the nail must be extraarticular but in line with the femoral shaft on the medial femoral condyle. After reaming, a 12-mm nail (maximum 13 mm) is driven across the fracture site with the bow in the coronal plane. The nail is then rotated 90° to the sagittal plane (2). When locking is required to stabilize a comminuted fracture, a Universal tibial nail is recommended. The locking screw holes in the Universal tibial nail are located distally and will lie in the proximal femur in the AP plane. In the presence of an open knee wound, the starting point for standard femoral nailing is made in the intercondylar notch and the nail is inserted retrograde in the normal orientation (Fig. 4). Femoral plating does not delay mobility because weight-bearing during the

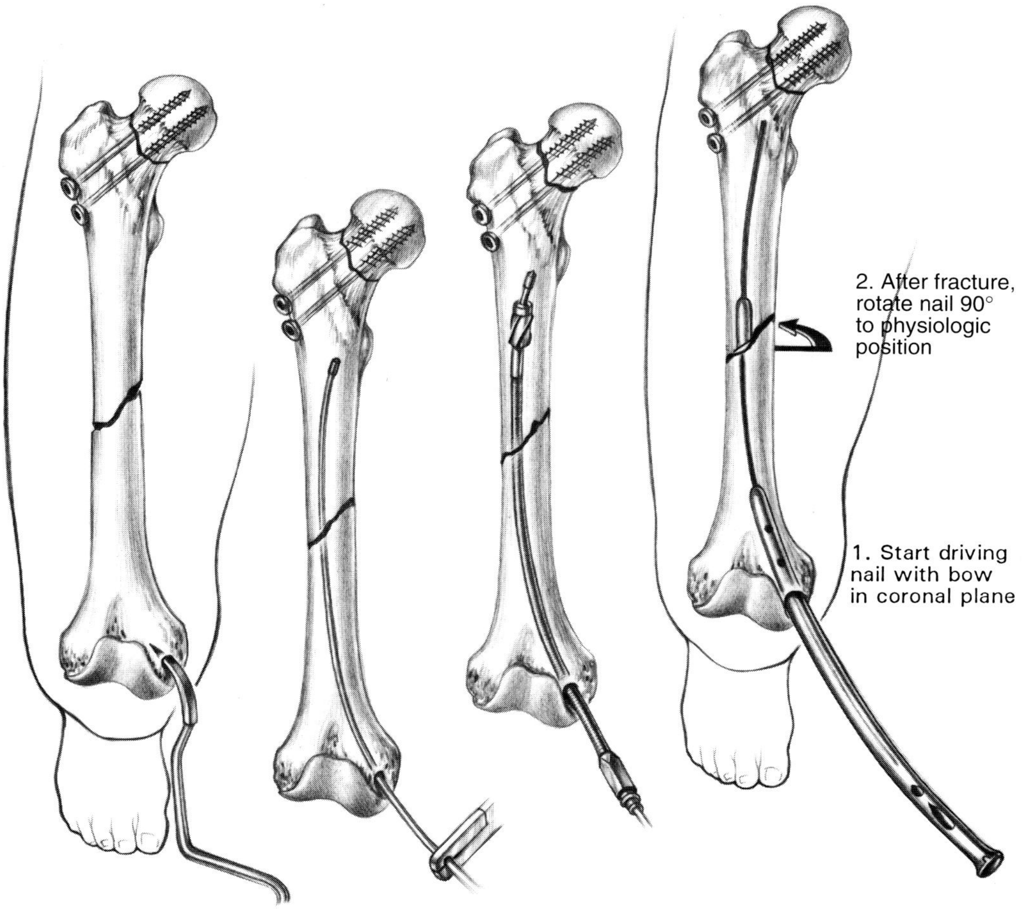

FIG. 4. After capsulotomy and screw fixation of the femoral neck fracture, an option is to stabilize the shaft fracture with a retrograde nail. The starting point is in the medial femoral condyle in line with the shaft (**A**). The ball-tipped guide is pushed across the reduced fracture (**B**), and reaming is sequential as for standard antegrade nailing (**C**). The nail insertion is initiated with the bow in the coronal plane and then is rotated into the sagittal plane **(D)**. This nail rotation can be avoided if a tibial locking nail is substituted.

postoperative phase of femoral neck stabilization is limited to touch-down weight-bearing for 3 months. Patients treated by retrograde nailing are limited to touch-down weight-bearing for 12 weeks.

COMPLICATIONS

Nonunion of femoral neck fractures is rare with appropriate treatment. Posttraumatic osteonecrosis occurs in 5% to 10% of combination fractures. This low rate of complications is attributed to the dissipation of energy through the femoral shaft fracture.

SKELETALLY IMMATURE PATIENTS

Double-level fractures are uncommon in children. When they occur, the femoral neck fracture component is considered an emergency and must be treated by capsulotomy, reduction, and fixation with lag screws; the femoral shaft fracture component can be treated initially with traction but is replaced by casting after 2 to 4 weeks. Plating or external skeletal fixation should be considered in children over the age of approximately 10 years to avoid prolonged hospitalization and to allow early motion of the knee and the hip. Weight-bearing must be delayed for 10 to 12 weeks regardless of the type of treatment used.

REFERENCES

1. Veith RG, Winquist RA, Hansen ST. Ipsilateral fracture of the femur and tibia. *J Bone Joint Surg* 1984;66A:991–1002.
2. Swiontkowski MF, Hansen ST, Kellam J. Ipsilateral fracture of the femoral neck and shaft: a treatment protocol. *J Bone Joint Surg* 1985;66A:260–8.
3. Swiontkowski MF. Ipsilateral femoral shaft and hip fractures. *Orthop Clin North Am* 1987;18:73–84.

Orthopaedic Trauma Protocols, edited by
Sigvard T. Hansen and Marc F. Swiontkowski,
Raven Press, Ltd., New York, ©1993.

CHAPTER 30

Soft-Tissue Injuries in the Lower Extremity

Sigvard T. Hansen, Jr.

NEURAL INJURIES

Lumbar and Sacral Plexus Injuries

Lumbar and sacral plexus injuries are usually the result of Malgaigne fractures with significant displacement of the hemipelvis. The resultant deficit can be widespread and may include paralysis, or it can be limited to the nerve roots located between L-5 and S-1 and result in a drop-foot deformity. Treatment of lumbar and sacral plexus injuries consists of early anatomic stabilization of the sacroiliac joint fracture–dislocation and possible decompression of the nerve roots, followed by observation. Myelography to rule out root lesions is not as reliable in the lower extremity as it is in the upper extremity. Attempts at high sciatic nerve repair indicate that repair of plexus injuries in the lower extremities is usually unsuccessful. Return of function after neuropraxia, which may take up to 6 months, can be further enhanced by tendon transfers and joint fusions.

Sciatic Nerve Injuries

Sciatic nerve injuries usually occur secondary to hip dislocations or fracture–dislocations. Treatment consists of early relocation, using care to avoid entrapping the nerve. In general, neuropraxia in the tibial portion of the sciatic nerve resolves with good function. Sciatic nerve injuries associated with pelvic and acetabular fractures can be caused by entrapment of the nerve between bony fragments and require surgical visualization and fracture reduction. The peroneal nerve portion is most vulnerable to injury. Good, although incomplete, eventual recovery of neural function is expected. If adequate peroneal nerve function does not return, tendon transfers, such as transfer of the posterior tibialis to the dorsum of the foot, can be done to enhance mobility.

Distal Nerve Injuries

Nerve injuries distal to the popliteal fossae may occur after knee dislocations and are treated by reduction and stabilization of the knee. The peroneal nerve can be injured by fibular dislocation, lateral ligamentous rupture, or severe varus angulation of the knee. Other mechanisms include excessive pressure from casts or splints or even from body weight in comatose patients. A suspected peroneal nerve injury in a previously comatose patient must be carefully differentiated from a compartmental syndrome. Return of neural function may take from 3 to 6 months after initial correction of the bony and ligamentous problems. If adequate function does not return after splinting and observation, muscle transfers and limited fusions can be done.

The posterior tibial nerve may occasionally be injured at the ankle level by fracture–dislocations of the pilon, ankle, or subtalar joints, particularly in open injuries with severe displacement. The nerve is explored by tracing it from normal tissue proximal to the injury to injured tissue. When neural function is disrupted by neuropraxia the limb can usually be salvaged. However, complete interruption concurrent with other severe injuries may be an indication for amputation in adults.

Department of Orthopaedics. Harborview Medical Center, University of Washington, Seattle, Washington 98104

VASCULAR INJURIES

Iliac Artery and Veins

Iliac artery injuries are rarely seen in trauma patients who survive their injuries. However, the artery can be disrupted in a so-called "wishbone" injury, in which one leg is violently abducted at the hip with partial lateral–superior dislocation of the hemipelvis. Occasionally the limb is completely avulsed at this level.

The iliac vein or its major branches are occasionally injured in severe hemipelvic injuries, such as Malgaigne fractures. The superior gluteal artery may be disrupted by a posterior pelvic ring fracture or during the exposure for reduction. Bleeding in this major artery must be controlled by embolization or by direct exposure and ligation. Torn pelvic arterial vessels may warrant angiographic embolization. More often, bleeding originates from small presacral veins or at the fracture surfaces, and the earliest possible reduction and stabilization with pelvic clamps, external skeletal fixation, or ORIF are indicated to control hemorrhage.

Femoral Artery

The femoral artery is occasionally injured in femoral shaft fractures, especially in distal fractures with long oblique fracture patterns. Early diagnosis and repair are important (1). Disruption usually occurs in Hunter's canal, which is located near the distal-third junction. Distal circulation can be quickly restored by a shunt followed by rapid stabilization of the femur, usually by plating. Definitive treatment of femoral artery disruptions is provided by primary suture or vein grafting. When an injury is discovered very early and collateral circulation is not disrupted, the artery can be temporarily clamped, the bone stabilized, and the artery repaired if these procedures are done quickly. A major concern during this procedure is prophylactic release of compartmental fascia in the injured leg. Compartmental release should be strongly considered when much of the circulation has been interrupted for 3 hours or longer and when significant swelling is anticipated. When circulation has not been extensively disrupted, the compartments should be monitored carefully during the postoperative phase.

Popliteal Artery

Disruption of the popliteal artery may occur with a knee dislocation, particularly an anterior dislocation: a partial tear involving the intima may be present in the absence of clinical symptoms at the time of the initial presentation if the knee has relocated spontaneously. A high index of suspicion must be maintained when an acute unstable knee injury is examined. A noninvasive duplex scan or a Doppler study should be done and, if arterial integrity is in doubt, angiographic studies must be performed to rule out intimal tears. In most hospitals these tests should be conducted on acutely injured patients in the operating room rather than in an angiographic suite. Although the quality of the angiogram taken in the operating room will be somewhat diminished, it will still be adequate, and the patient's other problems can be continuously monitored and managed. Like femoral artery injuries, popliteal artery injuries that significantly interrupt circulation to the leg for longer than 4 h warrant prophylactic compartmental releases in the leg and possibly in the foot. Alternatively, the compartments must be closely monitored in the postrepair phase.

Vessels in the Proximal Tibial Region

Arterial and venous injuries are often seen in the trifurcation area after high-energy displaced fractures of the proximal tibial metaphysis. The anterior tibial artery branches off the popliteal artery and travels through the tibiofibular interosseous membrane between the fibular head and the lateral tibial condyle approximately 2 cm to 3 cm below the articular facet. The tibioperoneal trunk runs 2 cm to 4 cm farther before branching into the peroneal and the posterior tibial arteries. The large posterior tibial artery enters the deep posterior compartment through a groove located posterior to the posterior tibial muscle and between the flexor hallucis longus laterally and the flexor digitorum longus medially. At the ankle, the tendons of the posterior tibialis and the flexor digitorum longus muscles lie medial and anterior to the posterior tibial artery, vein, and nerve and just behind the medial malleolus. After rounding the malleolus, the posterior tibial artery divides to provide circulation to the sole of the foot.

Depending on the level of the proximal injury, one or more of these vessels may be lacerated. The posterior tibial artery is occasionally explored and repaired when circulation is inadequate. The main casualty of posterior tibial artery disruption is the deep posterior compartmental musculature. In some cases, differentiating a posterior tibial artery injury from a deep posterior compartmental syndrome is difficult, just as differentiating a deep peroneal nerve injury from an anterior compartmental syndrome may require careful evaluation.

In young patients the collateral circulation can maintain foot viability if the anterior and peroneal vessels are intact. In warm climates, adequate treatment of one-vessel injuries in proximal fractures may consist of ligation of the vessel. However, the situation is quite different when only one vessel, usually the anterior tibial artery, remains uninjured. The leg in which arterial circulation is supplied by a single major vessel is very feeble because circulation is inadequate for cold weather, heavy activity and, occasionally, even for healing of distal fractures.

Similar considerations apply to vessels damaged by high-energy injuries in the tibial shaft. A posterior tibial artery laceration can often be repaired. Major considerations in this area are the zone of injury and the potential for the "freeway syndrome" (see Chapter 1). A vein graft traversing a large zone of injury becomes, in essence, a freeway carrying blood to the foot and ankle but provides no circulation to the damaged soft tissues in the region it traverses. When the injury is caused by laceration or a bullet injury, few complications are expected to develop after arterial repair. However, crushing injuries with large zones of injury (6 inches ± 2 inches), in which considerable muscle has been lost and in which a vein graft of at least 4 inches is required, can pose major problems with regard to regional soft-tissue viability and even bone viability. The sequelae of inadequate muscular and bony viability are manifested as progressive necrosis, chronic infection, failure of bony union and, eventually, amputation.

Posterior Tibial Artery

Injury to the posterior tibial artery may occur at the ankle level with fracture–dislocations of the pilon, ankle, talus, or subtalar joints. In many fracture–dislocations the posterior tibial artery simply follows a lateral ankle dislocation through a tear in the deep posterior compartment without sustaining any damage, but the artery is likely to be damaged in a lateral subtalar dislocation.

Like dissection for posterior tibial nerve injuries, dissection of the posterior tibial artery should proceed from more normal anatomy to more damaged anatomy, and the torn area should be visualized if it is not already exposed. The vessel may not actually be damaged but merely trapped between bony fragments or between the tibia and the fibula, or the area may be shredded or crushed and not amenable to repair. A large zone of injury containing crushed or divided muscles, nerves, and tendons or multiple fractures may warrant early amputation instead of repair and salvage. In contrast, injuries caused by sharp lacerations may heal well after the artery is tied off if the collateral circulation has not been disrupted and other structures are not severely injured. Direct suture repair or vein grafting is done for injuries of intermediate severity. The consequences of arterial injuries are not particularly significant in the foot. Postinjury necrosis in the forefoot is often blamed on arterial injuries when, in fact, it is caused by compartmental syndrome, which is easily treatable.

COMPARTMENTAL SYNDROMES

Compartmental syndromes present a potential threat to the limb and must always be ruled out in blunt high-energy injuries. Compartmental syndromes can occur in any muscle but are most common in muscle that is confined in a limited space between fascia and bone. An insult such as hemorrhage, postischemic edema, restricted venous flow, or muscle contusion may increase the volume of soft tissue in the compartment and inhibit incoming arterial circulation. As a result, the cycle of ischemic injury and edema progresses until cell death occurs. Muscle and then nerve may die, with grave consequences for residual function.

In the lower extremity, compartmental syndromes occur most commonly in the most restrictive compartments, the deep posterior and anterior compartments in the calf musculature. The fascia of the lateral (peroneal) compartment is less restrictive and is less commonly involved. The superficial posterior compartment containing the gastrocnemius and soleus muscles is the least restrictive and is rarely involved.

Deep Posterior Compartmental Syndrome

Deep posterior compartmental syndromes can occur after high-energy talar and calcaneal fractures as well as tibial fractures, and are difficult to diagnose. This compartment is neither superficially palpable nor easily measurable by manometric techniques, and the compartmental syndrome may involve only certain muscles in the compartment. Diagnosis of a compartmental syndrome in the deep posterior compartment can be made by stretching the toes passively into dorsiflexion. This maneuver results in inordinate pain if the compartmental syndrome is in the ischemic phase. However, the posterior tibialis muscle cannot be easily tested by active motion or passive stretch when it is splinted or casted. Because the intrinsic muscles in the foot can mimic toe flexion exactly, the status of the flexor digitorum communis and the flexor hallucis longus muscles cannot be established. For these reasons, compartmental syndromes here are easily missed during the acute phase.

The first symptoms of deep posterior compartmental syndrome may appear as slowly increasing contractures of the involved muscles during the recovery phase. Sepsis and limb loss are uncommon in the acute phase. When the posterior tibialis muscle is not involved, compartmental syndrome is manifested only as flexion contracture in the toes. With posterior tibial muscle involvement the foot becomes internally rotated, inverted on the lateral border with weight-bearing, and generally stiff. It should be noted that tethering of these muscles at the fracture site by scarring can produce very similar symptoms. These sequelae can be treated successfully by opening the deep posterior compartment, isolating the involved muscles, and debriding the scarred and contracted muscles and their tendons. Significant early necrosis often produces inflammation around the tendon and the area distal to it. Tendinous adhesions that prevent the foot from becoming supple and relaxed require complete removal of the tendon (2,3). Deep posterior compartmental syndromes may occur in the postischemic phase as the result of injury to a more proximal vessel.

Anterior Compartmental Syndrome

The anterior compartment contains the massive muscle bellies of the anterior tibial muscle and the toe extensors. The sequelae of compartmental syndrome are more severe in this compartment, but fortunately, diagnosis is not as difficult here as it is in the deep posterior compartment. The anterior compartment is accessible to direct palpation and is easily measured by manometric techniques. On physical examination, stretching the toes into plantarflexion through the full range of passive range of motion (ROM) causes intense pain during the ischemic phase. Because the intrinsic foot muscles allow flexion and extension through a short range, the ability to wiggle the toes does not rule out a compartmental syndrome. Another sign of impending compartmental syndrome that is sometimes unrecognized is increased pain with elevation of the leg above the level of the heart. Elevation of the leg increases the arterial pressure needed to push oxygenated blood into the compartment. By the time myoglobin can be detected in urine, which confirms muscle cell death, it is usually too late to salvage significant function. Full functional recovery is achieved through early detection and compartmental release without regard for cosmetic deficits from significant scarring or skin grafting. A scar can be revised with good results by plastic surgery, but a compartmental syndrome in the anterior compartment causes permanent functional disability.

Standard incisions (a single long lateral incision or combined lateral and medial incisions) are used for fasciotomy (Fig. 1). Fibulectomy through the lateral incision has been advocated in the past but is no longer recommended. The fibula is an important structure in the lower extremity for partial weight-bearing and as the attachment of the peroneal tendons and muscles to the great toe, and these functions must not be sacrificed. The lateral incision is made first to expose the lateral peroneal compartment. At this point in the operation the distal superficial peroneal nerve must be protected. The anterior compartment is reached by undermining the anterior flap at the muscle fascia-to-fat interface. The length of the fasciotomy must extend the full length of the compartment. The posterior compartment is also accessible from the lateral approach. The incision for the release begins distally and extends proximally more than halfway up the leg after the compartment is located in front of the fatty tissues anterior to the heel cord. A second medial incision can be made to release the deep posterior compartment. Release of any compartment associated with a fracture mandates concurrent stabilization of the fracture. The lateral surface of the tibia can be plated through the fasciotomy incision or the tibial fracture can be stabilized by nonreamed locked intramedullary nailing. An unstabilized fracture exposes the soft tissues to contact with bony edges and increases morbidity.

Sepsis can develop in a compartmental syndrome that is missed, opened late, or contaminated by an open fracture or by diagnostic needles. The consequence of sepsis occurring in conjunction with necrosis or after a significant fracture may be amputation. Even without sepsis, necrosis results in drop-foot deformity with serious functional deficits that will require bracing or muscle transfers for adequate function. The deep posterior tibial muscle and tendon can be rerouted to the dorsum of the foot, but this transfer is only partially successful and does not allow full ankle motion. The goals of fasciotomy are to completely release the compartment while avoiding damage to nerves and major vascular structures. Every trauma surgeon should practice compartmental releases on cadavers and become proficient in this technique. Inexperience is the most common reason for delaying fasciotomy and, subsequently, for losing muscle tissue. The sequelae of missed compartmental syndromes (necrosis, sepsis, and possible amputation of the limb) are poorly defensible from the standpoint of malpractice.

Proximal Compartmental Syndromes

Compartmental syndromes in the buttocks and thighs are rare. Compartmental syndromes may occur in the gluteus maximus and, occasionally, in the gluteus medius secondary to pressure from sitting for a long time in a drug-induced stupor or from poor surgical positioning. Other causes include major blunt injuries to the area resulting in concurrent pelvic or acetabular fractures. High-energy injuries, in which a pedestrian is struck by a vehicle on the lateral or anterolateral thigh musculature, can produce compartmental syndromes at the level of impact. Such injuries usually produce large closed contusions which are associated with massive swelling after the compartments are released and which may be responsible for secondary muscle loss. Symptoms of massive swelling in the thigh and intense pain from ischemia are indicative of a compartmental syndrome and should be investigated. In comatose patients, diagnosis is made by palpation and direct measurement. Pressures of 35 to 50 mm Hg that are sustained for over 2 h indicate the need for compartmental release. Opening the fascia longitudinally is sufficient treatment as long as the incision extends the full length of the muscle compartment. The anterior and posterior thigh compartments can be released through a single lateral incision. A second medial incision must be added for release of the adductor compartment.

Compartmental Syndromes in the Foot

Compartmental syndromes can occur in foot compartments, particularly in the proximal plantar compartment, after high-energy calcaneal fractures. They are also seen here in association with Lisfranc's or combination Lisfranc's and metatarsal fractures that involve intrinsic muscle compartments in the forefoot. Other causes include soft crushing injuries (e.g., a tire rolling over the foot) not associated with fractures but only with generalized massive swelling. In such cases the skin may be the limiting factor and may function as the restrictive compartment.

Compartmental syndromes in the proximal plantar compartment that are associated with calcaneal fractures can be released by making an incision along the abductor hallucis,

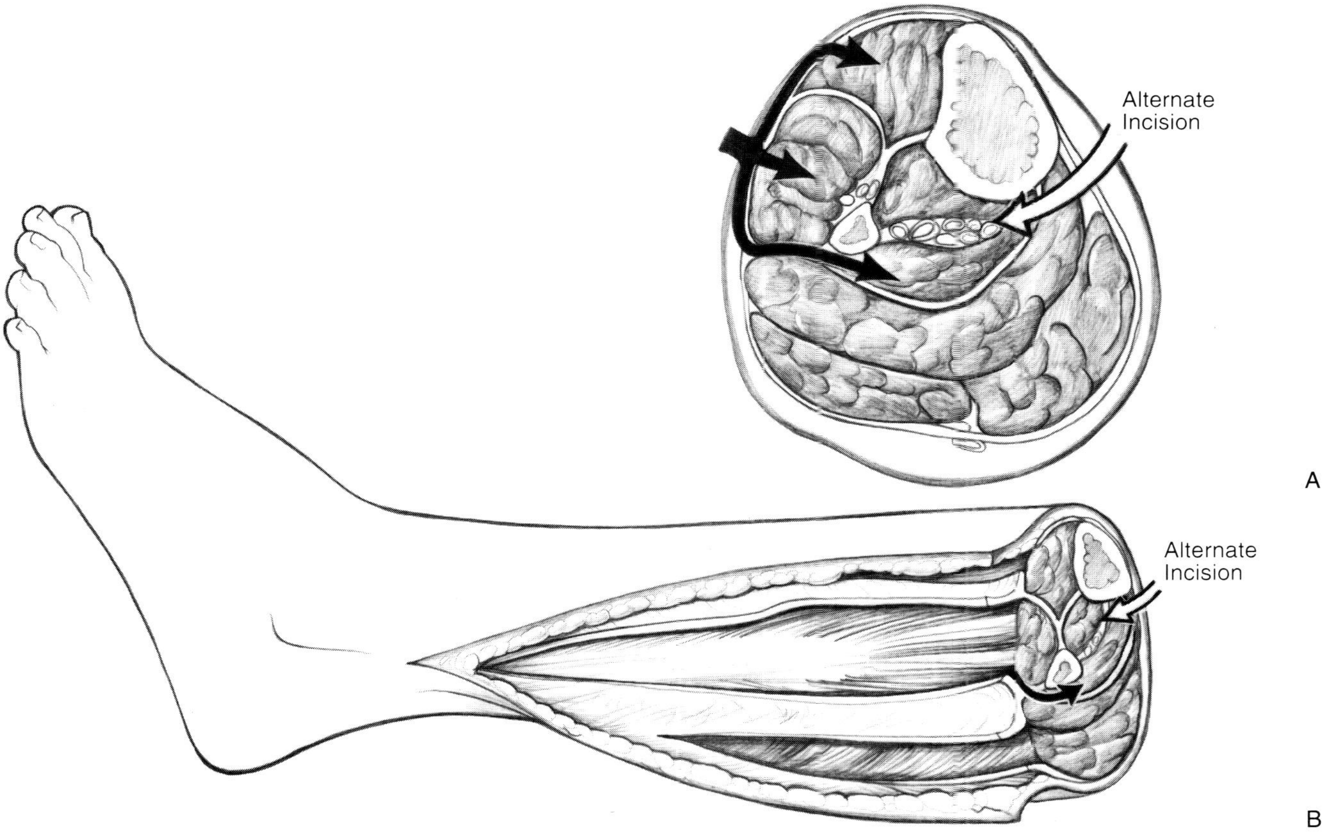

FIG. 1. Release of compartmental syndrome. **A:** The relative positions of the muscles in the middle part of the leg. **B:** The incisions that are made to release the compartments—a long lateral incision or, alternatively, a lateral medial incision—are seen in cross-sectional representations. When making a long lateral incision, the peroneal nerve that angles anteriorly from its exit to the distal third of the muscle must be identified and protected. The anterior flap is lifted forward to identify the anterior compartment. An incision made blindly may miss the anterior compartment. Separate incisions must be made in the fascia for the lateral and anterior compartments. The deep posterior compartment can be easily located in the distal part of the wound and the incision is run proximally from there. Attempts to keep the incision short, and thus more cosmetic, may simply result in continuation of intercompartmental necrosis. Compartmental syndromes released late complicate the assessment of tissue viability. Necrosis often starts centrally or deep inside the muscle. Muscle that looks viable on the surface may, in fact, be markedly necrotic in the deep compartment. Evidence of myoglobinuria and increased temperature are symptomatic of necrosis. Skin grafts should never be placed over superficially viable muscle with deep necrosis .

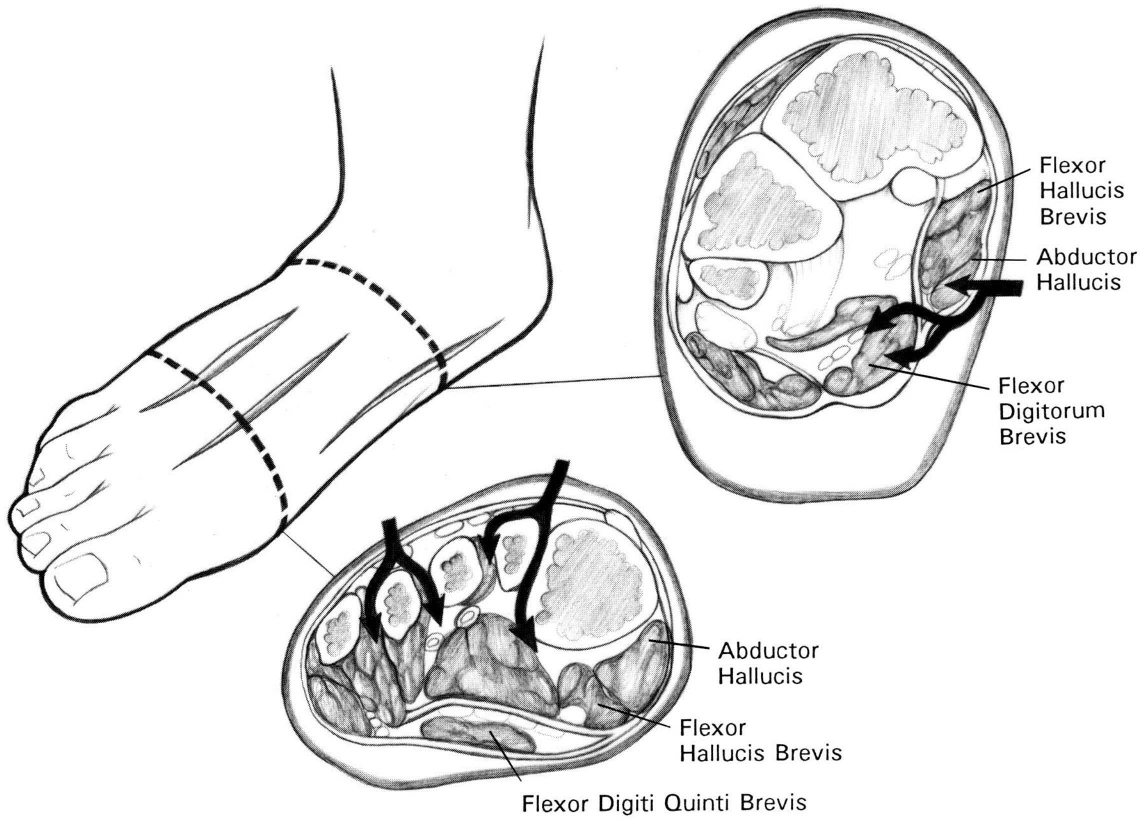

FIG. 2. Incisions for plantar or subcalcaneal compartmental syndromes and forefoot compartmental syndrome. The incision for a plantar compartmental syndrome, most commonly associated with calcaneal fractures, is made directly over the abductor hallucis. Compartment syndromes in the forefoot are more commonly associated with Lisfranc's fracture–dislocations or Lisfranc's dislocations with associated metatarsal shaft fractures. Two incisions are recommended: one between the first and second metatarsals and the other over the fourth metatarsal. These incisions also are ideal for repairing fracture–dislocations, which should be done whenever a compartment is released. Opening the skin relieves a significant amount of pressure and using a small straight clamp to release the deeper tissues under the fascia releases additional compartmental pressures. In a calcaneal fracture, the compartmental release and open reduction of the calcaneal fracture are done through separate incisions.

retracting it upwards, and carefully opening the deep compartments (Fig. 2) (4). Sharp or blunt dissection is carried out with hemostats until hemorrhage and edema are relieved. The calcaneal fracture can be repaired at the same time through a lateral incision, or it can be stabilized later through the same lateral approach.

Forefoot compartments are released through two dorsal longitudinal incisions (see Fig. 2). A medial incision is started over the first web space and extended over the mid-tarsus, and a parallel lateral incision is placed in the region dorsal to the fourth metatarsal and extended over the tarsus. These incisions allow release of the intrinsic muscle compartments between each of the metatarsals. They also allow immediate reduction and fixation of a Lisfranc's dislocation and associated metatarsal fractures, which must be stabilized in the acute phase. These fractures are diagnosed from plain radiographs and do not require CT scanning or other diagnostic studies that might delay fixation. Closure of the fasciotomy wounds is postponed for approximately 5 days until compartmental release and fixation have been accomplished; skin grafts can be applied if edge-to-edge skin closure is not possible.

Diffuse swelling in the foot associated with soft-tissue roll-over injuries can be treated by the "pie-crust" or Böhler technique (Fig. 3). Multiple 2–5-mm longitudinal incisions are made on the dorsal and lateral aspects of the skin, allowing egress of edema fluid and hematoma and expansion of the skin. The incisions are not deep and penetrate only the skin, avoiding injury to deeper veins, nerves, and arteries. The resulting pattern is similar to a meshed graft.

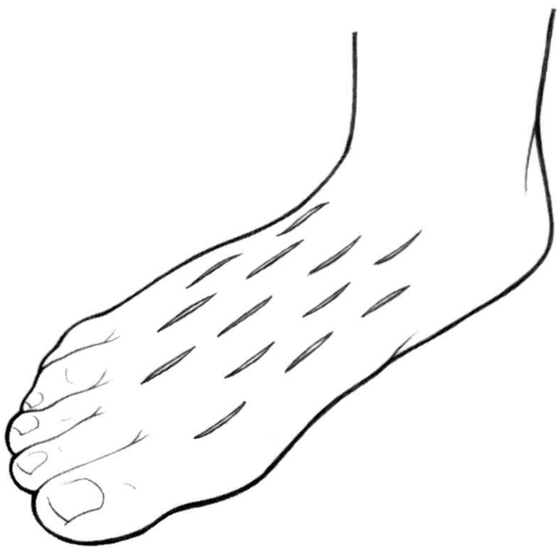

FIG. 3. The Böhler technique for releasing pressure under the skin of the foot. The incisions are made linearly through the skin and the fascia, carefully avoiding nerves, tendons, and vessels. This technique allows the skin to expand and the edema to be released. The incisions heal with minimal elevation and compression dressings.

INTEGUMENTARY INJURIES

Laceration, Contusion, and Crushing

When a skin laceration resembles a surgical incision it may do very little harm, especially when the skin is not separated from underlying fat and muscle. The zone of injury may be very narrow and closure may be possible with minimal debridement. Lacerations occurring from the inside out or those caused by blunt objects may produce larger areas of contusion and crushing or irregular margins at the skin edges and require thorough debridement. Inadequate debridement can lead to slower healing, greater scarring, partial or complete necrosis of the skin edges, and compromised protection to the underlying tissues. In general, the margins of debridement can be determined by close examination of the skin edges, noting color, consistency, and separation of skin from underlying soft tissues. The amount of necrosis increases with greater crushing and separation of tissue layers.

The viability of closed contused or crushed skin is more difficult to evaluate. A superficial area of skin may become necrotic and covered with blackened eschar while the underlying dermal tissue and epidermal islands regenerate new integument. This process is desirable in a small area. The prognosis for adequate regeneration is poor when shearing from the underlying tissue or degloving has occurred.

Degloving

Degloving injuries are familiar to all traumatologists but are so varied in presentation that little has been written about their etiology, prognosis, treatment, or outcome (Fig. 4). This type of injury may involve a very large area, such as the entire lateral buttock and flank, or it may be confined to a small area, such as the distal extremity near the knee or the lateral calf. The lesions can be either closed or open, and they can occur with or without significant fracture. In closed injuries degloving consists of a separation of skin and subcutaneous fat from deeper muscles at the muscle fascial level.

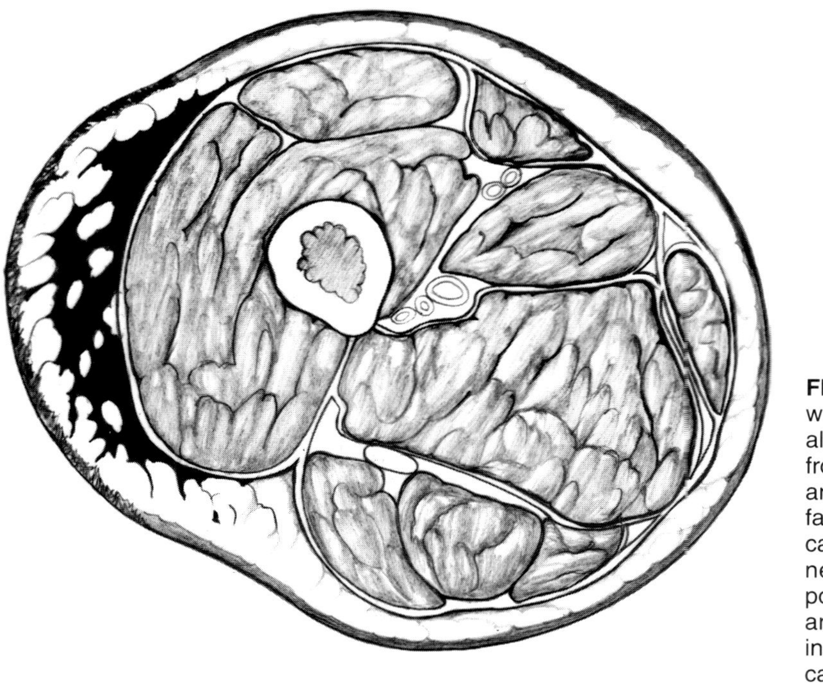

FIG. 4. Cross-sectional representation of the thigh with a closed degloving injury over the vastus lateralis. This injury can result from a very hard fall or from being struck by a moving vehicle. The large area of separation of the deep fat in the muscle fascia and subsequent hematoma and tension can cause necrosis of the overlying skin and subcutaneous fat. The hematoma and the free fat are potential culture mediums. Sufficiently defining the area of necrosis or draining the area to prevent infection and necrosis is an important aspect of care in multiply traumatized patients.

In a closed injury the resultant defect is filled with hemorrhage and free fat. Most closed degloving injuries are caused by high-energy blunt trauma with a shear component. Large, closed degloving injuries are more common in patients with a thick layer of subcutaneous fat. A large fatty hematoma may become necrotic and possibly infected in a closed space, and skin in the center of the area may become necrotic and slough, leaving a large open wound. Open degloving injuries are often seen with fractures in the lower extremities, where a significant area of the detached and devascularized skin may eventually become necrotic and expose the underlying fracture and other injured tissues to infection.

Treatment of closed degloving injuries with small hematomas and a high likelihood of skin viability consists of cool compressive dressings to slow the progress of bleeding, followed by compression after 48 h. The volume of some hematomas increases over time, requiring either aspration or open drainage to enable the fat and fascial layers to adhere together. However, the value of routine aspiration of liquified hematomas with large-bore needles several days after injury is unclear because this procedure poses a threat of contaminating and infecting this excellent culture medium.

In large areas of degloving, we recommend opening and evacuating the large hematoma, followed by fluorescein and Wood's light examinations to evaluate the viability of the skin circulation. Skin in the center of the degloved area can be removed superficially with a skin-graft knife, noting the presence of bleeding points. This technique is particularly useful in the foot (5). Bleeding in the area of degloving is an indication that the area will survive and that the underlying tissue can be left untouched. Areas that do not bleed with the skin-graft removal technique should be resected early and the removed split-skin graft placed immediately on viable tissue under the debrided area. This technique is especially useful in dark-skinned patients, in whom fluorescein is unreliable, and in areas where degloved skin is clearly nonviable. It is an excellent source of split-thickness skin grafts and eliminates the need for harvesting tissue from normal areas of the body.

All devitalized skin in areas larger than 3 cm in diameter should be excised and replaced with skin grafts or muscle flaps. These areas should not be left to demarcate spontaneously because large areas of necrotic or septic tissue are detrimental to patients' overall health. However, small areas of devitalized skin may spontaneously heal across surrounding live tissue. Eschar develops over the area and, after several weeks, gradually contracts and becomes detached. If the eschar becomes moist, macerated, or clearly infected underneath, it should be debrided back to healthy tissue.

Finally, making an accurate diagnosis and prognosis of these injuries can be significant from a medicolegal standpoint. If unexpected wound slough results in unsightly scarring, the quality of surgical care may come into question. When patients are warned early that this eventuality may occur as part of the natural progression of their injuries, such criticism is far less likely.

MUSCLE INJURIES

Crushing, Laceration, and Separation from Bone

Muscle does not heal by tissue regeneration but by scarring, and major transection or crushing injuries are associated with significant functional deficits. Muscle is virtually impossible to suture back to its original length or into its original position after it has been lacerated or crushed. Lacerated or crushed muscle also deprives regional vessels, nerves, and bone of protective cover and blood supply, leaving them vulnerable to drying or desiccation. This eventuality poses even greater problems immediately after repair of vessels, nerves, or bone, when muscle coverage is virtually essential for healing. Evaluation of muscle viability is difficult because no quantitative data exist to predict tissue survival. Normal color, consistency, and contractibility are the standards by which muscle is evaluated, but these qualities are subjective in every case. Inadequate debridement promotes infection; radical debridement creates large areas of dead space without coverage for bone, vessels, and nerves and requires early free-tissue composite grafting. Transplanted tissue is functional only as a replacement for missing coverage, not for motor function.

The general protocol for grading muscles that are divided, crushed, stripped, or detached from bone is similar to that used for grading soft-tissue injuries in general. When an entire muscle or an entire compartment (especially the anterior compartment) is transected or debrided, the advantages of attempted salvage must be carefully weighed against the advantages of immediate amputation. The treatment decision must be based not only on the limb's potential for survival but also on the quality of its potential function compared to the function of a well-designed modern prosthesis. Prosthetic replacements are extremely functional in the lower leg but are far less functional in the thigh, where salvage is desirable. In elderly or severely injured patients, attempted salvage of a limb with a large volume of damaged or nonviable muscle may threaten the patient's survival. In this case, amputation is a life-saving procedure that assumes priority over functional considerations.

Soft-Tissue Grading

Soft-tissue grading is necessary in all open and closed injuries, with or without fracture, for providing a prognosis, as a guide to treatment, and for research purposes. The criteria for grading can be fairly general or minutely detailed. The simplest schemes are noncomprehensive and inexact but are most likely to be used. Detailed schemes, although they are ideal for research, are awkward to use routinely in hurried circumstances. The system we have used for several years lies somewhere in between the two extremes. It consists of Tscherne's four grades of closed injuries (C-0, C-I, C-II, C-III) and a revised version of Gustilo's five grades of open injuries (O-I, O-II, O-IIIA, O-IIIB, and O-IIIC). The parameters for grading include the amount of energy that caused the injury, the type of force that was applied (indirect or direct), the size of the zone of injury, and the amount of fracture comminution. With these criteria, injuries of similar severity and prognosis are grouped together in numerical grades corresponding to treatment. Clearly, no open injury is as benign as a C-0 injury and virtually no closed injury is as severe or as difficult to manage as a grade O-IIIB or O-IIIC injury. High-grade injuries require skin or free-tissue grafting for wound closure and are often best treated by amputation. The basic parameters and criteria for each grade are found in Chapter 1. A more sophisticated but comparable system is proposed in a companion text to this book (6). Although it is slightly more difficult to use, the system described there is more exacting and should be used to document data for research.

OPEN FRACTURES

Initial management of open fractures is usually provided by emergency medical technicians or paramedics, the first medically trained personnel to arrive at the scene of the accident. The patient's wound should be covered with a sterile dressing and the limb aligned in a Thomas splint, even though splinting might retract exposed and contaminated bone back into the soft tissues. Although reinserting open bone ends into the soft tissues is controversial, soft tissues are damaged less when the bone is aligned in traction and splinted during transport to the hospital. The wound will be thoroughly opened, cleansed, and debrided in the operating room, and the most urgent consideration is to protect blood supply to the bone, not to decrease the amount of contamination. The rare exception is a patient with an entrapped nerve, when aligning the leg is more painful than leaving it in a deformed position.

In the emergency department, the wound should be inspected by a senior house officer who can accurately describe and tentatively grade the wound. After this examination the leg should remain splinted and again be covered with a sterile dressing. The wound should not be examined again in the emergency department, but only in the operating room after anesthesia has been administered. The senior surgeon should carefully examine the wound and amend the grading on the basis of the grading criteria described earlier. This information is integrated with an analysis of the patient's overall history, including age, the presence of other injuries, and any previous other medical problems, especially vascular disease. The treatment decision is made on several levels: grading the injury between O-I, a low-risk injury, to O-IIIC, a very high-risk injury; establishing the goal of treatment as life-saving, limb-saving, or aimed at maximal rehabilitation; and choosing the most appropriate fixation device from a number of possible alternatives, including external skeletal fixation, plates and screws, nonreamed interlocking nails, and prereamed nails. Finally, the injury is graded definitively for documentation.

The primary reason for immediate skeletal stabilization is preservation and protection of soft-tissue viability. Fixation techniques that help promote bony union are desirable but are not as important at this stage as protection of the soft tissues. Fortunately, these techniques are not mutually exclusive. In high-grade injuries with extremely contaminated wounds, the leg is draped (without a tourniquet) and irrigated again, and preliminary sharp debridement is carried out to remove all crushed, contused, or devitalized tissue. The leg is then prepped again for more precise debridement, high-volume irrigation, and internal fixation. In less severely contaminated wounds of lower grades, a single prep with careful sharp debridement is sufficient before proceeding with fixation using indirect reduction techniques (7). Indirect reduction techniques are used to align and provisionally stabilize the fracture with the least possible direct manipulation of the bone ends, particularly manipulations that would further separate muscle and fascial attachments from the bone. Elevators and bone clamps that encircle the bone and strip soft tissue are not used. Intramedullary devices with locking capability, whether reamed or nonreamed, are ideal for indirect reduction of open fractures. These devices produce minimal damage to the intramedullary blood supply in the femur, even though they present a significant risk in high-grade tibial fractures

After all necrotic tissue, including detached and degloved skin and muscle, has been debrided and provisional fixation has been performed, the limb is evaluated for realistic salvage. Salvage should be attempted if all the following criteria are met: (i) adequate circulation remains in the foot and in all the regional tissues in the wound area; enough muscle remains to provide function and local coverage and protection of vessels and nerves; (ii) enough skin and subcutaneous tissue remains intact to provide reasonable venous and lymphatic return; and (iii) the amount of injury in the limb does not overwhelm the patient's capacity for healing. If one of these criteria is not met, especially in an injury below the mid-leg, amputation should be seriously considered.

The skin covering the open wounds should be left open in all cases. In deep lacerations, some suturing of fascia, tendons, and muscles will be required to hold the soft tissues in place over neurovascular structures and to restore anatomy. Care must be taken to avoid leaving loculated dead spaces in which hematoma and seroma can collect and to avoid strangulation of soft tissues with large sutures, which creates necrotic tissue and a culture medium. The exudate that is produced during the first 3 to 5 days after injury must have easy egress from the wound. Occasionally a counter-incision must be made in a dependent location, or a suction drain must be enclosed within the wound. After these precautions have been taken, the wound is covered with a sterile dressing (with or without Betadine or another antibacterial solution), casted, and elevated slightly for 3 to 5 days. During this time monitoring is conducted for compartmental syndrome and other systemic problems, even though any evidence of infection in the wound is highly unlikely during this short period.

In injuries with extensive soft-tissue loss, vascularized rotational free-tissue grafting can be done at 3 to 5 days. The vascular pedicle must make contact with a vessel outside the zone of injury. In lower grade injuries, a split-thickness skin graft is applied in the operating room during the first cast and dressing change at 4 to 6 days. Injuries that received inadequate initial debridement and those with questionable vascularity or serious contamination are returned to the operating room after 36 to 48 h for debridement and reevaluation. In most cases this intermediate step is unnecessary after adequate initial treatment. If the decision is made to proceed with reevaluation, wound coverage must be delayed until 3 or 4 days after the resolution of any problems. Once secure soft-tissue coverage has been obtained, patients are gradually mobilized with gentle isometric exercises in cast to assist circulation. After 3 or 4 weeks bony union is assessed, and the need for an additional procedure is ascertained. By this time the soft tissues should be well stabilized and clearly viable. When cortical bone or vascularity has been lost at the bone ends, a stimulating bone-graft procedure can be considered after 4 to 6 weeks. Although cancellous bone graft can be applied at the time of delayed primary closure without significant morbidity or additional hospitalization, early grafting has a lower incidence of success than grafting done 4 to 6 weeks postinjury.

REFERENCES

1. Sher MH. Principles in the management of arterial injuries associated with fracture/dislocations. *Ann Surg* 1975;182:630–33.
2. Hansen ST Jr. Chronic sequelae of leg compartment injury. In: Jahss MH, ed. *Disorders of the foot and ankle. Medical and surgical management.* 2nd ed. Philadelphia: WB Saunders Company; 1991:2586–90.
3. Manoli A II, Weber TG. Fasciotomy of the foot: an anatomical study with special reference to release of the calcaneal compartment. *Foot Ankle* 1990; 10:267–75.
4. Fakhouri AJ, Manoli A II. Acute foot compartment syndromes. *J Orthop Trauma* 1975;6:223–8.
5. Ziv I, Zeligowski A, Mosheiff R, et al. Split-thickness skin excision in severe open fractures. *J Bone Joint Surg* 1988;70B:23–.
6. Border JR, Allgöwer M, Hansen ST, Rüedi TP. Evaluation of extremity injuries. In: Border JR, Allgöwer M, Hansen ST, Rüedi TP, eds. *Blunt multiple trauma. Comprehensive pathophysiology and care.* New York: Marcel Dekker; 1990:441–56.
7. Mast J, Jakob R, Ganz R, eds. *Planning and reduction techique in fracture surgery.* Berlin: Springer-Verlag; 1989.

Subject Index

A

Accident, process of, 23
Accident-prone individual, 23
Acetabular dysplasia, in pelvic fracture, 234, *235*
Acetabulum, fracture of, 243–254
  anatomic considerations in, 243–247, *244, 245, 246, 247*
  assessment of, 247–250, *249*
  both-column, 251–253, *251, 252*
  in children, 254
  classification of, 247, *248*
  columnar, 250
  complications of, 253–254
  deep venous thrombosis in, 250, 253–254
  definitive management of, 250–253, *251, 252,* 253(t)
  emergent management of, 250
  heterotopic ossification in, 253
  infection in, 254
  intraabdominal injury with, 243
  mechanisms of, 243
  physical therapy for, 68–69
  positioning considerations in, 252–253
  preoperative planning in, 251–252
  radiographic evaluation in, 248, *249*
  secondary congruence in, 251, *251*
  traction in, 250
  transverse, 250
  vascular injury in, 254
  wall, 250
Acetaminophen, in pain management, 34(t)
Acromioclavicular, injury to, 80–83
  anatomic considerations in, 80, *80*
  assessment of, 80–82
  in children, 83
  classification of, 80, *81*
  complications of, 83
  definitive management of, *82,* 82–83
  emergent management of, 82
  mechanisms of, 80
Acromion, fracture of, 84
Addiction
  iatrogenic, 35
  opioid, 35
  pain management and, 41–42
Adult respiratory distress syndrome
  incidence of, 28
  nursing assessment of, 19
  risk factors for, 28
Airway, establishment of, 13, 27–28
Alcohol
  anesthesia and, 30
  trauma and, 23
Amputation
  lower extremity
    occupational therapy in, 53–54, *54*
    rehabilitation in, 48
  upper extremity
    occupational therapy in, 55–59, *57, 58*
    prosthesis for, 59
Analgesia, 31–42. *See also* Pain, management of
Anesthesia, 27–30
  alcohol and, 30
  cocaine and, 30
  in head injury, 29
  patient position and, 30
Ankle, fracture of, 339–343
  anatomic considerations in, 339
  assessment of, 339, 341
  in children, 343
  classification of, 339, *340*
  complications of, 343
  definitive management of, 341, *341*
  emergent management of, 341
  mechanisms of, 339
  physical therapy for, 70–71
Ankylosis, in acetabular fracture, 253
Anterior cord syndrome 193, *194*
Antishock clamp, pelvic, 230, *230*
Arm. *See* Humerus; Radius; Ulna
Arrhythmia, hypothermia and, 29
Aspirin, in pain management, 34(t)
Atlanto-dens interval, 203
Atlanto-occipital joint, dislocation of, 198–203
  anatomic considerations in, 198, *198, 199*
  assessment of, 200–201
  in children, 203
  classification of, 200, *201*
  complications of, 203
  definitive management of, 201, *202*
  emergent management of, 201, *202*
  mechanisms of, 198
  radiographic evaluation of, 200–201
Atlas, fracture of, 203–206
  anatomic considerations in, 203
  assessment of, 203–204
  in children, 206
  classification of, 203, *204*
  complications of, 206
  definitive management of, 205
  emergent management of, 204–205
  mechanisms of, 203
Avascular necrosis, in femoral neck fracture, 261
AVPU system, 14

B

Bed rest, complications of, 61
Behavior management, 24–25
Bennett's fracture, 153–156
  anatomic considerations in, 153
  assessment of, 153–154
  classification of, 153
  complications of, 156
  definitive management of, 154–155, *154, 155*
  emergent management of, 154
  mechanisms of, 153, *153*
Brace, in spinal fracture management, 70–71
Brachial plexus, injury to, 187–188
  assessment of, 187
  management of, 187
Brown-Séquard's syndrome, 193–194, *194*
Bupivacaine, for epidural analgesia, 39
Burst fracture, of thoracolumbar spine, 215, *217, 218,* 223

C

C–1. *See* Atlas
C–2. *See* Odontoid process
Calcaneus, fracture of, 354–359
  anatomic considerations in, 354, *354*
  assessment of, 356–357, *357*
  in children, 359
  classification of, 354, *355*
  complications of, 359

Calcaneus, fracture of, *continued*
computed tomography in, 356–357, *357*
definitive management of, 358–359, *358, 359*
emergent management in, 357–358
mechanisms of, 354
physical therapy for, 70–71
Calcar femorale, 263, 271
Capitate, fracture of, 150–151
anatomic considerations in, 150
assessment of, 150
complications of, 151
emergent management of, 150
management of, 150–151, *151*
mechanisms of, 150, *150*
Carpus, instability of, 133–139
anatomic considerations in, 133–134, *133*
assessment of, *135*, 135–137, *136*
in children, 139
classification of, 134, 134(t)
complications of, 139
definitive management of, 137–139, *137, 138*
emergent management of, 137
lunate, volar, 138–139
lunate-triquetral, 138
mechanisms of, 133
perilunate, dorsal, 138–139
scapholunate, 137–138, *137, 138*
Central cord syndrome, 193, *194*
Cerebrospinal fluid (CSF), epidural opioid injection into, 38–39, *38*
Chance fracture of thoracolumbar spine, 220, *221*, 224
Chopart's joint, dislocation of, 345
Circulation, injury to, 5
Clavicle, fracture of, 77–79
anatomic considerations in, 77, *77*
assessment of, 78
in children, 79
classification of, 77
complications of, 79
definitive management of, 78–79, *78, 79*
emergent management of, 78
mechanisms of, 77
physical therapy for, 66–67
Coagulation, hypothermia and, 29
Coagulation factors, administration of, 29
Cocaine, anesthesia and, 30
Codeine, bioavailability of, 36(t)
Cold
contraindications to, 47
in rehabilitation, 46–47
Colloid solution, administration of, 28
Communication skills in occupational therapy, 53
Compartmental syndromes, 188–190, 377–380
anterior, 377–378, *379*
diagnosis of, 188, *188*
in foot, 378, 380–381, *380, 381*
management of, 188–190, *189*
in open fracture, 190
posterior, 377
proximal, 378
Condyle, occipital, fracture of, 198–203
anatomic considerations in, 198, *198, 199*
assessment of, 200–201
classification of, 200, *200*
complications of, 203
definitive management of, 201, *202*
emergent management of, 201, *202*
mechanisms of, 198
Continuous passive motion
for acute physical therapy, 63, *64*
for elbow, *64*
for finger, *58*
for hip, *64*
for knee, *64*
for shoulder, *64*
Contracture, prevention of, 43–44, *44*
Contusion, 381
Coping, modes of, 21
Cortical ring sign, *136*
Coumadin, in intertrochanteric femoral fracture, 267
Crushing
of muscles, 382
of skin, 381
Crystalloid solution, administration of, 28
Cuboid, fracture of, 363–364, *364*
Cultural beliefs, recovery and, 22
Cuneiform, fracture of, 365–367
anatomic considerations in, 365
assessment of, 365
in children, 365
complications of, 365
definitive management of, 365–367, *366, 367*
emergent management of, 365
mechanisms of, 365

D

Death, fear of, 24
Deep venous thrombosis
in acetabular fracture, 250, 253–254
prevention of, 43
Degloving injury, 381–382, *381*
Diathermy, in rehabilitation, 46
Dislocation. *See also specific locations, e.g.,* Elbow
atlanto-occipital, 198–203
Chopart's, 345
elbow, 97–100
facet, of cervical spine, 211, 212, 213
Galeazzi, 119–121
glenohumeral, 86–87
hip, 237–242
interphalangeal
distal, 184–185
proximal, 178–183
lunate, volar, 138–139
metacarpophalangeal, 162–168
patellofemoral, 293–294
perilunate, dorsal, 138–139
phalangeal, 162–168
radiocarpal, 131–132
sternoclavicular, 75–76
subtalar, 343–344
tibiofemoral, 291–293
Disuse weakness, rehabilitation for, 47, *47, 48*
Dysplasia, acetabular, in pelvic fracture, 234, *235*

E

Edema
in occupational therapy, 52
in upper extremity injury, 56
Elbow. *See also* Humerus; Olecranon; Radius; Ulna
continuous passive motion of, *64*
dislocation of, 97–100
anatomic considerations in, 97
assessment of, 97–98, *98*
in children, 100
classification of, 97, 97(t)
complications of, 100
definitive management of, 98–100, *99, 100*
emergent management of, 98
mechanisms of, 97
splint for, *57*
Embolism, pulmonary, in acetabular fracture, 253
Emergency medical technician, 4
Endotracheal tube, placement of, 27–28
indications for, 27
technique for, 27–28
Energy, fracture absorption of, 5
Epidural opioid analgesia, 38–39, *38*, 41–42
Erythrocytes, administration of, 28–29
Exercises
in glenohumeral dislocation management, 63
in hip dislocation management, 62–63
in intraarticular fracture management, 62
in muscle atrophy, 61, *62*
in physical therapy, 65
in spinal injuries, 63
Extremity. *See also specific structures, e.g.,* Humerus; Tibia
lower, occupational therapy for, 53–54
upper
occupational therapy for, 55–59, *57, 58*
prosthesis for, 59

F

Family management, 23–24
Femoral artery, injury to, 376
Femur
fracture of
intertrochanteric, 263–270
anatomic considerations in, 263, *263*

    assessment of, 265
    in children, 269
    classification of, *264,* 265
    complications of, 267, *268*
    Coumadin therapy in, 267
    definitive management of, 265–267, *266*
    emergent management of, 265
    ipsilateral, 371, 372
    mechanisms of, 263
    nonunion of, 267
  ipsilateral, 369–371
    anatomical considerations in, 369
    in children, 371
    complications of, 371
    definitive management of, 369–371, *370*
    emergent management of, 369
    mechanisms of, 369
  physical therapy for, 68–69
  subtrochanteric, 271–277
    anatomic considerations in, 271, *272*
    assessment of, 274
    in children, 277
    classification of, 271, *272, 273*
    complications of, 277
    definitive management of, 274–277, *275, 276*
    emergent management of, 274
    mechanisms of, 271
    95° condylar blade plating in, 275, 277
    second-generation intramedullary nailing in, 274–275, *275, 276*
    sliding hip screw in, 277
    standard intramedullary nailing in, 274
  supracondylar, 294–308
    anatomic considerations in, 294, *295*
    assessment of, 295, 297, *297*
    in children, 308
    classification of, 294–295, *296*
    complications of, 306
    definitive management of, 297–306
    emergent management of, 297
    extraarticular (type A), 297–298, *297*
    intercondylar (type C), 301–306, *301–307*
    mechanisms of, 294
    radiographic evaluation of, 296, *297*
    unicondylar (type B), 298, *299, 300*
head of, fracture of, 237–242
  anatomic considerations in, 237
  assessment of, 237, 239
  in children, 242
  classification of, 237, *238,* 239(t)
  complications of, 242
  definitive management of, 239, *240, 241,* 242
  emergent management of, 239
  mechanisms of, 237
neck of, fracture of, 255–261
    anatomic considerations in, 255, *256*
    assessment of, 256–258
    avascular necrosis in, 261
    in children, 261
    classification of, 255–256, *257*
    complications of, 261
    definitive management of, 258–261, *259, 260*
    displaced, 258–261, *259, 260*
    emergent management of, 258
    impacted, 258
    ipsilateral, *372,* 373–374, *373*
    mechanisms of, 255
    nondisplaced, 258
    nonunion of, 261
  shaft of, fracture of, 279–290
    anatomic considerations in, 279
    assessment of, 279–280
    in children, 289–290, *289*
    classification of, 279, *280*
    complications of, 288
    definitive management of, 281–288, *281*
    emergent management of, 280–281
    external fixation of, 288, 289
    intramedullary nailing in, 281–286, *282, 283, 284, 285, 286,* 288
    ipsilateral, 371–374
      anatomic considerations in, 371
      in children, 374, *374*
      classification of, 371
      complications of, 374
      definitive management of, 371–374, *372, 373, 374*
      emergent management of, 371
      mechanisms of, 371
    mechanisms of, 279
    plating of, 287–288, *287,* 288
Fentanyl, for epidural opioid analgesia, 39
Fingers. *See* Phalanx (phalanges)
Flexion-distraction injury, of thoracolumbar spine, 215, *219,* 220, 223–224
Fluid, replacement of, 13, 28–29
Foot. *See also specific structures, e.g.,* Ankle; Talus; Tarsometatarsa joint
  physical therapy for, 70–71
  splints for, 52, *52,* 53, *53*
Forearm. *See also* Radius; Ulna
  compartments of, 188, *188. See also* Compartmental syndromes
Fracture. *See also specific structures, e.g.,* Acetabulum
  acetabular, 243–254
  acromial, 84
  ankle, 339–368
  Bennett's, 153–156
  burst
    of cervical spine, 211, *211,* 212, 213 *213*
    of thoracolumbar spine, 215, *217,* 223
  C-1, 203–206
  calcaneal, 354–359
  capitate, 150–151
  Chance, of thoracolumbar spine, 220, *221,* 224
  clavicular, 77–79
  closed, 5
    classification of, 5, 5(t), 6
  compression, of thoracolumbar spine, 215, *216,* 220, 223
  condylar, occipital, 198–203
  cuboid, 363–364
  cuneiform, 365–367
  early stabilization of, 7
  energy absorption of, 5
  femoral
    head, 237–242
    intertrochanteric, 263–270
    ipsilateral, 369–374
    neck, 255–261
    shaft, 279–290
      ipsilateral, 371–374
    subtrochanteric, 271–277
    supracondylar, 294–308
  Galeazzi, 119–121, *120, 121*
  glenoid, 84, *85*
  grading of, 4, 5, 5(t)
  hangman's, 206–210
  hip, ipsilateral, 371–374
  humeral
    distal, 100–107
    proximal, 87–90
    shaft, 91–95
  Jefferson's, 203, 205
  metacarpal
    of fingers, 156–162
    of thumb, 153–156
  metatarsal, 367–368
  Monteggia, 117–119
  navicular, 360–362
  odontoid, 206–210
  olecranon, 110–114
  open, 5, 190–192
    classification of, 5, 5(t), 6, 190, 190(t)
    management of, 190–192, *191,* 383–384
    of upper extremity, 190–192, 190(t), *191*
  patellar, 308–313
  pattern of, 5
  pelvic, 225–235
  phalangeal
    distal, 176–178
    middle, 168–176
    proximal, 168–176
  physical therapy for, 62, 66–71
  radial, 107–110, 122–124
    distal, 125–130
  Rolando's, 153–156
  scaphoid, 143–146
  scapular, 83–85

Fracture, *continued*
spinal
cervical, 210–214
thoracolumbar, 214–224
talar, 350–353
teardrop, 211
tibial
eminence, 326–329
ipsilateral, 369–371
plafond, *342,* 343
proximal, 313–315
shaft, 331–338
trapezial, 146–148
triquetral, 148–149
ulnar, 122–124
isolated, 115–117
proximal, 110–114
Fracture board, *48*
Fracture-dislocation
Galeazzi, 119–121, *120, 121*
anatomic considerations in, 119–120
assessment of, 120, *120*
in children, 121
classification of, 120
complications of, 121
management of, 120–121, *121*
mechanisms of, 119
Lisfranc's, 346–349
anatomic considerations in, 346
assessment of, 347, *347*
in children, 349
classification of, 346, *346*
complications of, 349
definitive management of, 348–349, *348, 349*
emergent management of, 347
mechanisms of, 346
metacarpal, 159, *159*
Freeway syndrome, 4

G

Gait retraining, in physical therapy, 70
Galeazzi fracture-dislocation, 119–121
anatomic considerations in, 119–120
assessment of, 120, *120*
in children, 121
classification of, 120
complications of, 121
management of, 120–121, *121*
mechanisms of, 119
Gardner-Wells tongs, in spinal cord injury, 196, *197*
Glasgow coma scale, 14, 14(t), 29
Glenohumeral joint, dislocation of, 86–87
assessment of, 86
complications of, 87
management of, 86
mechanisms of, 86
Glenoid, fracture of, 84, *85*

H

Habituation, to opioids, 35
Haemonetic Cell Saver, 28–29
Halo vest, in hangman's fracture, 209–210
Hand. *See also* Carpus; Metacarpals; Phalanx (phalanges)
in occupational therapy, 56–59, *57, 58*
physical therapy for, 66–67
splints for, 53, *53*
Hangman's fracture, 206–210
anatomic considerations in, 206
assessment of, 206–207
in children, 210
classification of, 206
complications of, 210
emergent management of, 207
halo vest application in, 209–210
management of, 208–210, *209*
mechanisms of, 206
Harborview Medical Center, musculoskeletal traumatology at, 3–8
Head injury, anesthetic management in, 29
Heat
contraindications to, 47
loss of, 29–30
prevention of, 30
in rehabilitation, 46–47
Hemorrhage, control of, 13, 28–29
Hip
continuous passive motion of, *64*
dislocation of, 237–242
acute physical therapy for, 62–63
anatomic considerations in, 237
assessment of, 237, 239
in children, 242
classification of, 237, *238,* 239(t)
complications of, 242
definitive management of, 239, *240, 241,* 242
emergent management of, 239
mechanisms of, 237
fracture of, ipsilateral, 371–374
anatomic considerations in, 371
assessment of, 371
in children, 374, *374*
classification of, 371
complications of, 374
definitive management of, 371–374, *372, 373, 374*
emergent management of, 371
mechanisms of, 371
rehabilitation of, 45, *45*
replacement of, self-care with, 54, *54*
Humerus
distal, fracture of, 100–107
anatomic considerations in, 100
assessment of, 102
capitellar, 103, *103*
in children, 107
classification of, 100, *101*
complications of, 107
emergent management of, 102
intercondylar, *104,* 105, *105, 106*
management of, 102–107, *102–106*
mechanisms of, 100
supracondylar, 102, *102*
unicondylar, 103, *103*
physical therapy for, 66–67
proximal, fracture of, 87–90
assessment of, 88
in children, 89–90
classification of, 88, *88*
complications of, 89
definitive management of, 88–89, *89, 90*
emergent management of, 88
management of, 88–89, *89, 90*
mechanisms of, 87
shaft of, fracture of, 91–95
anatomic considerations in, 91
assessment of, 91
in children, 95
classification of, 91, *92*
complications of, 95
definitive management of, 93–95, *93, 94, 95*
emergent management of, 91
mechanism of, 91
Hydraulic principle, of orthoses, 49
Hydromorphone, bioavailability of, 36(t)
Hypothermia, 29–30
prevention of, 30

I

Ibuprofen, in pain management, 34(t)
Iliac artery, injury to, 376
Iliac vein, injury to, 376
Infection
in acetabular fracture, 254
in intertrochanteric femoral fracture, 267
in metacarpal fracture, 156
nursing diagnosis of, 19
in open fracture, 190
in subtrochanteric femoral fracture, 277
Innominate bone
soft tissues about, 244, *245, 246–247*
trabecular architecture of, 243, *244*
Instability, carpal, 133–139
anatomic considerations in, 133–134, *133*
assessment of, 135–137, *135, 136*
in children, 139
classification of, 134, 134(t)
complications of, 139
definitive management of, 137–139, *137, 138*
emergent management of, 137
lunate, volar, 138–139
lunate-triquetral, 138
management of, 137–139, *138*
mechanisms of, 133
perilunate, dorsal, 138–139
scapholunate, 137–138, *137, 138*
Integument, injury to, 381–382, *381*
Interphalangeal joint
distal, subluxation of, 184–185
anatomic considerations in, 184

  assessment of, 184
  with avulsion fracture, 184–185, *185*
  in children, 185
  classification of, 184, 184(t)
  complications of, 185
  definitive management of, 184–185, *184, 185*
  emergent management of, 184
  mechanisms of, 184
  without avulsion fracture, 184, *184, 185*
 proximal, dislocation of, 178–183
  anatomic considerations in, 178–179
  in children, 183
  classification of, 179, 179(t)
  complex, 180–181, *180*
  complications of, 183
  definitive management of, 179–183, *180, 181, 182, 183*
  emergent management of, 179
  ligament injury with, 182, *183*
  mechanisms of, 178
  simple, 179, *180*
  volar, 181–182, *182, 183*

J

Jefferson's fracture, 203, 205

K

Ketorolac, in pain management, 34
Knee. *See also* Femur; Patella; Tibia
 continuous passive motion of, *64*
 patellofemoral dislocation of, 293–294
 tibiofemoral dislocation of, 291–293, *292*

L

Laceration
 of muscles, 382
 of skin, 381
Ligament(s)
 pelvic, 225, *226*
 of radioulnar joint, 139
 transverse, rupture of, 203–206
 anatomic considerations in, 203
 assessment of, 203–204
 management of, 206
 mechanisms of, 203
Lisfranc's fracture-dislocation, 346–349
 anatomic considerations in, 346
 assessment of, 347, *347*
 in children, 349
 classification of, 346, *346*
 complications of, 349
 definitive management of, 348–349, *348, 349*
 emergent management of, 347
 mechanisms of, 346
Lumbar plexus, injury to, 375
Lunate, dislocation of
 dorsal, 138–139
 volar, 138–139
Lunate-triquetral instability, 138

M

Major Trauma Outcome Study, 12
Malleolus, fracture of, physical therapy for, 70–71
Meperidine, bioavailability of, 36(t)
Metacarpals
 fracture-dislocation of, 159, *159*
 fracture of, 153–162
  anatomic considerations in, 153, 156–157, *157*
  assessment of, 153–154, 157
  avulsion, 159, *159*
  in children, 156, 162
  classification of, 153, 157, 157(t)
  complications of, 156, 162
  definitive management of, 154–156, *154, 155, 156, 158*, 158–162, *159, 160, 161, 162*
  emergent management of, 154, 157
  extraarticular, 158, *158*
  head, 161–162, *161, 162*
  impaction, 158, *158*
  intraarticular, 158–159, *158, 159*
  joint stiffness and, 162
  mechanisms of, 153, *153, 154,* 156
  multiple, 160, *160*
  neck, 160–161, *161*
  shaft, 160, *160*
Metacarpophalangeal joint, dislocation of, 162–168
 anatomic considerations in, 163, *163*
 assessment of, 164
 in children, 167–168
 classification of, 163, 163(t)
 collateral ligament injury and, 167
 complications of, 167
 definitive management of, 164–167 *165, 166, 167, 168*
 dorsal, 167, *167, 168*
 emergent management of, 164
 mechanisms of, 162
Metatarsals, fracture of, 367–368
 anatomic considerations in, 367
 assessment of, 367
 classification of, 367
 management of, 367–368, *368*
 mechanisms of, 367
Methadone, bioavailability of, 36(t)
Methylprednisolone
 in spinal cord injury, 196, 197
 in thoracolumbar fracture, 220
Military antishock trousers, 13
Minimum effective analgesic concentration (MEAC), 34, *34*
Mobility, 7
 in lower extremity injury, 54
 nursing assessment of, 18
 in occupational therapy, 52–53, *53*
 in upper extremity injury, 55, 56
Monteggia fracture, 117–119
 anatomic considerations in, 117
 assessment of, 117, *118*
 in children, 119
 classification of, 117
 complications of, 119, *119*
 definitive management of, 118–119, *118*
 emergent management of, 117
 mechanism of, 117
Morphine
 bioavailability of, 36(t)
 for epidural opioid analgesia, 39, 39(t)
Mortality
 emotional factors in, 21–22
 preventable, 15
Motion, resisted, 55
Muscles
 atrophy of, 61, *62*
 injury to, 382–383

N

Nalorphine, 35
Naproxen, in pain management, 34(t)
Narcotics Anonymous, pain management philosophy of, 42
Navicular, fracture of, 360–362
 anatomic considerations in, 360
 assessment of, 360
 in children, 362
 classification of, 360, *361*
 complications of, 362
 definitive management of, 360–362, *362*
 emergent management of, 360
 mechanisms of, 360
Near-death experience, 24
Nerve, injury to, 375
Nerve block
 continuous
  in pain management, 40–41, *41*
  protocol for, 41
  side effects of, 40
 in pain management, 40–41, *41*
Neuraxial opioid analgesia, 38–39, *38*, 41–42
Neurological assessment, 14, 14(t)
 by nursing staff, 18
Nonunion
 in femoral neck fracture, 261
 in intertrochanteric femoral fracture, 267
 in odontoid fracture, 207
 in pelvic fracture, 234
 in scaphoid fracture, 146, *146*
 in subtrochanteric femoral fracture, 277
Nursing diagnosis
 of impaired mobility, 18
 of ineffective coping, 19
 of infection, 19
 of neurovascular complications, 18
 of pain, 17
 of respiratory complications, 19
 of self-care deficit, 18
 of skin breakdown, 18–19
Nursing pain management flowsheet, *32*
Nursing staff, 4, 11

O

Occipital condyle, fracture of, 198–203
Occipital condyle, fracture of, *continued*
  anatomic considerations in, 198, *198, 199*
  assessment of, 200–201
  classification of, 200, *200*
  complications of, 203
  definitive management of, 201, *202*
  emergent management of, 201, *202*
  mechanisms of, 198
Occipitocervical articulation, injury to, 198–203
  anatomic considerations in, 198, *198, 199*
  assessment of, 200–201
  in children, 203
  classification of, 200, *200, 201*
  complications of, 203
  definitive management of, 201, *202*
  emergent management of, 201, *202*
  mechanisms of, 198
Occupational therapy, 51–59
  in amputations, 53–54
  edema in, 52, 56
  hand function in, 56–59, *57, 58*
  in intensive care unit, 51–53, *52*
  in lower extremity injuries, 53–54
  mobility in, 52–53, *53*
  mobility restrictions in, 55, 56
  patient communication skills in, 53
  patient management for, 51–53, *52*
  precautions in, 51
  pressure restrictions in, 55
  range of motion in, 56
  resistance restrictions in, 55
  self-care in, 53
  sensory evaluation in, 56
  skin assessment in, 56
  skin protection in, 52, *52*
  in spinal injuries, 53–54
  strength evaluation in, 56
  in upper extremity injury, 55–59, *57, 58*
  weight-bearing restrictions in, 55
Odontoid process, fracture of, 206–210
  anatomic considerations in, 206
  assessment of, 206–207
  C–1 ring fracture and, 208
  in children, 210
  classification of, 206
  complications of, 210
  definitive management of, 207–208, *208*
  emergent management of, 207
  mechanisms of, 206
Olecranon, fracture of, 110–114
  anatomic considerations in, 110
  assessment of, 111
  in children, 114
  classification of, 111, *111*
  complications of, 114
  definitive management of, 111–112, *112, 113*
  emergent management of, 111
  mechanism of, 110
  physical therapy for, 66–67
Opioids
  addiction to, 35
  epidural, 38–39, *38*
  habituation to, 35
  intramuscular, 36–37
  intravenous, 37
  neuraxial, 38–39, *38*
  oral, 35–36, 36(t)
  in pain management, 34–37, *34,* 36(t)
  side effects of, 35
  systemic, 34–35, *34*
  tolerance to, 35
Orthoses
  hydraulic principle of, 49
  in spinal injury, 54
Os magnum. *See* Capitate
Ossification, heterotopic, in acetabular fracture, 253
Oxycodeine, bioavailability of, 36(t)

P

Pain
  components of, 31, *31*
  definition of, 31, *31*
  management of, 7, 25, 31–42
    barriers to, 33, 33(t)
    dependence on, 44
    epidural local anesthetic in, 39–40
    failures in, 32, 32(t)
    Ketorolac in, 34
    for lower extremity, 42(t)
    minimum effective analgesic concentration in, 34, *34*
    neuraxial opioid injection in, 38–39, *38,* 41–42
    nonopioid, 33–34, 34(t)
    nonpharmacologic, 33
    opioid, 34–37, *34,* 36(t)
    opioid addiction and, 41–42
    pain cocktail in, 36, *36,* 44
    patient-controlled, 37, *37*
    for pelvis, 42(t)
    peripheral nerve block in, 40–41
    for spine, 42(t)
    Toradol in, 7
    for upper extremity, 42(t)
  measurement of, 31–33, *32,* 32(t)
  morbidity of, 32–33
  nursing diagnosis of, 17
  nursing pain management flowsheet for, *32*
  phantom, local anesthetic infusion in, 41
  quantity of, 32
Pain cocktail, 36, *36,* 44
Patella, fracture of, 308–313
  anatomic considerations in, 308
  assessment of, 308
  in children, 313
  classification of, 308
  complications of, 313
  definitive management of, 308–313, *309, 310, 311, 312*
  emergent management of, 308
  mechanisms of, 308
  physical therapy for, 70–71
Patellofemoral joint
  dislocation of, 293–294
    anatomic considerations in, 293
    assessment of, 293–294
    in children, 294
    classification of, 293
    complications of, 294
    definitive management of, 294
    emergent management of, 294
    mechanisms of, 293
  quadriceps exercise effect on, 47, *47, 48*
Pelvis
  fracture of, 225–235
    assessment of, 225, 229, *229, 230*
    in children, 234, *235*
    classification of, 225, *227,* 227(t), *228, 229*
    complications of, 234, *234*
    definitive management of, 231–234, *231, 232, 233*
    emergent management of, 230, *230*
    mechanism of, 225
    physical therapy for, 68–69
    postoperative care for, 234
    type A1, 231
    type A2, 231
    type B1, 231, *232, 233*
    type B2, 231, 233, *233*
    type B3, 231, 233
    type C1, 233
    type C2, 233
    type C3, 233–234, *233*
  ligaments of, 225, *226*
Peroneal nerve, injury to, 375
Personality, coping style and, 21
Phalanx (phalanges). *See also* Metacarpals
  dislocation of, 162–168
    anatomic considerations in, 163
    assessment of, 164
    in children, 167–168
    classification of, 163, 163(t)
    collateral ligament injury and, 167
    dorsal, 167, *167, 168*
    management of, 164, 167, *167, 168*
    mechanisms of, 162
  distal, fracture of, 176–178
    anatomic considerations in, 176
    assessment of, 176, *176*
    avulsion, 177, *177*
    classification of, 176, 176(t)
    definitive management of, 177–178, *177, 178*
    emergent management of, 177
    mechanisms of, 176
    shaft, 177, *178*
    tuft, 177
  extension splint for, *57*
  middle, fracture of, 168–176

anatomic considerations in, 168–169
assessment of, 169, *169*
in children, 175
classification of, 169, 169(t)
comminuted, 175
complications of, 175
condylar, 175, *175*
definitive management of, 174–175, *175*
emergent management of, 170
extraarticular, 174
intraarticular, 174
mechanisms of, 168
oblique, 174, *175*
transverse, 174
proximal, fracture of, 168–176
anatomic considerations in, 168, *169*
assessment of, 169, *169*
bicondylar, 174, *175*
in children, 175
classification of, 169, 169(t)
comminuted, 172–173, *172*
complications of, 175
condylar, 173, *173*
definitive management of, 170–174, *170, 171, 172, 173, 174*
emergent management of, 170
extraarticular, 170, *170, 171*
intraarticular, 171, *171*
mechanisms of, 168
oblique, 172
transverse, 172
range of motion of, *58*
Physeal bar, in pelvic fracture, 234, *235*
Physical therapist, 4
Physical therapy
acute, 61–64, *62, 64*
continuous passive motion in, 63, *64*
for glenohumeral dislocations, 63
for hip dislocations, 62–63
for intact spinal injuries, 63
for intraarticular fractures, 62
traction in, 63
nonacute, 65–72
exercises in, 65
gait retraining in, 70
for spinal fracture, 70–72
Pilon, fracture of, physical therapy for, 70–71
Piroxicam, in pain management, 34(t)
Popliteal artery, injury to, 376
Position, patient
anesthesia and, 30
for contracture prevention, 43–44, *44*
Preoperative instruction, recovery and, 22–23
Pressure sores, prevention of, 44
Pressure wraps, in upper extremity injury, 55
Prosthesis
for lower extremity injury, 54
for upper extremity amputation, 59
Psychiatric illness, nursing assessment for, 19
Pulmonary embolism, in acetabular fracture, 253

Q

Quadriceps board, *48*
Quadriceps muscle, exercise of, patellofemoral joint effect of, 47, *47, 48*

R

Radiocarpal dislocation, 131–132, *132*
anatomic considerations in, 131
assessment of, 131
in children, 132
classification of, 131
complications of, 131–132
definitive management of, 131, *132*
emergent management of, 131
mechanism of, 131
Radiology technician, 11
Radioulnar joint
distal, injury to, 139–142, *140, 141, 142*
anatomic considerations in, 139–140, *140*
assessment of, 140–142, *141*
in children, 142
classification of, 140
complications of, 142
definitive management of, 142, *142*
emergent management of, 142
mechanisms of, 139
Radius
distal, fracture of, 125–130
anatomic considerations in, 125–126, *126*
assessment of, 126
in children, 130
classification of, 126, *127*
complications of, 128, 130
definitive management of, 127–128, *128, 129, 130*
emergent management of, 126–127
mechanisms of, 125, *125*
fracture of, 122–124
anatomic considerations in, 122–123, *122*
assessment of, 123 *123*
in children, 124
classification of, 123
complications of, 124
definitive management of, 123–124, *124*
emergent management of, 123
mechanism of, 122
physical therapy for, 66–67
head of, fracture of, 107–110
anatomic considerations in, 107
assessment of, 107–108
in children, 110
classification of, 107, *108*
complications of, 110
definitive management of, 108–110, *108, 109*
emergent management of, 107–108
mechanism of, 107
Range of motion
for fingers, *58*
in rehabilitation, 45
in upper extremity injury, 56
Rectus femoris muscle, stretching of, 45–46, *46*
Red blood cells, administration of, 28–29
Rehabilitation, 7, 25
acute physical therapy in, 61–64. *See also* Physical therapy, acute
adaptive devices in, 48–49
in bed-bound patient, 43
cold in, 46–47
contracture prevention in, 43–44, *44*
in disuse weakness, 47, *47, 48*
function enhancement in, 48
function restoration in, 44–46, *45*
heat in, 46–47
nonacute physical therapy in, 65–72. *See also* Physical therapy, nonacute
occupational therapy for, 51–59. *See also* Occupational therapy
pain dependence in, 44
pressure sore prevention in, 44
range of motion in, 45
in regional trauma care system, 16
secondary disability prevention with, 43–44
thrombosis prevention in, 43
treatment strategies for, 43–49
ultrasound in, 45, *45*
Respiratory distress
epidural opioid analgesia and, 38–39
incidence of, 28
nursing assessment of, 19
risk factors for, 28
Respiratory technician, 11
Resuscitation, 13–14, 14(t)
Rolando's fracture
anatomic considerations in, 153
assessment of, 153–154
classification of, 153
complications of, 156
definitive management of, 155
emergent management of, 154
mechanisms of, 153, *154*

S

Sacral plexus, injury to, 375
Sarmiento humeral splint, *57*
Scaphoid, fracture of, 143–146
anatomic considerations in, 143, *143*
assessment of, 143–144, *144*
in children, 146
classification of, 143
complications of, 146, *146*
definitive management of, 144–145, *145*

Scaphoid, fracture of, *continued*
emergent management of, 144
mechanisms of, 143
Scapholunate instability, 137–138, *138*
Scapula, fracture of, 83–85
anatomic considerations in, 83
assessment of, 83–84
in children, 84
classification of, 83
complications of, 84
management of, 84, *85*
mechanisms of, 83
physical therapy for, 66–67
Sciatic nerve, injury to, 253, 375
Secondary congruence, in acetabular fracture, 251, *251*
Self-care
in lower extremity injury, 54, *54*
nursing assessment of, 18
in occupational therapy, 53
Self-image, trauma and, 22
Sensation, in upper extremity injury, 56
Shoulder. *See also specific structures, e.g.,* Scapula; Sternoclavicular joint
acute physical therapy for, 63
continuous passive motion of, *64*
rehabilitation of, 45, *45,* 46
Skin
crush injury of, 381
nursing assessment of, 18–19
in occupational therapy, 52
in thoracolumbar injury, 18–19
in upper extremity injury, 56
Spinal cord, injury to, 193–198
anatomic considerations in, 193
assessment of, 194–196
in children, 197
classification of, 193–194, *194*
complications of, 197
definitive management of, 196–197
emergent management of, 196
Gardner-Wells tongs in, 196, *197*
mechanisms of, 193
methylprednisolone in, 196
physical examination in, 194
radiographic evaluation in, 194–196, *195*
traction in, 196
Spine
cervical
extension injury of, 210–214
anatomic considerations in, 210
assessment of, 212
in children, 214
classification of, 212
complications of, 214
definitive management of, 213–214
emergent management of, 212
mechanisms of, 210
facet dislocations of, 210–214
anatomic considerations in, 210
assessment of, 212
in children, 214
classification of, 211
complications of, 214
definitive management of, 213
emergent management of, 212
mechanisms of, 210
fracture of, 210–214
anatomic considerations in, 210
assessment of, 212
burst, 211, *211,* 212, 213, *213*
in children, 214
classification of, 210–212, *211*
complications of, 214
definitive management of, 212–214
emergent management of, 212
mechanisms of, 210
minor, 210–211, 212
physical therapy for, 71–72
occupational therapy and, 53–54
physical therapy for, 63, 70–72
thoracolumbar
burst fracture of, 215, *217, 218,* 223
Chance fracture of, 220, *221,* 224
compression fracture of, 215, *216,* 220, 223
flexion-distraction injury of, 215, *219,* 220, 223–224
flexion-distraction injury to, 223–224
injury to, 214–224
anatomic considerations in, 214
assessment of, 220
in children, 224
classification of, 215–220, *215*
complications of, 224
definitive management of, 220, 223–224
emergent management of, 220
mechanisms of, 214
skin breakdown and, 18–19
translational injury to, 220, *222,* 224
Splints
elbow, *57*
finger, *57*
foot, 52, *52,* 53, *53*
hand, 53, *53*
upper extremity, *57*
wrist, *57, 58*
Sternoclavicular joint, dislocation of, 75–76
anatomic considerations in, 75, *76*
assessment of, 75–76
in children, 76
classification of, 75
complications of, 76
management of, 76
mechanisms of, 75
Stiffness, hand fracture and, 162
Strength, in upper extremity injury, 56
Subluxation. *See also* Dislocation
interphalangeal, distal, 184–185
anatomic considerations in, 184
assessment of, 184
in children, 185
classification of, 184, 184(t)
complications of, 185
definitive management of, 184–185, *184, 185*
emergent management of, 184
mechanisms of, 184
Subtalar joint, dislocation of, 343–344
anatomic considerations in, 343
assessment of, 344
classification of, 344
complications of, 344
management of, 344
mechanisms of, 343
Support systems, recovery and, 22

T

Talus, fracture of, 350–353
anatomic considerations in, 350
assessment of, 351
in children, 353
classification of, *350,* 351
complications of, 353
definitive management of, 351–353, *351, 352, 353*
emergent management of, 351
mechanisms of, 350
physical therapy for, 70–71
Tarsometatarsal joint, fracture-dislocation of, 346–349
anatomic considerations in, 346
assessment of, 347, *347*
in children, 349
classification of, 346, *346*
complications of, 349
definitive management of, 348–349, *348, 349*
emergent management of, 347
mechanisms of, 346
Teardrop fracture, 211
Thrombosis, deep-vein
in acetabular fracture, 250, 253–254
prevention of, 43
Thumb
dislocation of, 162–168
anatomic considerations in, 163, *163*
assessment of, 164
in children, 167–168
classification of, 163, 163(t)
definitive management of, 164–167, *164, 165, 166*
dorsal, 166–167
emergent management of, 164
mechanisms of, 162
radial collateral ligament injury and, 166
ulnar collateral ligament injury and, 164, *164*
fracture of, 153–156
anatomic considerations in, 153
assessment of, 153–154
in children, 156
classification of, 153

complications of, 156
management of, 154–156, *154, 155, 156*
mechanisms of, 153, *153, 154*
pin-track infection in, 156
shaft, 155–156, *156*
Tibia
eminence of, fracture of, 326–329
anatomic considerations in, 326
assessment of, 326, *327*
in children, 329
classification of, 326
complications of, 329
definitive management of, 327–329, *327, 328*
emergent management of, 326–327
mechanisms of, 326, *326*
ipsilateral fracture of, 369–371
anatomical considerations in, 369
in children, 371
complications of, 371
definitive management of, 369–371, *370*
emergent management of, 369
mechanisms of, 369
physical therapy for, 70–71
plafond fracture of, *342,* 343
proximal, fracture of, 313–325
anatomic considerations in, 313, *314*
assessment of, 313, 315
bicondylar, 321, 323, *323*
with metaphyseal extension, 323–324, *324, 325*
in children, 324–325
classification of, 313, *315*
complications of, 324
definitive management of, 315–324
depression, 318, 320, *320*
emergent management of, 315
mechanisms of, 313
medial plateau, 321, *322*
split, *316,* 317, *317*
split depression, 317–318, *318, 319*
shaft of, fracture of, 331–338
anatomic considerations in, 331, *332*
assessment of, 331–332
casting for, 334
in children, 338
classification of, 331, *333*
complications of, *337,* 338
definitive management of, 332, 334–338
emergent management of, 332
external skeletal fixation for, 334, *335*
intramedullary nailing for, 335–338, *337*
mechanisms of, 331
plate fixation for, 335, *336*
reduction for, 334
Tibial artery, injury to, 376–377
Tibial nerve, injury to, 375
Tibiofemoral joint, dislocation of, 291–293
anatomic considerations in, 291, *292*
assessment of, 291–292
in children, 293
classification of, 291
complications of, 293
definitive management of, 292–293
emergent management of, 292
mechanisms of, 291
Tolerance, to opioids, 35
Toradol, in pain management, 7
Traction
in acetabular fracture, 250
in acute physical therapy, 63
in cervical spinal cord injury, 196, 197
Translational injury, of thoracolumbar spine, 220, *222,* 224
Trapeze, in rehabilitation, 48–49
Trapezium, fracture of, 146–148
anatomic considerations in, 145
assessment of, 146–147
in children, 148
classification of, 146
complications of, 148
definitive management of, 147–148, *147, 148*
emergent management of, 147
mechanisms of, 146
Trauma
classification of, 5, 5(t), 6
documentation of, 8
emotional response to, 21–23
evaluation of, 5, 5(t)
pain management in, 7
preventable death from, 15
psychological response to, 23–25
rehabilitation after, 7
self-image and, 22
support services for, 7–8
three-phase response to, 15–16
treatment of, 7
Trauma center
classification of, 11–12
mortality rates and, 15
regional, 15–16
Trauma registry, 12
Trauma surgeon, 9–12, *10,* 10(t)
Trauma team, 7
captain of, 10, *10,* 10(t)
members of, 10–11, 10(t)
organization of, 4, 9–12, *10,* 10(t)
preassignment of, 11, *11*
quality assurance of, 11–12
Traumatology, musculoskeletal, 3–8
Triage, 12–13
Triple response of Lewis, 187
Triquetrum, fracture of, 148–149
anatomic considerations in, 148, *149*
assessment of, 149
classification of, 148
complications of, 149
management of, 149
mechanisms of, 148, *149*

U

Ulna
fracture of, 115–117, 122–124
anatomic considerations in, 122–123, *122*
assessment of, 123, *123*
in children, 124
classification of, 123
complications of, 124
definitive management of, 123–124, *124*
emergent management of, 123
isolated, 115–117, *115, 116*
anatomic considerations in, 115
assessment of, 115–116
in children, 117
classification of, 115
complications of, 117
management of, 116
mechanisms of, 115, *115, 116*
mechanism of, 122
physical therapy for, 66–67
proximal, fracture of, 110–114
anatomic considerations in, 110
assessment of, 111
in children, 114
classification of, 111, *111*
complications of, 114
definitive management of, 111–112, *112, 113*
emergent management of, 111–112, *112, 113*
mechanism of, 110
Ultrasound, in rehabilitation, 45, *45*
Upper extremity. *See also specific structures, e.g.,* Humerus
assessment of, 56–59, *57, 58*
brachial plexus injury of, 187–188
splints for, *57*

V

Vascular assessment, by nursing staff, 18
Vena caval filter, 234, *234*
Ventilation, 13, 28
Volume resuscitation, 28

W

Weight-bearing
orthosis for, 49
in upper extremity injury, 55
Wrist. *See also* Carpus; Radius; Scaphoid
physical therapy for, 66–67
splint for, *57, 58*